Applications of

Noninvasive Vascular Techniques

Amil J. Gerlock, Jr., MD

Professor of Radiology
Chief, Angiography and Noninvasive Vascular Laboratory
Louisiana State University Medical Center
Shreveport, Louisiana

Vishan L. Giyanani, MD

Associate Professor of Radiology
Chief, Ultrasound and CT Sections
Louisiana State University Medical Center
Shreveport, Louisiana

Carol Krebs, RT, RDMS, RVT

Department of Radiology
Ultrasound Section
Louisiana State University Medical Center
Shreveport, Louisiana

W. B. SAUNDERS COMPANY
Harcourt Brace Jovanovich, Inc.

Philadelphia / London / Toronto / Montreal / Sydney / Tokyo

W. B. SAUNDERS COMPANY
Harcourt Brace Jovanovich, Inc.

The Curtis Center
Independence Square West
Philadelphia, PA 19106

Library of Congress Cataloging-in-Publication Data

Gerlock, Amil J.

Applications of noninvasive vascular techniques.

1. Diagnosis, Noninvasive.   2. Blood-
   vessels—Diseases—Diagnosis.   3. Diagnosis,
   Ultrasonic.   I. Giyanani, Vishan L.   II. Krebs,
   Carol.   III. Title. [DNLM: 1. Ultrasonic Diagnosis. 2.
   Vascular Diseases—diagnosis. WG 500 C371a]

RC691.6.N65G47   1988   616.1'3075   87–26605

ISBN 0–7216–2335–2

Designer: W. B. Saunders Staff
Production Manager: Bill Preston
Manuscript Editor: Mark Crowe
Illustration Coordinator: Brett MacNaughton
Indexer: Mark Crowe

Applications of Noninvasive Vascular Techniques   ISBN 0–7216–2335–2

Last digit is the print number: 9   8   7   6   5   4   3

Dedication

To my beloved mother, Harriet.
A.J.G.

To my beloved wife, Suzanne, and lovely daughter, Rachel.
V.L.G.

To all those individuals devoted to their respective professions
and to the teaching of others.
C.A.K.

Preface

Armed with the philosophy that although vascular disease is painful its diagnosis should be painless, we began to take on the challenge of doing noninvasive vascular examinations. One of the first hurdles was to gain some knowledge about these procedures so that they could be performed and interpreted with confidence. There were already several excellent books available in 1982 when we began planning the noninvasive vascular laboratory, all of which were a great help to us. Several other factors were even more important to us in gaining an understanding of this emerging field. They centered around the fact that our situation was unique because the angiographic and ultrasound suites were located next door to each other, and all the personnel in these two quite different modalities worked together extremely well. Our patients were also most cooperative in granting us permission to study their vessels with ultrasound after their angiographic procedures. These two factors gave us the opportunity to correlate the ultrasound findings with the angiographic abnormalities in a large group of patients with known vascular disease. Vessels were scanned and re-scanned until the maneuvers necessary to show the angiographic pathology by ultrasound were learned.

Initially, this was facilitated by placing a film from the angiogram on a viewbox in the ultrasound room to be used as a guide during the examination. A member of the angiographic section went over the normal and pathologic angiographic anatomy shown on the angiogram with the sonographer before the patient was brought into the room and the ultrasound examination begun. Often both the angiographic and ultrasound personnel could be seen putting their heads together in an attempt to figure out how to demonstrate by ultrasound the various abnormalities seen on the angiograms. It soon became obvious that this correlative process was a good way to learn how to perform and interpret noninvasive vascular procedures, and this is why there are so many angiographic-ultrasound correlative illustrations in this book. They were so instructive for us that we decided to combine them together into a format that could be used by anyone beginning to learn this exciting modality.

AMIL J. GERLOCK, JR., M.D.
VISHAN L. GIYANANI, M.D.
CAROL KREBS, R.T., R.D.M.S., R.V.T.

Foreword

Applications of Noninvasive Vascular Techniques is a comprehensive text that skillfully correlates angiography with real-time sonography and noninvasive vascular technology to provide anatomical and hemodynamic information for a wide variety of pathological conditions. For those physicians and technologists who are just beginning their study of this exciting imaging modality, the book offers extensive information concerning examination techniques and protocols, normal values, and reporting methods for the various types of noninvasive procedures. The anatomical diagrams of the vascular system combined with the angiographic correlation permit the reader to rapidly gain familiarity with the basic principles and imaging findings of these noninvasive vascular techniques. The more experienced reader will appreciate the opportunity to see the many excellent examples of vascular pathology that are illustrated with a wealth of correlated figures from both angiography and sonography.

RONALD L. EISENBERG, M.D.
Professor and Chairman of Radiology
Louisiana State University School of Medicine
Shreveport, Louisiana

Acknowledgments

We were extremely fortunate throughout this project to have had so many wonderful, dedicated people to work with. Each and every one of them played a major role in this work, and we would like to take this opportunity to thank them all officially:

To those individuals, including Keith Mauney and Michael Rush, who allowed us to come into their facilities and learn the methods for performing various examinations.

To our Chairman, Ronald L. Eisenberg, M.D., who inspired us and acquired the equipment we needed to do the job.

To Robert Pool, R.T., R. Kent Walker, R.T., and Terri Glover, R.T., outstanding special procedures technologists who took all the angiograms illustrated in this book. We also remember the hours you spent in the darkroom making all those subtractions and copy films.

To Linda Nall, M.D., and Sandra Ratcliff, R.T., R.D.M.S., for the extra workload they took on so that others could learn the noninvasive procedures. They also participated in the Noninvasive Vascular Diagnostic Symposium that ultimately led to the production of this book.

To Mrs. Connie Monette for working in both angiography and ultrasound to provide us with the film jackets we needed, for pushing all those huge cartloads of film folders back and forth to the File Room, and for pulling all of those articles and getting our reference material together too.

To Julie A. Swain, M.D., Chief of Cardiovascular Surgery, for organizing the Vascular Conference that provided informative discussions between us and our surgical colleagues concerning the role of noninvasive vascular testing in the management of their patients. These included Edward Benzel, M.D., Chief of Neurosurgery; Charles Knight, Jr., M.D., Clinical Consultant to the Department of Surgery; and Travis Phifer, M.D., Assistant Professor of Surgery.

To Mrs. Florence Johnston for making us find the right spelling for each of the new words we encountered from the very beginning. She was most instrumental in seeing that words like plethysmography were always spelled correctly in our reports. We may have floundered in our diagnoses, but she made sure that we did not flounder in our vocabulary.

To Jim Wilson, a truly exceptional artist and medical illustrator who did all the line drawings used in this book. Photography was carried out under the direction of the L.S.U. Medical Communications Department by Ron Aldin, Cindy Payton, Stan Carpenter, and Glen Bundrick. The expertise of these medical photographers was used in getting all the clinical photographs used in this book.

To Mrs. Betty Digrazia, Radiology Department Administrative Assistant, and Jeff Weissmann, M.D., Radiology Resident, for allowing us to use them as models.

To the Radiology resident and staff of L.S.U. School of Medicine for their assistance and support in this endeavor.

Finally, to Mrs. Rhoda Lancaster for letting her fingers do the walking through the whole darn thing—not only for typing the whole manuscript but also for holding the thing together against all odds.

Contents

Part I • Instrumentation and Doppler Principles

1 • Sound Spectral Analysis of Arterial

Blood Flow

Sound Spectral Analysis Instrumentation

Sound spectral analysis is the electronic transformation of sound into an image that can be seen on a television screen. To understand how it works, one must first review the two basic components of sound and how they are created.

Sounds are created by vibrations from objects. These vibrations travel through the air as sinusoidal waves with different frequencies. An object vibrating with a frequency of one cycle per second (cycle/second) would emit a sound with the sinusoidal waveform shown in Figure 1–1. The unit of measurement for a sound wave with a frequency of one cycle per second is the *hertz* (Hz). The various Hz units used in medical diagnosis are given below:

1 cycle/second = 1 Hz (hertz)
1,000 cycles/second = 1 kHz (kilohertz)
1,000,000 cycles/second = 1 MHz (megahertz)

Sound waves are further categorized as infrasonic (less than 20 Hz), audible (20 Hz to 20 kHz), and ultrasonic (greater than 20 kHz).

A continuous 1 Hz frequency sound, like the one in Figure 1–1, could be electronically converted into a television (TV) image that would look like Figure 1–2. It would appear as a gray line located at a 1 Hz level above the zero baseline. This line would indicate that a 1 Hz sound is being perceived by the sound spectral analyzer.

Components of Sound

Pitch is the first component of sound to be examined. Increasing the frequency of a sound increases its pitch. A sound with a frequency of 2 Hz would have a higher pitch than a sound with a frequency of 1 Hz. The electronic trans-

formation of this 2 Hz sound would present the image in Figure 1–3 on the TV screen. Again, there is a gray line going across the screen, only this time it is placed higher, at the 2 Hz level. The 1 Hz sound can now be eletronically discriminated from the 2 Hz sound.

The second component of a sound is its *volume*. The electronic transformation of sound volumes into black and white TV images is obtained through the use of shades of gray. An extremely soft sound may not be seen at all, whereas a moderately soft sound would appear as a dark shade of gray. Extremely loud sounds would have a brilliant white appearance. The different sound volumes are then displayed on black-and-white TV monitors through the use of a "gray scale."

Spectral Analyzer

The spectral analyzer listens to a sound and projects an image of that sound frequency and volume onto a TV screen. Simply stated, 400 spectral lines/second are generated across the TV screen. For illustration purposes, only ten spectral lines/second were used in Figure 1–4. Each spectral line in this illustration is calibrated to detect sounds ranging in frequency from 0 to 4 Hz. When a sound is detected by one of these spectral lines, it is displayed on the TV screen as a flash of light or scintillation, which appears at the calibrated hertz level of its frequency (Fig. 1–4). The brightness of these flashes depends upon the sound volume level detected by each spectral line. Generally, a gray scale generator containing 16 different shades of gray is used for black-and-white TV displays.

Consider the spectral analysis of the loud sound in Figure 1–5. It is a simple sound and will appear on the TV screen through the process of spectral analysis as shown in Figure 1–4. Two brilliant white lines, one above the other, will

3

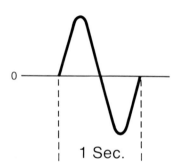

Figure 1–1. Diagram of a 1 cycle/second (1 Hz) sound wave frequency.

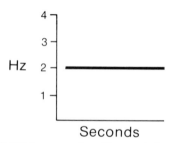

Figure 1–3. TV image produced by spectral analysis of a 2 Hz sound wave frequency.

traverse the TV screen. One line is at the 1 Hz level; the other is at the 2 Hz level. Both lines are white because the sound was loud. There will be only two lines because the sound was composed of two frequencies, one at 1 Hz and the other at 2 Hz. This completes the spectral analysis of this particular sound. It looks nothing like the TV image of blood flowing through a blood vessel. However, it did serve a purpose, which was to introduce how sound is analyzed and displayed as a TV image.

The Conversion of Blood Flow into Sound

Blood flow must be converted into a sound because a sound must be available for the spectral analyzer to analyze. This conversion is accomplished through the application of the Doppler principle and the use of the Doppler probe.

Doppler Principle

The Doppler principle was formulated by the Austrian physicist Christian Johann Doppler (1803–1853). He demonstrated that the frequency of light or sound emitted by a source

traveling toward the observer is perceived as higher than its transmitted frequency and that the perceived frequency is lower when the source is moving away from the observer. An often cited example is the pitch of a train whistle, which seems higher as the train approaches and lower as the train recedes into the distance. The sound waves, therefore, are compressed into higher frequencies as the sound from the train whistle moves toward us and expanded into lower frequencies as it moves away from us.

Application of this principle allows three observations to be made about the train:

1. The fact that the train is moving.
2. The direction in which it is going.
3. How fast it is moving.

No change in the whistle sound frequency would mean that the train is standing still (Fig. 1–6A). A steadily increasing, higher-pitched whistle sound would mean that the train is moving toward us. A rapidly increasing, higher-pitched whistle sound would mean that we were in the path of a fast-moving train.

Doppler Probe

It would be nice to know all of these factors about blood flow. Unfortunately, there are no whistles in the blood stream, and blood flow cannot be heard under normal circumstances.

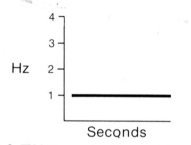

Figure 1–2. TV image produced by spectral analysis of the sound diagrammed in Figure 1–1. The vertical axis shows the calibration in hertz; the time duration of the sound is shown on the horizontal axis in seconds.

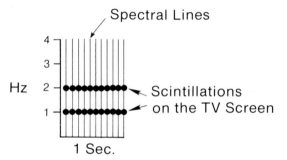

Figure 1–4. Illustration of spectral lines used in the TV display of two different sound wave frequencies.

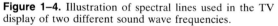

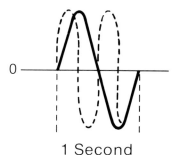

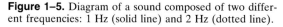

1 Second

Figure 1–5. Diagram of a sound composed of two different frequencies: 1 Hz (solid line) and 2 Hz (dotted line).

The blood stream, however, does contain many "trains" in the form of red blood cells (RBCs). All that is needed is to give these trains "whistles." The Doppler principle could then be applied to blood flow to determine its movement, the direction of its movement, and how fast it is moving or its velocity. A Doppler probe can be thought of as an instrument that does just this. It gives the RBC a whistle. How this is accomplished is illustrated in Figure 1–7.

A continuous-wave Doppler probe is used to transmit a 1 Hz frequency sound from *Point Source 1* into a blood vessel. The sound strikes a RBC located at position A. This RBC now has a 1 Hz frequency sound whistle. As the RBC moves to position B, it moves closer to the probe face, where the 1 Hz sound bounces back to the probe and is received at *Point Source 2*. According to the Doppler principle, the frequency of sound emitted by a source traveling toward the observer is perceived as higher than its transmitted source. The RBC is the source in this case, and Point Source 2 in the probe face is the observer. Point Source 2 in Figure 1–7 will then perceive a sound from the RBC at position B with a higher frequency than its transmitted sound of 1 Hz. For illustration purposes, the higher frequency sound of the RBC is 2 Hz.

The Doppler probe was able to give the RBC a 1 Hz transmitting frequency from Point Source 1 and to perceive an increase in this frequency to 2 Hz with Point Source 2 as the RBC moved toward the probe face. Point Sources 1 and 2 are actually piezoelectric crystals. Piezoelectricity is the physical phenomenon by which the 1 to 10 MHz sound waves used in the medical diagnosis of vascular diseases are generated. A piezoelectric crystal is one that vibrates and emits a sound in response to an applied voltage (Point Source 1). It can also vibrate in response to a sound and emit a voltage (Point Source 2). This voltage can then be used to project the changing sound frequency of an RBC moving toward the probe

face through a loudspeaker, as illustrated in Figure 1–7. A sound is now available from blood flow for sound spectral analysis.

As previously mentioned, this process analyzes a sound and displays its two basic components, pitch and volume, onto a TV screen. In other words, one does not hear a sound through sound spectral analysis but perceives its image on a TV screen. The changing frequency of an RBC moving either toward or away from the probe face is electronically displayed on a TV screen as the RBC Doppler shift frequency. The RBC Doppler shift frequency is the difference between its transmitting 1 Hz frequency at position A and its perceived increase to a 2 Hz frequency at position B in Figure 1–7. A loudspeaker would project this as an audible sound with increasing pitch; the sound spectral analyzer would display it on a TV screen as a 1 Hz Doppler shift frequency.

Factors Affecting the Doppler Shift Frequency

The various factors that may either increase or decrease the Doppler shift frequencies are shown by the relationship in Figure 1–8. Here it can be seen that the Doppler shift frequencies increase when the transmitted Doppler probe frequency increases, the velocity of the RBC increases, or the angle (theta) between the transmitted Doppler probe beam and the direction of blood flow carrying the RBC decreases. Notice that if the emitted probe frequency and the scanning angle (Θ) are kept constant, only the velocity (v) of the RBC will significantly affect the Doppler shift frequency.

Although it is possible to keep the probe emitting frequency constant, it is difficult to keep the scanning angle constant because of the tissue characteristics and tortuosity of the vessels under examination. This angle is critical, as demonstrated in Figure 1–8. For example, placing the probe beam perpendicular to the blood flow with a scanning angle of 90° would yield no Doppler shift at all. This would make it appear that the vessel under investigation is occluded when it is actually patent. In practice, the probe beam is usually oriented to make a 30° to 60° scanning angle with the vessel lumen. These scanning angles are obtainable under most clinical situations.

The Doppler shift frequency is then used by the sound spectral analyzer to display on the TV screen how fast the RBC is moving. A fast-moving RBC would have a higher Doppler shift

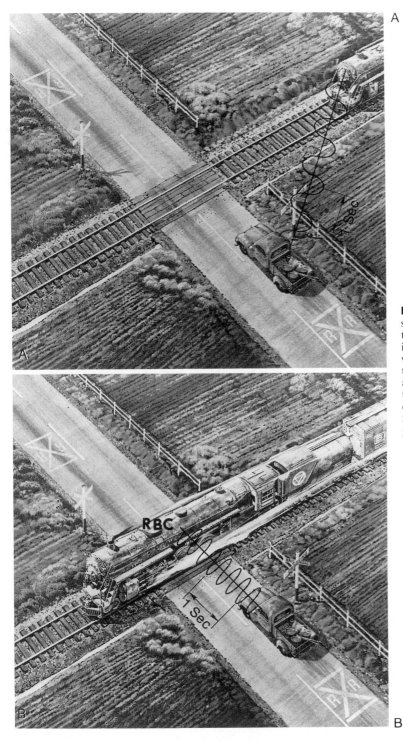

Figure 1–6. No change in the whistle sound frequency *(A)* would mean that the train is standing still. A steadily increasing higher-pitch, high-frequency whistle sound would mean that the train in *B* is moving towards the truck at the railroad crossing. In these illustrations the trains represent red blood cells (RBCs). (Illustration courtesy of Sonicaid, Inc., Fredericksburg, Virginia.)

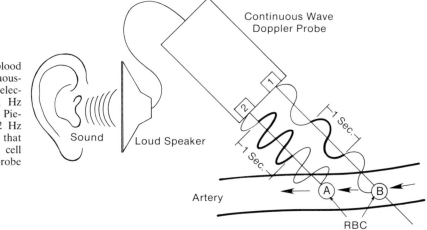

Figure 1–7. Conversion of blood flow into sound with a continuous-wave Doppler probe. *1*, Piezoelectric crystal transmitting a 1 Hz sound (heavy dark line). *2*, Piezoelectric crystal receiving 2 Hz sound (heavy dark line) that bounced off a red blood cell (RBC) moving towards the probe face.

frequency than would a slow-moving RBC because the Doppler shift frequency is proportional to the velocity of the RBC.

Bi-directional Doppler Probes

A red blood cell moving toward the probe face will have an increase in its Doppler shift frequency, whereas one moving away from the probe face will have a decrease in its Doppler shift frequency according to the Doppler principle. This change in frequency can be used to determine the direction in which the RBC is going in relation to the probe face. A bi-directional Doppler probe indicates whether or not the frequency shift is upward or downward from

the transmitted probe frequency. For example, the bi-directional continuous-wave Doppler probe in Figure 1–9*A* is transmitting a 10 Hz sound wave, which bounces off a moving RBC and is received by the probe as a 15 Hz sound wave. This represents a 5 Hz frequency shift upward from the transmitted frequency, meaning that the RBC is moving toward the observer or receiving crystal in the probe face. A downward 5 Hz frequency shift is illustrated in Figure 1–9*B* by an RBC moving away from the observer or receiving crystal. An analog waveform tracing either above or below a zero blood flow velocity baseline may be used to display this graphically (Fig. 1–9*A* and *B*). A positive blood flow waveform above the zero baseline would then mean that the RBC is moving toward the probe face

Figure 1–8. Technical factors affecting the Doppler shift frequencies.

A, Upslope of line indicates that the Doppler shift frequency increases as the Doppler probe emitting frequency increases.

B, Upslope of line indicates that the RBC velocity (cm/sec) increases as the Doppler shift frequency increases.

C, Downslope of line indicates that the Doppler shift frequency decreases as the probe angle θ to the blood flow in the vessel increases.

D, Diagram illustrating probe angle θ to the blood flow in a vessel. Arrow denotes blood flow directed towards the probe face.

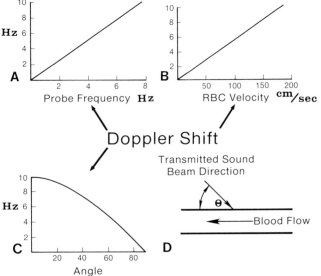

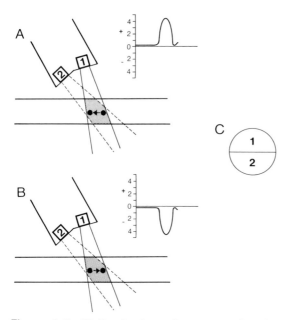

Figure 1–9. Bi-directional continuous-wave Doppler probe. *A,* Doppler probe detecting direction of a red blood cell moving towards it. *B,* Doppler probe detecting direction of a red blood cell moving away from it. *C,* Frontal view of probe showing how the piezoelectric crystals are cut into two semicircles—*(1)* output and *(2)* receiving crystals—to conform to probe face.

(Fig. 1–9*A*). Blood flow carrying RBCs away from the probe face would cause a negative deflection below the zero baseline (Fig. 1–9*B*).

The transducer design in Figure 1–9 is used for most continuous-wave, bi-directional Doppler probes. Two separate, inclined piezoelectric crystals are placed in the probe face. One is used to transmit ultrasonic waves (*Transmitting Crystal 1*), while the other is used to receive them (*Receiving Crystal 2*). A frontal view of the probe (Fig. 1–9*C*) shows how the piezoelectric crystals are cut into the shape of semicircles to conform to the circular probe face configuration.

The sound beams transmitted by Crystal 1 and received by Crystal 2 are directional as illustrated by the lines extending from these crystals in Figure 1–9*A* and *B*. Inclining the crystals in the probe face causes these lines to overlap, forming a zone in which the Doppler shift frequency of a moving RBC can be detected. This zone is depicted as the shaded area in Figure 1–9*A* and *B*. The RBC in Figure 1–9*A* is moving from right to left through this zone. As the RBC enters the right side of this zone, it comes into contact with the 10 Hz sound wave being transmitted by Crystal 1. The RBC continues to move across the zone, producing an ever-increasing higher frequency sound wave as it travels toward Re-

ceiving Crystal 2. This increase in frequency reaches a peak of 15 Hz as the RBC leaves the left side of the zone. A 5 Hz Doppler shift upward from the 10 Hz transmitted frequency is now recorded by the probe.

Figure 9–1*B* illustrates how the inclined crystals in the probe face are used to detect the movement of an RBC in the opposite direction. The RBC in this figure is moving from left to right. It enters the left margin of the zone, where it comes into contact with the 10 Hz sound wave being transmitted by Crystal 1. The RBC reflects sound waves with ever-decreasing lower frequencies to Crystal 2 because it is traveling away from it. This decrease in frequency reaches a maximum of 15 Hz as the RBC leaves the right side of the zone. A 5 Hz Doppler shift downward from the 10 Hz transmitted frequency is now recorded by the probe.

Laminar Blood Flow

Placing the concepts of instrumentation aside for the moment, one must define some of the properties of blood flow itself before its sound spectral analysis can be further understood. These properties may be explained by describing Newtonian fluid flow through a rigid pipe at a steady rate. Admittedly, this is somewhat removed from the complexities of non-Newtonian blood flow in a flexible artery at a pulsatile rate. But it does serve as a model for examining the spectral analysis of blood flow under certain conditions. These conditions assume that the blood flow in a vessel has a laminar profile consisting of multiple flow patterns of RBCs moving in straight lines parallel to the walls of the vessel (Fig. 1–10). The flow patterns are further organized into multiple concentric layers, with the innermost layers of RBCs moving more rapidly than the layers next to the vessel walls. The many different sounds from the Doppler shifts of these multiple layers of RBCs moving at varying velocities could be rather confusing to both the spectral analyzer and the observer. Pulsed Doppler systems have been devised in an attempt to eliminate some of this confusion.

Laminar Flow Profile

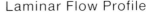
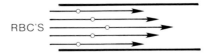

Figure 1–10. Laminar blood flow.

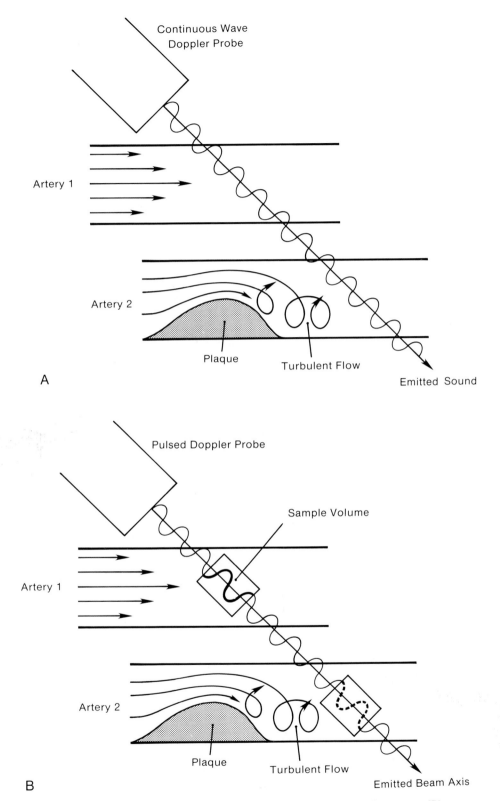

Figure 1–11. Continuous wave-system *(A)* and pulsed Doppler probe systems *(B)*.

Pulsed and Continuous-Wave Doppler Systems

A pulsed Doppler system makes it possible to "listen" to the sound arising from a discrete sample volume located at a specific distance from the probe face. Why this is important is further illustrated in Figure 1–11. Figure 1–11 also illustrates the blood flow sound sampling differences between a continuous-wave and a pulsed Doppler probe. The continuous-wave Doppler probe in Figure 1–11A is in a position to receive sound information from all of the RBC flow velocities across the laminar flow profiles of two arteries. Attempts to examine only Artery 1 could be a problem because it is now lying adjacent to Artery 2, which has a turbulent flow pattern. The pulsed Doppler system solves this problem by range gating. With range gating, only those sounds in a sample volume are received by the probe. Sounds originating from outside this sample volume are completely ignored by the probe (Figure 1–11B). The sample volume, which may be as small as 1 to 2 mm³, can be moved up and down the long axis of the probe's emitted beam. Moving the sample volume downward would allow the turbulent flow in Artery 2 to be distinguished from the laminar flow in Artery 1.

The pulsed Doppler system, therefore, not only allows the sound sample to be taken from the midstream blood flow position where, according to the Newtonian flow model, most RBCs are moving at nearly the same velocity but also permits the blood flow in one vessel to be distinguished from the blood flow in another adjacent vessel. Coupling the pulsed Doppler system with a real-time B-mode ultrasound image of the vessel being examined completes the instrumentation needed to obtain blood flow sound information for spectral analysis. The real-time B-mode image allows precise placement of the sample volume within the vessel lumen so that sounds from its flow patterns can be studied accurately. This successful marriage of real-time B-mode ultrasound imaging with pulse-gated Doppler ultrasound has resulted in a happy offspring known as *duplex scanning*.

Placing a duplex scanning probe over an artery will produce an entirely different spectral analysis image on the TV screen than the one shown in Figure 1–4. A review of this figure reveals two brilliant white lines, one above the other, traversing the TV screen. Two lines appeared on the screen because a continuous sound with only two different hertz frequencies was being analyzed. Blood flowing in an artery presents many different sound frequencies to the spectrum ana-

lyzer. This can be readily appreciated by comparing the spectral analysis TV image in Figure 1–4 with the spectral analysis TV image of arterial blood flow provided in Figure 1–12. Instead of two straight lines traversing the TV screen, multiple flashes of light or scintillations are seen following the contours of the cardiac cycle. These scintillations reflect the rapid Fourier transformational spectral analysis sound frequencies from groups of RBCs at each point in the cardiac cycle. There, Doppler shift frequencies in kHz are shown on the vertical axis, time in relationship to the cardiac cycle on the horizontal axis, and their sound amplitude or volumes by a gray scale. Amplitude or volume relates to the number of RBCs present in the emitted beam moving at a given velocity bouncing the sound back to the probe face. The sound volume increases as the number of RBCs increases and decreases as the number of RBCs decreases.

The same thing would happen if two trains were moving toward you at the same speed with their whistles blowing at the same volume. In other words, two trains are twice as loud as one train. Even though the combined sound of these two train whistles is louder, the increases in their Doppler shift frequencies would remain the same because the two trains are moving at the same speed.

For example, if a large proportion of RBCs within the sound beam are moving at a certain velocity (X), the TV image will be white at the Doppler shift level corresponding to that velocity. If a moderate number of RBCs are traveling at velocity X, the TV image will be a light gray, and if only a small number of RBCs are moving at velocity X, the image will be a dark shade of gray.

A color-coded format may also be used to display these various sound volume changes on a color TV monitor. The instrumentation is then essentially the same for analyzing the arterial blood flow as it was for the analysis of the two simple, continuous sounds described at the beginning of this chapter and shown in Figure 1–4. Only the methods by which the sounds were obtained and the fact that they are originating from the blood flow in an artery make Figure 1–12 different from Figure 1–4.

The Sound Spectral Analysis Image Format

A closer inspection of the TV image obtained during the real-time duplex scanning of blood flow in an artery will now be described. The

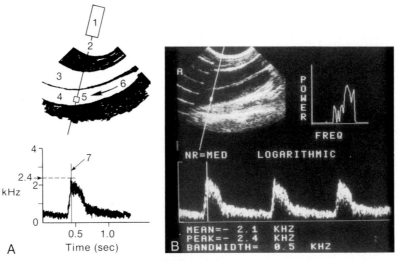

Figure 1–12. Freeze-frame TV image of an arterial duplex scan.

A, Representation. *1*, Duplex scanning probe angled towards the head. *2*, Direction of emitting and receiving probe beams. *3*, Jugular vein. *4*, Common carotid artery. *5*, Sample volume. *6*, Blood flow direction. *7*, Cursor for measuring Doppler shift frequencies at various points in the cardiac cycle.

B, Actual freeze-frame sound spectral analysis image of a common carotid artery.

example shown in Figure 1–12 is typical of that obtained during the examination of a normal common carotid artery (CCA) without associated disease in either the internal carotid artery (ICA) or the external carotid artery (ECA). It is presented in the freeze-frame mode with a *B*-mode *ultrasound image* of the CCA showing placement of the pulsed Doppler range gate sample volume within the midportion of the CCA lumen. Below is the *sound spectrum analyzer waveform* showing the Doppler shift frequency sounds of pulsatile blood flow within the sample volume. The sound spectral analysis waveform has been electronically manipulated to project in a positive, upward direction away from the zero hertz baseline.

A close inspection of the probe face angle in Figure 1–12 will show that the blood flow direction is away from the probe face. This occurred because the probe face had to be angled toward the head in order to obtain a satisfactory B-mode image of the CCA. On the real-time examination, the waveform showed a negative, downward deflection away from the zero hertz baseline. This bi-directional function of the Doppler probe showed that the blood flow in the CCA was in a normal direction away from the probe face and into the cerebral circulation.

Because an inverted waveform is sometimes difficult to read, it is customarily electronically flipped upward to a positive deflection for freeze-frame imaging and interpretation, as was done in this case. Frequency levels in kHz of the different RBC velocities moving through the sample volume are displayed on the vertical axis, and the duration of each cardiac cycle is given on the horizontal axis in seconds. As previously described, the amplitude or volume of the Doppler signal sound at any given frequency is displayed in shades of gray on the sound spectral analysis waveform. A movable cursor may be adjusted to measure the frequency at any horizontal level on the waveform. The cursor in Figure 1–12 is measuring the hertz frequency on a horizontal level corresponding to the systolic peak Doppler frequency shift, which is 2.4 kHz in this case. This measurement appears as a digital read-out depicted at the bottom of the TV screen freeze-frame image (Peak = 2.4 kHz).

The sound spectral analysis format in combination with duplex scanning instrumentation offers a powerful tool to be used in the diagnosis of vascular disease.

Part II • Noninvasive Assessment of the Extracranial Carotid Arteries

2 • Sound Spectral Analysis Blood Flow
Patterns of the Extracranial Carotid Arteries

Introduction

The different extracranial carotid artery blood flow patterns displayed by the sound spectral analyzer may be studied by breaking them down into the events occurring during three periods of the cardiac cycle: *systole, early diastole,* and *late diastole.* The sound spectral analysis image of a normal common carotid artery (CCA) blood flow pattern containing each of these three components is shown in Figure 2–1*A*.

The systolic component shown in Figure 2–1*B* begins with left ventricular contraction, which causes the pressure in the left ventricle to rise and closes the mitral valve. As the left ventricular pressure continues to rise, the aortic valve is opened. Immediately, blood begins to pour out of the left ventricle into the ascending aorta, causing a sharp increase in both the pressure and blood flow velocity within the CCA. This blood flow velocity increase is detected by the sound spectral analyzer as a sharp increase in the Doppler shift frequencies as the red blood cells (RBCs) rapidly accelerate from point (a) to point (b) (Figure 2–1*B*). Since most of the RBCs are moving at the same velocity through the sample volume of the pulsed Doppler probe during systole, they will have similar Doppler shift frequencies. The sound spectral analyzer displays these similar Doppler shift frequencies as a thin, narrow line extending upward from point (a) to point (b). The brightness or amplitude of this line will depend on the number of RBCs passing through the sample volume of the pulsed Doppler probe. An increased number of RBCs passing through the sample volume increases its brightness, whereas a smaller number of RBCs passing through the sample volume decreases its brightness.

At the end of systole, ventricular relaxation begins suddenly, allowing the intraventricular pressures to fall rapidly. The elevated pressure in the blood-filled, distended large arteries begins to immediately push blood back toward the left ventricle, which snaps the aortic valve closed. During systole, the RBCs gained momentum as they were ejected from the left ventricle. As this momentum decreases during the latter part of systole, the kinetic energy of the momentum is converted into pressure in the aorta. Blood pushed out of the aorta by this pressure enters the large systemic arteries, causing their walls to distend and stretch and their pressure to rise.

The RBCs begin to decelerate at different velocities during the end of systole and at the beginning of early diastole. This causes the RBCs to have many different Doppler shift frequencies during this deceleration phase. The sound spectral analyzer displays these different deceleration Doppler shift frequencies as a wide line extending down from point (b) to point (c) (Figure 2–1*C*). Again, the brightness of this line will depend upon the number of RBCs passing through the sample volume of the pulsed Doppler probe. Point (b) is important because it denotes the region during systole where the RBCs have reached their maximum velocities or Doppler shift frequencies. This maximum value is termed the *systolic peak* and is the point at which the systolic Doppler peak frequencies are measured on the sound spectral analysis blood flow image. The RBCs, having reached their maximum velocities at point (b), decelerate rapidly until the aortic valve closes at point (c), marking the end of early diastole.

The entry of blood into the arteries during systole causes the walls of these arteries to stretch and the pressure to rise. Then, at the end of systole, after the left ventricle stops ejecting blood and the aortic valve closes, the elastic recoil of the arteries maintains a high pressure in the arteries during late diastole. This recoil also forces the blood flow out of the arteries into the capillary bed. The sound spectral analyzer re-

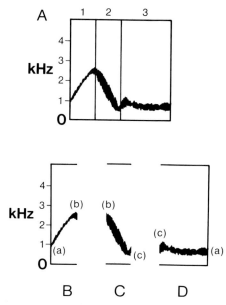

Figure 2–1. Sound spectral analysis pattern of arterial Doppler sounds broken down into three periods of the cardiac cycle.

A, Normal common carotid artery blood flow pattern. *1*, Systole. *2*, Early diastole. *3*, Late diastole.

B, Systolic component point *(a)*. The aortic valve opens and the red blood cells accelerate to the systolic peak *(b)*.

C, Early diastole point *(b)*. Having reached maximum velocity, the red blood cells decelerate to the point of aortic valve closure *(c)*.

D, Late diastolic component *(c-a)*.

cords late diastolic blood flow as a gradual downward-sloping wide line of diminishing Doppler shift frequencies extending from point (c) to point (a). This line remains wide because the RBCs continue to decelerate at different velocities. Late diastole begins with aortic valve closure at point c and ends at point a, where the aortic valve opens and the RBCs accelerate once again.

Putting all three of these components together gives one the sound spectral analysis image blood flow pattern in Figure 1–1*A*. It represents the many different Doppler shift frequencies arising from numerous RBCs moving at various velocities in the CCA throughout the cardiac cycle.

Image patterns of this type are then used to diagnose a wide variety of abnormalities in many different arteries. All the sound spectral analyzer does is apply the Doppler principle to groups of RBCs as they move through the sample volume of the pulsed Doppler probe during each of the three components of the cardiac cycle and determines:

1. Whether or not the RBCs are moving (*movement*).

2. How fast the RBCs are moving (*velocity*).

3. Whether or not all of the RBCs in a sample

volume are moving at the same or different speeds (*turbulence*).

4. In which direction the RBCs are moving (*direction*).

5. Whether or not a large or small number of RBCs is moving through the sample volume of the pulsed Doppler probe (*amplitude*).

Therefore, it is the various combinations of movement, velocity, turbulence, direction of movement, and amplitude of RBCs for each of the three components of the cardiac cycle that make up the blood flow sound spectral analysis pattern seen on the television (TV) screen.

Normal Extracranial Carotid Artery Blood Flow Patterns

The sound spectral analysis patterns of the external carotid artery (ECA), internal carotid artery (ICA), and common carotid artery (CCA) should all be examined together as a unit. Approximately 80% of the blood flowing from the CCA goes through the ICA into the brain, whereas 20% goes through the ECA into the facial musculature (Fig. 2–2). The relative de-

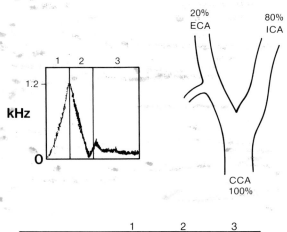

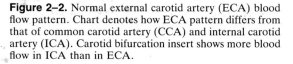

	1	2	3
MOVEMENT	Yes	Yes	Yes
VELOCITY	▲	▼	Low
TURBULENCE	None	None	None
DIRECTION	Normal	Normal	Normal
AMPLITUDE	Low	Low	Low

Figure 2–2. Normal external carotid artery (ECA) blood flow pattern. Chart denotes how ECA pattern differs from that of common carotid artery (CCA) and internal carotid artery (ICA). Carotid bifurcation insert shows more blood flow in ICA than in ECA.

crease in blood flow through the ECA will cause it to have a lower amplitude gray scale waveform throughout all three components of the cardiac cycle than that found in either the ICA or the CCA. This is noted in the charts in Figures 2–2 and 2–3 as a low amplitude for the ECA and a high amplitude for the CCA and ICA.

The ECA carries blood into the high-resistance facial musculature circulation; the ICA carries blood into the low-resistance brain circulation. As a result, the ECA has a steep systolic upward slope, a spiked systolic peak, and a steep early diastolic downward slope (Fig. 2–2). Both the CCA and the ICA, which are carrying blood to a lower-resistance circulation, have a gradual systolic upward slope, a rounded systolic peak, and a gradual early diastolic downward slope (Fig. 2–3). Because the ICA is a high flow–low resistance system, it has a higher systolic peak Doppler shift frequency (2.5 kHz) (Fig. 2–3) than does the ECA (1.2 kHz) (Fig. 2–2), which is a low flow–high resistance system.

A comparison of the late diastolic component of the ECA (Fig. 2–2) and the CCA and ICA (Fig. 2–3) shows some distinct differences between these vessels. The ECA late diastolic blood flow is low because of the decreased run-off of blood into the high-resistance vascular bed of the facial musculature. This results in the low, late diastolic Doppler shift frequencies, which approach the zero baseline (Fig. 2–2). The CCA and ICA late diastolic blood flows are increased as compared with the ECA late diastolic blood flow because there is a greater run-off of blood from these vessels into the low-resistance vascular bed of the brain. This results in the elevated late diastolic Doppler shift frequencies above the zero baseline as shown in Figure 2–3. A low, late diastolic blood flow velocity is recorded in the ECA chart, whereas it is recorded as high in the CCA and ICA charts. Movement of the RBCs in a normal direction is present because none of these vessels are occluded.

Turbulence is usually found in the flow patterns of abnormal vessels. Therefore, it is not expected to be encountered, except at specific sites, in the normal extracranial carotid arteries.

Turbulent Blood Flow Patterns

The projection of an atheromatous plaque into the arterial lumen disrupts the smooth laminar flow of RBCs through the vessel, producing a turbulent flow pattern. As the RBCs meet the projecting margin of the plaque, they are thrown into eddy currents composed of RBCs moving at

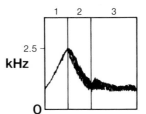

	1	2	3
MOVEMENT	Yes	Yes	Yes
VELOCITY	▲	▼	High
TURBULENCE	None	None	None
DIRECTION	Normal	Normal	Normal
AMPLITUDE	High	High	High

Figure 2–3. Normal common carotid artery and internal carotid artery blood flow pattern.

different speeds and in different directions. These are similar to the eddy currents formed by the rippling waters of a mountain stream. The invasion of these eddy currents into the central arterial lumen introduces the random movement of the RBCs into the sample volume (Fig. 2–4). This causes a large number of many different Doppler shift frequencies to be detected by the pulsed Doppler probe. The sound spectral analyzer displays these on the TV screen as randomly placed scintillations at many different frequency levels.

Normally, the RBC Doppler shift frequencies are grouped together, forming a spectral line that is narrow in systole and wide in early and late diastole (Fig. 2–1A). The zone between the spectral line and the zero hertz (OHz) frequency baseline is black because there are no scintillations in this zone. This black zone is called the *spectral window* (Fig. 2–5A).

When the random movement of RBCs flowing over and around plaques causes scintillations to fall outside their normal limits, the spectral line becomes broad, as shown in Figure 2–5B. The term *spectral broadening* is used to describe this phenomenon. As the random movements of the RBCs increase, the differences in their Doppler shift frequencies also increase, causing scintillations to fall outside the broadened spectrum and into the spectral window zone (Figs. 2–5C and D). Initially, there may be only a few speckles of scintillation in this zone. But as the random motion of the RBCs increases, more and more scintillations appear and begin to fill in the spec-

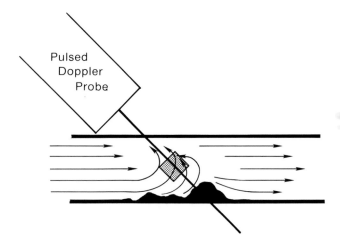

Figure 2–4. Plaque causing random movement of red blood cells (RBCs), which are entering the sample volume at varying speeds. Square indicates sample volume of the pulsed Doppler probe.

tral window. The amount of spectral broadening also continues to increase throughout all of the periods of the cardiac cycle. Finally, the spectral window is totally obliterated (Fig. 2–5E), and no distinction can be made between the original spectral line and the original spectral window.

The turbulent sound spectral image in Figure 2–5E indicates a complete saturation of the sample volume with multiple eddy currents filled with RBCs moving at many different random speeds. It is important to note that the spectral line contour has remained unchanged throughout Figure 2–5A to E. This is because the plaque did not produce a significant stenosis or narrowing of the vessel lumen. It, therefore, caused only turbulent flow without an increase in the blood flow velocity.

Unfortunately, there are other conditions that may produce turbulent blood flow patterns similar to those caused by plaque formation. Some of these represent potential pitfalls in the diagnosis of plaque disease because they are found in completely normal arteries (Fig. 2–6A). For example, it is quite normal to find turbulence at the site of branching vessels.

Turbulence may occur at two specific sites in

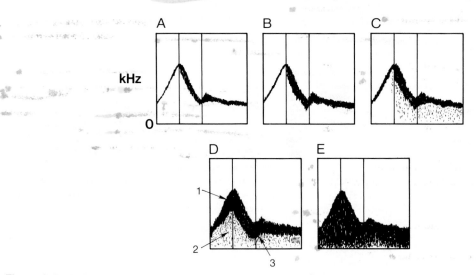

Figure 2–5. Turbulent blood flow patterns.
   A, Normal ICA flow pattern with absence of scintillations in the spectral window.
   B, Spectral flow pattern broadening in early and late diastole with absence of scintillations in the spectral window.
   C, Speckled scintillations beginning to fill in the spectral window during systole, early diastole, and late diastole.
   D, Spectral broadening of all three cardiac cycle components *(1)*. Increased spectral window scintillations *(2)*. A distinction can still be made between the original spectral line and spectral window zone *(3)*.
   E, Turbulent spectrum with obliterated spectral window. No distinction can be made between the original spectral line and the spectral window zone.

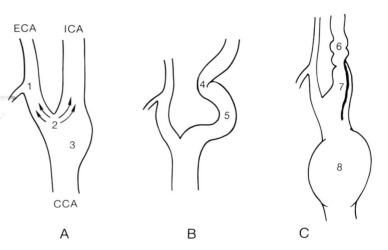

Figure 2–6. Normal carotid bifurcation (A), kinked and tortuous internal carotid artery (ICA) (B), and non-atheromatous causes of turbulent blood flow (C).

1, Origin of superior thyroid artery from external carotid artery (ECA). 2, Origins of ECA and ICA adjacent to carotid bulb (separation zone). 3, Normal carotid bulb. 4, Kink in ICA. 5, Tortuous ICA. 6, Fibromuscular dysplasia without significant stenosis. 7, ICA wall dissection. 8, Common carotid artery (CCA) aneurysm.

the region of carotid bifurcation. First, there is the site where the CCA branches into the ECA and ICA. Second, there is the site where the superior thyroid artery branches off of the ECA. Turbulence may also be found at sites where there is an abrupt change in the diameter of a vessel. This explains why turbulence may be encountered in a normal carotid bulb where the CCA terminates in a localized area of dilatation as it divides into the ECA and ICA.

Elderly patients who present with a long history of hypertension often have bizarre, tortuous carotid bifurcations that are quite capable of producing a turbulent flow pattern in the absence of plaque disease (Fig. 2–6B). Isolated kinks in the ICA will also induce turbulence (Fig. 2–6B). Some other non-atheromatous causes of turbulent blood flow in the extracranial carotid arteries include aneurysms, arterial wall dissections, and fibromuscular dysplastic abnormalities unassociated with significant stenotic lesions (Fig. 2–6C). A correlation of the sound spectral analysis with the B-mode image of the arteries being examined is used in the diagnosis of these non-atheromatous causes of turbulence.

Another concept in the formation of turbulent blood flow patterns concerns the *Reynolds number,* the equation for which is given in Figure 2–7. The Reynolds number has no units and defines the point at which turbulent blood flow occurs. When the Reynolds number rises above 200 to 400, turbulent flow will occur in some branches of vessels, but the turbulence will disappear along the smooth, nonbranching portions of the vessel. However, when the Reynolds number rises above approximately 2,000, turbulence will usually occur even in the straight, smooth, nonbranching portion of the vessel.

As shown in Figure 2–7, the tendency for turbulent flow patterns to occur increases in direct proportion to the velocity of blood flow. This may account for the presence of turbulent flow patterns observed in collateral arteries circumventing a total arterial occlusion. For example, turbulence can be observed in normal ECAs, vertebral arteries, and contralateral CCAs and ICAs when they are acting as collaterals to circumvent the cerebral blood flow around a totally occluded ICA. The increased velocity of blood flow may also account for the turbulence sometimes observed in the normal extracranial carotid arteries of young patients with normal cardiac outputs or in the patient who is in a high cardiac output state.

Turbulence is also seen in arteries supplying arteriovenous fistulas and arteriovenous malformations. The Reynolds number equation demonstrates that the tendency for turbulent flow increases in direct proportion to the increase in the vessel diameter, thus explaining why turbulence is encountered in the carotid bulb and in aneurysms with expanded lumens. Changes in either the density or viscosity of blood also may induce turbulence, as is shown by this equation.

There are numerous causes for the turbulent blood flow pattern observed on the sound spectral analysis image of both the extracranial carotid and vertebral arteries. The sound spectral analysis can detect the turbulence, but it cannot define the etiology of the turbulence without the help of the B-mode image. This is especially true in the evaluation of arteries in the presence of atherosclerotic plaque formation.

$$\text{REYNOLDS' NUMBER} = \frac{\text{VELOCITY} \times \text{DIAMETER} \times \text{DENSITY}}{\text{VISCOSITY}}$$

Figure 2–7. The Reynolds number equation.

High-Velocity Blood Flow Patterns

The overall concept of high-velocity blood flow can be best understood by simply observing the flow of water in a mountain stream. At a point in the stream where the flow of water is quiet and serene, one will observe that the water is deep and the banks along the stream are wide. Walking down the shoreline, however, one will invariably hear the sound of rapids originating from a source in the distance downstream. Approaching the source of this sound, one observes that the speed of the water flow begins to gradually increase. Walking still further downstream, one will encounter a swift current and notice that the sound of the rapids begins to get louder. Finally, at the source of the sound, one finds two large boulders projecting into the stream, reducing its diameter by 50%. Here the current is extremely swift, and as the water rushes through the narrowing created by the protruding boulders, it has numerous white, foaming, bubbling rapids. Walking downstream, one notes that the rapids begin to turn into multiple swirling eddy currents and that the sound of rushing water begins to fade away. The flow of the water gradually begins to slow down as one progresses further downstream, and the banks widen, and the flow of the mountain stream becomes quiet and serene once again.

This journey through a narrowing in a mountain stream is quite similar to that of the course taken by red blood cells flowing through an arterial stenosis. The velocities of the RBCs increase as they approach and traverse the stenosis, which is recorded on the sound spectral analyzer as an increase in the RBC Doppler shift frequencies. The RBCs passing through a tight stenosis will have higher Doppler shift frequencies than RBCs passing through a mild stenosis because of the greater velocities of the former. Like the water in the mountain stream, the velocities will begin to increase as the RBCs approach the stenosis, remain high in the stenosis, and decrease downstream past the stenosis. The RBCs also undergo considerable turbulence (like the mountain stream rapids in between the two boulders) as they pass through the stenosis. This turbulence is detected in the sample volume of the pulsed Doppler probe and recorded on the sound spectral analysis image as spectral broadening. The velocity increase and the spectral broadening of the Doppler shift frequencies of the RBCs make up the patterns used in the diagnosis of mild and tight arterial stenoses.

Any atherosclerotic plaque that protrudes into the vessel lumen will create an arterial stenosis. The stenosis may be so mild (e.g., 5 to 15% vessel diameter reduction) that it does not increase the blood flow velocity. Instead, it only creates turbulence as shown in Figure 2–4 and 2–5. Attempts to diagnose these mild stenoses by sound spectral analysis alone may be misleading, as indicated by Jacobs and colleagues.[1] They observed that the minimal turbulence present in such cases is easily mimicked by "pseudoturbulence" caused by slight adjustments in gain settings and other technical factors. A real-time B-mode image of the plaque causing the turbulent blood flow must be obtained to eliminate this potential pitfall.

Mild stenoses are diagnosed most accurately by real-time B-mode imaging in both the cross-sectional and sagittal planes in the area of turbulent blood flow rather than by the amount of turbulence present on the sound spectral analysis alone. This is also true for moderate stenoses resulting in less than a 50% reduction in the vessel diameter. Again, these stenoses produce turbulence without a significant increase in the blood flow velocity, making their diagnosis by sound spectral analysis difficult.

Stenoses causing a greater than 50% diameter reduction of the vessel lumen begin to establish a high-velocity blood flow pattern. This pattern is quite distinct from the turbulent blood flow patterns shown in Figure 2–5. An example of the high-velocity blood flow pattern is shown in Figure 2–8. Initially, the blood flow velocity increase in the stenosis may exist only during systole and may return to normal during diastole (Fig. 2–8). With progressively more severe stenosis, the blood flow velocity will be increased throughout the entire cardiac cycle (Fig. 2–9).

The precise Doppler shift frequencies denoting increased velocities throughout the cardiac cycle must be individualized for each noninvasive laboratory. The reasons for this are illustrated in Figure 1–7. A review of this figure will show that the Doppler shift frequencies vary according to the output Doppler probe frequency and the scanning angle used in performing the examinations.

The detection of a stenosis is very operator-dependent, and the results obtained in one laboratory may be different from the results obtained in another laboratory. The Doppler shift frequencies in Table 2–1 used to describe the high-velocity blood flow patterns in this chapter and throughout this text were obtained with a pulsed Doppler repetition frequency of 4.5 MHz

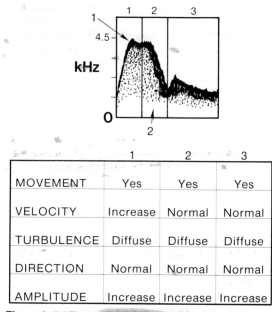

	1	2	3
MOVEMENT	Yes	Yes	Yes
VELOCITY	Increase	Normal	Normal
TURBULENCE	Diffuse	Diffuse	Diffuse
DIRECTION	Normal	Normal	Normal
AMPLITUDE	Increase	Increase	Increase

Figure 2–8. High-velocity blood flow pattern in ICA with 50 to 60% diameter reduction stenosis. *1*, Broad, round systolic peak with systolic peak frequency of 4.5 kHz. *2*, Increase in spectral broadening with speckling near zero baseline.

and a probe beam angle of 30 to 60° to the blood flow in the vessel, as is shown in Figure 1–7.

The second spectral analysis blood flow pattern in Figure 2–8 represents that of an ICA critical stenosis. It is characterized by an increase in the systolic peak frequency of 4.5 kHz. A critical stenosis is defined as the degree of narrowing of a vessel required to produce a detectable pressure gradient or reduction in blood flow.[2] Experimentally, appreciable changes in pressure and flow do not occur until the cross-sectional area of a vessel has been reduced by more than 75% (usually 80 to 95%).[2] If we assume that the stenosis is symmetric, this reduction in cross-sectional area corresponds to at least a 50% reduction in diameter. The presence of a critical stenosis in the ICA is an important diagnosis to make because it may be an indication for surgical intervention in either the symptomatic or asymptomatic patient.[3]

In an ICA critical stenosis, both early and late diastolic peak frequencies remain normal, as is indicated in the chart for Figure 2–8. Turbulence creates a diffuse spectral broadening throughout all three phases of the cardiac cycle. A sound spectral analysis image of this flow pattern is displayed in brilliant white on a black-and-white TV monitor because its amplitude is increased throughout all three phases of the cardiac cycle as a result of the intense amount of spectral broadening present. The amplitude is also increased because the RBCs are compressed together as they pass through the stenosis. This compacted mass of RBCs bounces back an increased number of echoes to the receiving crystal in the Doppler probe face.

The sound spectral analysis image changes as

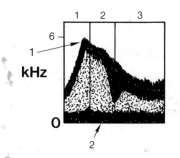

Figure 2–9. High-velocity blood flow pattern in ICA with 60 to 80% diameter reduction stenosis. *1*, Broad, flattened systolic peak with systolic peak frequency of 6 kHz. *2*, Increased spectral broadening and speckling near zero baseline.

	1	2	3
MOVEMENT			
VELOCITY	Increased	Increased	Increased
TURBULENCE	Yes/Low	Yes/Low	Yes/Low
DIRECTION			
AMPLITUDE	Increased	Increased	Increased

Table 2–1. Systolic Peak Frequencies and Percentage of Stenosis

Doppler Shift (kHz)	Diameter Reduction (%)
<3.5	0–40%
4–5	50–60%
5.5–6	60–80%
>6	80–95%

the percentage of stenosis increases. An example of the high-velocity blood flow pattern in a 60 to 80% stenosis is illustrated in Figure 2–9. The systolic peak frequencies range from 5.5 to 6 kHz (Table 2–1), and an increase in the blood flow velocity is present throughout all three phases of the cardiac cycle. This increase in velocity produces extremely severe turbulence and a concentration of low-level Doppler shift frequencies adjacent to the zero baseline. Again, there is an increase in the amplitude caused by the intense spectral broadening.

When considering the hemodynamics and anatomy of a stenosis, one must take care to distinguish blood flow volume rate from blood flow velocity and the percentage of diameter reduction from the percentage of cross-sectional area reduction. These are all quite different quantities, which are used to define a given stenosis, as is shown in Figure 2–10.

The percentage of diameter reduction is a common measurement used to express the severity of an arterial stenosis. This measurement is usually taken from a selective common carotid arteriogram obtained in the plane showing the maximal stenosis. No correction is made for magnification, and the percentage of diameter reduction is calculated according to the formula in Figure 2–10A.

It is now possible to measure the percentage of cross-sectional area reduction in an artery with the use of B-mode imaging. A cursor is used to outline both the outside circumference of the artery and the inside circumference of the stenosis from a freeze-frame cross-sectional B-mode image of the vessel on the TV screen (Fig. 2–10B). The appropriate computer program uses these cursor measurements to calculate the percentage of cross-sectional area reduction. This method is extremely user-dependent because it relies heavily on the operator's skill to accurately define both the outside surface of the vessel and the inside residual vascular lumen.

It is important to realize that two entirely different numerical values are used to define a critical stenosis for each of these two methods. As stated previously, a critical stenosis is defined

in the cross-sectional area reduction method as 80 to 95%, whereas with the diameter reduction method it is defined as 50%.

Volume blood flow rate may be confused with blood flow velocity. These are two quite different parameters for expressing blood flow measurements. Volume blood flow rate is the amount of blood passing a point in a vessel per unit of time expressed in milliliters per minute (ml/min). Blood flow velocity is the speed at which blood is flowing past a point in a vessel expressed in centimeters per second (cm/sec). It is important to realize that as either the percentage of diameter reduction or the cross-sectional area reduction of the stenosis increases, the blood flow volume rate decreases, whereas the blood flow velocity increases (Fig. 2–10C).[4] Utilizing Doppler technology as described in Chapter 1, the Doppler shift frequencies obtained from moving RBCs are used to detect blood flow velocity (cm/sec). The Doppler shift frequencies increase as the velocity of the RBCs increases.

Computer programs are available in some du-

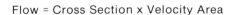

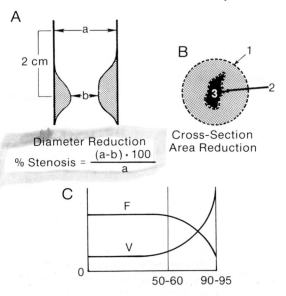

Figure 2–10. Methods for expressing the anatomy and hemodynamics of a stenosis.

A, Percentage of diameter reduction: *(a)* is the diameter in millimeters of the first normal part of the artery at 2 cm distal to the stenosis and *(b)* is the diameter in millimeters of the maximal stenosis.

B, Cross-sectional area reduction. *1,* Outside vessel circumference. *2,* Inside stenosis circumference. *3,* Vessel lumen.

C, Increase in percent diameter stenosis causes the blood flow volume rate *(F)* to decrease and the blood flow velocity *(V)* to increase.

plex scanning units, which allow an approximation of the blood flow volume rate to be made at a point in a vessel or graft conduit carrying blood. These units use both the blood flow velocity and the B-mode image cross-sectional area measurements to calculate the instantaneous volume blood flow rate at any point in the cardiac cycle according to the equation:

$$\text{Volume blood flow rate} = \text{cross-sectional area} \times \text{average velocity.}$$

Because of the pulsatile nature of blood flow, the instantaneous volume flow changes during each phase of the cardiac cycle. The average volume blood flow rate can be obtained by averaging the instantaneous values in one or more cardiac cycles. A simple way to check the accuracy of these measurements is to take the sum of the volume flow rates of the external and internal carotid arteries and compare it with the volume flow rate in the CCA. If the measurements are accurate, the sum of the external plus the ICA

volume flow rates should roughly equal the volume flow rate through the CCA (Fig. 2–11).

Slow Flow/No Flow Patterns

The analogy of building a dam across a mountain stream provides an opportunity to understand some of the characteristics of the slow flow/no flow patterns created in an artery by either a severe stenosis or a total occlusion. As the sand is shoveled onto the banks and into the stream to build the dam, the flow of water will undergo quite a few changes before it is completely stopped.

Begin by piling up the sand so that it extends from each bank towards the middle of the stream. This causes the water flow to become turbulent while both its velocity and volume flow rate remain constant. Shoveling more and more sand onto the dam narrows the stream, producing an increase in both its turbulence and velocity. The volume flow rate remains constant.

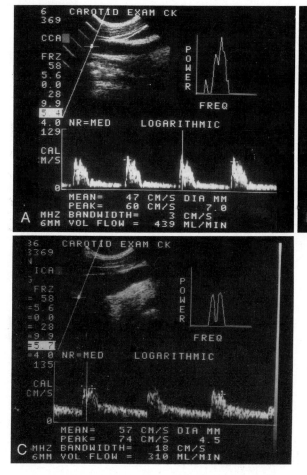

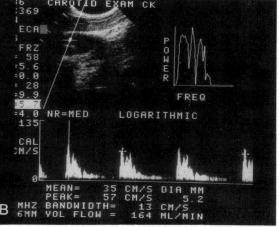

Figure 2–11. Accuracy testing of volume flow rate measurements of extracranial carotid vessels. Note that external carotid artery (ECA) and internal carotid artery (ICA) roughly equal common carotid artery (CCA). *A,* Volume flow rate in CCA using continuous-wave Doppler (439 ml/min). *B,* Volume flow rate in the ECA using pulsed Doppler (164 ml/min). *C,* Volume flow rate in the ICA using pulsed Doppler (310 ml/min).

Continuing to throw shovel loads of sand onto the dam narrows the stream even further. This causes both the velocity and turbulence of the water flow in the stream to increase while its volume flow rate begins to decrease. Adding still more sand towards the middle of the dam dramatically decreases the turbulence, velocity, and volume flow rate of the water flow as it slowly passes through the very small opening left in the middle of the dam.

Now only a few handfuls of sand are necessary to reduce this slow flow to a mere trickle of water passing over the dam. The water's turbulence, velocity, and volume flow rate have just about disappeared. Looking upstream, you notice that the water flow, velocity, and turbulence have decreased there too but the volume flow rate still remains the same. Unlike blood, which is contained within the confines of an artery, the water in the mountain stream soon spills over the banks, forming a small lake behind the dam. Because the blood is confined to a closed space, its volume flow rate is drastically reduced as the artery begins to become occluded by a severe stenosis.

The slow flow/trickle flow phenomenon described in the mountain stream analogy can cause two potential pitfalls in the sound spectral analysis of a severely stenosed artery. A slow, turbulent blood flow pattern may be mistakenly assumed to result from mild plaque disease without a significant stenosis when, in reality, it is caused by a marked amount of plaque disease and a severe stenosis. As stated previously, the progressive decrease in the cross-sectional area of an artery causing a critical stenosis is initially accompanied by a proportional increase in the systolic peak Doppler shift frequencies, as illustrated by the high-velocity blood flow pattern in Figure 2–9.

As the stenosis increases in severity, however, the resistance created by the stenotic zone causes a dramatic decrease in the number of RBCs to pass through the stenosis at high velocities. The sound spectral analyzer will display the diminished number of high-velocity RBCs as low-amplitude scintillations, which may be such a dark shade of gray that they may be difficult to see on the TV screen. When they are seen, they appear as a ghost waveform composed of sparsely speckled, low-amplitude scintillations superimposed above a waveform containing higher-amplitude scintillations with lower Doppler shift frequencies (Fig. 2–12).

The presence of these low-amplitude, weak scintillations in the ghost waveform makes it difficult to measure the precise point of the maximum systolic peak frequencies. This is further complicated by the fact that as the stenosis progresses in severity, even the ghost waveform is lost as the RBCs begin to move slowly or trickle through the stenosis. Now only the lower

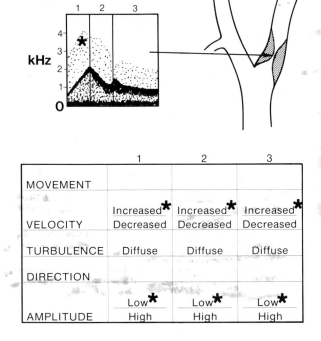

	1	2	3
MOVEMENT			
VELOCITY	Increased* Decreased	Increased* Decreased	Increased* Decreased
TURBULENCE	Diffuse	Diffuse	Diffuse
DIRECTION			
AMPLITUDE	Low* High	Low* High	Low* High

Figure 2–12. Sound spectral analysis of severe stenosis greater than 90% diameter reduction, producing low-amplitude, increased-velocity ghost waveform (asterisk) superimposed above a high-amplitude, low-velocity waveform. As the ghost waveform disappears, it leaves behind the waveform below with a systolic peak frequency of 2 kHz that underestimates the severity of the illustrated stenosis (arrow).

waveform containing the high-amplitude scintillations with lower Doppler shift frequencies is visible on the TV screen.

The sound spectral analysis of the blood flow through the stenotic zone under these conditions will be misleading because it will either underestimate or completely fail to detect the severity of the stenosis. One method of avoiding this particular pitfall consists of obtaining a real-time B-mode image of the arterial anatomy in the region of the turbulent blood flow. This image should reveal the presence of a severe stenosis as the cause of the turbulent blood flow pattern. Another method consists of using the sound spectral analyzer to observe how far along the artery the turbulent flow pattern extends. Small, nonobstructive plaques usually cause turbulent flow patterns to exist in short arterial segments, whereas turbulent flow patterns extending throughout long arterial segments should always arouse the suspicion that an underlying occult severe stenosis is present. The detection of a reversed blood flow in the periorbital arteries, indicating the presence of ECA collateral blood flow around a severe ICA stenosis, may also assist in avoiding this pitfall.

The collateral blood flow through the ECA can also be evaluated by the sound spectral analysis of this vessel at the carotid bifurcation in the neck. Here the ECA diastolic blood flow is normally low because of the decreased run-off of blood into the high-resistance vascular bed of the facial musculature. This results in the low diastolic Doppler shift frequencies, which approach the zero baseline level, as shown in Figure 2–2. However, this pattern changes when the ECA acts as a collateral pathway around either a severe stenosis or a total occlusion in the ICA. Under these circumstances, the peripheral arterioles in the terminal ECA branches dilate, allowing an increase in the volume blood flow rate through the ECA into the cerebral vessels. This causes an elevation in the ECA diastolic Doppler shift frequencies, as illustrated in Figure 2–13A. This figure shows the changes in the normal ECA high-resistance, low-volume blood flow rate pattern when it is converted into one of a low-resistance, high-volume blood flow rate pattern.

The close scrutiny of the CCA sound spectral analysis waveform will also help in the diagnosis of an occult, severe stenosis in the ICA. If we recall what happened to the flow of water upstream as the dam was being built across the mountain stream, the water flow velocity upstream began to diminish as the sand was shoveled onto the dam, blocking the flow of water

downstream. The same thing happens in the CCA when a severe stenosis in the ICA diminishes cerebral blood flow.

Normally, the diastolic peak Doppler shift frequencies associated with the CCA are above the zero baseline level because of the run-off of blood flow into the low-resistance vascular bed of the brain. A severe ICA stenosis converts the normal CCA low-resistance, high-volume blood flow pattern into an abnormal, high-resistance, low-volume blood flow pattern like the one shown in Figure 2–13B. This pattern is characterized by a decrease in the blood flow velocity during early and late systole and either a greatly diminished or totally absent flow velocity throughout the diastolic components of the cardiac cycle.

A more quantitative and sensitive method of measuring the common carotid flow characteristics is the resistivity index (RI) described by Planilo and associates.[5] The resistivity index is derived from the equation

$$RI = A - B/A.$$

Markers were placed on Figure 2–13B to denote the locations on the sound spectral analysis waveform used to measure peak systolic Doppler shift

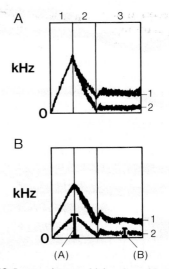

Figure 2–13. Low-resistance, high-volume blood flow rate pattern in ECA *(A)* and high-resistance, low-volume blood flow rate pattern CCA *(B)*.

A, Collateral blood flow through the ECA increases diastolic Doppler shift frequencies *(1)*, which are above the normal level at *(2)*.

B, Severe stenosis in ICA decreases the CCA normal elevated diastolic Doppler shift frequencies *(1)* to abnormal ones *(2)* close to the zero baseline levels. Markers denote sites for measuring A and B in order to obtain the resistivity index.

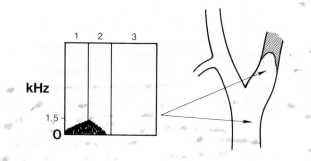

	1	2	3
MOVEMENT			None
VELOCITY	Decreased	Decreased	None
TURBULENCE	Diffuse	Diffuse	
DIRECTION			
AMPLITUDE	High	High	

Figure 2–14. CCA and ICA stump flow patterns in the presence of an occluded ICA.

frequency (A) and diastolic Doppler shift frequency (B). The normal common carotid RI, as determined by Courbier and others,[6] ranges from 0.5 to 0.75. With hemodynamically significant ICA stenosis, defined by these investigators as greater than a 90% decrease in diameter or as complete occlusion, the RI exceeded 0.75 in all cases, with a mean value of 0.93 for stenosis and 0.96 for occlusion.

Trickle flow produces another pitfall that will be encountered during the sound spectral analysis of a severe stenosis (greater than 95% diameter reduction). The trickle of RBCs through these extremely tight stenoses may be so small that their Doppler shift frequencies are too low to be detected by the sound spectral analyzer. A severe stenosis may be mistaken for a total occlusion in an artery under these circumstances.[7] An error of this type may have considerable clinical significance because a totally occluded ICA is usually inoperable, whereas a normal circulation can be restored in an ICA containing a severe stenosis. Unfortunately, the use of Doppler noninvasive methods will require further investigation and research before this error can be avoided with a high degree of accuracy.

The use of a reversal in the periorbital blood flow is of no diagnostic help because ECA collateral flow may occur in either a severe stenosis or a total occlusion and is therefore not useful in distinguishing the two. Slow infusion or "trickle" angiography using contrast media injected at flow rates of 3 to 4 ml/sec for a total volume of 10 to 12 ml, combined with prolonged serial film sequences of 1 frame/sec for 10 to 15 seconds, remains the method of choice in distinguishing a severe stenosis from a total occlusion.

Finally, the last shovel load of sand is placed on the dam, and the flow of water downstream past the dam is stopped. There is, however, a flow of water still coming from upstream towards the dam. This analogy simulates what happens in a totally occluded ICA rather nicely. The absence of water flow downstream past the dam represents the absence of blood flow in the fresh clot or thrombus-filled occluded arterial segment, whereas the water flowing from upstream towards the dam represents blood flow in a patent stump leading to the occluded arterial segment. Again, unlike the blood flow confined within the stump, the flow of water coming down from upstream continues to spill over the stream's banks, forming a lake. It will continue to flow at a relatively constant rate.

Because the flow of blood into the occluded stump segment has nowhere to go, blood flow velocity will be absent or greatly decreased. The pulsatile expansion of the elastic stump arterial walls may allow minimal blood flow to enter it during left ventricular contraction. Stump flow of this type audibly sounds like a dull thud with each systole and has a sound spectral analysis image pattern as that shown in Figure 2–14. This same pattern may also be obtained in a patent

CCA when the ICA is occluded with or without a patent stump segment.

As shown by the chart in Figure 2–14, the stump flow pattern is characterized by a greatly decreased early and late systolic blood flow velocity and absent blood flow velocity throughout diastole. Turbulence within the flat systolic waveform is diffuse, and the amplitude remains high. The sound spectral analysis waveform over the clot or thrombus-filled occluded arterial segment will be flat because no Doppler shift frequency signals exist from the RBCs that are not moving.

The most common pitfall in the sound spectral analysis of a totally occluded ICA is to mistake a patent ECA or one of its branches for the ICA. This type of error arises when the ECA acts as a major collateral pathway around the occluded ICA and its normally high-resistance, low–blood flow pattern is converted into an abnormal low-resistance, high–blood flow ECA pattern, which may then be mistaken for an ICA normal blood flow pattern.

A comparison of the waveforms in Figure 2–13A and B will demonstrate how easy it is to make this error. The B-mode image may also be confusing. For instance, examine the lateral view of the selective common carotid arteriogram in Figure 2–15. At first glance, the stenosis appears proximal to the carotid bifurcation. This, of course, is incorrect because the stenosis is located in the proximal ECA and because the ICA is totally occluded. The pseudobifurcation formed by the enlarged ECA branches could easily be mistaken for a true carotid bifurcation on the B-mode image.

A periorbital bi-directional Doppler examination is most helpful in avoiding this pitfall because it may identify the ECA as a collateral pathway around a diseased ICA. Once this is known, occlude or tap on the superficial temporal artery with your finger while observing the sound spectral analysis waveform of the unidentified vessel in the neck. A change in the sound spectral analysis waveform made by these maneuvers will

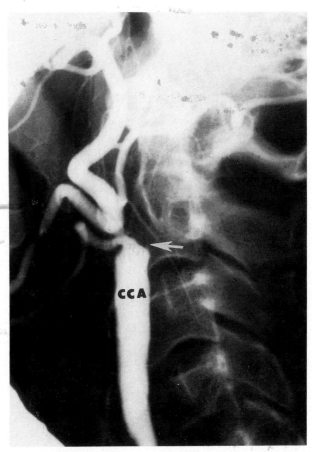

Figure 2–15. Pseudobifurcation formed by enlarged external carotid artery (ECA) branches as shown on lateral view of selective common carotid artery (CCA) arteriogram. Arrow denotes internal carotid artery (ICA) occlusion site.

identify the unknown vessel as the ECA, and the pseudobifurcation formed by its branches will not be mistaken for the true carotid bifurcation.

References

1. Jacobs NM, Grant EG, Schellinger D, Byrd MC, Richardson JD, Cohan SL. Duplex carotid sonography: criteria for stenosis, accuracy, and pitfalls. Radiology 1985; 154:385–391.
2. May AG, Van de Berg L, De Weese JA, et al. Critical arterial stenosis. Surgery 1963; 54:250–259.
3. Ricotta JJ, Holen J, Schenk E, Plassche W, Green RM, Gramiak R, De Weese JA. Is routine angiography necessary prior to carotid endarterectomy? J Vasc Surg 1984; 1:96–102.
4. Spencer MP. Hemodynamics of carotid stenosis. *In* Spencer MP, Reid JM (eds). Cerebrovascular evaluation with Doppler ultrasound. The Hague, Martinus Nijhoff, 1981: 113–132.
5. Planiol T, Pourcelot L, Pottier JM, et al. Etude de la circulation carotidienne par les méthodes ultrasoniques et la thermographie. Rev Neurol (Paris) 1972; 126:127–141.
6. Courbier R, Reggi M, Jausseran JM. Exploration of carotid arteries and vessels of the neck by Doppler techniques. *In* Diethrich ED (ed). Noninvasive cardiovascular diagnosis: current concepts. Baltimore, University Park Press, 1978: 61–73.
7. Zwiebel WJ, Crummy AB. Sources of error in Doppler diagnosis of carotid occlusive disease. AJR 1981; 137:1–12.

3 • Examination of the Extracranial Cerebrovascular System

Introduction

Doppler ultrasound has been used for many years in vascular examinations. The addition of real-time imaging with high-resolution arrays and high-performance electronics has greatly increased the sensitivity and accuracy of the procedure. Therefore, the popularity of these examinations has also increased, especially in the evaluation of cerebrovascular disease.

The noninvasive examination of the extracerebral vascular system requires approximately one hour of time, utilizing a duplex scanner. The length of time will depend on the protocol, patient difficulties, and the extent of disease involvement. Speed is not the prime consideration; the emphasis is placed on precise evaluation of each vascular structure. The Doppler sounds from each vessel must be correlated with fine-quality imaging for a definitive diagnosis. As in any type of sonographic examination, the key to fine imaging is a complete understanding of the anatomical components and their many variations. An ideal way to study the extracranial system is to match the anatomical diagrams with the clinical sonographic scans and review these with the angiographic studies, which may be used as the "gold standard." Figures 3–1 through 3–4 demonstrate the primary anatomy of the extracerebral vascular system and the intracerebral circulation from which collateral pathways arise.

Anatomy of the Extracerebral Vascular System

Arising from the aortic arch are the brachiocephalic vessels, as seen in Figures 3–1 and 3–2. The innominate or brachiocephalic artery arises from the aortic arch and divides into the right subclavian and right common carotid arteries. The subclavian artery supplies blood to the arm and gives rise to its first branch, the vertebral artery. Variations may include the absence of the innominate artery, with the right subclavian and the right common arteries arising from the aorta.[1]

On the left, the subclavian artery and the common carotid artery are separate branches, with the vertebral being the first branch of the subclavian artery. In some cases, there may be a left innominate artery, or the aorta may arch to the right, reversing the normal arrangement.

The vertebrals arise as the first branch of the subclavian arteries and ascend through the foramina in the transverse processes of the upper six cervical vertebrae. The right and left vertebral arteries enter the skull through the foramen magnum and join to form the basilar artery, which is a major blood supply for the brainstem and cerebellum. Figure 3–3 outlines the vertebral pathways, which can be difficult to image because of overlying bony structures.

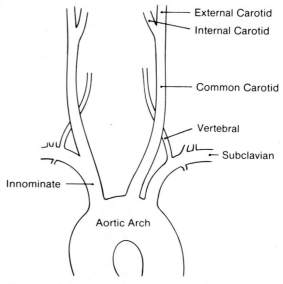

Figure 3–1. Diagram of extracranial cerebrovascular arteries.

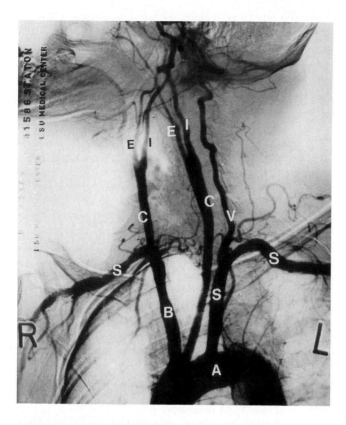

Figure 3–2. Angiogram of extracranial cerebrovascular system. A = Aortic arch; B = brachiocephalic (innominate) artery; S = subclavian artery; C = common carotid artery (CCA); V = vertebral artery; E = external carotid artery (ECA); I = internal carotid artery (ICA).

The right common carotid artery (CCA) arises from the innominate artery, and the left CCA arises directly from the aortic arch (Fig. 3–1). They pass cephalad into the anterolateral aspect of the neck, slightly behind the thyroid gland (Fig. 3–4A and B). An enlarged thyroid may cause posterior displacement of the CCAs. Each CCA passes obliquely upward to the superior border of the thyroid cartilage. At this level it divides into the external carotid artery (ECA) and the internal carotid artery (ICA), at a point commonly termed the *carotid bifurcation*.

The level of the carotid bifurcation may vary and affect the examination technique. Figure 3–5 demonstrates the various levels in relation to the thyroid cartilage. In most patients, the ICA is posterior and lateral to the ECA. However, this also varies, depending on the anatomical structure and position of the examination. The ECA has low branches that supply blood to the neck, face, and scalp. The ECA branches may be used to distinguish it from the ICA, whereas the ICA has no branches until it enters the base of the skull. The ICA supplies blood to the eyes

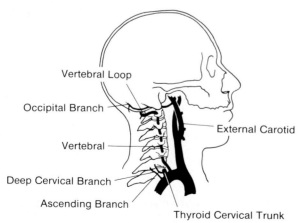

Figure 3–3. Diagram of the vertebral artery.

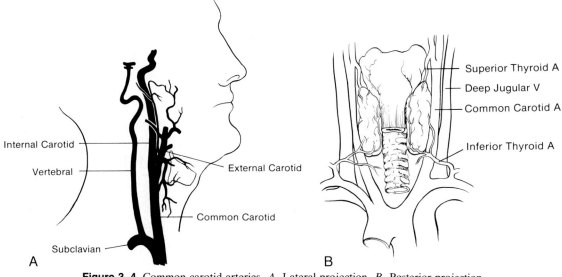

Figure 3–4. Common carotid arteries. *A*, Lateral projection. *B*, Posterior projection.

and cerebral hemispheres. Variations may include (1) the right common carotid arising directly from the aorta, (2) the left common carotid arising from the innominate artery, and (3) the absence of subdivisions (ICA, ECA) of the common carotid artery or the absence of the common carotid artery, with the ICA and ECA arising from the arch.[1]

Collateral pathways play an important role in cases of severe stenosis and occlusion. The normal anatomy and the collateral pathways must be clearly understood for diagnosis of cerebrovascular disease. The two major pathways are the circle of Willis and the ICA–ECA network. These major pathways are diagrammed in Figures 3–6 and 3–7 and will be referred to in the subsequent text.

Scanning and Positioning

Once the appropriate history has been obtained, the patient is placed in a recumbent, supine position with the mandible hyperextended. In cases of extreme obesity, the shoulder can be placed on a pillow, elongating the neck and extending the mandible. With patients who are taut and have limited neck movement, slant the body by placing a sponge wedge under the thoracolumbar region. This allows the head to be placed in a lateral position. Other considerations might be the use of dental chairs and multipositional stretchers.

Scanning usually begins with the head turned away from the side being examined. This places the vessels more perpendicular to the transducer

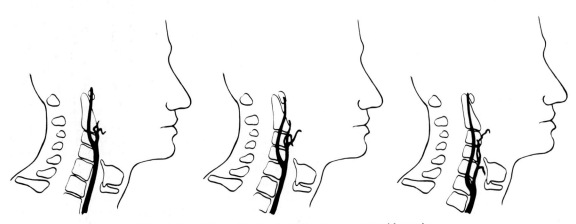

Figure 3–5. Bifurcation levels of the common carotid arteries.

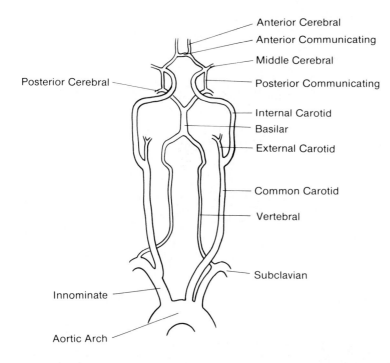

Figure 3–6. The circle of Willis collateral pathways.

for maximum reflection. Anatomical configuration is highly variable, and patients will require various degrees of rotation. A problem often encountered in the oblique position is the overlying jugular vein, which may interfere with carotid visualization. Rotating the neck back to the neutral anterior position will remove the jugular vein from the area of interest. Figure 3–8A and B illustrates the jugular vein and its location with various positions of the head.

Transverse views are obtained from the suprasternal level to the bifurcation, including views of the ECA and ICA. If possible, first view the branches of the brachiocephalic vessels from the aortic arch (Fig. 3–9). If these lower vessels cannot be viewed, one should demonstrate the proximal carotid artery and subclavian artery in a longitudinal plane (Fig. 3–10). Every effort should be made to visualize secondary sites (e.g., vertebral and subclavian arteries). An example of plaque in the subclavian artery is seen in Figure 3–11.

Transverse scan views are then obtained at multiple levels of the CCA and the carotid bifurcation (Fig. 3–12A and B). Blood flow spectral analysis is not obtained in the transverse cross-sectional projection because the angle of incidence cannot be accurately determined. Plaque may be located on the lateral wall of the vessel, and this should be demonstrated in both transverse and longitudinal views. When lateral wall plaque is present, a single plane may give the false impression of an occlusion or other artifactual appearances (Fig. 3–13).

It takes special imaging techniques to define plaque characterization properly. One method uses variable power levels. Another method utilizes various digital processing techniques to enhance high-level echoes (calcifications), low-level echoes (fresh clot), or medium-level echoes (thrombus). If the plaque creates acoustical shadowing, limiting the lumen from view, multiple transducer positions will often eliminate the shadowing. If visualization of plaque is poor because of improper penetration, this can be corrected by decreasing the transducer frequency (e.g., 10

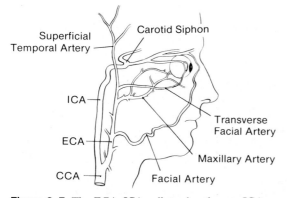

Figure 3–7. The ECA–ICA collateral pathways. ICA = Internal carotid artery; ECA = external carotid artery; CCA = common carotid artery.

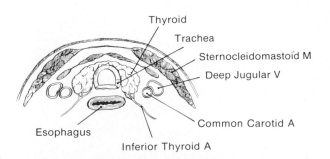

Figure 3–8. Jugular vein anatomy. *A*, Cross-sectional diagram of neck. *B*, Changes in position of jugular vein with head rotation. J = Jugular vein; C = carotid artery.

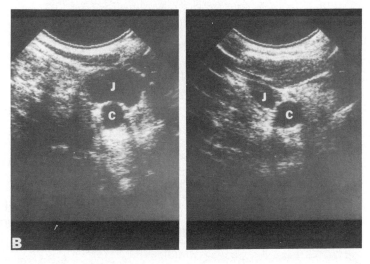

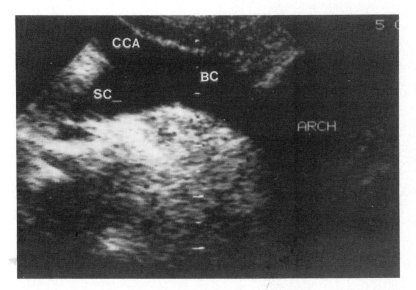

Figure 3–9. Brachiocephalic artery arising from the aortic arch. BC = Brachiocephalic artery; CCA = common carotid artery; SC = sub-clavian artery.

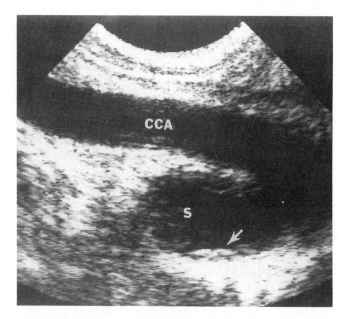

Figure 3–10. Longitudinal view of the proximal CCA and the subclavian artery. CCA = Common carotid artery; S = subclavian artery; arrow = plaque formation.

to 7.5 MHz). Figures 3–14 and 3–15 demonstrate these special imaging techniques.

Longitudinal duplex scan views are thereby obtained. Flow characteristics with spectral analysis are obtained in this projection because the correct angle of incidence can be achieved and correct calculations can be obtained. When pathology is present, sample volumes at multiple positions are obtained to identify the various changes in flow characteristics. Figure 3–16 rep-

resents multiple positioning of the sample volume to obtain the highest Doppler frequency shift. The frequency range then denotes the percentage of stenosis. Area and percentage calculations are used to further verify the degree of stenosis. Electronic cursors are used to outline the internal lumen and the outside vessel diameter. The duplex system computes the area and circumference of the outlined cross-sectional regions. The two areas are then compared, with the system auto-

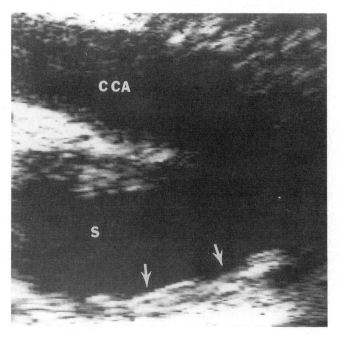

Figure 3–11. Longitudinal view of the proximal CCA and subclavian artery with plaque formations. CCA = Common carotid artery; S = subclavian artery; arrows = plaque formation.

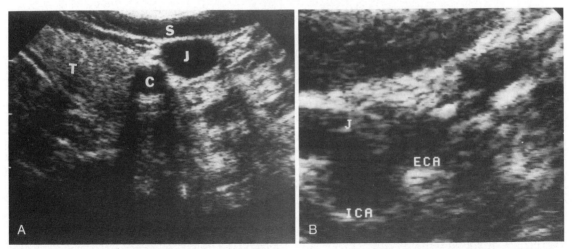

Figure 3–12. Transverse views of the common carotid artery (CCA). *A*, Thyroid level. T = Thyroid; C = CCA; J = jugular vein; S = sternocleidomastoid muscle. *B*, Bifurcation level. J = Jugular vein; ICA = internal carotid artery; ECA = external carotid artery.

matically computing the percentage difference or percentage of cross-sectional area stenosis (Fig. 3–17).

The Scanning Sequence

Our longitudinal viewing sequence follows.
Proximal Portion of the Common Carotid Ar-

tery. Identify the subclavian and common carotid arteries (Fig. 3–10).

Long Axis of the Entire Common Carotid Artery. Identify the echogenic wall, the sonolucent blood-filled vessel lumen, and any associated abnormalities. The normal measurement of the wall and of fatty deposits is no more than 1 mm. Figure 3–18 demonstrates the CCA with wall measurements. To obtain the laminar flow spec-

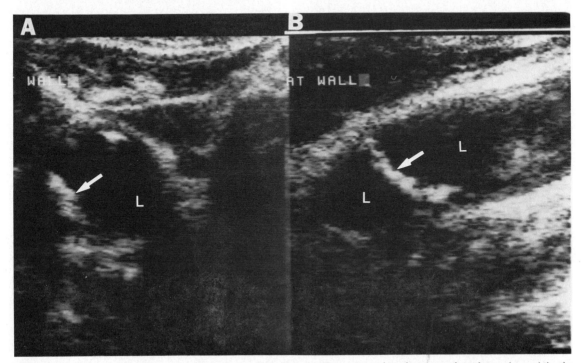

Figure 3–13. Lateral wall plaque with artifactual appearance. *A*, Transverse view demonstrating plaque (arrow) in the lateral wall with patent lumen (L). *B*, Longitudinal view in the lateral plane with plaque (arrow) artifact crossing the lumen (L).

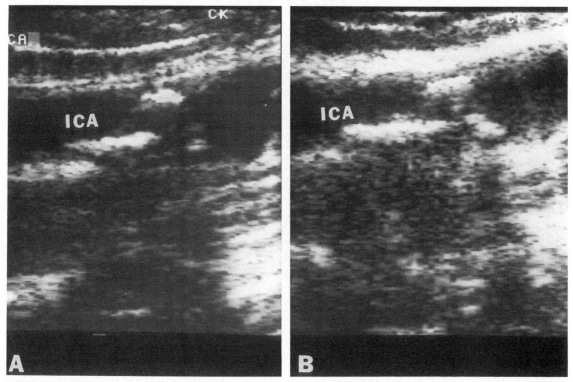

Figure 3–14. Power enhancement. *A*, Longitudinal view of the internal carotid artery (ICA) with normal power settings. High-level echoes from echogenic structures are seen with a loss of low-level echoes owing to attenuation. *B*, Longitudinal view of the internal carotid artery (ICA) with increased power settings. The increased power enhances the back wall and identifies soft tissue components.

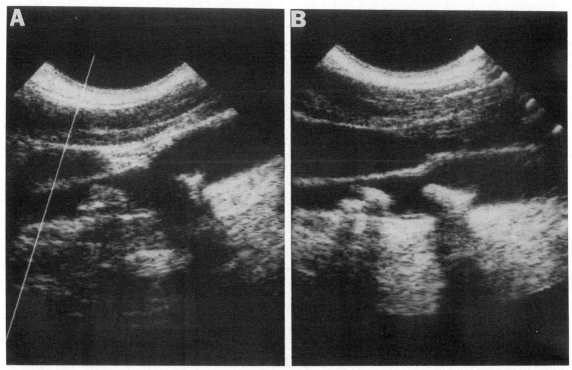

Figure 3–15. Transducer positioning for increased vessel definition. *A*, Anterior view of the ICA with loss of visibility due to acoustical shadowing from plaque. *B*, Lateral view of the ICA enhances the posterior walls and better defines the plaque.

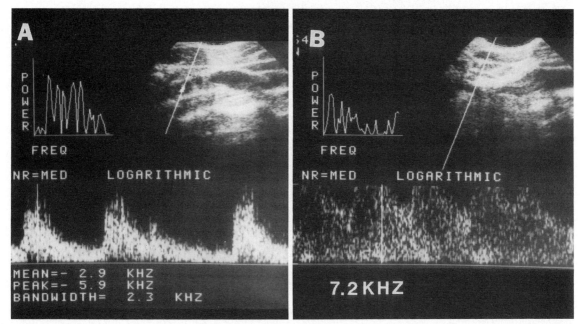

Figure 3–16. Multiple sample volume positioning for obtaining the highest frequency shift. *A*, Demonstrates a frequency shift of 5.9 kHz. *B*, Repositioning of the sample volume demonstrates a frequency shift of 7.2 kHz.

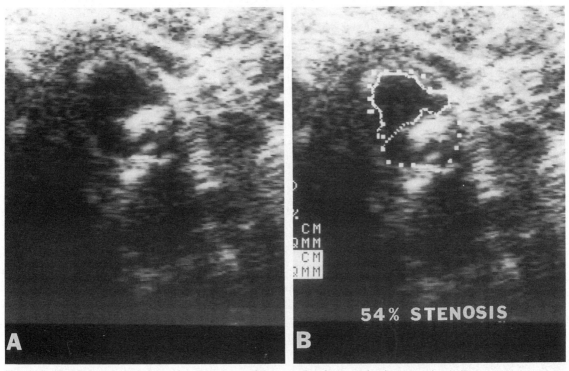

Figure 3–17. Method for obtaining the percentage of cross-sectional area reduction stenosis. *A*, Transverse view of the vessel containing plaque. *B*, Cursor measurements with computer calculation of the percentage of stenosis.

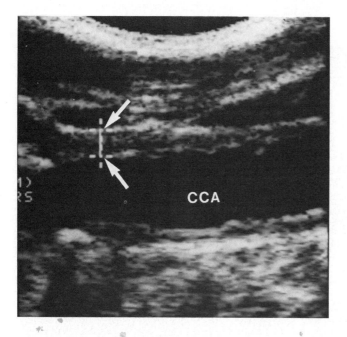

Figure 3–18. Enlarged view of the common carotid arterial wall with cursor measurement (arrows). CCA = Common carotid artery.

trum (Fig. 3–19), the pulsed Doppler with the sample volume is taken in the center of the CCA. The CCA normally is pulsatile, with a prominent diastolic flow resting above the zero baseline. Characteristically, it is similar to the ICA, which is a high-flow and low-resistance vessel and receives approximately 80% of the common carotid flow. It has been established that significant disease of the ICA affects the CCA, resulting in a reduction of the diastolic velocity and a change in the systolic and diastolic ratios. Compare the normal CCA spectral analysis in Figure 3–20A

with the CCA spectral analysis proximal to an ICA occlusion in Figure 3–20B.

Many investigators have utilized special formulas to evaluate the normal parameters, and these are available on some duplex scanners. Particular emphasis is placed on the peak systolic velocity, peak diastolic velocity, and/or Doppler frequency shifts. The bandwidth histogram and resting zero baseline level are also included.

The Carotid Bulb and Bifurcation. The predominant areas of pathology are the carotid bulb, and bifurcation. Cadaver specimens (Figs. 3–21

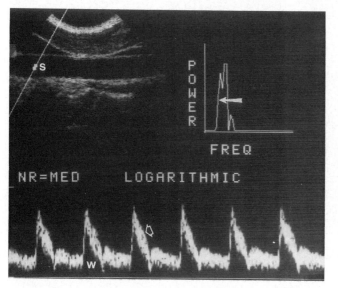

Figure 3–19. CCA with spectral analysis waveform. Sample volume placement at a 30 to 60° angle in midstream of the vessel to obtain the laminar flow profile. Open arrow demonstrates the narrow frequency distribution of the normal CCA with the open spectral window. Closed arrow demonstrates the level of bandwidth measurement in the histogram. S = Sample volume; W = open spectral window.

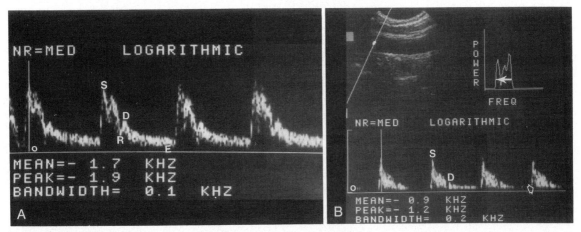

Figure 3–20. CCA waveform.

A, Normal CCA spectral analysis waveform exhibits a pulsatile waveform with a prominent diastolic flow resting above the zero baseline. 0 = Zero baseline; S = peak systolic velocity; D = peak diastolic velocity; R = reverse flow with aortic valve closure; E = end diastolic velocity.

B, CCA proximal to ICA occlusion. The waveform becomes dampened owing to a drop in the Doppler shift, and the diastolic portion of the waveform returns to the zero baseline. There will be some spectral broadening (solid arrow) with filling in of the spectral window (open arrow). 0 = Zero baseline; S = peak systolic velocity; D = peak diastolic velocity.

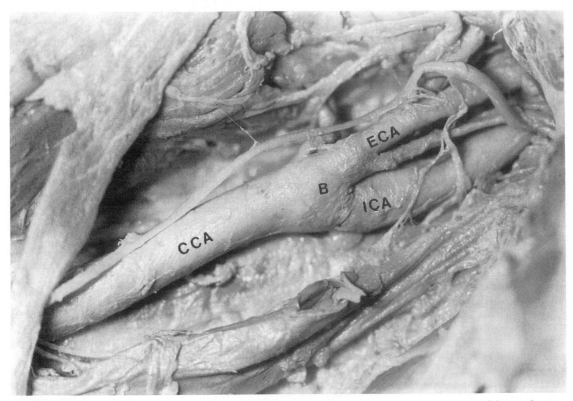

Figure 3–21. Cadaver specimen. Longitudinal view of the CCA, the bifurcation, and the branches. CCA = Common carotid artery; B = carotid bulb; ECA = external carotid artery; ICA = internal carotid artery.

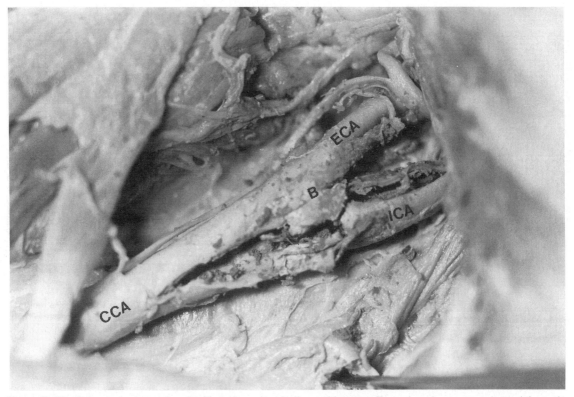

Figure 3–22. Cadaver specimen. Longitudinal view of excised carotid artery. Extensive plaque was removed from the bulb with clotted blood and ulcerations present. CCA = Common carotid artery; B = carotid bulb; ECA = external carotid artery; ICA = internal carotid artery.

and 3–22) demonstrate these areas for clarity. It is preferable to view the carotid bulb and bifurcating vessels in a single plane, as seen in Figure 3–23A. If this is not possible, the bulb, ECA, and ICA must be viewed selectively (Figs. 3–23B and C). Characteristically, the carotid bulb exhibits a bulbous effect with a slight widening. Spectral analysis of the blood flow through this region may show slight frequency drops and turbulence. This type of pseudoturbulence should not be confused with pathology. Figure 3–24 displays the spectral analysis of a normal carotid bulb. Frequently, the complete bifurcation is not seen in one projection because it may bifurcate at various levels and may be thrown out of view when the neck is rotated. It is mandatory that both the ICA and ECA be localized and examined. As a rule, the ECA lies more anterior and medial to the ICA; however, in some instances, this may be reversed.

Other criteria for distinguishing the ECA and ICA are as follows:

1. Comparison of vessel size will identify the ICA as being the larger of the two vessels.

2. Branches of the ECA may often be low-lying, supplying the facial circulation. Because the ICA has no branches extracranially, this aids in distinguishing the ICA from the ECA. Figure 3–25 identifies the ECA and its branch.

3. The Doppler signals should clearly identify the vessel in question. The ICA exhibits a high pitch (frequency) with a high diastolic flow (approximately one half of the systolic peak). In contrast, the ECA exhibits a strong multiphasic signal with a high-peak systolic frequency, which rapidly drops off and remains low in diastole. Figures 3–26 and 3–27 demonstrate the spectral analysis waveforms of the ICA and ECA for comparison.

The ICA characteristically is a high-flow/low-resistance vessel with a prominent diastolic flow and a high-pitched sound. The spectral analysis will define the characteristics as well as the audible sound. Confusion may arise in the presence of turbulence that is caused by plaque or stenotic areas; therefore, multiple areas should be examined. It is also important to evaluate the vessel as superiorly as possible because the pathology may be present in the distal portions (Fig. 3–28).

The ECA in contrast is a low-flow/high-resis-

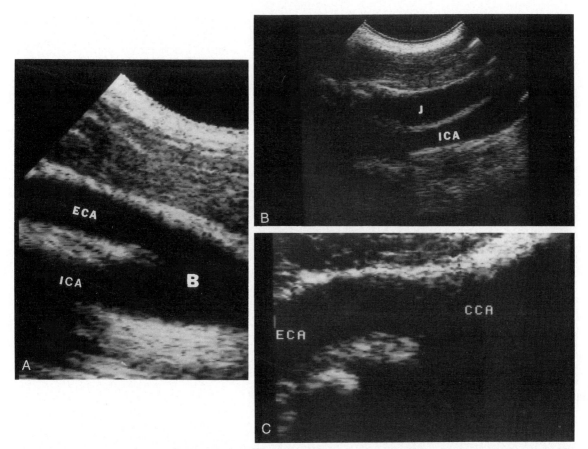

Figure 3–23. Carotid artery views. *A*, CCA with bifurcation. B = Carotid bulb; ECA = external carotid artery; ICA = internal carotid artery. *B*, Selective ICA view. J = Jugular vein; ICA = internal carotid artery. *C*, Selective ECA view. CCA = Common carotid artery; ECA = external carotid artery.

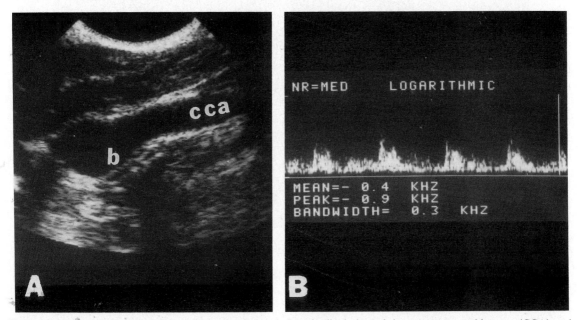

Figure 3–24. Carotid bulb spectral analysis waveform. *A*, Longitudinal view of the common carotid artery (CCA) and the carotid bulb (b). *B*, Spectral analysis of the normal carotid bulb demonstrates a slight frequency drop and mild turbulence.

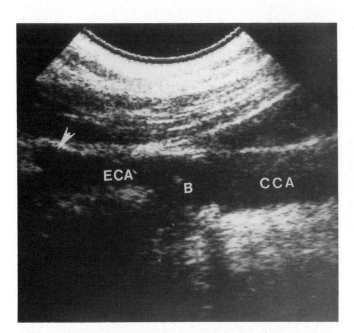

Figure 3–25. ECA identified by branch vessel. CCA = Common carotid artery; B = carotid bulb; ECA = external carotid artery; closed arrow = ECA branch.

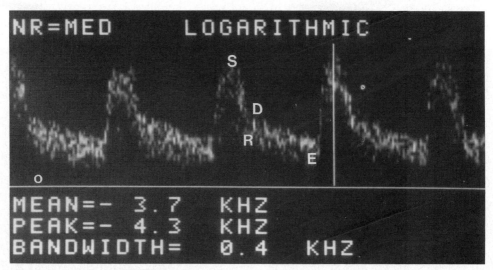

Figure 3–26. ICA spectral analysis waveform. 0 = Zero baseline; S = peak systolic velocity; D = peak diastolic velocity; R = reverse flow with aortic valve closure; E = end diastolic velocity.

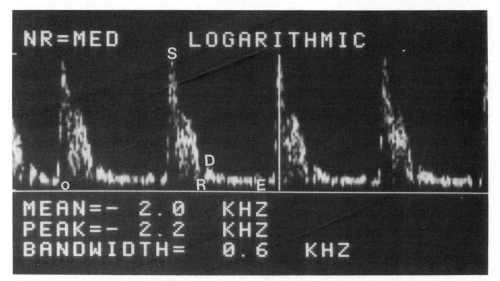

Figure 3–27. ECA spectral analysis waveform. 0 = Zero baseline; S = peak systolic velocity; D = peak diastolic velocity; R = reverse flow with aortic valve closure; E = end diastolic velocity.

Figure 3–28. ICA with distal multisegmental disease and plaque in distal ICA (arrows). J = Jugular vein.

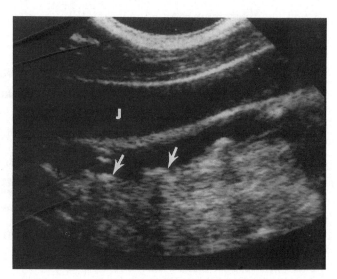

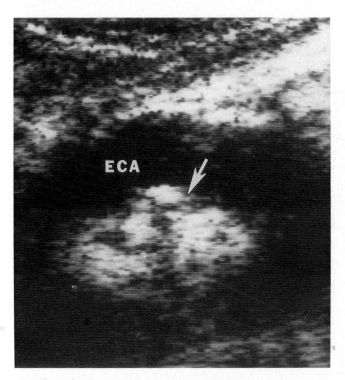

Figure 3–29. External carotid artery plaque (arrow). ECA = External carotid artery.

tance vessel with a strong multiphasic sound.[2] The ECA has a low diastolic flow, displayed as resting on the zero baseline. In some instances, pathology may be present in the ECA with altered waveforms. Figure 3–29 illustrates plaque in the ECA. In cases of ICA occlusion, the ECA Doppler waveforms may mimic the ICA because of the re-routing of the blood flow. It is of prime importance to identify both vessels with their specific characteristics. If the ICA is not identified, the zero flow is documented along with the ECA, bulb, and CCA waveforms.

Noninvasive Vascular Examination of the Vertebral Arteries. This should be attempted on all extracranial examinations. Identification of the subclavian steal is of primary consideration and can be diagnosed by using Doppler or duplex techniques. Future efforts will be made to both image and evaluate the blood flow in these vessels.

Examination of the vertebral arteries has not been associated with the success that has occurred with the carotid artery examination. This has been due to several factors:

1. The origin of the vertebral arteries, which lie low in the neck and in close proximity to the thyrocervical trunk, thus making it difficult to identify the vertebral artery.

2. The vertebral artery ascends through the foramina in the transverse process from C6 to C2 and is obscured by bone, making visualization and examination difficult.

3. The vertebral artery makes a loop at the level of the atlas as it enters the foramen magnum. This loop can produce confusing results on the Doppler examination, as the blood flow may be either towards or away from the probe face, depending on placement of the probe over the artery.

Doppler examination of the vertebral arteries at the base of the skull has been described by Pourcelot.[3] This method remains in use today primarily for the diagnosis of subclavian steal.

The patient is placed in the supine position, with the head turned away from the side being examined. The Doppler probe is placed behind the mastoid bone at the base of the skull. Using a medial superior angle towards the foramen magnum will identify the vertebral artery (Fig. 3–30). Pressure is applied by the probe to compress the occipital artery and to eliminate mistaking the occipital artery for the vertebral artery. The vertebral waveform exhibits a low pulsatility with a high diastolic flow.

Presently, duplex sonography offers the best method for evaluating the vertebral artery. There are generally two areas used to localize the vertebral artery. One is low in the neck at its origin, and the other is midlevel between the transverse processes of the cervical vertebrae.

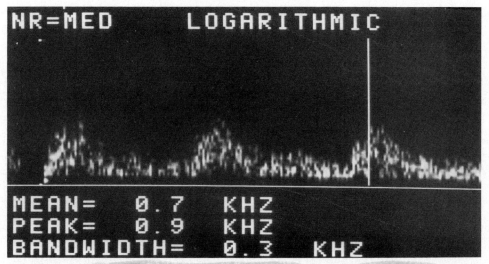

NR=MED   LOGARITHMIC

MEAN=   0.7   KHZ
PEAK=   0.9   KHZ
BANDWIDTH=   0.3   KHZ

Figure 3–30. Vertebral artery waveform exhibiting low pulsatility and high diastolic flow.

To locate the proximal segment of the vertebral artery, the transducer is moved laterally from the common carotid artery in a longitudinal plane. A slight caudal angle identifies the vertebral artery arising from the subclavian (Fig. 3–31). The sample volume is placed in the vertebral artery lumen by rotating the transducer face in a cephalad position. Figure 3–32 demonstrates plaque and stenosis in the proximal vertebral artery.

The transducer is then moved upward and slightly posterior to the midcervical region to identify the vertebral artery ascending between the transverse processes.[4] In the longitudinal plane, multiple acoustical shadows identify the cervical vertebral processes with the vertebral artery in between. The sample volume is then taken between these vertebral processes to identify the blood flow characteristics of the vertebral artery. Normally, the blood flow pattern is low-resistance/high-volume, similar to that in the cerebrovascular circulation (e.g., CCA and ICA).

Bilateral blood pressures are obtained, completing the extracranial vascular examination. The two brachial pressures should be within 10 mm Hg. If there is greater than 10 mm Hg difference, subclavian steal or upper extremity pathology should be suspected.[5]

Doppler supraorbital examination is an indi-

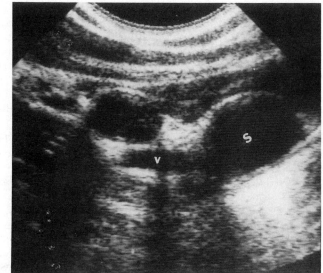

Figure 3–31. Vertebral artery originating from subclavian artery. S = Subclavian; V = proximal portion of vertebral artery.

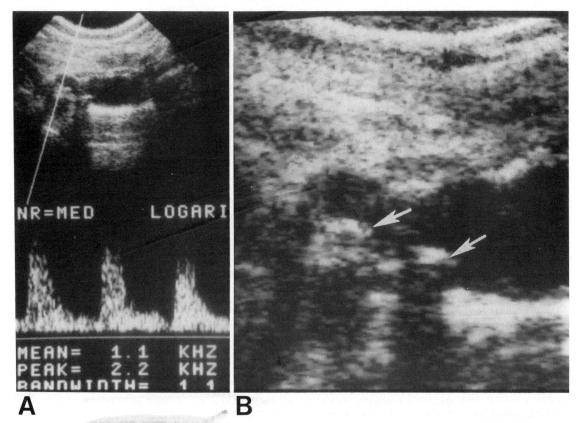

Figure 3–32. Vertebral artery stenosis. *A*, Vertebral artery spectral analysis with increased frequency, filling of the spectral window, and spectral broadening. *B*, Longitudinal view of the vertebral artery with multiple plaque formations (arrows).

rect method of evaluating stenosis and occlusion of the ICA. Although this method by no means achieves the accuracy and sensitivity of the duplex scan, it provides important information about the cerebrovascular system, as is presented in Chapter 8.

A worksheet is used to record the various findings during the examination. It is important to record all of the examination findings along with the clinical history for correlation. The worksheet should provide the actual record, in addition to any Doppler waveforms not present on the film format. For example, the duplex examination may not identify the supraorbital recordings. The Doppler supraorbital waveforms should be attached to the worksheet. It is also helpful to document the pathological sites on a graphic form, which can be coordinated with the film documentation. An example of the worksheet is seen in Figure 3–33.

The accuracy of the extracranial vascular examination can be determined by comparison with angiography. This is an excellent method to eval-uate the findings and to assist in setting up the standards. Comparison of these examinations will enhance the examiner's understanding of the many anatomical variants, as well as identify pathological conditions. After sufficient examinations have been performed, statistical information can be gathered to judge the sensitivity and specificity of the examination, as shown in the chapter on accuracy measurements.

Sonographic Equipment

The extracranial cerebrovascular system can be assessed by several ultrasound methods. The simplest of these is the bi-directional continuous-wave Doppler unit (Fig. 3–34). With these units is a chart strip recorder displaying the analog waveform simultaneously with the sound emission. To use this unit, however, requires a great deal of expertise in the recognition of sound characteristics of specific vascular structures. Extensive disease processes and hemodynamic sig-

CAROTID VASCULAR EXAMINATION

Patient Number_____   Patient History_____

Patient Name_____   _____

Date_____   _____

BLOOD PRESSURE (Normal value less than   _____
10 mm/hg)

Right_____   Left _____   _____

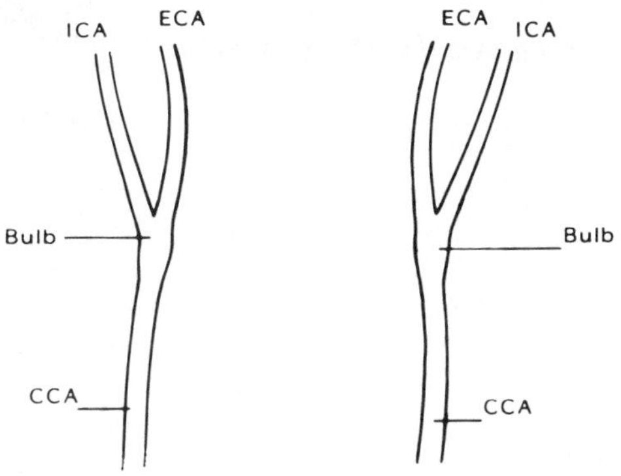

Figure 3–33. Vascular worksheet.

ICA   ECA   ECA   ICA

Bulb ——   —— Bulb

CCA ——   —— CCA

DOPPLER FREQUENCY VALUES   NORMAL VALUES

Right		Left			
				0 – 20%	< 3.0 khz
CCA	____khz	CCA	____khz	20 – 40%	< 3.0 khz
ICA	____khz	ICA	____khz	40 – 60%	3.0 – 4.5 khz
ECA	____khz	ECA	____khz	60 – 80%	4.5 – 6.5 khz
Vertebral	____khz	Vertebral	____khz	80 – 99%	> 6.5 khz
Stenosis	_____	Stenosis	_____		
	_____		_____		

SUPRAORBITAL DOPPLER

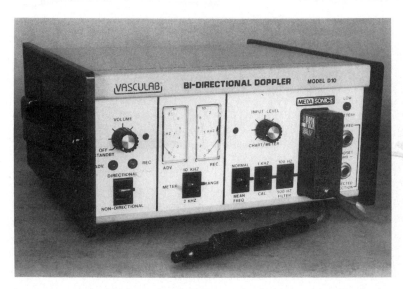

Figure 3–34. Bi-directional continuous-wave Doppler unit. (Courtesy of Medasonics Corporation.)

nificant stenosis will be readily detected, but small plaque formations and minimal disease may not be diagnosed.

A slightly more complex unit is the Doppler unit, which forms images by ultrasonically mapping out the vascular structures. This is not the image that we see with a real-time scanner but, rather, a gross anatomical depiction of the vessels with its corresponding Doppler evaluation. This unit does not produce the sensitivity or specificity of the current duplex scanners, and in most instances the diagnosis rests on the Doppler evaluation.

There are a multitude of small, inexpensive real-time units available that employ real-time imaging only. A separate Doppler system must be used to interrogate the vessels by sound. This is certainly not state-of-the-art, but is a method of achieving results that are comparable to those produced by the duplex systems. There are multiple problems associated with using separated systems:

1. The examination is performed twice: once with the real-time imager and again with the continuous-wave Doppler. This not only increases the operator's time but requires additional patient cooperation.

2. Localizing specific sites of disease in the vessel with both units for correlation may be difficult and in some cases impossible.

3. Using a continuous-wave, bi-directional unit without spectral analysis may not demonstrate low-grade lesions or minimal disease.

Currently, the state-of-the-art rests with the duplex scanner, which is the best of both worlds. These units combine a high-resolution real-time imager with a 7 to 10 MHz transducer frequency and a 3 to 5 MHz transducer frequency for Doppler analysis. The lower-frequency transducers (5 MHz) can image the vessel structure but are unable to differentiate ulcerations, thrombi, and soft plaque formations. It takes at least a 7 MHz transducer to provide adequate tissue characterization and, preferably, a 10 MHz transducer.

Figures 3–35 and 3–36 compare the 5 MHz and 10 MHz image quality. No smaller frequency than 5 MHz should be employed because of the extreme loss of resolution. The higher frequencies offer an axial resolution of 0.2 mm and a lateral resolution of 0.8 mm. Doppler capabilities on the duplex system should include analysis of both the pulsed and continuous-wave beams with spectral analysis processing of their resultant waveforms. The pulsed Doppler should be equipped with a variable sample volume that can be range-gated or placed at varying depths within the tissue under investigation. The pulsed Doppler analyzes specific sites within the vessel and produces a clearer signal than the continuous-wave Doppler, which interrogates the entire vessel. However, the vessel must be seen on the real-time B-mode image in order to place the sample volume of the pulsed Doppler wave within its lumen. Because the continuous-wave Doppler does not have to be placed at a specific point within the vessel lumen, it is used to obtain the signal from a vessel when it cannot be seen with real-time B-mode imaging. An example is the high carotid bifurcation that cannot be seen on the real-time B-mode image. Here the continuous-wave Doppler beam may be used to identify the CCA, ICA, and ECA. The signals from each of these vessels are then analyzed by spectral

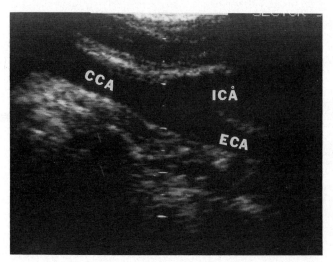

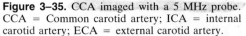
Figure 3–35. CCA imaged with a 5 MHz probe. CCA = Common carotid artery; ICA = internal carotid artery; ECA = external carotid artery.

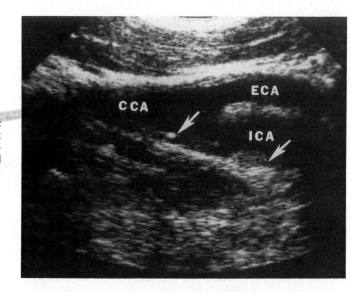

Figure 3–36. CCA imaged with a 10 MHz probe. Note the clear demonstration of soft tissue and calcifications (arrows). CCA = Common carotid artery; ICA = internal carotid artery; ECA = external carotid artery.

analysis to provide the diagnosis that would otherwise be lost with the inability to view these vessels.

The spectral analyzer converts the Doppler signal into a waveform composed of multiple Doppler shift frequencies. A normal waveform has a narrow frequency distribution (bandwidth), which creates a window where no frequencies are displayed. Abnormalities within the vessel lumen may produce a wide variety of Doppler shift frequencies. These expand the bandwidth and may ultimately broaden the waveform until its window is completely filled in. Figures 3–37 and 3–38 compare the normal and abnormal waveforms. The bandwidth, which is displayed on the histogram, demonstrates the distribution of frequencies. The bandwidth measurement is obtained at the 50% level of the amplitude or power axis, as is seen in Figure 3–39. The display can be obtained at any point in the cardiac cycle for assessment of the frequency range. The various changes in waveforms are used to diagnose disease in the vessel being examined.

The Doppler computer also provides multiple calculations, which include mean frequency, peak frequency, bandwidth, the Doppler shift in fre-

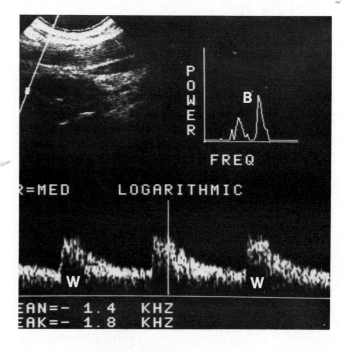

Figure 3–37. Normal ICA waveform with narrow range of bandwidths (B) and opened spectral window (W).

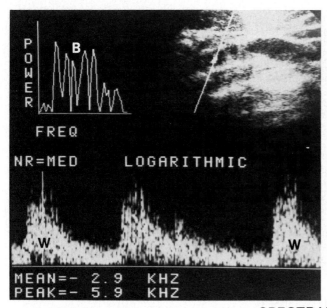

Figure 3–38. Waveform of ICA stenosis demonstrating a wide range of bandwidths (B) and a filled-in spectral window (W).

SPECTRAL DISPLAY (HISTOGRAM)

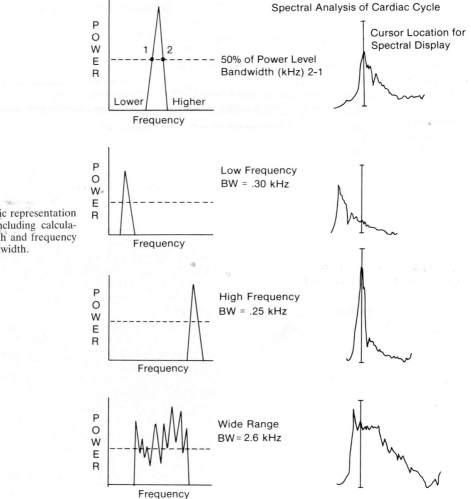

Figure 3–39. Graphic representation of the histogram, including calculation of the bandwidth and frequency ranges. BW = Bandwidth.

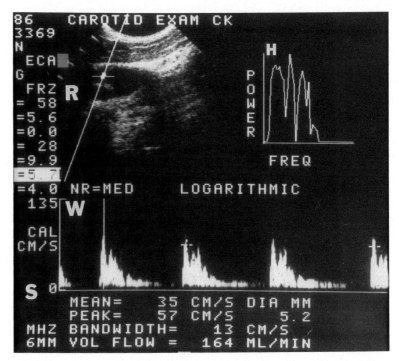

Figure 3–40. Statistical calculations are displaced along with the Doppler waveform, the real-time image, and the histogram. H = Histogram displays range of bandwidths; S = statistical computer calculations; W = waveform; R = real-time image.

quency (hertz) or velocity (cm/sec) (Fig. 3–40), and volume flow.

Recording and Documentation

There are various methods of recording and documenting the vascular examination. Ideally, permanent recordings are made and stored for a 5-year period or whatever legal time period is required by state law. This not only provides data in the event of any legal proceedings but also provides an image that can be seen by the referring clinicians and utilized for conferences, rounds, and so forth.

The most popular recording methods are (1) *video tape recording,* (2) *strip recording,* (3) *Polaroid prints,* and (4) *film format cameras.*

Video Tape Recording

Video tape recording is ideal for studying the vascular structures in motion. It captures both the sound analysis and the real-time B-mode scan images when the duplex system is used. The limitations of this type of recording include:

1. Cost of the equipment to record and play back the recordings.

2. Cost of the video tapes, which can be very expensive for large departments performing a large number of examinations.

3. Storage problems when all of the examinations are to be stored permanently.

Most laboratories that use video taping exclusively do not store all of the examinations on tape permanently. Instead, they make hard copy film for storage and re-use the same video tape over again during their daily examinations.

Paper Strip Recording

Paper strip recording is available on all Doppler units for permanent storage and is the method of choice for recording all vascular examination parameters except B-mode imaging studies. In this method heat pens are used to burn a graphic representation of the vascular sound profile. In some laboratories this type of permanent record may not be used. Instead, the sound is heard by the examiner, who analyzes it and records the result on a worksheet. If the examination is interpreted after the fact or without the physician being present during the examination, however, permanent documentation becomes a necessity. "If we hear it, we should see it," which gives a dual method of confirming results. It also gives a permanent recording for comparison on follow-up studies. Additionally, the strip recording provides a means of teaching.

Polaroid Prints

The Polaroid print has been around for quite some time. A distinct advantage is that major equipment, such as processors and expensive cameras, are not required to produce a permanent recording. There are inexpensive Polaroid cameras that attach to the cathode ray tube (CRT) and television (TV) monitors or to a "gun-type" device to hold up to the CRT or monitor for instant prints. These prints are excellent for documenting areas of pathology, attaching to the chart, or sending to the clinician with the patient's report. The disadvantages of Polaroid prints include:

1. The cost per print is about three times higher than film format cameras.
2. The prints fade.
3. If documentation of the complete examination is required, numerous prints become cumbersome.

Film Format Camera

The film format camera is the method of choice when duplex scanning is used. A film processor and the initial investment of a camera are necessary. Film format cameras are more economical than any other method of image recording, and they provide multiple images on one sheet of film, making viewing easier. They maintain their quality and are easily stored. Care should be exercised in selecting a format camera because vascular imaging with high-frequency transducers necessitates a high-resolution camera monitor to reproduce the quality of the image. Portability, ease of use, and relatively little maintenance are also desired features.

Photography

Photography is a specialty coupled to the use of format cameras. It is an art in itself and is easily mastered with relatively little time and study. The quality of the image is often judged by the film produced. Nothing is more detrimental than producing a fine-quality examination and having poor recordings that do not reflect the good diagnostic quality of the examination.

The first requirement is a good processor, the best being a 90-second instant-on processor for quick use and easy maintenance. Become familiar with the operation of the processor and set up the chemicals compatible with your film. The chemicals, replenishment levels, and temperatures are adjusted to produce the desired results. Usually, a single-emulsion film of medium speed and fairly wide latitude is used to produce a wide range of gray shades for various tissue densities. We do not want a high-contrast image but rather one that will display multiple shades of gray for various tissue characteristics.

Once the processor and film choice are established, set up the cameras. Start with the monitor settings, which demonstrate the anatomic structures and various shades of gray for various tissue characteristics. White on black is usually preferable, but this is often debatable and so becomes a personal choice. However, white images on a black background are easier to calibrate and to maintain standard reproducible settings. Once the viewing monitor is adjusted, set up the camera to achieve identical results with the viewing monitor. Most cameras function similarly. Begin calibration with the brightness setting for the black background. Set the camera so that the finished film background reads 1.8 density value on a standard densitometer. Then set the contrast to show multiple shades of gray as seen on the viewing monitor. It is helpful to set up a Quality Assurance (QA) Program to ensure that the quality is continuously maintained. Using these methods will standardize the technique and keep the scans reproducible.

References

1. Gray H. Anatomy of the human body. Philadelphia, Lea & Febiger, 1954.
2. Rutherford RB, Jones DN. Carotid velocity waveform analysis. *In* Kempczinski RM, Yao JST (eds). Practical noninvasive vascular diagnosis. Chicago, Year Book Medical Publishers, Inc, 1982: 215–225.
3. White DN. Vertebral ultrasonography. *In* Zwiebel WJ (ed). Introduction to vascular ultrasonography. New York, Grune and Stratton, 1982: 188–190.
4. Poehlmann HW, Bigongiari LR. An introduction to carotid duplex sonography. J Diag Med Sonography 1986; 2:2–11.
5. Bridges RA, Barnes RW. Segmental limb pressures. *In* Kempczinski RM, Yao JST (eds). Practical noninvasive vascular diagnosis. Chicago, Year Book Medical Publishers, Inc, 1982: 91.

4 • B-Mode Image Patterns of
Atherosclerotic Plaques

Introduction

Two concepts are used to explain the etiology of transient ischemic attacks (TIAs) and strokes:

One is the hemodynamic concept, which states that a critical stenosis produces symptoms by reducing cerebral blood flow. It was proposed in 1954, when Eastcott, Pickering, and Rob described their successful repair of a carotid artery stenosis in a patient with intermittent attacks of hemiplegia.[1] This was followed by the development of one of the current criteria for carotid endarterectomy, which requires the reduction of a vessel's diameter by at least 50%.[2]

The second concept states that TIAs and strokes are the result of cerebral emboli coming from irregular atherosclerotic plaques frequently located in the common carotid artery bifurcation, as described by Fisher in 1952.[3]

Both of these concepts are important in B-mode imaging because they define the site and type of lesions most commonly examined during duplex scanning of the extracranial carotid arteries: critical stenosis and the ulcerative plaque located either in the common carotid artery (CCA) or in the internal carotid artery (ICA), or the external carotid artery (ECA) at the site of the CCA bifurcation.

Morphology

Before either the B-mode ultrasound or the sound spectral analysis images of these lesions can be thoroughly understood, some knowledge of their gross and microscopic pathological morphology is required. The basic structure of an uncomplicated, clinically significant atherosclerotic plaque is illustrated in Figure 4–1. It consists of two basic parts: the fibrous cap, and the lipid core, both of which are located in the intima of the artery.

The connective tissue fibrous cap is made up of collagen and varying numbers of smooth muscle cells. Contained within the lipid core are cholesterol, cholesterol clefts, and cellular debris. The uncomplicated, clinically significant plaques vary in the amount of fibrous tissue, smooth muscle cells, and lipid material they contain. Some are composed predominantly of smooth muscle and fibrous tissue, whereas others contain large amounts of lipid materials.

Complications of Plaque

Atherosclerotic plaques are considered clinically significant because they may spontaneously undergo a series of changes, the complications of which lead to TIAs and strokes. It is of considerable diagnostic importance that all of these complications may be observed on the B-mode image of the plaque. These complications include (1) intraplaque hemorrhage, (2) surface ulcerations, and (3) intraluminal thrombus formation.

"Significant" intraplaque hemorrhage is most frequently found in association with symptomatic plaques causing focal neurological defects and is less frequently found in asymptomatic plaques.[4] The hemorrhage results from rupture of the thin-walled capillaries that vascularize the endothelium, smooth muscle, and fibrous connective tissue adjacent to the lipid core (Fig. 4–1). Hemorrhage can dissect and extend into the media muscularis, rupture into the lipid core, and elevate the fibrous cap, causing it to protrude into the arterial lumen, as shown in Figure 4–2A. This figure shows one cause for the development of a critical stenotic arterial lesion. As the hemorrhage elevates the fibrous cap, it tears the overlying thin endothelial surface, which soon becomes ulcerated. These ulcers erode down into the fibrous plaque, exposing its surface to the blood stream. The ulcers may also extend down

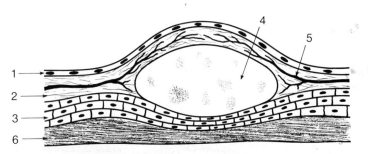

Figure 4–1. Components of a clinically significant atherosclerotic plaque. *1*, Endothelium. *2*, Fibrous cap. *3*, Media muscularis. *4*, Lipid core and cholesterol clefts. *5*, Thin-walled capillaries. *6*, Adventitia.

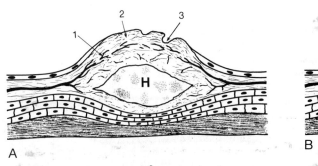

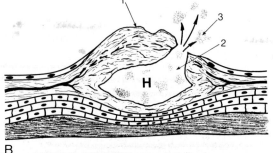

A

B

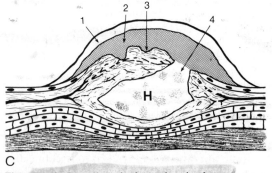

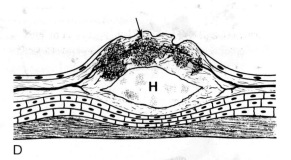

C

D

Figure 4–2. Complicated atherosclerotic plaques.

   A, Intraplaque hemorrhage (H) from ruptured capillaries *(1)*, causing elevation of fibrous cap *(2)* and endothelial ulcerations *(3)*.

   B, Loss of normal endothelial surface *(1)*, ulceration extending into hemorrhage of lipid core *(2)*, releasing microemboli of fibrin platelet aggregates and lipid core contents into the blood stream *(3)*.

   C, Red clot *(1)* and gray or pink thrombus *(2)* covering ulcerated fibrous plaque *(3)* and hemorrhagic lipid core *(4)*.

   D, Calcifications (arrow) in fibrous plaque protruding into artery lumen as a result of hemorrhage beneath it.

into the hemorrhagic lipid core, which now acts as a nidus for the microembolization of lipid debris, fibrin, and platelets into the blood stream (Fig. 4–2*B*).

Both the non-endothelialized surfaces of the fibrous plaque and the exposed hemorrhagic lipid core act to stimulate thrombus formation. The thrombus may be either gray, pink, or red. Gray or pink thrombus is initiated by the adherence of fibrin and platelets to the plaque surface. It is microscopically characterized by the lines of Zahn, representing alternating bands of platelets and fibrin with relatively few trapped red blood cells. This type of thrombus occurs over plaque surfaces in arteries when there is rapid blood flow.

Red clot forms in arteries with either sluggish or absent blood flow. For example, it may be seen distal or proximal to a tight stenosis or in a totally occluded artery. It is microscopically characterized by an absence of the lines of Zahn and contains all of the blood elements with numerous trapped red blood cells.

As shown in Figure 4–2*D*, the complicated ulcerated plaque can be covered with both gray or pink thrombus and red clot. The proliferation of gray or pink thrombus can cause further stenosis of the artery until it becomes totally occluded. It then becomes completely filled with fresh red clot. Within a matter of weeks, the fresh clot becomes a densely organized thrombus within the vessel lumen. The transition period between a fresh red clot and an organized thrombus explains why some totally occluded arteries appear anechoic, whereas others show dense areas of echoes on the B-mode image.

Recently clotted blood has little inherent echogenicity, and even a totally occluded artery can appear surprisingly normal on the B-mode image (Fig. 4–3*A*).[5] This may be explained by the fact that a fresh clot is composed of blood elements, mainly red blood cells, and lacks an organized matrix of fibrous connective tissue (collagen). A careful adjustment of the gain settings to enhance low-amplitude signals may be helpful in demonstrating these clots. If this fails, other parameters that can be used to diagnose an occluded artery caused by a fresh clot include (1) pulsed Doppler sonography to detect absent blood flow, and (2) real-time imaging to detect absent arterial pulsations and a decrease in the diameter of the occluded artery as compared with the contralateral patent artery of the same size.

Internal echoes begin to appear as the clot becomes an organized thrombus. Areas of liquefaction often appear as anechoic, cystic spaces

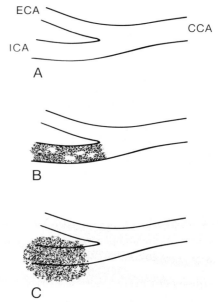

Figure 4–3. Patterns of clot and thrombus formations in occluded arteries. *A,* Non-echogenic fresh clot. ECA = External carotid artery; ICA = internal carotid artery; CCA = common carotid artery. *B,* Echogenic thrombus with cystic spaces. *C,* Echogenic thrombus in occluded artery surrounded by an inflammatory reaction.

scattered throughout the echogenic thrombus (Fig. 4–3*B*). Old thrombosed arteries incite an inflammatory-like reaction in the surrounding soft tissues. This causes intraluminal echoes from the organized thrombus of the occluded ICA to blend in with the surrounding adjacent soft-tissue, inflammatory-like reaction.[6] The result is a loss in the normal acoustical interface between the occluded artery and the surrounding soft tissues (Fig 4–3*C*). A B-mode image of the chronically occluded artery cannot be obtained under these circumstances. The inability to visualize the ICA with the B-mode scan then offers another clue that it is occluded.

Calcification is another complication that may occur in the intimal plaque. Almost always, atheromas in advanced disease undergo patchy or massive calcification. Hemorrhage beneath a calcified plaque may cause it to protrude into the lumen, resulting in an arterial stenosis[7] (Fig. 4–2*D*). This is similar to the stenosis produced when hemorrhage occurs beneath a dense fibrous cap, as shown in Figure 4–2*A*.

As illustrated in Figures 4–2 and 4–3, the atherosclerotic plaque can undergo quite a few complications that have the potential of insulting the cerebral circulation. Cerebral ischemia can occur from either interference with blood flow through the cerebral vessels in the neck because

Table 4–1. B-Mode Echoes of Plaque Morphology

Anechoic
Fresh clot in lumen
Fresh hemorrhage in plaque
Low Echogenicity
Thrombus in artery lumen
Thrombus (old hemorrhage in plaque)
Soft fibrous plaque
High Echogenicity (Acoustic shadowing absent)
Hard fibrous plaque (collagen)
High Echogenicity (Acoustic shadowing present)
Calcification

of high-grade stenoses or obstructions or because of either or both atheromatous and platelet emboli to the cerebral arteries.[4]

Although the exact pathogenesis for plaque formation and its complications remains unclear, the theories proposed in Figures 4–1, 4–2, and 4–3 serve to illustrate some of the patterns seen on the B-mode images of these lesions. They also help explain why all atherosclerotic plaques do not look alike on the B-mode scans. Their appearance depends on whether or not they contain calcium, a dense fibrous cap, ulcerations, hemorrhage, or organized thrombus with associated fresh clot formation. It is then the amount and arrangement of these various pathological abnormalities that determine the B-mode image of the plaque under investigation. Whether or not these patterns are predominantly echogenic, anechoic, or a complex combination of both will depend upon the composition of the plaque and its complications. The various echogenic characteristics of the components of plaque are given in Table 4–1. These are also shown in the following illustrations: fibrous plaques, Figures 4–4 through 4–18; calcified plaques, Figures 4–19 through 4–21; and occluded vessels, Figures 4–22 through 4–25. These characteristics are important because the morphology of plaque seems to play an important role in the development of cerebral insufficiency symptoms and in the prediction of stroke risk. Ultrasonographic scanning can be used to assess plaque morphology and distinguish between heterogeneous and homogeneous plaques with an accuracy of 82%.[8] This is important because the heterogeneous plaque is associated with a statistically greater incidence of pathological plaque hemorrhage and ulceration features that correlate with a greater incidence of TIAs or stroke.[8] The noninvasive ultrasound determination of carotid plaque histology may be of considerable value in identifying clinically significant carotid artery lesions and may ultimately aid in the choice of therapy.

Text continued on page 68

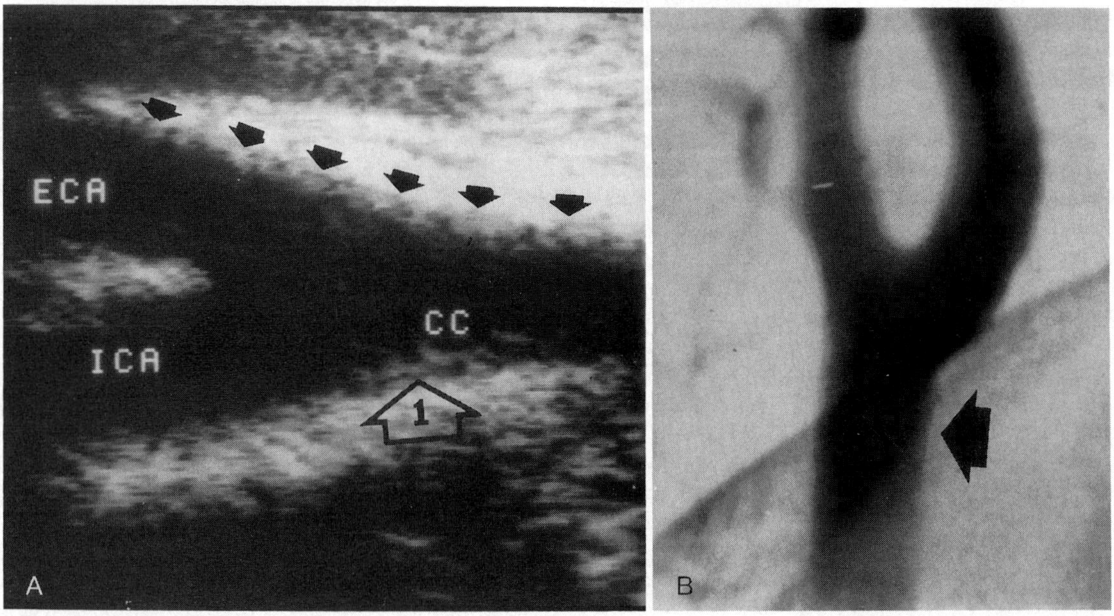

Figure 4–4. Carotid bifurcation artifacts simulating soft fibrous plaque formations. *A,* Diffuse wall thickening (black arrows). Intraluminal echoes are due to low gain setting (arrow *1*). ECA = External carotid artery; ICA = internal carotid artery; CCA = common carotid artery. *B,* Arteriogram showing no abnormality in the region of intraluminal echoes (arrow).

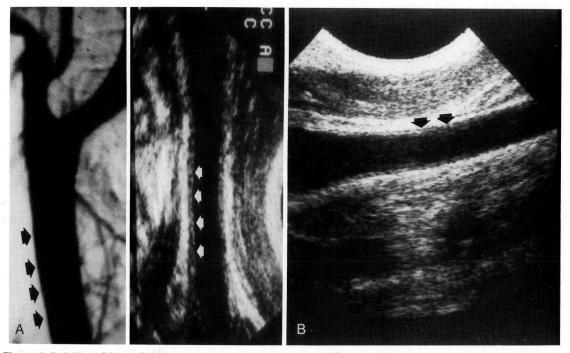

Figure 4–5. Diffuse CCA wall thickening simulating fibrous plaque in 79-year-old hypertensive patient. *A,* Arteriogram shows normal CCA lumen (black arrows) and CCA. B-mode image shows diffuse wall thickening (white arrows). *B,* Low gain setting also produced intraluminal, low-level echoes on B-mode image of this CCA (arrows).

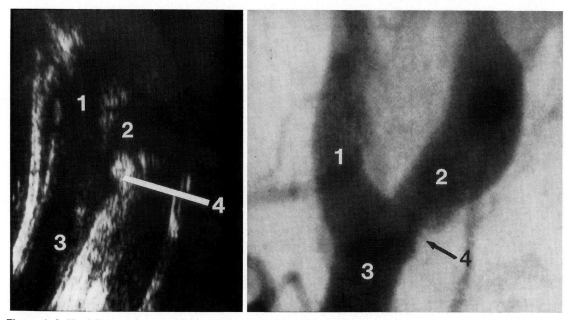

Figure 4–6. Hard fibrous plaque exhibiting high echogenicity with absence of acoustic shadowing. *1,* ECA. *2,* ICA. *3,* CCA. *4,* Hard fibrous plaque.

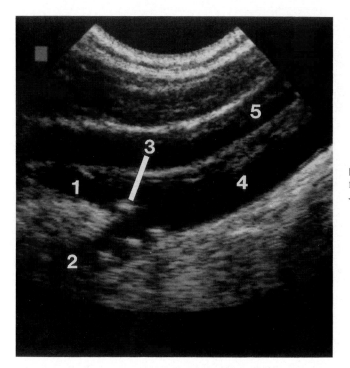

Figure 4–7. Fibrous plaques that appear to be floating within the vessel lumen. *1*, ECA. *2*, ICA. *3*, Fibrous plaque. *4*, CCA. *5*, Jugular vein.

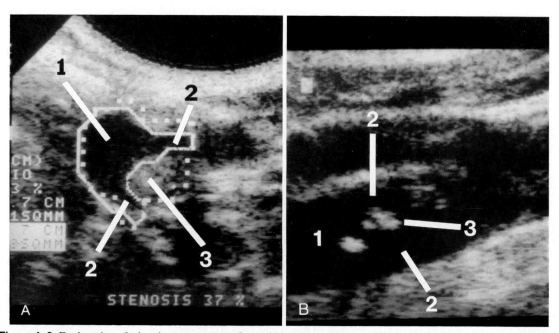

Figure 4–8. Explanation of why plaques appear to float within vessel lumen. *A*, Transverse B-mode image shows plaque projecting into vessel lumen with luminal recesses extending on both sides of plaque. *B*, Sagittal B-mode image shows plaque projecting into lumen and surrounded by luminal recesses, which causes the plaque to appear as though it were floating free in vessel lumen. *1*, Lumen. *2*, Luminal recesses. *3*, Fibrous plaque.

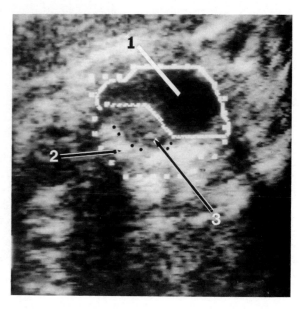

Figure 4–9. Transverse B-mode image showing ulcer crater in hard plaque filled with thrombus. Ulcer crater margins defined by row of black dots. *1*, Lumen. *2*, Hard plaque (high echogenicity). *3*, Thrombus (low echogenicity and containing cystic spaces).

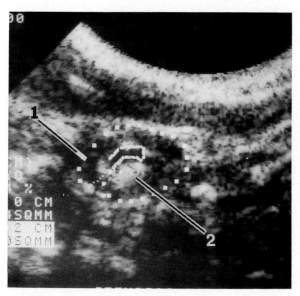

Figure 4–10. Transverse B-mode image showing hard plaque surrounded by hemorrhage. White dots define outer vessel surface. Solid white line defines narrowed vessel lumen. *1*, Plaque hemorrhage (anechoic). *2*, Hard plaque (high echogenicity).

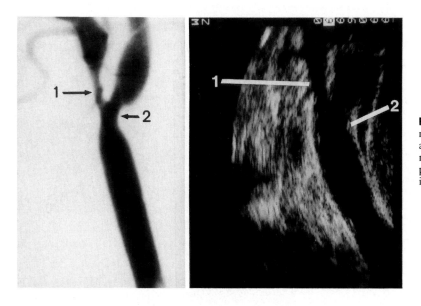

Figure 4–11. Soft fibrous plaque narrowing carotid bulb and ECA and ICA lumens. *1*, Soft plaque narrowing ECA lumen. *2*, Soft plaque (low echogenicity) narrowing carotid bulb and ICA lumens.

Figure 4–12. Close-up view of B-mode carotid bifurcation image shown in Figure 4–11. This image was obtained with a gain setting to enhance the low echogenicity characteristics of the soft fibrous plaques. The low-level echoes of these plaques are outlined by white arrow markers. White dash markers were used to obtain lumen diameter measurements. *1*, ECA soft plaque outlined by arrows. *2*, Carotid bulb and ICA soft plaque outlined by arrowheads.

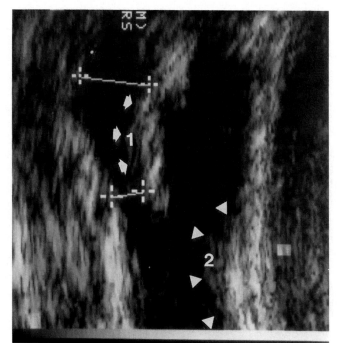

Figure 4–13. Gross carotid bifurcation endarterectomy specimen from patient shown in Figures 4–11 and 4–12. Markers placed on outer specimen surface for orientation. Note sagittal incision made through long axis of common carotid and internal carotid arteries. CC = Common carotid artery; EC = external carotid artery; IC = internal carotid artery; P = fibrous plaque surrounding IC and carotid bifurcation.

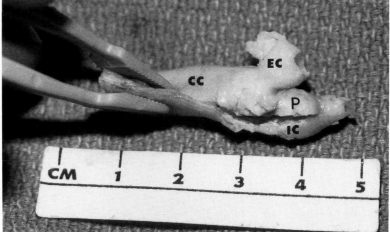

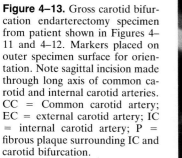
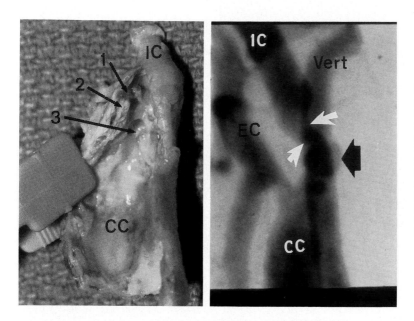

Figure 4–14. Gross specimen wall and inner surface compared with arteriogram. *1*, Intraplaque hemorrhage. *2*, Hard fibrous plaque in endarterectomy specimen wall. *3*, Ulcer crater. White arrows = Internal carotid artery stenosis caused by hard fibrous plaques *(2)*; black arrow = ulcer crater; vert = superimposed vertebral artery; IC = internal carotid artery; CC = common carotid artery; EC = external carotid artery.

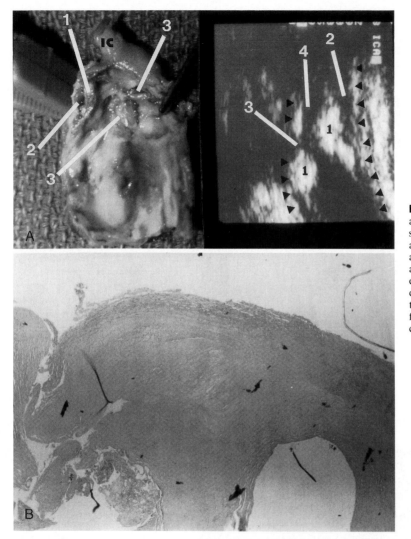

Figure 4–15. Gross specimen wall and inner surface compared with sagittal B-mode image *(A)*. Black arrowheads define internal carotid artery (IC) margins on B-mode image. *1*, Hard fibrous plaque (high echogenicity). *2*, Hemorrhage under plaque (anechoic). *3*, Ulcer craters. *4*, ICA stenosis caused by hard fibrous plaques. *B*, Plaque microscopy showing dense fibrous tissue.

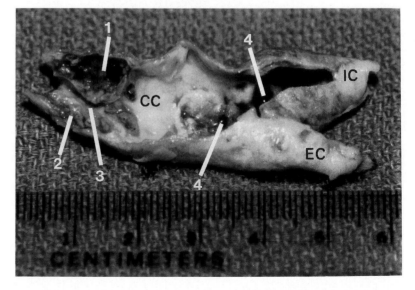

Figure 4–16. Gross carotid bifurcation endarterectomy specimen cut sagittally through common carotid (CC) and internal carotid (IC) arteries to expose inner surface and wall. *1*, Large intraplaque hemorrhage. *2*, Small intraplaque hemorrhage. *3*, Stenosis caused by plaques. *4*, Clot in ulcer craters. EC = External carotid artery.

Figure 4–17. Anteroposterior view *(A)* and lateral view *(B)* arteriograms showing CCA stenosis (arrow) caused by the plaques in Figure 4–16. B-mode image with histological correlation of this case are shown in Figure 4–18.

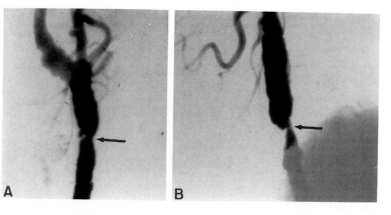

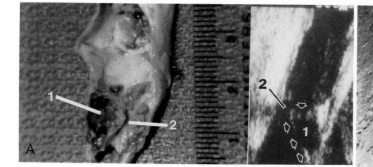

Figure 4–18. Gross endarterectomy specimen compared with B-mode image *(A)*. Arrows outline large intraplaque hemorrhage on B-mode image. *1*, Large intraplaque hemorrhage. *2*, Stenosed CCA lumen. *B*, Plaque microscopy showing hemorrhage. Angiograms of this case are shown in Figure 4–17.

HEMORRHAGE

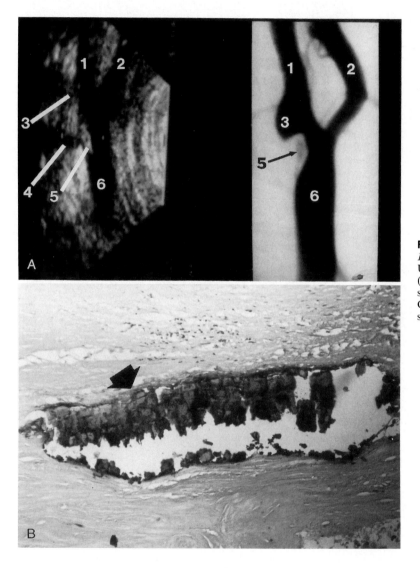

Figure 4–19. *A*, Calcified plaque. *1*, ICA lumen. *2*, ECA lumen. *3*, Ulcer crater containing thrombus (low echogenicity). *4*, Acoustical shadowing. *5*, Calcified plaque. *6*, CCA lumen. *B*, Plaque microscopy showing calcification (arrow).

Figure 4–20. Complex ulcerated hard fibrous and calcified plaque. *1,* Calcified plaque. *2,* Ulcer crater. *3,* Acoustical shadowing. *4,* Hard fibrous plaque.

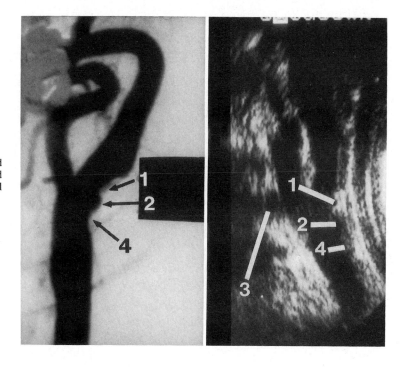

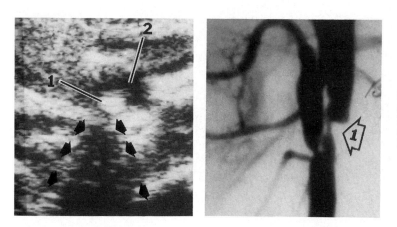

Figure 4–21. Transverse B-mode image of calcified plaque projecting into ICA lumen. Arrows denote acoustical shadowing. *1,* Calcified plaque. *2,* ICA lumen.

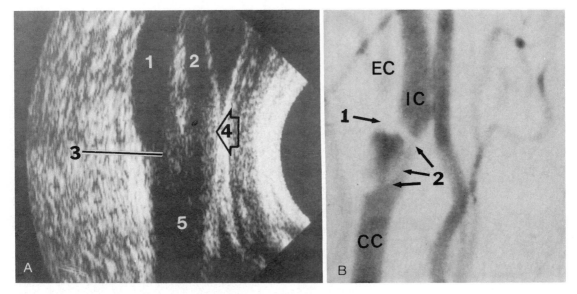

Figure 4–22. Carotid bifurcation, fresh clot, and thrombus formation.

A, B-mode image showing low echogenicity or thrombus. The ECA and ICA appear patent because the fresh clot obstructing these vessels is anechoic. *1,* ICA lumen. *2,* ECA lumen. *3,* Thrombus (low echogenicity) in ICA. *4,* Thrombus (low echogenicity) in ECA. *5,* CCA lumen.

B, Carotid bifurcation arteriogram shows total occlusion of ECA and an extremely tight ICA stenosis. *1,* Fresh clot in ECA. *2,* Large thrombus and fresh clot formation extending from carotid bulb into ICA lumen. EC = External carotid artery; IC = internal carotid artery; CC = common carotid artery.

Figure 4–23. Thrombus occluding CCA. *1,* Thrombus (low echogenicity). *2,* Hard fibrous plaque (high echogenicity). *3,* Hemorrhage (anechoic).

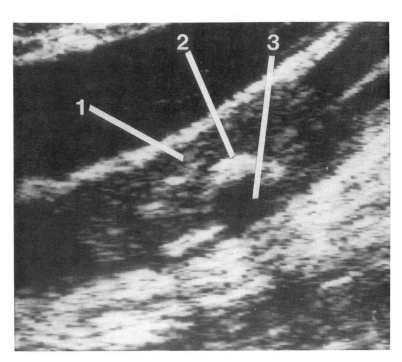

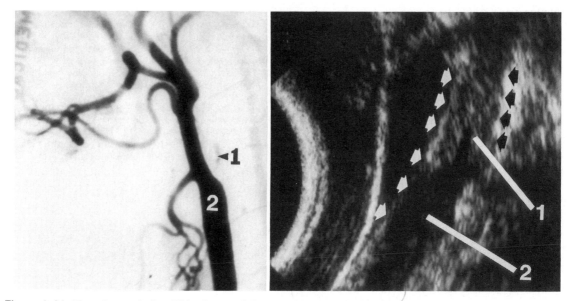

Figure 4–24. Thrombus occluding ICA. Arrows define carotid bulb and ICA margins on the B-mode image. *1*, Small ICA stump surrounded by thrombus. *2*, Carotid bulb. The ECA is not included on this B-mode image of the ICA.

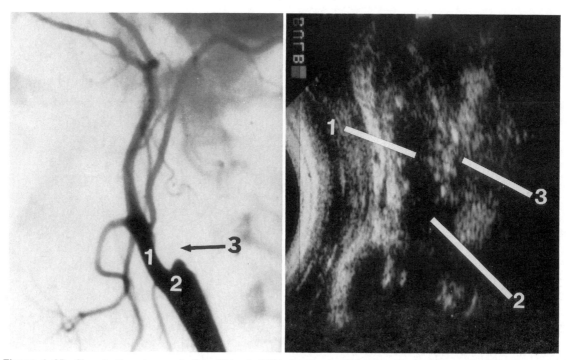

Figure 4–25. Chronic thrombus occluding ICA. *1*, ECA lumen. *2*, Carotid bulb. *3*, ICA unidentified because of surrounding soft tissue inflammations caused by the chronic thrombosis of ICA.

References

1. Eastcott HHG, Pickering GW, Rob GC. Reconstruction of the internal carotid artery in a patient with intermittent attacks of hemiplegia. Lancet 1954; 2:994–999.
2. Crawford ES, DeBakey ME, Blaisdell FW, Morris GC Jr, Fields WS. Hemodynamic alterations in patients with cerebral artery insufficiency before and after operation. Surgery 1960; 48:76–82.
3. Fisher CM. Transient monocular blindness associated with hemiplegia. Arch Ophthalmol 1952; 47:167–172.
4. Imprato AM, Riles TS, Gorstein F. The carotid bifurcation plaque: pathologic findings associated with cerebral ischemia. Stroke 1979; 10(3):238–242.
5. Wing V, Scheible W. Sonography of jugular vein thrombosis. AJR 1983; 140:333–339.
6. Gooding GAW, Effeney DJ. Static and real-time B-mode sonography of arterial occlusions. AJR 1982; 139:949–954.
7. Persson AV, Robichaux WT, Silverman M. The natural history of carotid plaque development. Arch Surg 1983; 118:1048–1052.
8. Reilly LM, Lusby RJ, Hughes L, et al. Carotid plaque histology using real-time ultrasonography. Am J Surg 1983; 146:188–193.

5 • Sound Spectral Analysis of Extracranial Carotid Artery Plaques

Introduction

This chapter shows the serial changes that occur in sound spectral analysis patterns ranging from normal to stenotic. Because most of these pattern changes have already been described in the previous chapter, they will not be repeated here. Correlative angiograms are included to display the anatomy of the plaques producing the sound spectral analysis patterns.

Patterns of Atherosclerotic Plaques

Figure 5–1 allows the serial changes in the sound spectral analysis pattern to be studied as they progress from normal to stenotic. A normal internal carotid artery (ICA) baseline pattern is shown in Figure 5–1A, which correlates with the angiogram in Figure 5–2A. A narrow bandwidth of Doppler shift frequencies is present throughout all three phases of the cardiac cycle, and scintillations are absent in the spectral window. The introduction of a smooth plaque causes spectral broadening in early and late diastole, as shown in Figure 5–1B. This sound spectral analysis pattern was obtained from the segment of a common carotid artery containing the plaque shown in Figure 5–2B. Rough, ulcerative plaques seem to cause further spectral broadening throughout all three phases of the cardiac cycle, as shown in Figure 5–1C. This figure also shows some scintillations beginning to appear in the spectral window during systole and during early and late diastole. It was obtained from the area of ulcerative plaque formation seen on the angiogram in Figure 5–2C. Another example of the sound spectral analysis pattern of ulcerative plaque disease is shown in Figure 5–1D. This figure shows further progression of the findings in Figure 5–1C. It was obtained from the ulcerated segment of ICA in Figure 5–2D.

A comparison of Figure 5–1A through D reveals little change in the peak systolic Doppler shift frequencies in any of the arterial segments examined. Instead, these frequency shifts only varied between 2.0 to 3.0 kHz. The main abnormality is not an increase in frequency shift but an increase in the amount of spectral broadening present. Minimal spectral broadening like that observed in Figure 5–1B may be difficult to distinguish from the normal pattern seen in Figure 5–1A. However, the patterns in Figure 5–1C and D are quite distinctive and characteristic of rough plaque formations that do not cause a significant narrowing of the arterial lumen.

As the plaque encroaches upon the arterial lumen, it creates a stenosis like the one in Figure 5–2E. How sound spectral analysis is used to grade the severity of a stenosis will not be discussed here because this subject is described in detail in a subsequent chapter. This type of stenosis is included here only to illustrate the serial progression on the sound spectral analysis from a nonstenotic plaque to one that is stenotic. The pattern caused by this stenosis is shown in Figure 5–1E. It is distinguished from the previous patterns in Figure 5–1 because its Doppler frequency shifts are increased throughout all three phases of the cardiac cycle. This can be appreciated by comparing the height of the scintillations above the zero baseline in this figure with those in the previous figures. The systolic peak Doppler frequency shift is increased to 6.6 kHz, and the velocity of the blood flow is increased through the stenosis in all three phases of the cardiac cycle. This velocity increase causes turbulence, which produces a wide band of different Doppler shift frequencies.

A comparison of the bandwidth histogram in Figure 5–1E with the one in Figure 5–1A shows the former to be composed of numerous different frequency spikes, whereas the histogram in Figure 5–1A contains only two frequency level

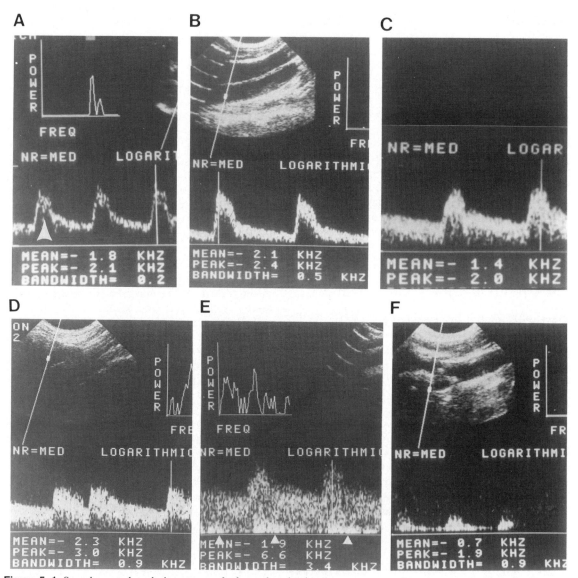

Figure 5–1. Sound spectral analysis patterns of atherosclerotic plaques.

A, Normal ICA flow pattern with narrow bandwidth (arrowhead) and scintillations absent in spectral window.

B, Spectral broadening in early and late diastole with scintillations absent in spectral window.

C, Speckled scintillations beginning to fill in spectral window in systole and early and late diastole.

D, Spectral broadening of all three cardiac cycle components. A distinction can still be made between the original spectral line and the spectral window zone.

E, Doppler shift frequencies increased in systole and early and late diastole. Scintillations fill in spectral window. Note the increased number of low Doppler frequency shift scintillations adjacent to zero baseline (arrows).

F, High Doppler shift frequencies are absent and only the low Doppler shift frequencies remain adjacent to the zero baseline.

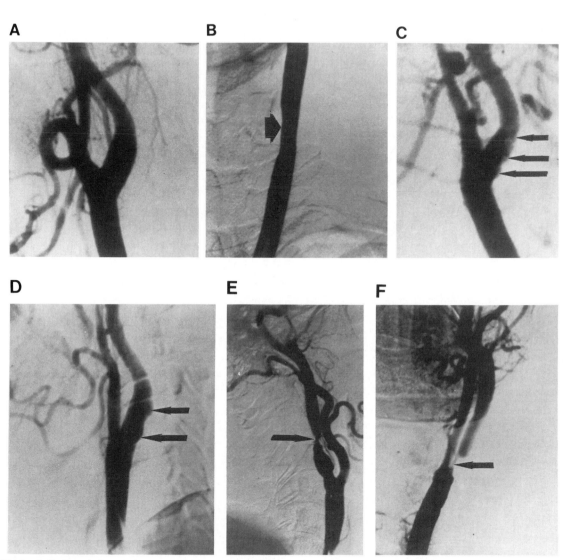

Figure 5–2. Correlative angiograms. *A*, Normal carotid bifurcation. *B*, Smooth common carotid artery plaque (arrow). *C*, Ulcerative internal carotid artery plaque (arrows). *D*, Ulcerative internal carotid artery plaque (arrows). *E*, Internal carotid artery stenosis (arrow). *F*, Extremely tight stenosis (arrow).

spikes. This wide bandwidth of different Doppler shift frequencies is best appreciated by a complete filling in of the spectral window by numerous, randomly placed scintillations. There is now no demarcation between the normal-appearing spectral line in Figure 5–1A and the spectral window zone in Figure 5–1E. This is the sound spectral analysis pattern of a severe stenosis. It is quite distinct from those of plaque formations without associated stenosis, as shown in the previous figures. A close inspection of Figure 5–1E will also reveal an increase in the brightness or amplitude of the low Doppler shift frequencies as compared with the higher Doppler shift frequencies. The high Doppler shift frequencies are about to be lost from this sound spectral analysis because of the severity of the stenosis shown in Figure 5–2E.

As the stenosis increases in severity, the velocity of the blood flow through it will continue to decrease until only a trickle remains or until all blood flow is stopped and the artery is totally occluded. No blood flow or Doppler shift frequencies will be seen by sound spectral analysis under these circumstances. Before the blood flow is reduced to a trickle or stopped, however, the high-frequency Doppler shift frequencies are lost, as shown in Figure 5–1F. This figure represents the last stage in the progression of an atherosclerotic plaque before it results in a vessel occlusion. Note that if the high Doppler shift frequencies in Figure 5–1E are eliminated, only the low Doppler shift frequencies in Figures 5–1E and F remain. Blood flow velocity in Figure 5–1F is decreased in systole and is almost absent in late diastole. Only a few "ghost" high Doppler frequency shift scintillations remain to indicate the existence of high-velocity blood flow through this extremely tight stenosis. The angiogram of this stenosis is shown in Figure 5–2F.

6 • Duplex Scanning of Extracranial Carotid Artery Stenoses

Introduction

This chapter provides a pictorial atlas of the B-mode freeze-frame images and sound spectral analysis waveform patterns of extracranial carotid artery stenoses. The B-mode images were obtained with a 10 MHz transducer; the sound spectral analysis waveforms were obtained with a 4.5 MHz pulsed Doppler signal angled 30 to 60° to the blood flow in the vessel lumen.

The illustrations are organized into five diagnostic categories according to the severity of the stenosis characterized by the duplex scan. These tegories include:

- I. Normal internal carotid artery
- II. Stenosis causing < 50% diameter reduction
- III. Stenosis causing 50 to 60% diameter reduction
- IV. Stenosis causing 60 to 80% diameter reduction
- V. Stenosis causing 80 to > 95% diameter reduction

Correlative angiograms are included to provide a better understanding of the arterial abnormalities and stenoses seen on the duplex scans.

Diagnostic Categories

Category I: Normal Internal Carotid Artery

The two parts of the duplex scan used in the diagnosis and characterization of extracranial carotid artery stenoses are shown in Figure 6–1. These are the sound spectral analysis waveform (Fig. 6–1A) and the B-mode image (Fig. 6–1B). The waveform has a thin line of Doppler shift frequencies in its systolic component, a 2.1 kHz systolic Doppler peak frequency, and a gradual downward-sloping wide line of diminishing Doppler shift frequencies throughout the early and late diastolic periods of the cardiac cycle. Its spectral window contains no scintillations, and the diastolic components of the waveform are in their normal positions above the baseline.

The 2.1 kHz systolic peak frequency indicates the absence of a stenosis causing a 50% or greater diameter reduction in the internal carotid artery (ICA) (Table 6–1). It does not rule out the presence of a stenosis causing less than a 50% diameter reduction in the ICA at the site of measurement. This is possible because Doppler criteria are far less sensitive to stenoses measuring less than 50% than to those measuring greater than 50%.[1-3] Turbulence may be the only abnormality noted on sound spectral analysis to indicate the presence of a stenosis measuring less than 50%. However, the minimal turbulence caused by stenoses of 5 to 15% can easily be mimicked by "pseudoturbulence" resulting from slight adjustments in gain and from other technical factors. Turbulence is also commonly found in the normal ICA at its origin from the carotid bulb (Fig. 6–2).[4] It is caused in part by boundary layer separation of the blood flow as it passes from the common carotid artery (CCA) into the ICA and external carotid artery (ECA). Flow disturbances of this type have also been implicated as a factor in the pathogenesis of carotid bifurcation atherosclerosis in humans.[5] They are most commonly encountered in young patients, and are not usually characterized by an increased systolic Doppler peak frequency shift.

Because the systolic Doppler peak frequency shifts cannot accurately detect stenoses of less than 50% and because pseudoturbulence as well as turbulence may be seen in normal vessels, the real-time B-mode ultrasound part of the duplex scan examination is more useful in determining whether or not a vessel is normal. A freeze-frame B-mode image from a real-time ultrasound examination of a normal carotid bifurcation is shown in Figure 6–1B. The vessel lumens are

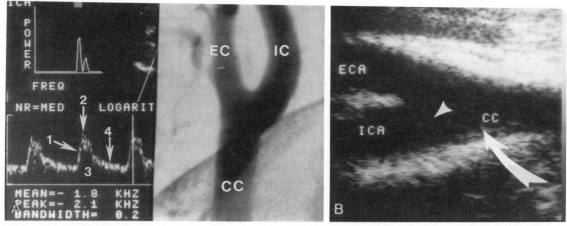

Figure 6–1. Normal ICA duplex scan.

A, Left: Normal ICA sound spectral analysis waveform. *1,* Thin line of Doppler shift frequencies in systolic component. *2,* Systolic peak. *3,* Spectral window. *4,* Gradual downward-sloping wide line of early and late diastolic component diminishing Doppler shift frequencies.

Right: Normal carotid bifurcation angiogram. EC. = External carotid artery; IC = internal carotid artery; CC = common carotid artery.

B, Normal carotid bifurcation B-mode image. Arrowhead indicates site where boundary layer separation turbulence occurs. Curved arrow points to low-level intraluminal echo artifacts, which should not be misinterpreted as atherosclerotic plaque formation.

wide and patent, and there is no evidence of obstructive atherosclerotic disease.

Category II: Stenosis Causing Less Than 50% Diameter Reduction

Examples of Category II stenoses are shown in Figures 6–3 and 6–4. The sound spectral analysis waveform of the ICA in Figure 6–3 should be compared with the one in Figure 6–1 to appreciate the turbulence caused by a plaque protruding into the ICA lumen. The plaque creates spectral broadening and speckling of scintillations in the spectral window. There is no increase in the systolic peak frequency because the stenosis has caused less than 50% diameter reduction of the ICA lumen (as determined by measurements obtained from the angiogram).

The sound spectral analysis in Figure 6–4 shows turbulence, but real-time ultrasound must be

Table 6–1. Systolic Peak (kHz) vs. Diameter Reduction (%) Stenosis

Systolic Peak*	Diameter Reduction
<4	<50
4–5	50–60
5–6	60–80
>6	80–>95

*Systolic peak (kHz) obtained with a 4.5 MHz Doppler probe at a 30 to 60° scanning angle.

used to define its cause. Ulcerative plaque was found to be the cause of turbulence, as is demonstrated in Figure 6–4*A.*

Category III: Stenosis Causing 50 to 60% Diameter Reduction

When a stenosis is encountered during duplex scanning, the sample volume must be carefully positioned to characterize it by sound spectral analysis, as is demonstrated in Figure 6–5. Both the beam angle and the sample volume were repositioned before this stenosis was fully characterized by sound spectral analysis. Initially, only turbulence was observed, without an increase in the systolic peak frequency; there was no increase in the late diastolic shift frequencies. These results occurred because the sample volume was placed against the arterial wall proximal to the stenosis. The arrows in the line drawing, Figure 6–6, show the direction of eddy currents in the blood flow moving against the arterial wall proximal to the stenosis, which explains why a sample volume placed in this position will not fully characterize the stenosis. A search must be made with the sample volume in order to position it within the plane of maximum blood flow passing through the orifice of the stenosis, as shown by the straight black arrow (Fig. 6–6). A re-positioning of the sample volume in Figure 6–5 did produce an increase in the systolic peak fre-

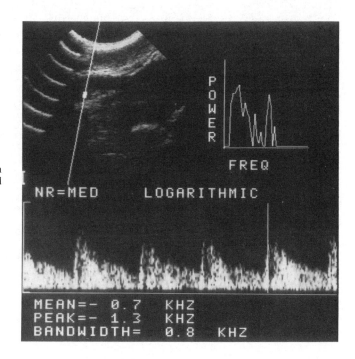

Figure 6–2. Normal carotid bulb turbulence with a 1.3 kHz systolic peak frequency. It was obtained from a young asymptomatic female.

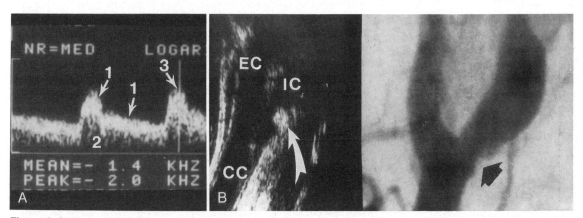

Figure 6–3. Plaque, 35% diameter reduction stenosis. *A,* ICA sound spectral analysis. *1,* Diastolic spectral broadening. *2,* Speckled scintillations in spectral window. *3,* 2.0 kHz systolic peak frequency. *B,* B-mode image and angiogram of plaque at IC artery origin (arrow). EC = External carotid artery; IC = internal carotid artery; CC = common carotid artery.

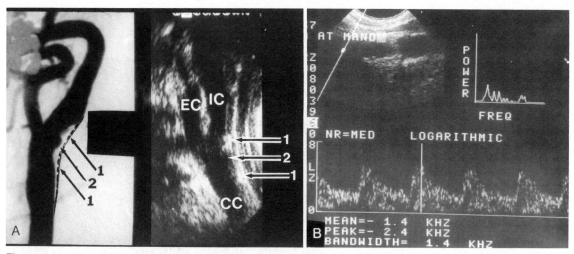

Figure 6–4. Ulcerative plaque, 28.5% diameter reduction stenosis. *A,* Angiogram and B-mode image of ulcerative plaque. Dotted line indicates area of lumen replaced by plaque. *1,* Plaque. *2,* Ulcer. EC = External carotid artery; IC = internal carotid artery; CC = common carotid artery. *B,* Sound spectral analysis of blood flow over ulcerative plaque with systolic peak frequency of 2.4 kHz.

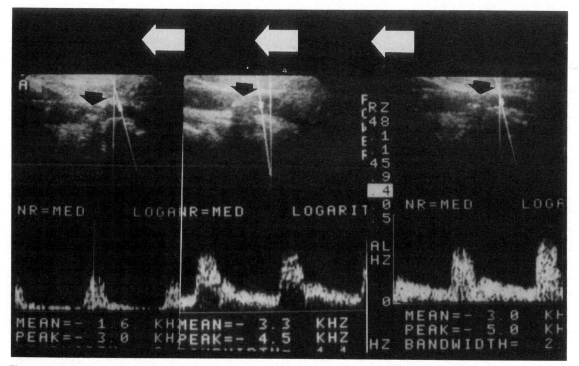

Figure 6–5. Probe angle and sample volume manipulations used to fully characterize a stenosis by sound spectral analysis. Serial white arrows indicate direction of blood flow through the stenosis (black arrows).

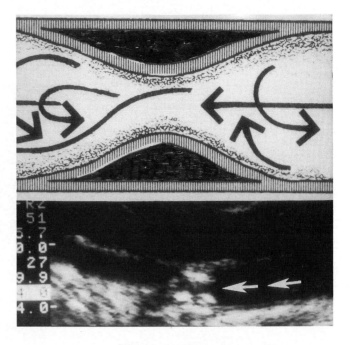

Figure 6–6. Line drawing of blood flow through stenosis. Curved black arrows denote eddy currents and turbulence both proximal and distal to stenosis. Straight black arrow shows plane of increased velocity, turbulent blood flow passing through stenosis orifice. White arrows indicate blood flow direction towards stenosis on B-mode image correlating with line drawing.

quency from 3.0 to 4.5 kHz, but it still did not define either the maximum systolic peak frequency or the maximum turbulence caused by the stenosis. Again, the sample volume and the beam angle were re-positioned until the stenosis was fully characterized by sound spectral analysis. Re-positioning resulted in a complete filling in of the spectral window, which was caused by turbulence and by a further increase in the systolic peak frequency from 4.5 to 5.0 kHz—a result of the increase in the velocity of the red blood cells (RBCs) traversing the stenosis. Manipulating both the probe angle and sample volume in this manner are most important in determining the

correct diagnosis. Examples of stenoses are shown in Figures 6–7 through 6–9. The example in Figure 6–7 is of particular interest because it demonstrates how both the B-mode image and the systolic peak frequency may be used to discriminate between normal and abnormal carotid bulb turbulence.

Category IV: Stenosis Causing 60 to 80% Diameter Reduction

Examples of Category IV stenoses are shown in Figures 6–10 through 6–12. Spectral broadening increases at the baseline, and there is pro-

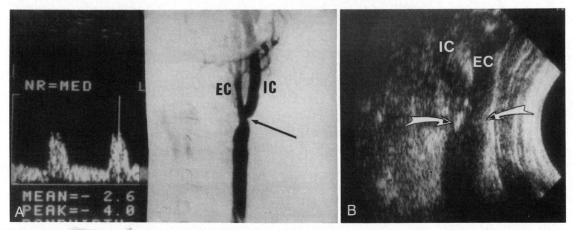

Figure 6–7. 57% diameter reduction stenosis. *A,* Carotid bulb stenosis on angiogram (arrow). Sound spectral analysis of carotid blood flow shows almost complete filling in of spectral window and a 4.0 kHz systolic peak frequency. *B,* Sagittal B-mode image of carotid bulb plaque (arrows). EC = External carotid artery; IC = internal carotid artery.

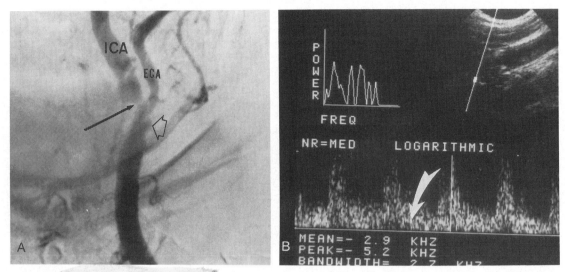

Figure 6–8. 60% diameter reduction stenosis. *A*, Angiogram of ulcerative plaque (open arrow) causing ICA stenosis (black arrow). ICA = Internal carotid artery; ECA = external carotid artery. *B*, Sound spectral analysis waveform of ICA stenosis showing increased scintillations near baseline (arrow) and a 5.2 kHz systolic peak frequency.

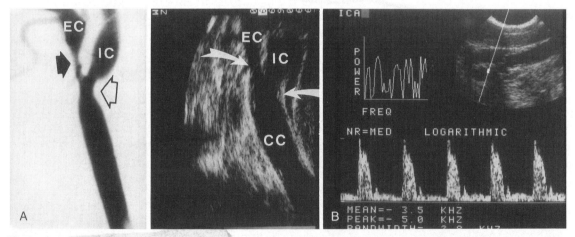

Figure 6–9. 60% diameter reduction stenosis. *A*, Angiogram of circumferential carotid bulb plaque stenosis (open arrow) and 60% diameter reduction stenosis of the external carotid artery (ECA) (solid arrow). B-mode image of stenoses (arrows). EC = External carotid artery; IC = internal carotid artery; CC = common carotid artery. *B*, ECA sound spectral analysis showing complete loss of spectral window and systolic peak frequency of 5.0 kHz.

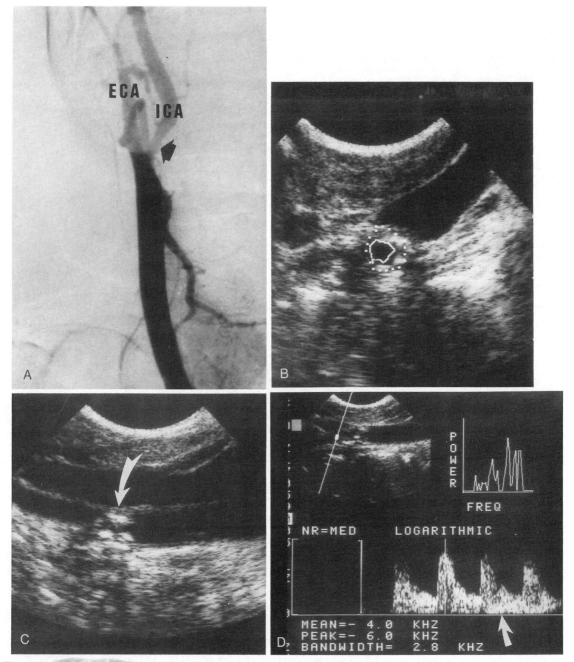

Figure 6–10. 62% diameter reduction stenosis. *A*, Angiogram of ICA stenosis (arrow). ECA = External carotid artery; ICA = internal carotid artery. *B*, Transverse ICA B-mode image of 76% cross-sectional area reduction stenosis. White dots outline outer ICA margin and solid white line outlines residual lumen. *C*, Sagittal B-mode image of ICA stenosis (arrow). *D*, ICA sound spectral analysis showing increased spectral broadening at baseline (arrow) and systolic peak frequency of 6.0 kHz.

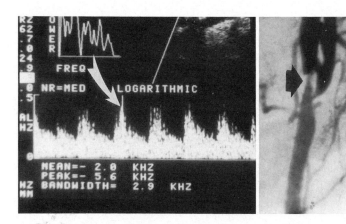

Figure 6–11. 75% diameter reduction stenosis. Sound spectral analysis of ICA stenosis on adjacent angiogram (arrow). There is complete homogeneous filling in of the spectral window owing to increased turbulence caused by this stenosis. White arrow indicates point at which systolic peak frequency of 5.6 kHz was obtained.

Figure 6–12. 72% diameter reduction stenosis. *A*, Angiogram of common carotid artery (CCA) stenosis (arrow) with 5.8 kHz systolic peak frequency. *B*, Transverse B-mode image of stenosis showing an 84% cross-sectional area reduction. White dots outline outer CCA margins, and solid white line outlines residual lumen.

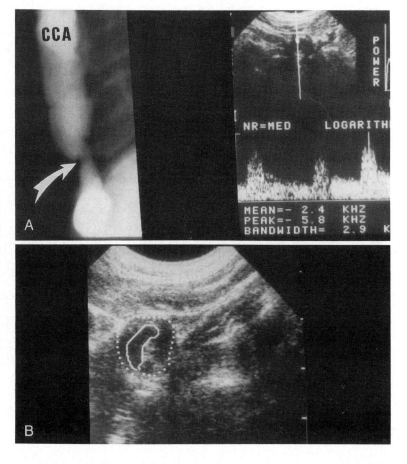

gressive filling in of the spectral window by homogeneous scintillations as the percentage of diameter reduction of the stenosis increases. The systolic peak frequency also continues to increase, as given in Table 6–1. Transverse B-mode images of some of these stenoses are included to illustrate the difference between the measurement of the percentage of diameter reduction and the percentage of cross-sectional area reduction. Measurements of the percentage of diameter reduction of the vessel lumen caused by the stenosis were made from the correlative angiograms given in the figures. A computer software program contained within the duplex scanner was used to make the cross-sectional area reduction measurements from the transverse B-mode images of the stenoses. These measurements were obtained from the regions outlined by the white dots indicating the outer circumference of the vessel containing the stenosis and by the solid white line outlining the circumference of the residual lumen left in the vessel by the plaque creating the stenosis. The zone between the white dots and the solid white line contains both the arterial wall and the intimal atherosclerotic plaque.

For cross-sectional area reduction measurements to be accurate, the operator first must obtain a good transverse image of the stenotic arterial segment and, second, must be able to outline the artery and its residual lumen with the dots and lines. Once these skills are mastered, the transverse B-mode image can be most useful in defining plaque morphology as well as determining the cross-sectional area reduction caused in the arterial lumen by the plaque. It will be noted in the subsequent figures that the cross-sectional area reduction measurement is greater than the measurement of the percentage of diameter reduction. These are not expected to be equal because they are two different quantities.

Category V: Stenosis Causing 80 to Greater Than 95% Diameter Reduction

Examples of Category V stenoses are shown in Figures 6–13 through 6–15. The systolic peak frequencies continue to increase as the percentage of diameter reduction of the vessel lumen becomes progressively greater. This is demonstrated in Figure 6–13, where the diameter reduction of the vessel lumen is shown to be 88% and the systolic peak has reached a frequency of >7 kHz. However, there is a point at which the number of RBCs moving at high velocities begins to decrease dramatically as the cells attempt to pass through an extremely tight stenosis like the one shown in Figure 6–14. The decrease in the number of RBCs passing through the stenosis produces high Doppler shift frequencies with such low amplitudes that their scintillations may not be detected by sound spectral analysis. If the scintillations are detected, they appear as a low-amplitude, ghost waveform superimposed above a high-amplitude waveform containing lower Doppler shift frequencies.

An example of this problem is shown by the sound spectral analysis waveform in Figure 6–14. It is impossible to accurately measure the systolic peak frequency in this waveform because the high Doppler shift frequencies have extremely low-amplitude scintillations. These low-amplitude scintillations create a problem because the severity of the stenosis will be misinterpreted by sound spectral analysis. The systolic peak frequency of the waveform in Figure 6–14 was obtained at the point indicated by the arrow and found to be 4 kHz. As shown in Table 6–1, this systolic peak frequency would indicate a stenosis with a reduction in diameter of only 50 to 60%, which is incorrect, as shown in the adjacent angiogram. Unfortunately, the B-mode image was of no help in this case because the stenosis was caused in part by a fresh clot containing no echoes. This is unusual, however, and the B-mode image may be of considerable importance in demonstrating the correct amount of stenosis present in a vessel containing low-amplitude, high Doppler shift frequency waveforms on sound spectral analysis.

Another cause of the severity of a stenosis being misinterpreted by sound spectral analysis is shown in Figure 6–15. Here the angiogram shows a tight ICA stenosis located so high above the carotid bifurcation that it could not be reached with the duplex scanning probe. The sound spectral analysis of the blood flow in the ICA at the carotid bifurcation proximal to the stenosis revealed a waveform with a decreased systolic peak of 1.9 kHz and late diastolic frequencies approaching the baseline. An ICA waveform pattern of this type may be obtained proximal to a tight stenosis or in the stump of a totally occluded ICA. Because there were no ICA intraluminal echoes present on the B-mode scan of the patient in Figure 6–15, the suspected diagnosis was either a tight ICA stenosis high above the bifurcation or an ICA occlusion by fresh clot formation.

It is difficult to avoid mistaking an extremely tight stenosis for one that is less severely stenosed

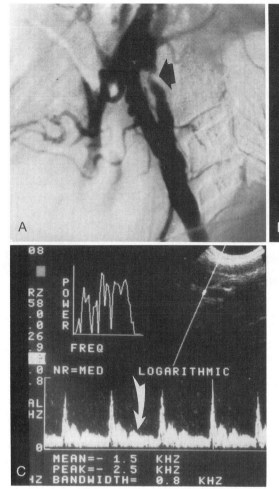

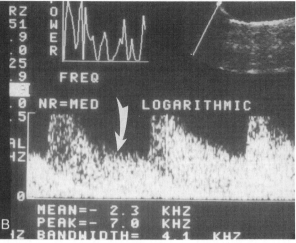

Figure 6–13. 88% diameter reduction stenosis. *A,* Angiogram of ICA stenosis (arrow). *B,* ICA sound spectral analysis showing systolic peak frequency of >7 kHz with elevation of diastolic Doppler shift frequencies high above baseline (arrow). *C,* Sound spectral analysis of ipsilateral ECA showing elevation of late diastolic frequencies above baseline (arrow). The ECA is acting as a collateral pathway around the tight ICA stenosis.

Figure 6–14. Greater than 95% diameter reduction stenosis. Sound spectral analysis of an extremely tight internal carotid artery (ICA) stenosis shown in adjacent angiogram (arrow). White arrow *1* points to a region of low-amplitude, high-frequency scintillations forming a ghost waveform superimposed above a waveform containing high-amplitude scintillations with lower Doppler shift frequencies as shown by white arrow *2*. ECA = External carotid artery; CCA = common carotid artery.

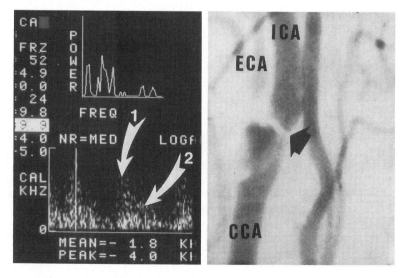

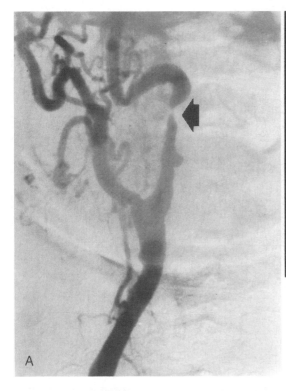

A

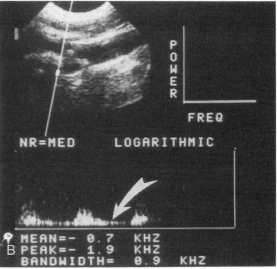

Figure 6–15. Greater than 95% diameter reduction stenosis. *A,* Angiogram of tight ICA stenosis (arrow) located high above the carotid bifurcation. *B,* Sound spectral analysis of ICA of carotid bifurcation shows decreased systolic peak frequency of 1.9 kHz and decreased late diastolic frequencies (arrow) close to baseline.

or mistaking a severe stenosis for an occlusion. External carotid artery collateral blood flow manifested by a reversal of the blood flow in the supraorbital arteries may occur either in severe stenoses or in occlusion and is, therefore, not useful in distinguishing the two. A reversal of the periorbital blood flow in the supraorbital arteries may be useful in indicating the presence of a tight stenosis when the sound spectral analysis shows a ghost waveform caused by low-amplitude scintillations, as demonstrated in Figure 6–14. Under these circumstances, the combination of a reversed periorbital blood flow and a low-velocity CCA waveform with diminished or absent late diastolic Doppler shift frequencies should arouse the suspicion that a tight stenosis is present in the ICA.

Summary

There are potential sources of error in the duplex scanning of carotid bifurcations for stenoses:

1. Anatomical configuration prohibits evaluation of the carotid bifurcation. Wetzner and associates reported that 3% of their patients could not be completely evaluated because of this problem.[6] In these patients, the bifurcation

or the stenosis may lie above the angle of the mandible or may be too deep for adequate visualization or the neck may be too short for proper placement of the transducer. Indirect tests, such as the detection of a reversed blood flow in the periorbital vessels with the bi-directional Doppler probe, can be useful in the evaluation of ICA stenoses and occlusions under these circumstances.

2. Acoustical shadowing secondary to calcification of the lumen walls limits visualization of the true vascular lumen. Figure 6–16 demonstrates how manipulating the duplex scanning probe can aid in preventing this problem.

3. Hypoechoic intraluminal lesions, such as fresh clot occlusions, may be difficult to differentiate from a normal, patent vascular lumen by real-time ultrasound imaging alone.

4. Low-amplitude, high-velocity sound spectral analysis scintillations not seen on the television screen may cause a tight stenosis to be misinterpreted as one of lesser severity.

5. Differentiating a tight stenosis from a complete occlusion—the diminished antegrade flow that results from a stenosis with a greater than 95% reduction in diameter—may be beyond the detection limits of the Doppler transducer. A tight stenosis and complete occlusion are both associated with abnormally damped common ca-

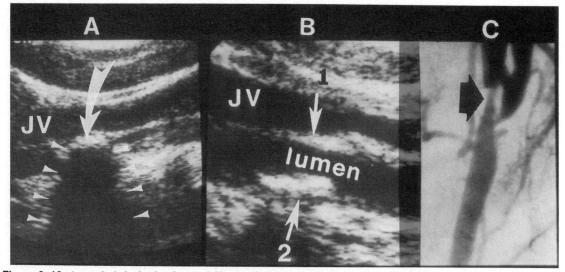

Figure 6–16. Acoustical shadowing from calcification limiting visualization of vascular lumen.

A, Acoustical shadowing from anterior wall calcified plaque (arrow) obscures lumen and posterior wall plaque. Arrowheads outline acoustical shadowing caused by calcified plaque. JV = Jugular vein.

B, A change in probe position detects both anterior and posterior wall plaques (arrows) on both sides of ICA lumen. *1,* Anterior wall plaque. *2,* Posterior wall plaque. JV = Jugular vein.

C, Angiogram of stenosis caused by plaques (arrow).

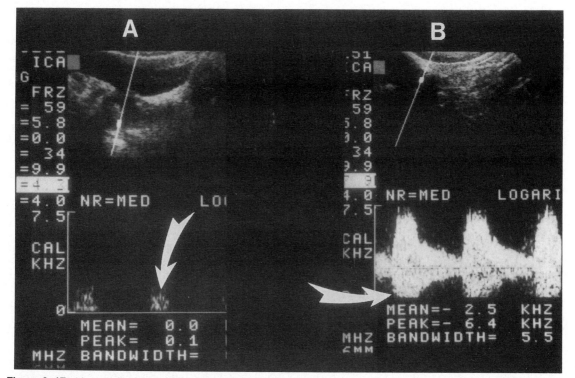

Figure 6–17. Abnormally damped ICA sound spectral analysis waveform.

A, Damped ICA waveform (arrow) proximal to a tight stenosis. It is characterized by a low systolic peak frequency and absence of diastolic Doppler frequency shifts.

B, Tight ICA stenosis causing "aliasing." Aliasing refers to the inability of some duplex scanning instruments to display the entire Doppler shift frequencies above the baseline because they exceed the kHz calibration scale. Instead, the higher frequencies are flipped below the baseline to produce an aliasing waveform (arrow). Most duplex scanners now allow for a recalibration so that the entire waveform may be examined above the baseline for precise measurements of their systolic peak frequencies.

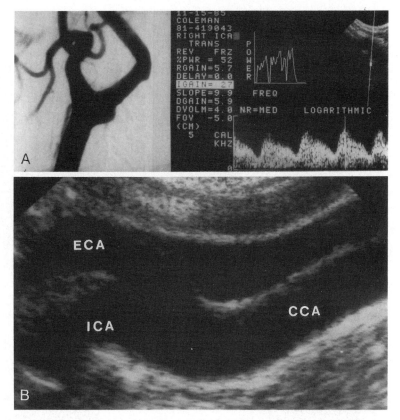

Figure 6–18. Tortuous internal carotid artery (ICA) causing bizarre sound spectral analysis waveform pattern. *A,* Angiogram of ulceration plaque in a tortuous ICA without a >50% diameter reduction stenosis. Sound spectral analysis waveform pattern compatible with >50% ICA diameter reduction stenosis. *B,* B-mode image of tortuous carotid bifurcation. ECA = External carotid artery; CCA = common carotid artery.

rotid artery waveforms as well as diminished wall pulsations, as observed on real-time B-mode scanning. Consequently, Wetzner and associates have recommended that angiography be performed in these circumstances, because ultrasonic evaluation cannot, as yet, consistently discriminate between the two conditions.[6]

6. An error may arise by misinterpreting the source of a damped ICA or CCA waveform as occurring proximal to a total occlusion rather than a tight stenosis. An example of a damped ICA waveform is shown in Figure 6–17A. Because this type of waveform is produced proximal to a high-resistance lesion, the vessel must be carefully examined to rule out a tight stenosis as was done in Figure 6–17B. A careful examination in this case showed a high-velocity waveform produced from a tight stenosis located above and more distal to the damped waveform produced from the proximal ICA (Fig. 6–17B).

7. Turbulence does not always mean that the vessel being examined is diseased; such turbulence may be either induced by technical factors or found in the normal carotid bulb.

8. Tortuous vessels may be difficult to evaluate by sound spectral analysis because they can produce bizarre waveform patterns. The sound spectral analysis waveform in Figure 6–18 shows turbulence and an elevation of both the systolic

and diastolic Doppler shift frequencies, indicating a tight ICA stenosis. However, only an ulcerative plaque in a tortuous ICA was seen on the angiogram, which demonstrated no evidence of a tight stenosis (Fig. 6–18). The B-mode image of this carotid bifurcation (Fig. 6–18) shows tortuosity of the extracranial carotid vessels. An increase in the Doppler shift frequencies may result from the tortuosity in the angle between the transmitted sound beam and the blood flow direction in the ICA. As shown in Figure 1–8, the Doppler shift frequencies increase as this angle increases and decrease as this angle decreases.

Turbulence and increased Doppler shift frequencies in non-tortuous vessels do not always indicate the presence of a stenosis caused by atherosclerotic plaque disease. For instance, an example of an ICA dissection causing a stenosis is shown in Figure 6–19. This stenosis produced both turbulence and an elevation in the systolic Doppler shift frequencies on the sound spectral analysis examination. The B-mode ICA image was used to determine that the cause of the stenosis was a result of dissection rather than an atherosclerotic plaque.

The accuracy of duplex ultrasound in the detection of hemodynamically significant stenosis is shown in Table 6–2.

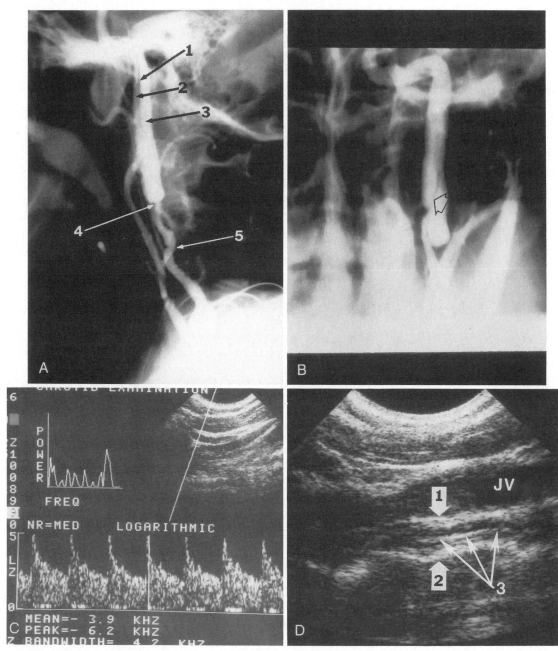

Figure 6–19. ICA dissection.

A, Lateral selective common carotid arteriogram. *1*, Intimal flap between true and false ICA lumen. *2*, True lumen. *3*, False lumen. *4*, ICA stenosis. *5*, Fibromuscular dysplastic ICA.

B, Anteroposterior view of ICA showing intimal flap (arrow).

C, Sound spectral analysis of blood flow through stenosis showing turbulence and 6.2 kHz systolic peak frequency.

D, B-mode image of ICA dissection. *1*, Anterior ICA wall. *2*, Posterior ICA wall. *3*, Intimal flap. JV = Jugular vein.

Table 6–2. Accuracy of Duplex Ultrasound in Detecting Hemodynamically Significant Stenosis (<50% Diameter Reduction)

Year	Investigator	Sensitivity	Specificity	Positive Predictive Value	Negative Predictive Value	Accuracy
1979	Blackshear et al. [7]	92% (24/26)	100% (8/8)	100% (24/24)	80% (8/10)	94% (32/34)
1981	Fell et al.[8]	100% (149/149)	57% (4/7)	98% (149/152)	100% (4/4)	98% (153/156)
1981	Clark and Hatten[9]	94% (63/67)	90% (75/83)	89% (63/71)	95% (75/79)	92% (138/150)
1982	Zbornikova et al.[10]	100% (24/24)	99% (75/76)	96% (24/25)	100% (75/75)	99% (99/100)
1982	Ackerstaff et al.[11]	100% (69/69)	13% (2/15)	84% (69/82)	100% (2/2)	85% (71/84)
1982	Chan et al.[12]	100% (139/139)	84% (47/56)	94% (139/148)	100% (47/47)	95% (185/195)
1982	Breslau et al.[13]	100% (79/79)	8% (1/12)	88% (79/90)	100% (1/1)	88% (80/91)
1982	Breslau et al.[13]	100% (33/33)	50% (4/8)	89% (33/37)	100% (4/4)	90% (37/41)
1982	Keagy et al.[14]	85% (82/97)	95% (130/137)	92% (82/89)	90% (130/145)	91% (212/234)
1982	Blasberg[15]	94% (32/34)	97% (65/67)	94% (32/34)	97% (65/67)	96% (97/101)
1983	Matsumoto and Rumwell[16]	93% (67/72)	90% (98/109)	86% (67/78)	95% (98/103)	91% (165/181)
1983	Garth et al.[17]	95% (39/41)	64% (28/44)	71% (39/55)	93% (28/30)	79% (67/85)
1983	Daigle et al.[18]	100% (30/30)	99% (96/97)	97% (30/31)	100% (95/96)	99% (126/127)
1983	Eikelboom et al.[19]	100% (60/60)	21% (3/14)	85% (60/71)	100% (3/3)	85% (63/74)
1984	Cardullo et al.[20]	99% (104/105)	81% (26/32)	95% (104/110)	96% (26/27)	95% (130/137)
1984	Glover et al.[21]	98% (40/41)	57% (12/21)	82% (40/49)	92% (12/13)	84% (52/62)
1985	Jacobs et al.[22]	96% (45/47)	90% (81/90)	83% (45/54)	98% (81/83)	92% (126/137)
1985	Flanigan et al.[23]	60% (21/35)	89% (108/122)	60% (21/35)	89% (108/122)	82% (129/157)
Total		96% (1100/1148)	86% (863/998)	89% (1100/1235)	94% (863/911)	91% (1963/2146)

References

1. Roederer GO, Langlois YE, Chan AR, et al. Ultrasonic duplex scanning of extra-cranial carotid arteries: improved accuracy using new features from the common carotid artery. J Cardiovasc Ultrasonography 1982; 1:373–380.
2. Fell G, Phillips DJ, Chikos PM, Harley JD, Thick BL, Strandness DE Jr. Ultrasound duplex scanning for disease of the carotid artery. Circulation 1981; 64:1191–1195.
3. Atkinson P, Woodcock JP. Doppler imaging of the extracranial cerebral arteries. *In* Doppler ultrasound and its use in clinical measurement. New York, Academic Press, 1982: 146–162.
4. Phillips DJ, Greene FM Jr, Langlois YE, Roederer GO, Strandness DE Jr. Flow velocity patterns in the carotid bifurcations of young, presumed normal subjects. Ultrasound Med Biol 1983; 9(1):39–49.
5. Fox JA, Hugh AE. Localization of atheroma: a theory based on boundary layer separation. Br Heart J 1966; 28:388–399.
6. Wetzner SM, Kiser LC, Bezreh JS. Duplex ultrasound imaging: vascular applications. Radiology 1984; 150:507–514.
7. Blackshear WM Jr, Phillips DJ, Thiele BL, et al. Detection of carotid occlusive disease by ultrasonic imaging and pulsed Doppler spectrum analysis. Surgery 1979; 86:698–706.
8. Fell G, Phillips DJ, Chikos PM, et al. Ultrasonic duplex scanning for disease of the carotid artery. Circulation 1981; 64(6):1191–1195.
9. Clark WM, Hatten HP. Noninvasive screening of extracranial carotid disease: Duplex sonography with angiographic correlation. AJNR 1981; 2:443–447.
10. Zbornikova V, Akesson JA, Lassvik C. Diagnosis of carotid artery disease—comparison between directional Doppler, duplex scanner and angiography. Acta Neurol Scand 1982; 65:335–346.
11. Ackerstaff RGA, Eikelboom BC, Hoeneveld H, et al. The accuracy of ultrasonic duplex scanning in carotid artery disease. Clin Neurol Neurosurg 1982; 84:213–220.
12. Chan A, Beach KW, Langlois Y, et al. Evaluation of extracranial carotid artery disease by ultrasonic duplex scanning: A clinical perspective. Aust NZ J Surg 1982; 52:562–569.
13. Breslau PJ, Knox RA, Phillips DJ, et al. Ultrasonic duplex scanning with spectral analysis in extracranial carotid artery disease: Comparison with arteriography. Vascular Diagnosis and Therapy 1982; 3:17–22.
14. Keagy BA, Pharr WF, Thomas D, et al. Comparison of oculoplethysmography/carotid phonoangiography with duplex scan/spectral analysis in the detection of carotid artery stenosis. Stroke 1982; 13(1):43–45.
15. Blasberg DJ. Duplex sonography for carotid artery disease: An accurate technique. AJNR 1982; 3:609–614.
16. Matsumoto GH, Rumwell CB. Screening of carotid arteries by noninvasive duplex scanning. Am J Surg 1983; 145:609–610.
17. Garth KE, Carroll BA, Sommer RG, et al. Duplex ultrasound scanning of the carotid arteries with velocity spectrum analysis. Radiology 1983; 147:823–827.
18. Daigle RJ, Gardner M, Smazal SF, et al. Accuracy of duplex ultrasound scanning in the evaluation of carotid artery disease. Bruit 1983; 7(3):17–21.
19. Eikelboom BC, Ackerstaff RGA, Ludwig JW, et al. Digital video subtraction angiography and duplex scanning in assessment of carotid artery disease: Comparison with conventional angiography. Surgery 1983; 94:821–825.
20. Cardullo PA, Cutler BS, Wheeler HB, et al. Accuracy of duplex scanning in the detection of carotid artery disease. Bruit 1984; 8:181–186.
21. Glover JL, Bendick PJ, Jackson VP, et al. Duplex ultrasonography, digital subtraction angiography, and conventional angiography in assessing carotid atherosclerosis. Arch Surg 1984; 119:664–669.
22. Jacobs NM, Grant EG, Schellinger D, et al. Duplex carotid sonography: Criteria for stenosis, accuracy, pitfalls. Radiology 1985; 154:385–391.
23. Flanigan DP, Schuler JJ, Vogel M, et al. The role of carotid duplex scanning in surgical decision making. J Vasc Surg 1985; 2(1):15–25.

7 • Duplex Scanning of Total Extracranial

Carotid Artery Occlusions

Introduction

This chapter provides a pictorial atlas of the B-mode freeze-frame images and sound spectral analysis waveform patterns of extracranial carotid artery occlusions. The B-mode images were obtained with a 10 MHz transducer; the sound spectral analysis waveforms were obtained with a 4.5 MHz pulsed Doppler signal angled 30 to 60° to the blood flow in the vessel lumen. For ease of comparison, the waveforms of each vessel are arranged around a line drawing showing the occlusion site in the extracranial cerebrovascular circulation. The arterial anatomy of the line drawing is shown in Figure 7–1. Correlative angiograms are included to provide a better understanding of the arterial occlusions seen on the duplex scans.

Total Extracranial Internal Carotid Artery (ICA) Occlusion

Figure 7–2 shows how high-resistance common carotid artery (CCA) velocity waveform patterns may be used to detect an ICA occlusion. Normally, the CCA has diastolic Doppler shift frequencies well above the zero baseline level because of the run-off of blood flow into the low-resistance vascular bed of the brain. An ICA occlusion converts this into an abnormal high-resistance/low-volume blood flow pattern characterized by a decrease in the blood flow velocity during systole, early diastole, and late diastole. This decrease in velocity reduces the Doppler shift frequencies and progressively lowers the amplitudes of waveforms during both systole and diastole as the blood flow in the CCA approaches the high resistance created by the occlusion site (Fig. 7–2). The CCA resistivity index (RI) is also increased. An RI of 0.92 was obtained from points A and B on the lower CCA waveform (Fig. 7–2).

The ICA occlusion shown on the angiogram in Figure 7–2 appears as internal echoes obliterating the lumen on the sagittal B-mode image. This occlusion has increased the resistance to blood flow in the CCA, as denoted by the sharply spiked systolic peaks with diminished Doppler shift frequencies and depression of diastolic waveform segments towards the zero baseline. These changes can be appreciated by a visual inspection of each individual CCA waveform or by comparing the right and left CCA waveforms with each other. These changes may also be measured using the resistivity index described by Planiol and associates.

The RI is a dimensionless ratio of the difference between the systolic and end-diastolic amplitudes divided by the systolic amplitude. This ratio is independent of the Doppler angle and is derived by the formula

$$RI = \frac{A - B}{A}$$

where A = systolic amplitude and B = end-diastolic amplitude. Because it is dimensionless, the measurement for A and B may be made from the CCA waveform using a standard centimeter ruler. An RI of 0.92 was obtained from points A and B on the CCA waveform (Fig. 7–2). A normal ratio is less than 0.75. A ratio above this level indicates either an ICA stenosis caused by a >90% diameter reduction or a total ICA occlusion. A total absence of diastolic flow in the CCA would cause the RI to equal 1.0 (RI = A/A = 1.0). This represents an obvious abnormality, which is readily appreciated by visual inspection of the waveform proximal to the ICA occlusion in Figure 7–2. Note that as the blood in the CCA flows towards the zone of increased resistance created by the ICA occlusion site, its RI increases from 0.92 to 1.0. The sharply spiked systolic peaks are rounded and flattened out towards the zero baseline because the velocity

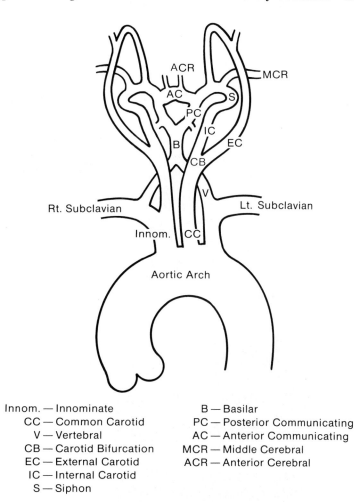

Figure 7–1. Artery nomenclature of line drawing.

Innom. — Innominate
CC — Common Carotid
V — Vertebral
CB — Carotid Bifurcation
EC — External Carotid
IC — Internal Carotid
S — Siphon

B — Basilar
PC — Posterior Communicating
AC — Anterior Communicating
MCR — Middle Cerebral
ACR — Anterior Cerebral

and Doppler shift frequencies also decrease as the CCA blood flow meets the resistance of the ICA occlusion site.

An unremarkable flow pattern is present in the external carotid artery (ECA) (Fig. 7–2). It normally has a sharply spiked systolic peak with late diastolic Doppler shift frequencies and a waveform segment that approaches the zero baseline level. The ECA is characterized by a high-resistance waveform pattern because it supplies the high-resistance vascular bed of the facial musculature. This pattern may change to one of low resistance when the ECA acts as a major collateral pathway around an ICA obstructing lesion. The fact that the ECA waveform pattern remains unchanged in Figure 7–2 is not unusual; generally, this means that the affected intracranial ICA is being compensated with blood flow through either the circle of Willis or the vertebrobasilar circulation or both. Under these circumstances, the normal high-resistance flow pattern is retained because the ECA is not required to func-

tion as a major collateral pathway around the obstructing lesion in the ICA. Whether or not the ECA is acting as a collateral pathway may be further evaluated by the periorbital Doppler examination.

Figure 7–3 shows how a comparison of the right and left CCA velocity waveforms is used to detect the ICA occlusion shown on the angiogram (Fig. 7–3A). This comparison was vital in this example because the ICA lumen was not obliterated by internal echoes on the B-mode image (Fig. 7–3B). The diastolic Doppler shift frequencies in the right CCA are well above the zero baseline level, indicating no increase in resistance to blood flow in this vessel. This is confirmed by the angiogram, which does not show a tight right ICA stenosis (Fig. 7–3A). Minimal spectral broadening exists because there are irregular plaque formations in the CCA, as shown on the angiogram. The diastolic Doppler shift frequencies in the left CCA approach the zero baseline level because there is increased

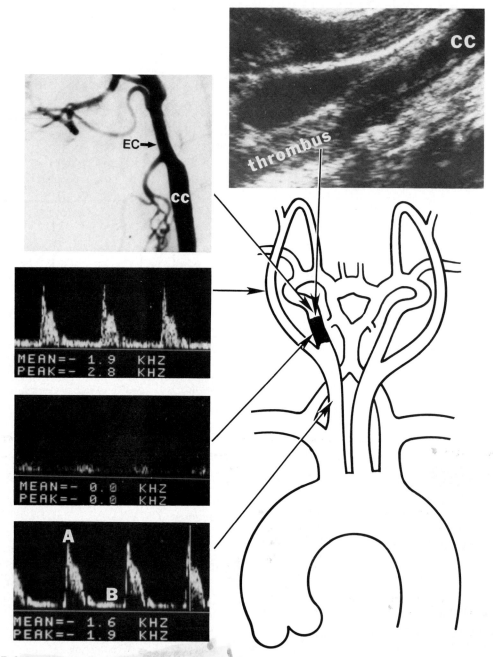

Figure 7–2. Internal carotid artery (ICA) occlusion on angiogram correlated with echogenic thrombus-obliterating lumen on B-mode image. High-resistance velocity waveforms in common carotid (CC) artery. Resistivity index (RI) increases from 0.92 to 1.0 as CCA blood flows towards ICA occlusion site. External carotid (EC) artery displays an unremarkable high-resistance flow waveform pattern. A = Systolic amplitude; B = end-diastolic amplitude.

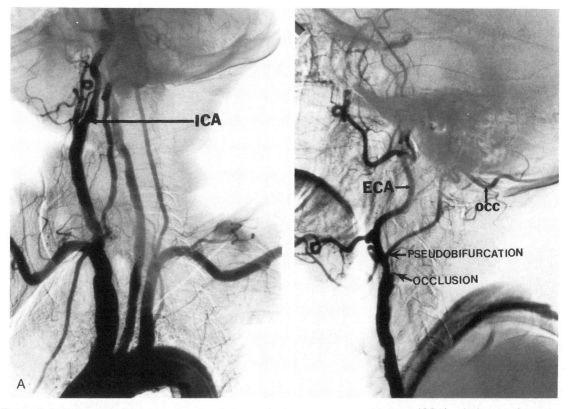

Figure 7–3. Illustration of how a comparison between the two common carotid artery (CCA) velocity waveforms may be used to detect internal carotid artery (ICA) occlusion. *A,* Nonhemodynamic significant right ICA stenosis and left ICA occlusion on angiogram. A left pseudobifurcation is formed by the occipital arterial branch (occ) of the external carotid artery (ECA).

Illustration continued on following page

resistance to blood flow in this vessel caused by the ICA occlusion.

The ECA velocity waveform is grossly abnormal in Figure 7–3*B* because it is acting as a major collateral pathway around the occlusion site. Normally, the ECA diastolic blood flow is low because of decreased run-off of blood into the high-resistance vascular bed of the facial musculature. This results in a low diastolic Doppler shift that approaches the zero baseline, as shown in Figure 7–2. However, this pattern changes when the ECA acts as a collateral pathway around an ICA obstruction. Under these circumstances, the peripheral arterioles in the terminal ECA branches dilate to allow more blood to flow into the low-resistance vascular bed of the intracranial vessels. This causes an elevation in the ECA diastolic Doppler shift frequencies, producing a waveform quite similar to that seen in either an ICA or CCA. Note the similarities between the right CCA and left ECA waveform in Figure 7–3*B.* Confusion between these two waveforms may be avoided by the periorbital Doppler ex-amination. A reversal of blood flow in either the ophthalmic or supraorbital arteries confirms that the ECA is acting as a major collateral pathway around the ICA obstruction, as shown in Figure 7–3*B.* Other examples of ICA occlusion are shown in Figures 7–4 through 7–7.

Total Occlusion of the Internal Carotid Artery with Contralateral Stenosis

Bilateral ICA obstructive lesions produce high-resistance velocity waveform patterns in both CCAs, as shown in Figure 7–8. A comparison of the CCA waveforms in this figure shows an absent late diastolic flow on the right and decreased diastolic flow on the left. The left CCA RI is 0.66. Even though a high-resistance velocity waveform pattern is present in both CCAs, it is more pronounced on the right than on the left. This indicates a more severe obstructive lesion in the right ICA than in the left ICA. The high-

Text continued on page 98

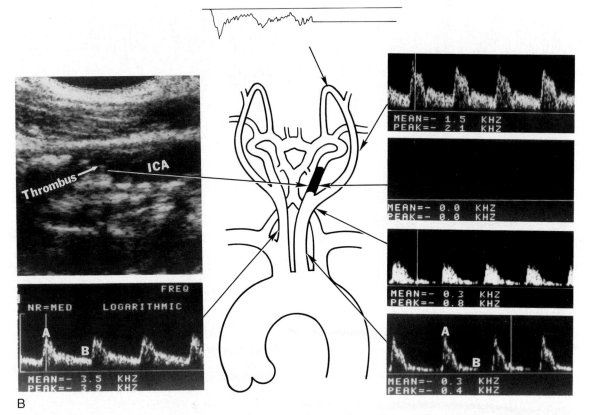

B

Figure 7–3 *Continued. B,* Comparison of low-resistance velocity waveform of right CCA with high-resistance velocity waveform of left CCA. Early and late diastolic waveform segments of left CCA depressed towards zero baseline level. Corresponding right CCA waveform segments not depressed towards zero baseline. Left CCA resistivity index (RI) = 0.9; right CCA (RI) = 0.6. Abnormal low-resistance ECA velocity waveform. Periorbital Doppler examination confirms reversed blood flow in ECA collateral pathway. Note how abnormal ECA waveform resembles normal right CCA waveform. Lumen obliterated by nonhomogeneous internal echoes on B-mode image of ICA occlusion site. A = Systolic amplitude; B = end-diastolic amplitude.

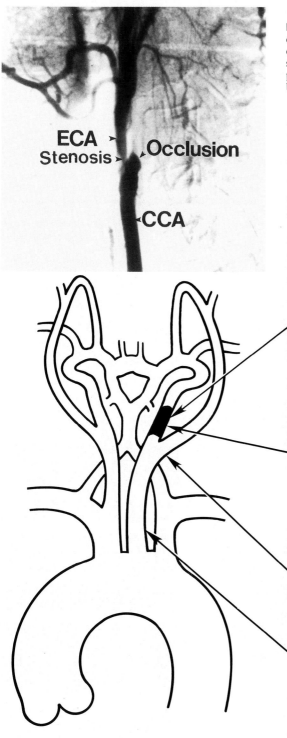

Figure 7–4. Internal carotid artery (ICA) occlusion and external carotid artery (ECA) stenosis. No intraluminal echoes on B-mode image and flow absent at occlusion site. Common carotid artery (CCA) high-resistance flow pattern; resistivity index increases from 0.8 to 1.0 as CCA blood flows towards the ICA occlusion site.

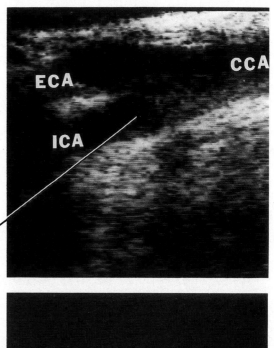

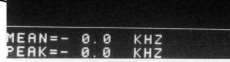

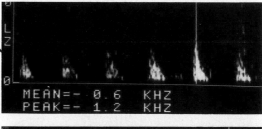

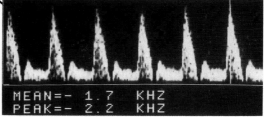

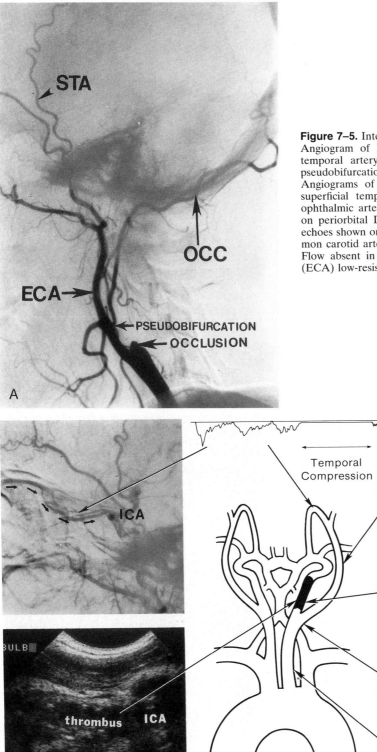

Figure 7–5. Internal carotid artery (ICA) occlusion. *A*, Angiogram of ICA occlusion. Note large superficial temporal artery collateral flow pathway (STA) and pseudobifurcation formed by occipital artery (OOC). *B*, Angiograms of reversed blood flow (arrows) in the superficial temporal artery through supraorbital and ophthalmic arteries into the intracranial ICA detected on periorbital Doppler examination. Soft intraluminal echoes shown on B-mode image of occlusion site. Common carotid artery (CCA) high-resistance flow pattern. Flow absent in occlusion site. External carotid artery (ECA) low-resistance flow pattern.

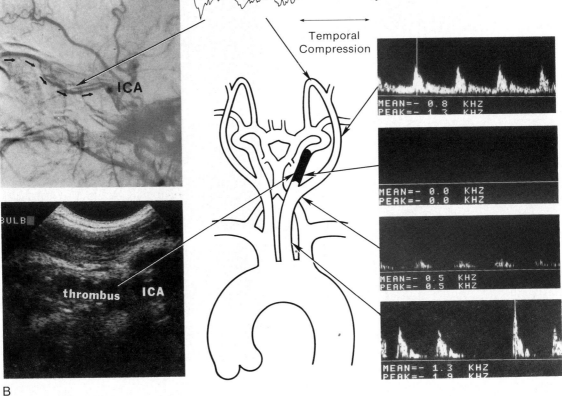

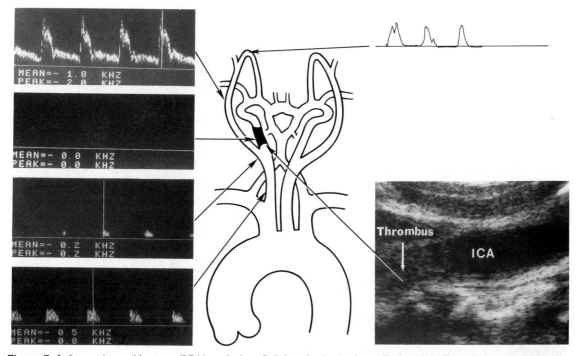

Figure 7–6. Internal carotid artery (ICA) occlusion. Soft intraluminal echoes displayed on B-mode image of occlusion site. Severe high-resistance flow pattern in common carotid artery (CCA). External carotid artery (ECA) low-resistance collateral velocity waveform simulating either ICA or CCA waveform. Positive compression test confirms potential ECA collateral pathway on periorbital Doppler examination even though the blood flow in the supraorbital artery is not reversed.

Figure 7–7. Internal carotid artery (ICA) occlusion. *A,* ICA occlusion with pseudobifurcation formed by enlarged external carotid artery (ECA) collateral arteries.

Illustration continued on following page

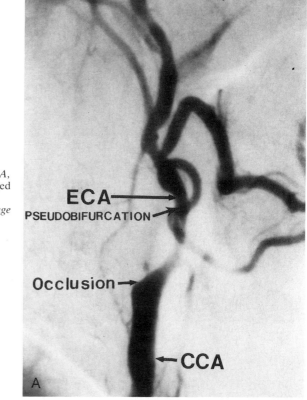

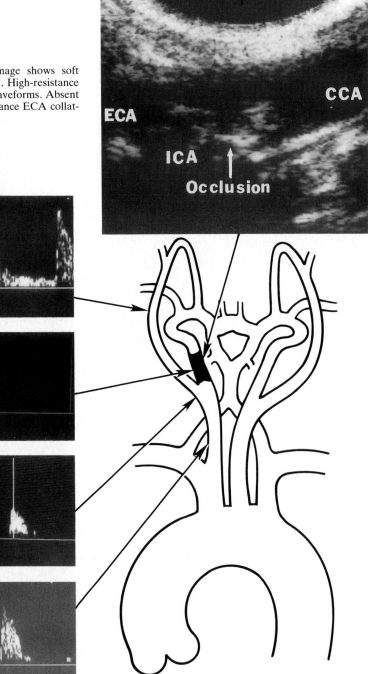

Figure 7–7 *Continued. B,* B-mode image shows soft intraluminal echoes at ICA occlusion site. High-resistance velocity common carotid artery (CCA) waveforms. Absent flow in occlusion site and mild low-resistance ECA collateral flow pattern.

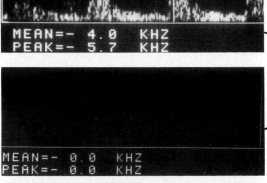

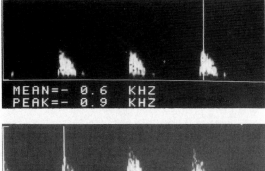

B

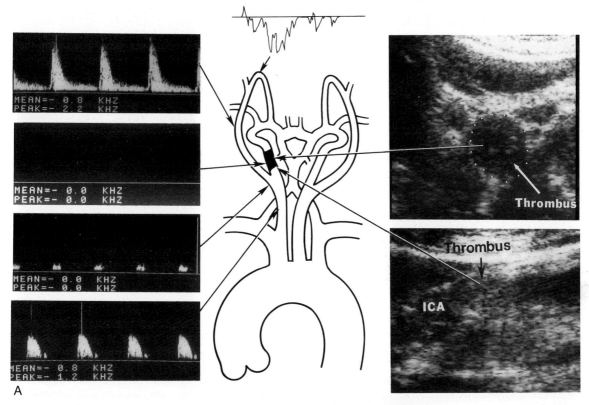

Figure 7–8. Total internal carotid artery (ICA) occlusion with contralateral ICA stenosis.

A, Right ICA occlusion with lumen obliterated by internal echoes on both cross-sectional and sagittal B-mode images. Common carotid artery (CCA) high-resistance flow patterns. Absent flow in occluded ICA segment. External carotid artery (ECA) low-resistance collateral flow pattern confirmed by reversed supraorbital blood flow on periorbital Doppler examination.

Illustration continued on following page

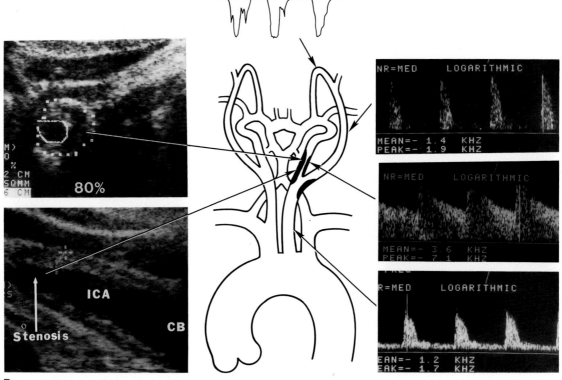

Figure 7–8 *Continued. B,* Left ICA stenosis. ICA cross-sectional B-mode image shows stenosis caused by heterogeneous plaque and 80% cross-sectional area reduction. Stenosis also seen on sagittal B-mode image. (+ − +) measures plaque thickness. High-velocity waveform with systolic peak frequency of 7.1 kHz obtained from the stenosis site seen on the B-mode image. Mild, low-resistance ECA flow pattern with reversal of supraorbital artery blood flow shown on periorbital Doppler examination. CB = Carotid bifurcation.

resistance flow pattern becomes even more pronounced as the transducer is moved towards the right ICA occlusion until there is no flow at all recorded in the right ICA. A B-mode image of the right ICA shows its lumen totally obliterated by internal echoes in both the cross-sectional and sagittal projections (Fig. 7–8A).

The duplex sonographic examination of the left ICA is shown in Figure 7–8B. It reveals a hemodynamically significant left ICA stenosis with systolic peak frequencies >7.1 kHz. The cross-sectional B-mode image at the site in the ICA where the maximum systolic peak frequency was obtained shows an 80% cross-sectional area reduction stenosis. The ICA stenosis is also seen on the sagittal B-mode image. Both ECAs are acting as collateral pathways around the obstructing lesions in the ICA, causing a reversal of the blood flow in both of the supraorbital arteries, as shown on the periorbital Doppler examination.

Middle Cerebral Artery Occlusion

An intracranial ICA occlusion may simulate an ICA occlusion at the carotid bifurcation on duplex sonography. An example is shown in Figure 7–9. Figure 7–9A shows a total occlusion of the right middle cerebral artery. A high-resistance velocity waveform is present in the right CCA. The RI in the proximal right CCA is 0.78. There is also a low-resistance/high blood flow waveform in the right ECA, which was confirmed as a collateral vessel on the periorbital Doppler examination. A left ICA stenosis is seen in this patient, as shown in Figure 7–9B. The stenosis measured less than a 50% diameter reduction on the angiogram, and an RI of 0.73 was present in the left CCA. A systolic peak frequency shift of 4.3 kHz was obtained at the stenosis site. The left ECA shows a low-resistance/high blood flow pattern.

The comparison of Figures 7–8 and 7–9 shows

Figure 7–9. Middle cerebral artery (MCA) occlusion. *A,* Angiogram of right middle cerebral artery occlusion. High, right common carotid artery (CCA) resistance flow pattern (resistivity index [RI] = 0.78), moderate, low-resistance right external carotid artery (ECA) flow pattern, and collateral flow seen on periorbital Doppler examination.

Illustration continued on following page

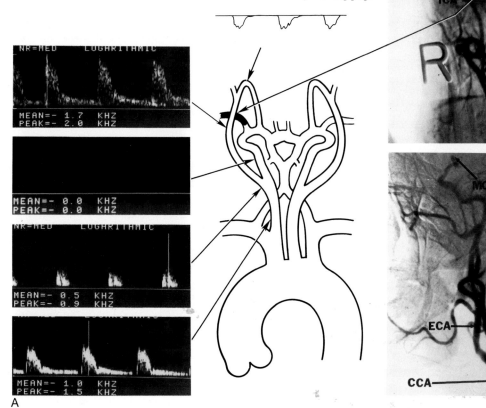

A

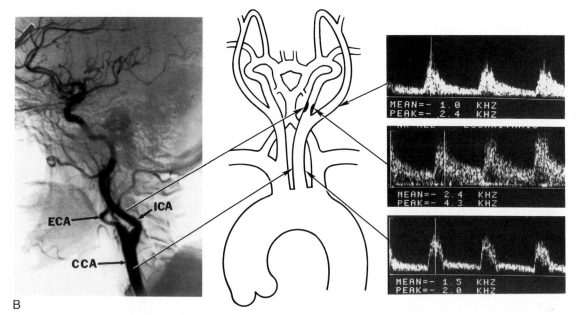

B

Figure 7–9 *Continued. B,* Stenosis causing less than 50% internal carotid artery (ICA) diameter reduction on angiogram. An RI of 0.73 in left CCA, systolic peak frequency shift of 4.3 kHz at stenosis site, and low-resistance collateral left ECA velocity waveform pattern were obtained.

how the middle cerebral artery occlusion mimics the cervical ICA occlusion on duplex sonography.

Total Common Carotid Artery Occlusions

Common carotid artery occlusion may produce duplex sonographic patterns that are quite different from those found with ICA occlusion. These patterns may also vary according to whether or not the ICA is occluded in addition to the CCA. To avoid this confusion, two types of CCA occlusion must be considered: Type I, ICA and CCA both occluded; and Type II, isolated CCA occlusion without ICA occlusion.

Type I Occlusion

An example of a Type I CCA occlusion is shown in Figure 7–10. The angiogram in Figure 7–10*A* shows no opacification of either the right CCA or ICA. Two large collateral pathways are shown bypassing the occlusions. They are formed from the right ECA and the vertebral arteries. In a Type I occlusion, the ECA can neither receive blood from the CCA nor supply blood to the ICA because its origin from the CCA is occluded. Blood flow through the ECA can then

flow in only one direction when it is acting as a major collateral pathway to the intracranial circulation. That direction is antegrade towards the brain through the periorbital and ophthalmic arteries into the intracranial ICA. Because the ECA cannot receive blood from the CCA, it must be filled with blood from the collateral vessels arising from the subclavian artery. These collateral vessels are generally supplied from the thyrocervical trunk, which arises from the subclavian artery. As shown in Figure 7–10*A*, the inferior thyroid branch of the thyrocervical trunk has enlarged and anastomosed with the superior thyroid artery to act as a collateral pathway to the right ECA. The arrows in Figure 7–10*A* indicate the blood flow direction through both the thyroid artery collaterals and ECA to the intracranial ICA.

There are circumstances that may cause a reversal of the blood flow from the intracranial ICA through the ECA and thyrocervical trunk collateral arteries to the subclavian artery. Of course, under these circumstances the ECA is no longer acting as a collateral pathway to supply the intracranial ICA with blood. Instead, it is stealing blood away from the intracranial ICA. This may occur when there is an occlusion of the innominate artery in addition to occlusions of the CCA and ICA. This is not a Type I CCA occlusion because the innominate artery is also

Figure 7–10. Type I common carotid artery (CCA) occlusion.
A, Angiogram shows both the right CCA and internal carotid artery (ICA) totally occluded. Dotted line denotes collateral pathway from right subclavian artery through the inferior and superior thyroid arteries to the external carotid artery (ECA). An enlarged right vertebral artery collateral pathway is also present. VERT = VERTEBRAL ARTERY.
B, Cross-sectional B-mode image of CCA showing intraluminal echoes. These extend into ICA on sagittal B-mode carotid bifurcation image. Blood flow absent in both CCA and ICA occluded segment. Low-resistance velocity waveforms in both the external carotid (EC) and vertebral arteries. Supraorbital blood flow, reversed on periorbital Doppler examination, confirmed by positive compression test. IJV = Internal jugular vein.

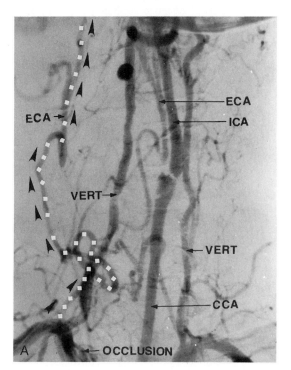

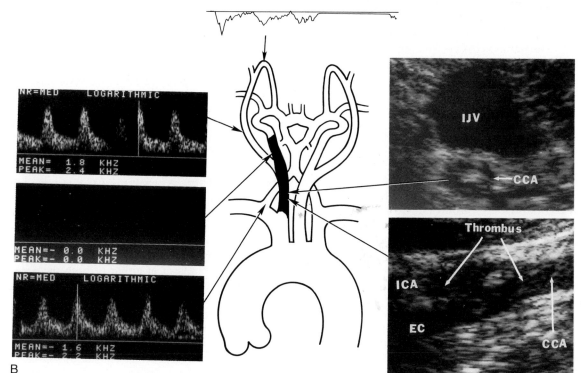

occluded. Instead, it represents an unusual form of innominate steal syndrome. This syndrome is described here because it may be encountered during the duplex sonographic examination of an occluded CCA. A systolic pressure difference >10 mm Hg between the two upper extremity brachial blood pressure measurements is used to distinguish a complicated innominate steal syndrome from a Type I CCA occlusion. Another finding that accompanies the innominate steal syndrome is a reversal of the blood flow direction in the right vertebral artery. This finding is also used to distinguish this unusual syndrome from a Type I CCA occlusion.

The duplex sonographic abnormalities of a Type I CCA occlusion are shown in Figure 7–10B. They are from the patient whose angiogram is shown in Figure 7–10A. The cross-sectional B-mode image shows an echogenic intraluminal CCA thrombus. A sagittal B-mode image of the carotid bifurcation again shows the CCA intraluminal echoes, but none are present in the ICA (Fig. 7–10B). An absence of blood flow Doppler shift frequencies from the ICA was used to detect the ICA occlusion in this case. A low-resistance velocity waveform exists in both the right ECA and the right vertebral artery, denoting that both of these vessels are acting as major collateral pathways around the Type I CCA occlusion. The periorbital Doppler examination also confirms the collateral pathway from the ECA through the supraorbital-ophthalmic system to the intracranial ICA.

Type II Occlusion

A line drawing illustrating the ECA blood flow pattern that may occur with a Type II CCA occlusion is shown in Figure 7–11. Because neither the ECA origin nor the ICA origin is occluded, the ECA may supply blood to the cervical ICA through the carotid bifurcation. The blood flow direction in the ECA is reversed as the blood flows in an antegrade manner around the carotid bifurcation into the ICA. The reversed ECA blood flow of the carotid bifurcation may appear to be in opposition to the reversal of the blood flow in the supraorbital-ophthalmic system on the periorbital Doppler examination. This confusion arises because the blood in the ECA is flowing in opposite directions at the same time and it is also unusual to find a reversal of the ECA blood flow at the carotid bifurcation. Figure 7–11 illustrates how this may occur with a Type II CCA occlusion. Only one potential collateral pathway is shown in this figure. There are, of course, many different collateral flow patterns that may exist with a Type II CCA occlusion. The flow pattern in Figure 7–11 shows collateral flow from the left ECA crossing over the forehead to anastomose with the right superficial temporal arterial branch of the right ECA. As the blood enters the superficial temporal artery, it flows in a reversed direction through the supraorbital and ophthalmic arteries into the intraluminal ICA. It also flows in a reversed direction down the superficial temporal artery to the carotid bifurcation to the cervical ICA.

Associated arterial obstructions that may potentiate these collateral pathways around a Type II CCA occlusion are shown by the dark-shaded areas in Figure 7–11. These lesions enhance the reversed ECA blood flow patterns because they further lower the pressure in the right intracranial ICA. For example, given a right Type II CCA occlusion, the pressure in the right intracranial ICA could be maintained by compensating blood flow from the left ICA through the anterior communicating artery into the right intracranial ICA. This compensating mechanism may be lost, however, when flow-limiting stenoses exist in the left ICA. These flow-limiting stenoses may occur in the left ICA at either the carotid bifurcation or carotid siphon (Fig. 7–11). A congenital absence of the anterior communicating artery can also prevent the blood flow from the left intracranial ICA from crossing over to the right intracranial ICA (Fig. 7–11).

The right intracranial ICA pressure may not drop even when these flow-limiting obstructions exist because the vertebrobasilar circulation is capable of supplying blood flow to the right intracranial ICA through the posterior communicating artery. The vertebrobasilar circulation becomes an important source of blood flow to the intracranial ICA when the CCA is occluded as shown in Figures 7–10 and 7–12. Unfortunately, it too may be lost when there are either flow-limiting stenoses at the vertebral artery origins or a congenital absence of the posterior communicating artery (Fig. 7–11). Because absence and hypoplasia of either or both the anterior and posterior communicating arteries are the most common anomalies of the circle of Willis, it is not unusual for these compensating collateral pathways to be absent with CCA occlusions. An absence of these collateral pathways traps the right intracranial ICA so that its major source of blood supply must come from the ECA (Fig. 7–11). When the right intracranial ICA is trapped by any of the combinations of flow-limiting lesions shown in Figure 7–11, the ECA blood flow of the carotid bifurcation should be reversed with Type II CCA occlusions. The ECA blood flow is not always reversed at the carotid bifurcation with Type II CCA occlusions because the associated flow-limiting lesions shown in Figure 7–11 may be absent.

In summary, the finding of a reversed blood flow in the ECA at the carotid bifurcation indicates a Type II CCA occlusion and an ipsilateral intracranial ICA that is not being fully compensated for by blood flow from the vertebrobasilar circulation and the contralateral ICA circulation. This reversed blood flow further indicates that the affected intracranial ICA is being compensated with blood flow from the ECA through the carotid bifurcation to the affected cervical ICA. Blood flow is then reversed in the affected ECA, but the blood flows in a normal direction through the affected ICA.

An angiographic demonstration of this phenomenon is shown in Figure 7–12. Because both vertebral arteries are patent and there is no hemodynamically significant stenosis in the right ICA, the lesions limiting flow to the left intracranial ICA were found to be hypoplastic communicating arteries. The brachiocephalic angiograms are shown to illustrate the hemodynamics of a Type II CCA occlusion that may be encountered on the duplex sonographic and periorbital Doppler examinations. These include (1) absent CCA

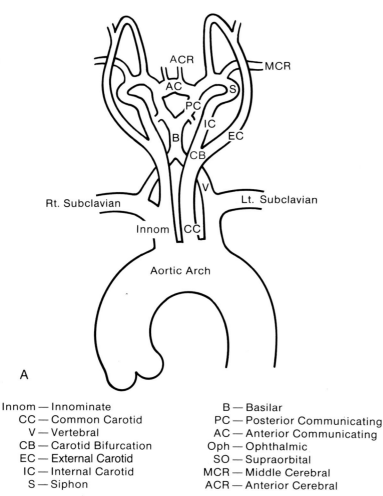

Innom — Innominate
CC — Common Carotid
V — Vertebral
CB — Carotid Bifurcation
EC — External Carotid
IC — Internal Carotid
S — Siphon

B — Basilar
PC — Posterior Communicating
AC — Anterior Communicating
Oph — Ophthalmic
SO — Supraorbital
MCR — Middle Cerebral
ACR — Anterior Cerebral

Figure 7–11. Line drawing of the blood flow hemodynamics of a Type II common carotid artery (CCA) occlusion. *A,* Nomenclature of arterial anatomy. *B,* Dark, shaded area in right CCA denotes occluded segment. Origins of both right ECA and ICA remain patent. Shaded areas in surrounding vessels denote sites of flow-limiting lesions, which trap the right intracranial ICA from collateral blood flow compensation. Arrows indicate blood flow direction from left ECA through the crossover forehead collateral anastomosing with right ECA. Note blood flow reversed in both supraorbital-ophthalmic systems and right ECA at the carotid bifurcation.

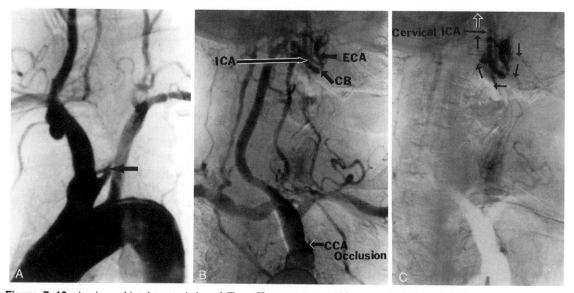

Figure 7–12. Angiographic characteristics of Type II common carotid artery (CCA) occlusion. *A,* Brachiocephalic angiogram: Right posterior oblique projection showing left CCA occlusion (arrow). *B,* Brachiocephalic angiogram: Left posterior oblique projection showing patent left carotid bifurcation (CB), external carotid artery (ECA) and internal carotid artery (ICA). *C,* Delayed brachiocephalic angiogram showing reversed collateral blood flow in ECA passing across the carotid bifurcation to flow in a normal direction through the cervical ICA (arrows).

Doppler shift frequencies, (2) reversed blood flow in the affected ECA at the carotid bifurcation, (3) bilateral reversed blood flow in the supraorbital-ophthalmic systems, and (4) blood flow in a normal antegrade direction through the affected ICA (Fig. 7–13).

Carotid Bifurcation Thrombosis

Obstruction of the ICA may be caused by abnormalities other than atherosclerosis. An example of an embolus partially occluding the ICA is shown in Figure 7–14. The high-resistance CCA velocity waveform pattern and B-mode images were used to identify the embolus. A follow-up B-mode image showed partial resolution of the carotid bifurcation embolus.

Limitations of Duplex Sonography

Some problems in the diagnosis of extracranial carotid artery occlusions include the following.

Pseudocarotid Bifurcation. Failure to recognize the true carotid bifurcation on B-mode imaging is a common source of error in the detection of carotid occlusions by duplex sonography.[2] This failure results when enlarged ECA collateral branches forming a pseudobifurcation are mis-

taken for the true carotid bifurcation. Several examples of pseudobifurcations are shown in the figures throughout this section and illustrate how readily these mimic true carotid bifurcations. The problem is further complicated by the fact that the true carotid bifurcation has numerous anatomical configurations[3] and its position in relation to the angle of the mandible varies considerably from patient to patient. The Doppler shift frequencies from pseudobifurcations cannot be relied on to differentiate them from true bifurcations. As shown in the figures, the Doppler shift frequencies from enlarged collateral ECA branches may be identical to those found in either the ICA or CCA.

Absence of Internal Echoes. Absence of internal echoes obliterating the vessel lumen on B-mode image may cause a totally occluded vessel to be misinterpreted as patent. As shown in the figures, there will be many cases in which the artery is totally occluded and the internal echoes do not obliterate the lumen on the B-mode image. The occlusion may be caused by fresh clot and hemorrhage, lying beneath fibrofatty plaques, that have echogenic properties identical to those of flowing blood.

A B-mode image of the occluded vessel segment will contain either low-level echoes or no echoes under these circumstances. Indeed, when the lumen is totally obliterated by internal echoes on both cross-sectional and sagittal B-mode images, occlusion is indicated.[4] Nonvisualization of an artery by B-mode imaging in a patient with a thin neck is also a useful index of total vessel occlusion: the inflammatory response surrounding the occluded vessel causes it to blend in with tissues of the neck. The occluded vessel is not seen because it cannot be distinguished from the surrounding inflamed tissues on the B-mode image.

The problems associated with pseudobifurcation and absence of intraluminal echoes may be solved by a close evaluation of the high-resistance CCA velocity waveform pattern, and an elevated RI above 0.75 should alert the examiner that an obstructive lesion exists somewhere in the ICA, even when it is not seen on the B-mode image. The reversal of the blood flow in the supraorbital-ophthalmic system on the periorbital Doppler examination and the failure to identify the normal, high-resistance ECA velocity waveform in either the pseudobifurcation or true carotid bifurcation vessels should also alert the examiner

that collaterals have formed around an obstructive lesion somewhere in the ICA. A search can then be made to identify the absent Doppler shift frequencies from the occluded arterial segment, even though it does not contain any intraluminal echoes on the B-mode image.

Complex Collateral Flow Patterns. Complex collateral flow patterns are confusing and often lead to a misidentification of the underlying obstructive vascular disease process. In order to overcome this dilemma, one must become a student of the numerous potential collateral pathways that develop around occlusion sites. The Type I and Type II classification of CCA occlusions is admittedly an oversimplification of the complex collaterals that may form around these obstructive lesions. However, it does serve to illustrate the concepts one must learn in order to understand what the collateral flow patterns mean on the duplex sonographic examination.

High-Resistance CCA Waveforms. High-resistance CCA waveforms may be present in the

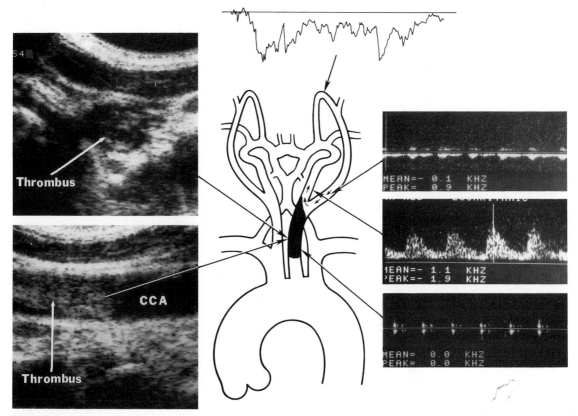

Figure 7–13. Type II common carotid artery (CCA) occlusion. Duplex scan shows bi-directional flow in the external carotid artery, which is predominantly in a reversed direction (arrows) as is noted by negative waveform deflection below the zero baseline. CCA "thump" pattern due to movement of thrombus during systole. Internal carotid artery blood flow is in normal direction. Intraluminal echoes, shown in CCA on both cross-sectional and sagittal B-mode images. Reversed left supraorbital blood flow shown on periorbital Doppler examination.

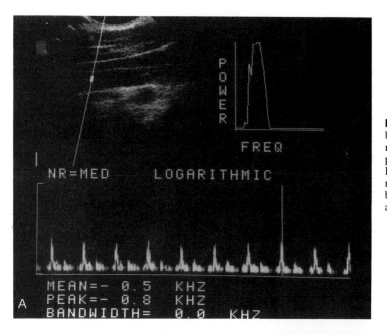

Figure 7–14. Carotid bifurcation embolus. *A,* High-resistance common carotid artery (CCA) velocity waveform pattern. *B,* Sagittal and cross-sectional B-mode images show reduction of internal carotid artery (ICA) lumen by embolus (arrows). ECA = External carotid artery.

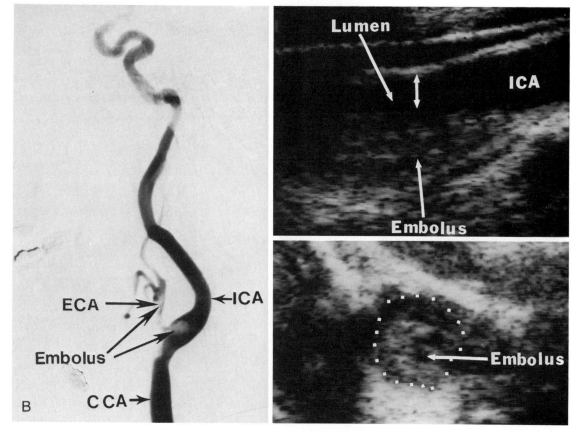

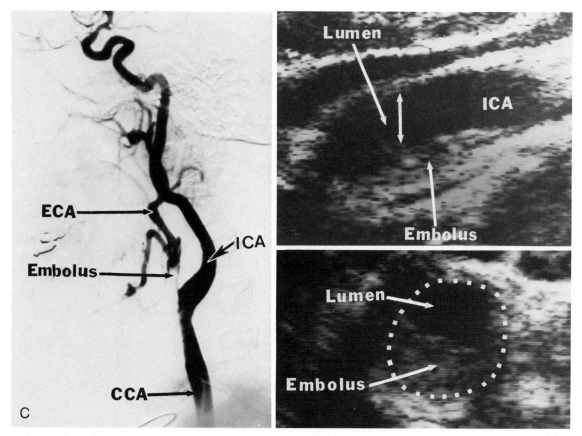

Figure 7–14 *Continued. C,* Six-week follow-up B-mode image shows partial resolution of carotid bifurcation embolus. Note increase in sagittal lumen diameter (arrows).

absence of ICA obstructive disease. Patients with hypertension or tachycardia may demonstrate elevated systolic peaks, whereas those with low cardiac states may have an absence of CCA diastolic blood flow.

Two limitations exist for which there are no readily available solutions: (1) velocity waveform distortions may be caused by dense plaque deposits that attenuate the ultrasound beam[5] and (2) a tight stenosis may be misinterpreted for a total occlusion.[6]

An example of a diseased vessel wall attenuating the sonographic beam is shown in Figure 7–15. The angiograms in Figure 7–15A show the severity of the atherosclerotic disease in the brachiocephalic vessels. Of considerable importance is the effect of the disease in the right CCA wall on the velocity waveform obtained from this vessel. A comparison of the two CCA velocity waveforms in Figure 7–15C shows a definite high-resistance flow pattern in the left CCA, but the right CCA velocity waveform appears to be damped. There is depression of the diastolic segments towards the zero baseline level, and the

systolic peak is blunted, producing a peak systolic Doppler shift frequency of only 1.0 kHz. This waveform is certainly misleading because it is compatible with an obstructive lesion located at the origin of either the innominate artery or the right CCA. However, not one of these lesions is present on the angiogram (Fig. 7–15A). The flat systolic peak also results in a CCA resistivity index of 0.50, which is also misleading because both an ECA stenosis and an 84% cross-sectional ICA reduction stenosis are seen on the angiogram in Figure 7–15A and the B-mode image in Figure 7–15B. These stenoses are not tight enough to produce a CCA RI greater than 0.75, but they are significant enough to cause a high-resistance CCA flow pattern similar to the one shown in Figure 7–8B. Placement of the pulsed Doppler probe sample volume close to the CCA wall offers one explanation of the absence of a high-resistance flow pattern in this vessel.

It is known that the velocity of the blood flow adjacent to the vessel wall is considerably slower than that in the midlumen region. Placement of the sample volume adjacent to the vessel wall

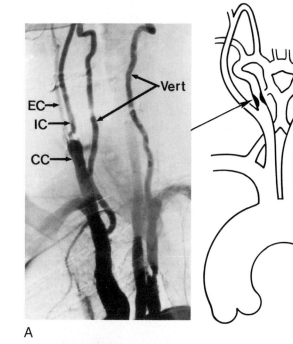

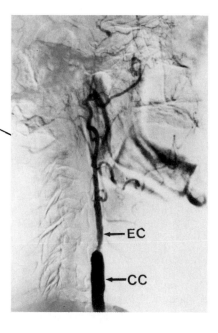

A

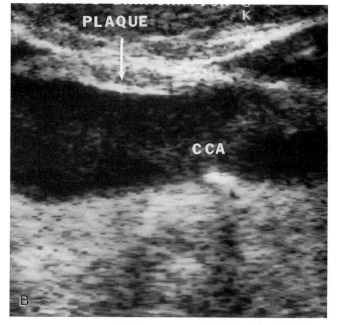

Figure 7–15. Sonographic beam attenuation caused by diseased vessel wall.

A, Brachiocephalic angiogram shows severely diseased common carotid (CC) artery and non-obstructed innominate artery. Stenoses are present in the right internal carotid (IC) artery, external carotid (EC) artery, bilateral vertebral (Vert) arteries, and left subclavian artery origin. Left selective CCA angiogram shows ICA occlusion and ECA origin stenosis. Note slow velocity flow in the left CCA on the brachiocephalic angiogram caused by the increased resistance of the ICA and ECA obstructive lesions.

B, Right sagittal B-mode image of dense CCA wall plaque causing attenuation of waveform from CCA.

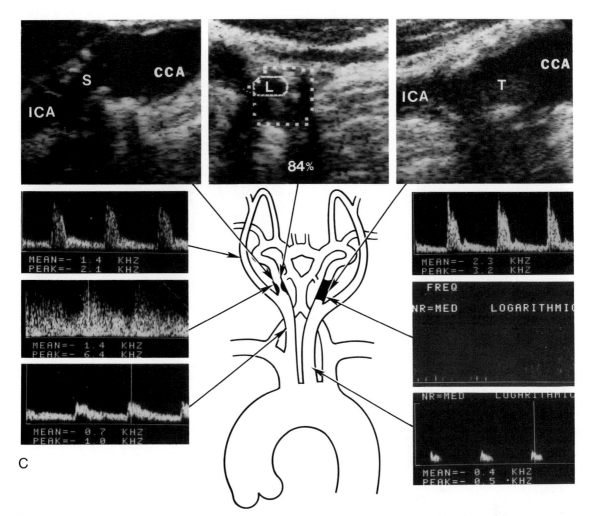

Figure 7–15 *Continued. C,* Right ICA stenosis causing cross-sectional area reduction of 84% on B-mode image and resulting in ICA systolic peak frequency shift of 6.4 kHz. Left ICA B-mode image of low-level echoes in occluding thrombus (T). High-resistance flow pattern in left CCA.

will result in low systolic velocity Doppler shift frequencies. However, this was not the problem in this particular case. The sagittal B-mode image of the CCA shows dense atherosclerotic plaque formation in the vessel wall (Fig. 7–15C). This plaque may attenuate the ultrasound beam and produce the confusing CCA waveform pattern seen in Figure 7–15C. When sampling the CCA for high-resistance waveform patterns and resistivity index analysis, use that portion of the vessel wall with minimal plaque deposits, if at all possible, to avoid this potential problem.

The misinterpretation of a tight stenosis for a total occlusion is one of the most serious problems confronting duplex sonography in the evaluation of the cerebrovascular circulation. An example of this problem is shown in Figure 7–16. The high-resistance CCA waveform pattern

indicates ICA obstructive disease. There is minimal flow detected in the ICA, and the systolic peak Doppler frequency shift is only 0.6 kHz. Whether or not the ICA obstructing lesion is either a tight stenosis or a total occlusion cannot be determined by the duplex sonographic findings in this case. A review of all the previously described abnormalities found on duplex sonography explains why this distinction remains beyond the scope of currently available techniques:

1. The *CCA resistivity index* will be abnormal (>0.75) in both >90% diameter reduction stenoses and total occlusions.

2. *High-resistance CCA velocity waveforms* will be abnormal (sharp systolic peaks with diastolic waveform segments depressed towards the zero baseline) in both >90% diameter reduction stenoses and total occlusions.

Figure 7–16. Example of how a tight stenosis may be misinterpreted as a total occlusion. Angiogram shows a tight internal carotid artery (ICA) stenosis containing low-level echoes on sagittal B-mode image. High-velocity waveform absent at ICA stenosis site. High-resistance common carotid artery (CCA) waveform is present. Mild external carotid artery low-resistance collateral blood flow pattern is also present.

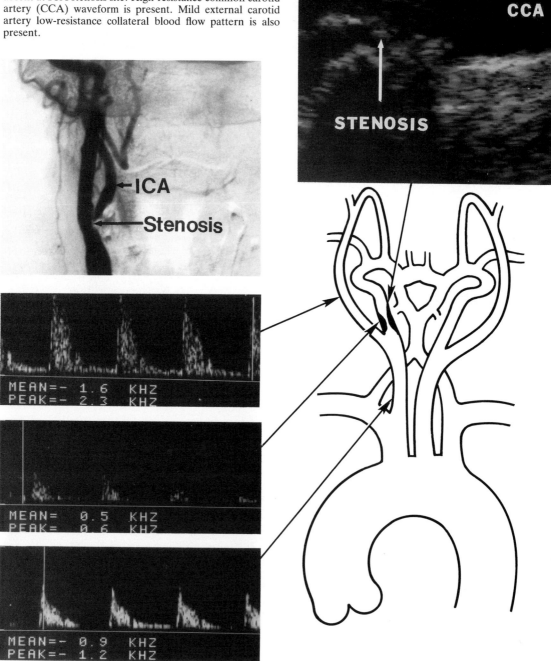

3. *B-mode image* lumen echoes may be absent when either tight stenoses or total occlusions occur.

4. *Low-resistance ECA velocity waveforms* may be absent when either tight stenoses or total occlusions occur because of the presence of other collateral pathways that are available through both the circle of Willis and the vertebrobasilar circulation. The periorbital Doppler examination may also be normal for the same reasons.

5. *Doppler shift frequencies* may be absent in both tight stenoses and total occlusions. The flow velocity in the residual lumen of a tight stenosis is too sluggish to yield a Doppler signal, which can distinguish it from a total occlusion.

6. *Real-time images of vessel pulsations* may be seen when the artery expands during systole and contracts during diastole. Vessel wall movements at right angles to the longitudinal axis are termed radial pulsations; those parallel to this axis are termed longitudinal pulsations. Neither of these has proved to be of major diagnostic use.

The tight stenosis remains the "Achilles heel" of cerebrovascular duplex sonographic examinations. Its significance is further intensified by the fact that a tight stenosis (Fig. 7–16) is a potentially correctable lesion whereas a total occlusion may only be corrected in selected cases.[7] Until this limitation can be resolved, arteriography will have to be used to distinguish between a tight stenosis and a total occlusion, even when a vessel is believed to be completely obstructed on the duplex sonographic examination.

References

1. Planiol T, Pourcelot L, Pottier JM, et al. Etude de la circulation carotidienne par les méthodes ultrasoniques et la thermographie. Rev Neurol (Paris) 1972; 126:127–141.
2. Zwiebel WJ, Crummy AB. Sources of error in Doppler diagnosis of carotid occlusive disease. AJR 1981; 137:1–12.
3. Prendes JL, McKinney WM, Buonanno FS, Jones AM. Anatomic variations of the carotid bifurcation affecting Doppler scan interpretation. JCU 1980; 8:147–150.
4. Gresham GE, Fitzpatrick TE, Wolf PA, McNamara PM, et al. Residual disability in survivors of stroke—the Framingham study. N Engl J Med 1975; 293:954–956.
5. Shung KK, Fei DY, Bronez MA. Effects of atherosclerotic lesions on ultrasonic beam and CW Doppler signals. JCU 1985; 13:11–18.
6. Spencer MP. Hemodynamics of carotid artery stenosis. *In* Spencer MP, Reid JM (eds). Cerebrovascular evaluation with Doppler ultrasound. The Hague, Martinus Nijhoff, 1980:113–131.
7. Hafner CD, Tew JM. Surgical management of the totally occluded internal carotid artery: a 10-year study. Surgery 1981; 89:710–717.

8 • The Periorbital Doppler Examination

Introduction

The periorbital Doppler examination is used to detect external carotid artery (ECA) collateral flow resulting from any disease process that obstructs the blood flow through the intracranial internal carotid arteries (ICAs) to the brain. For example, the total occlusion of the ICA in Figure 8–1 obstructs the blood flow to the intracranial ICA. The obstruction is bypassed by the collateral blood flow from the left ECA through the ophthalmic artery into the intracranial ICA. The detection of the ECA collateral blood flow offers an effective indirect method of diagnosing any obstructive disease process that is limiting blood flow to the intracranial carotid artery circulation.

Examination Methods

Two diagnostic methods are used: (1) the periorbital examination of Brokenbough[1] and (2) the posterior orbital study of Spencer.[2]

Periorbital Method

A bi-directional, continuous-wave pencil Doppler probe (10 MHz) is used to determine the blood flow direction in the supraorbital artery (SOA). The SOA lies in the supraorbital notch of the superior orbital rim (Fig. 8–2); the probe should be positioned over the artery as shown in Figure 8–3. Holding the probe between the tips of the fingers and thumb while resting the palm of the hand on the patient's forehead helps to keep the probe steady during the examination. This is important because even the slightest movement will alter the strength and character of the Doppler signal. With the probe in position, record a sample of the velocity waveform produced by the Doppler signal on the chart strip recorder for hard copy analysis. Each waveform strip must be labeled correctly as taken either from the right or left supraorbital artery.

Two other arteries—the frontal and the nasal—may be encountered with the periorbital method (Fig. 8–2). Like the signal from the supraorbital artery, a signal from the frontal artery may be used to assess the blood flow direction in the external carotid circulation. However, the signal from the nasal artery is not recommended for use because this artery is tortuous and might yield a confusing waveform that is difficult to interpret.

Posterior Orbital Method

A bi-directional, continuous-wave, pencil Doppler probe is placed in contact with the closed eyelid, as shown in Figure 8–4A. The ultrasound beam is directed into the orbit and angled approximately 10° towards the nose until a signal is obtained from the ophthalmic artery. Again the probe is grasped between the tips of the thumb and fingers while the palm of the hand rests on the forehead. To prevent the signal being attenuated by the lens of the eye, instruct the patient to look towards the side opposite that being examined. Once a good signal is obtained, record the velocity waveform for hard copy analysis.

Periorbital Hemodynamic Anatomy

The ophthalmic artery arises from the intracranial ICA, passes into the orbit, and terminates in three main branches that carry blood supply to the musculature of the face and scalp. These three branches are the *supraorbital, frontal,* and *nasal* arteries (Figs. 8–1, 8–2, and 8–4). The nasal artery becomes the angular artery, which descends along the lateral border of the nose to communicate with the facial branch of the ECA.

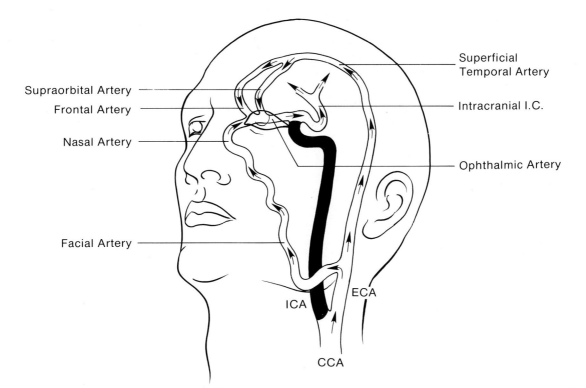

Figure 8–1. External carotid artery (ECA) collateral flow through the ophthalmic artery into the intracranial internal carotid artery (ICA) bypassing an ICA occlusion. CCA = Common carotid artery.

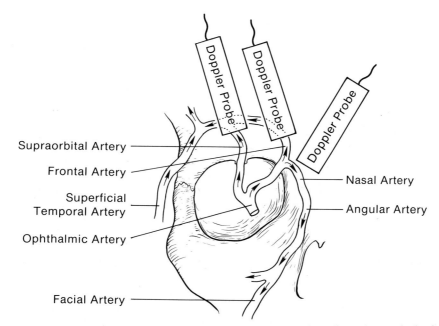

Figure 8–2. Locations of periorbital arteries. Arrows indicate normal blood flow directed towards the face of Doppler probes placed over the supraorbital and frontal arteries. Blood flow is directed away from the probe face placed over the nasal artery.

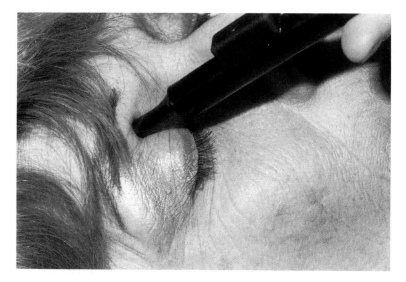

Figure 8–3. Probe positioning for supraorbital method.

The supraorbital and frontal arteries turn upward over the supraorbital rim and pass into the subcutaneous tissue of the forehead, where they communicate with the superficial temporal artery branch of the ECA (Fig. 8–2).

It is important to understand that the musculature of the face and scalp is normally supplied with blood from both the ICA and ECA. Figure 8–5 shows that the blood from the ICA joins with the blood from the ECA to flow out into the musculature of the face and scalp. The blood from the ICA passes through the ophthalmic, frontal, and supraorbital arteries; the blood from the ECA passes through the superficial temporal and facial arteries. Normally, the direction of blood flow in the supraorbital-ophthalmic system is towards the Doppler probe face. An upward, deflected, positive velocity waveform is then recorded on the chart strip for hard copy analysis (Fig. 8–5). For standardization purposes, any flow directed towards the probe face is recorded as a positive deflection above the zero baseline and flow away from the probe face is recorded as a negative deflection below the zero baseline.

Any obstructive lesion that reduces the flow and pressure in the intracranial ICA may cause the flow in the supraorbital-ophthalmic system to reverse its direction and pass from the ECA into the ICA. A negative velocity waveform below the zero baseline will be recorded because the flow is now directed away from the probe face (Fig. 8–6). Occlusive disease located in the innominate artery, the CCAs, the ICAs, or the carotid siphon may lower the intracranial ICA pressure, causing a reversal of the blood flow in the affected supraorbital-ophthalmic system. Persons with occlusive disease of the innominate

artery or subclavian arteries may "steal" blood from and lower the pressure in the intracranial ICAs. This gives a pattern of reversed flow with Doppler insonation that cannot be distinguished from the reverse flow pattern that occurs with occlusive disease of the ICA. Furthermore, a reversed flow in the affected supraorbital-ophthalmic system cannot be used to differentiate between a total occlusion and a hemodynamically significant stenosis because both are capable of decreasing the pressure in the intracranial ICA.

Even though a total occlusion or a hemodynamically significant stenosis exists in the ICA circulation, it may not reduce the pressure in the affected intracranial ICA. Blood flow and pressure from the opposite or contralateral ICA and ECA may compensate for any potential drop in pressure in the affected intracranial ICA. This is called the *compensating collateral pathway concept*, as illustrated in Figure 8–7.

No flow reversal in the left supraorbital-ophthalmic system is seen in Figure 8–7A because the left intracranial ICA pressure remains normal. It is being compensated by the pressure in the right ICA, which is transmitted across the anterior communicating artery to the left intracranial ICA. The anterior communicating artery acts as the compensating collateral pathway in this case. When the anterior communicating artery is small or does not exist, the uncompensated pressure drops in the affected intracranial ICA and the flow reverses in the affected supraorbital-ophthalmic system (Fig. 8–7B).

The compensating collateral pathway concept can be further understood by reviewing the angiograms of the two different patients with total occlusions of the left ICA. A selective CCA

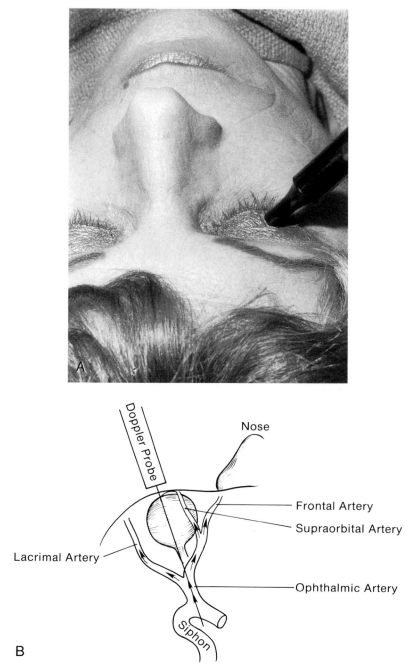

Figure 8–4. Probe positioning for posterior orbital method *(A)*. Line drawing *(B)* shows why probe is angled towards the nose to insonate the long axis of the ophthalmic artery. Normal blood flow direction (arrows).

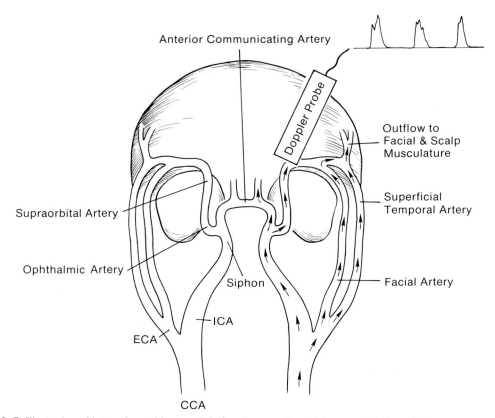

Figure 8–5. Illustration of internal carotid artery (ICA) and external carotid artery (ECA) supplying the face and scalp musculature. Ophthalmic artery blood flow directed towards the probe face causes an upward, positively deflected waveform above the zero baseline. CCA = Common carotid artery.

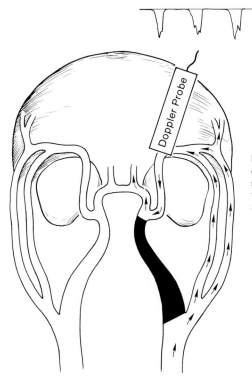

Figure 8–6. Total ICA occlusion reduces intracranial ICA pressure, causing a reversal of the blood flow direction in the ophthalmic and supraorbital arteries (arrows). A downward, negatively deflected waveform below the zero baseline is recorded from the supraorbital artery because the blood flow direction is away from the probe face.

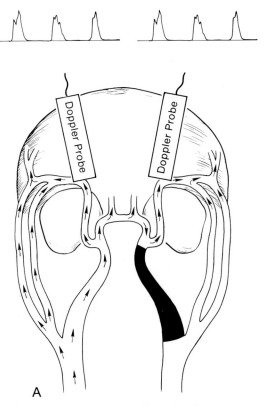

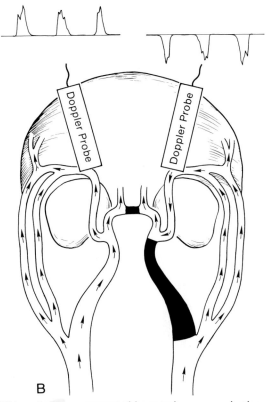

Figure 8–7. Compensating collateral pathway concept. *A,* Left ICA occlusion compensated by anterior communicating artery collateral pathway. Normal flow direction in both supraorbital and ophthalmic systems. *B,* Left ICA occlusion uncompensated by absent anterior communicating artery collateral pathway. Reversed flow in left supraorbital-ophthalmic system; normal flow direction in right arterial system.

angiogram of patient A shows a total left ICA occlusion with blood flow reversal in the left supraorbital and ophthalmic arteries (Fig. 8–8*A* and *B*). This indicates that the pressure in the left intracranial ICA is low and that it is not receiving adequate blood flow from the intracranial compensating pathways. The ECA branches then act as a compensating collateral pathway to carry blood flow through the supraorbital and ophthalmic arteries into the affected intracranial ICA.

Opacification of the reversed blood flow by contrast media in the facial, supraorbital, and ophthalmic arteries is shown in Figure 8–8*A*. There is also prompt opacification of the supraclinoid ICA intracranial segment because it is receiving blood flow from the ophthalmic artery. The cervical ICA is not seen because it is occluded. Figure 8–8*B* shows opacification of the reversed blood flow in the superficial temporal, supraorbital, and ophthalmic arteries. The intracranial ICA is again shown filled with opacified blood from the ophthalmic artery. This figure also illustrates why a bi-directional Doppler

probe placed over the supraorbital artery detected a downward deflected, negative waveform of reversed blood flow in this patient. A selective right CCA angiogram (Fig. 8–8*C*) shows good filling of the right middle cerebral arteries (MCA) and poor opacification of the left MCA. This angiogram clearly shows that the left intracranial ICA is not receiving an adequate amount of compensating blood flow from the right intracranial ICA. The reason for this inadequacy in this case is the presence of both a hypoplastic small anterior communicating artery and an A-1 segment of the left anterior cerebral artery. Because this compensation is inadequate, the low pressure in the left ICA is being compensated for by the blood flow from the left ECA.

The selective right CCA angiogram of patient B shows just the opposite situation (Figs. 8–9 and 8–10). Figure 8–9*A* and *B* show good filling of both the right and left MCAs from the contrast media injected into the right CCA. The right intracranial ICA is able to compensate for the blood flow lost to the left intracranial ICA—caused by left ICA occlusion—because the an-

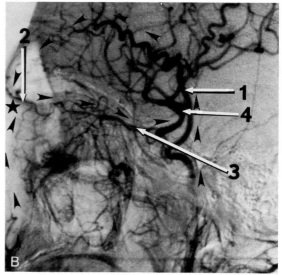

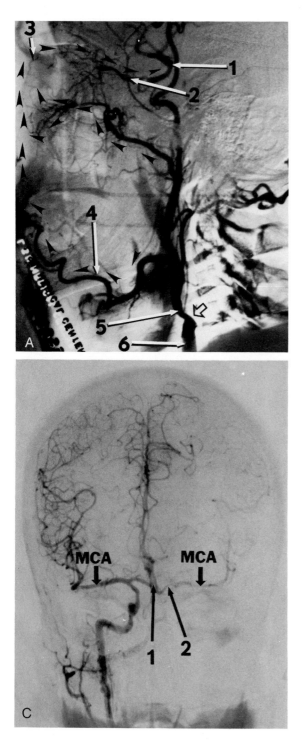

Figure 8–8. Left ICA occlusion without intracranial compensating pathway (Patient A).

A, Left CCA angiogram shows left ICA occlusion (open arrow). Arrowheads show blood flow direction in the following arterial segments: *1,* Supraclinoid ICA segment. *2,* Ophthalmic artery. *3,* Supraorbital artery. *4,* Facial artery. *5,* External carotid artery. *6,* Common carotid artery.

B, Arrowheads show blood flow direction in the following arterial segments: *1,* Superficial temporal artery. *2,* Supraorbital artery. *3,* Ophthalmic artery. *4,* Supraclinoid ICA segment. Asterisk denotes point where Doppler probe is placed to detect blood flow reversal in the supraorbital artery.

C, Right CCA angiogram showing good filling of the right middle cerebral artery (MCA) and poor opacification of left MCA. Blood flow from the right intracranial ICA cannot adequately compensate for the blood flow lost to the left intracranial ICA (a result of left ICA occlusion) because of the hypoplastic small anterior communicating artery (1) and A-1 segment of the left anterior cerebral artery (2).

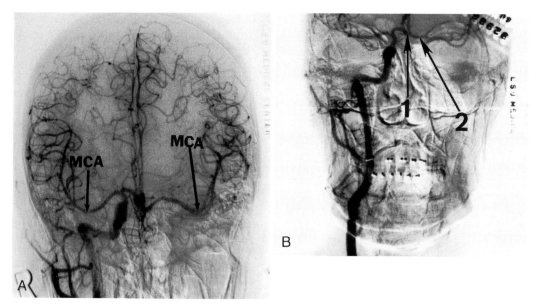

Figure 8–9. Left ICA occlusion with intracranial compensating pathway (Patient B). *A,* Right CCA angiogram shows good opacification of both middle cerebral arteries (MCA). *B,* Right CCA angiogram shows widely patent anterior communicating artery *(1)* and A-1 segment of left anterior cerebral artery *(2).*

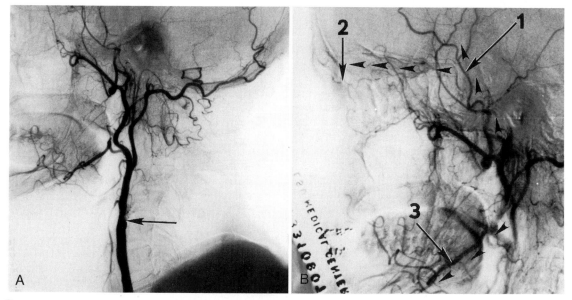

Figure 8–10. Left CCA angiogram (Patient B).

A, Early arterial phase showing ICA occlusion (arrow).

B, Late arterial phase showing no opacification of either the ophthalmic artery or the supraclinoid intracranial ICA segment. Arrows show blood flow direction in the following arteries: *1,* Superficial temporal artery. *2,* Supraorbital artery. *3,* Facial artery.

Compare the size of the superficial temporal artery in this figure with the one shown in Figure 8–8. It is smaller because it is not acting as a major collateral pathway to bypass the ICA occlusion.

terior communicating artery is widely patent, as shown in Figure 8–9B. There is then no need for the ECA to bypass the left ICA occlusion because the right intracranial ICA is acting as an adequate compensating collateral pathway. This is further confirmed by the selective left CCA angiogram in this patient (Fig. 8–10). The angiograms show normal blood flow direction in the supraorbital artery and no opacification of either the ophthalmic artery or the left supraclinoid intracranial ICA segment. No blood flow reversal in the supraorbital artery was demonstrated on the periorbital Doppler examination done without compression maneuvers. Blood flow reversal was detected in the left supraorbital artery by the Doppler probe when the right CCA was compressed.

Understanding the function of intracranial compensating collateral pathways is important because it helps to explain why all patients with an ICA obstruction do not exhibit a reversed blood flow pattern on their periorbital Doppler examinations. It also points out the importance of the various maneuvers used in association with the periorbital Doppler examination to diagnose ICA obstructions.

Another collateral pathway that may compensate for a potential drop in the intracranial ICA pressure is the vertebrobasilar circulation. Pressure is transmitted across the posterior communicating artery into the affected intracranial ICA in these instances. Zwiebel and Crummy reported that one third of patients with ICA occlusion will not exhibit a reversal of blood flow in the affected supraorbital-ophthalmic system because the compensating collateral pathways are well developed.[3]

The flow may not be reversed in the affected supraorbital-ophthalmic system even when these compensating pathways are absent, as shown in Figure 8–14B. Here the stenosis is located in the intracranial carotid siphon. The pressure in the affected intracranial ICA is not being compensated for by the pressure in the opposite ECA and ICA because the anterior communicating artery is absent. The carotid siphon stenosis is a hemodynamically significant lesion because it lowers the pressure in the affected left intracranial ICA. However, this pressure reduction is not low enough to cause a reversal of flow in the affected supraorbital-ophthalmic system. Instead, it only damps the velocity of the blood flow through the supraorbital-ophthalmic system, as indicated by the decrease in amplitude of the velocity waveform recorded from the affected system (Fig. 8–14B). The left ECA is now supplying most of the blood flow to the facial and scalp musculature as well as the ophthalmic artery vascular bed, as indicated by the thick arrows in Figure 8–14B.

The blood flow in the supraorbital-ophthalmic system is balanced between the blood flow in the ICA and ECA. As the disease progressively narrows the carotid siphon stenosis, the pressure in the affected intracranial ICA will drop even lower until there is no forward velocity flow in the affected supraorbital-ophthalmic system at all. At this point, the orbital, periorbital, facial, and scalp tissues, once supplied by the supraorbital-ophthalmic arterial system, will receive their total blood supply from the ECA. Blood will then begin to flow in a reversed direction through the supraorbital-ophthalmic system, and the affected intracranial ICA will receive its blood supply from the ECA.

In summary, there are three basic hemodynamic states that may be produced in the periorbital vasculature by an obstructing lesion in the ICA circulation:

1. Flow reversal in the supraorbital-ophthalmic system.

2. Absence of flow reversal in the supraorbital-ophthalmic system because of compensating collateral pathways.

3. Absence of flow reversal in the supraorbital-ophthalmic system when compensating pathways are absent because of the decreased severity of the obstructive disease process.

Compression Maneuvers

Compression maneuvers are not necessary when the bi-directional Doppler probe demonstrates reversal of blood flow in the supraorbital-ophthalmic system. This constitutes an examination with positive results, and the diagnosis of an obstructive lesion in either the carotid siphon or the extracranial carotid artery circulation can be inferred.

Compression maneuvers are used to reveal an obstructive lesion when blood flow reversal in the supraorbital-ophthalmic system is absent because of intracranial compensating collateral pathways. Compression maneuvers are also used to unmask disease that has not yet progressed to the point of causing a flow reversal in the affected supraorbital-ophthalmic system.

Common Carotid Artery Compression Maneuvers

Compression maneuvers of the CCA are used to detect an obstructive lesion when flow reversal

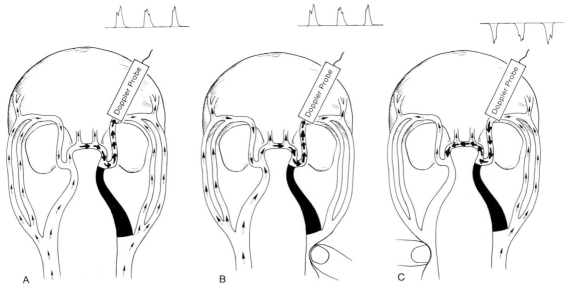

Figure 8–11. Common carotid compression maneuvers used to detect occlusion in compensated ICA with normal flow direction in the affected supraorbital-ophthalmic system. *A,* Compensated ICA occlusion. *B,* Flow in affected supraorbital-ophthalmic system unchanged by ipsilateral CCA compression. *C,* Flow in affected supraorbital-ophthalmic system reversed by contralateral CCA compression.

in the supraorbital-ophthalmic system is absent because of intracranial collateral compensation from the contralateral CCA. These maneuvers are illustrated in Figure 8–11. Figure 8–11A shows flow in a normal direction through the supraorbital-ophthalmic system and arising from a compensated intracranial ICA. The left ICA is totally occluded. Compressing the ipsilateral CCA may have no effect on the direction of the blood flow in the supraorbital-ophthalmic system under these circumstances. Compression of the contralateral CCA will reveal the compensated

ICA lesion by severely diminishing, terminating, or reversing the direction of the flow in the affected supraorbital-ophthalmic system, as shown in Figure 8–11C. No change in the affected supraorbital-ophthalmic system when either ipsilateral or contralateral CCA compression is performed denotes that the compensating collateral pathway has its origin from the vertebrobasilar circulation. The CCA compression site is shown in Figure 8–12.

Barnes and associates[4] and Brokenbough[1] have attested to the safety of the carotid compression

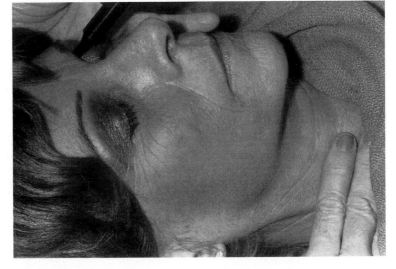

Figure 8–12. Common carotid artery (CCA) compression maneuver. The Doppler probe is placed over the ipsilateral supraorbital-ophthalmic system while digital compression is briefly applied to the contralateral CCA.

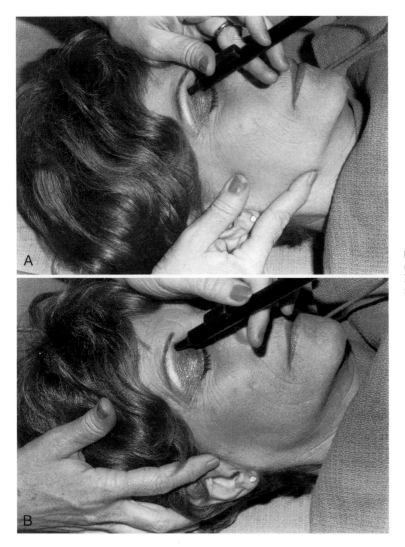

Figure 8–13. External carotid artery (ECA) compression maneuvers. *A,* Facial artery compressed. *B,* Superficial temporal artery compressed.

maneuver. In their experience only three transient neurologic deficits occurred in 5,000 patients subjected to carotid compression. Compression should be done by a physician rather than a sonographer and should be brief (only two or three heartbeats). Compressing the CCA at the base of the neck is used to prevent dislodging unknown atheromatous material from the carotid bifurcation vessels. The CCA compression maneuvers should not be done when the duplex scan reveals obvious disease present in either the carotid bifurcation vessels or the CCAs.

Figure 8–14. Responses to ECA compression maneuvers.

A, Normal response. Velocity waveform height increases as flow through the supraorbital-ophthalmic system from the intracranial ICA increases to make up for the blood lost from the ophthalmic, facial, and scalp vascular bed during ECA compression.

B, Uncompensated carotid siphon stenosis without reversal of flow in the affected supraorbital-ophthalmic system. Blood flow to the ophthalmic, facial, and scalp vascular bed is prodominantly from the left ECA (heavy arrows). Carotid siphon stenosis limits blood flow to these structures.

C, Abnormal response. Velocity waveform height decreases or becomes negative during ECA compression maneuvers (arrows).

D, A large cross-over collateral pathway between the right and left ECA requires compression of the right superficial temporal artery to elicit an abnormal response in the left supraorbital-ophthalmic system.

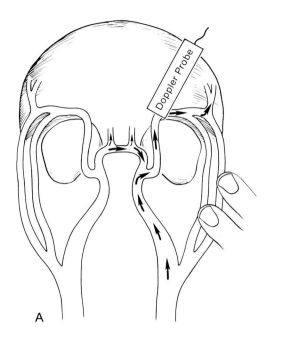

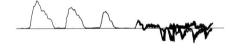

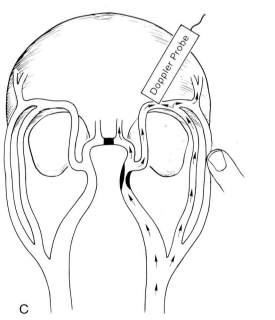

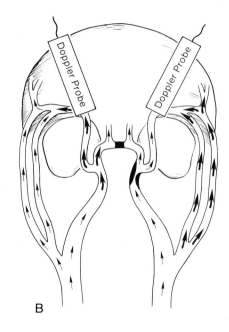

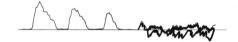

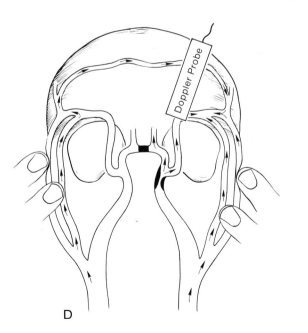

External Carotid Artery Compression Maneuvers

Compression maneuvers of the ECA are used to unmask uncompensated obstructive disease in the cerebrovascular circulation when there is no flow reversal in the affected supraorbital-ophthalmic system. The arteries compressed are the facial, as it passes across the mandible, and the superficial temporal, as it passes in front of the ear (Fig. 8–13). Each of these four compression points should be located before the examination is begun. Compressing one or more of the points reduces the blood flow from the ipsilateral ECA into the musculature of the face and scalp. This reduction is compensated for by an increase in the blood flow from the ipsilateral intracranial ICA into the ipsilateral supraorbital-ophthalmic system. The height of the recorded velocity waveform increases because more blood is flowing through the supraorbital-ophthalmic system towards the probe face during these compression maneuvers, as shown in Figure 8–14A. This is a normal response and implies that an uncompensated, hemodynamically significant lesion does not exist in the carotid siphon or extracranial carotid circulation. However, in patients with significant disease in the carotid arteries, there may be no flow reversal in the supraorbital-ophthalmic systems; compression maneuvers must be used to identify these patients. Disease may be suspected when orbital Doppler velocity waveforms are asymmetrical, as shown in Figure 8–14B. When the height of the velocity waveform on the side in question is reduced to half that of the opposite side, it is interpreted as abnormal (Fig. 8–14B). This parameter is important only in patients with unilateral carotid disease because those with bilateral lesions may show a bilateral and symmetric reduction in velocity waveform height.

The blood flow in the left supraorbital-ophthalmic system (Fig. 8–14B) is balanced between the blood flow in the left ICA and the left ECA. Compressing either or both of the left superficial temporal and facial arteries will reduce the blood flow to the left supraorbital-ophthalmic system from the left ECA. Because the carotid siphon stenosis limits the flow in the uncompensated intracranial ICA, it cannot increase its blood flow to make up for the blood lost from the ophthalmic, facial, and scalp vascular bed when the superficial temporal and facial arteries are compressed. This causes the height of the velocity waveform from the affected supraorbital-ophthalmic system to be further decreased or deflected downward below the zero baseline during the ECA compression maneuvers (Fig. 8–14C).

Compressing the ipsilateral superficial temporal and facial arteries may not elicit the abnormal response shown in Figure 8–14C. The absence of an abnormal response occurs when there is a large crossover collateral pathway between the right and left ECAs (Fig. 8–14D). The blood flow in the affected left supraorbital-ophthalmic system may now be balanced between the left intracranial ICA and the right ECA. Under these circumstances, compressing the left superficial temporal and facial arteries will have no effect on the amplitude of the velocity waveform from the affected left supraorbital-ophthalmic system. The right superficial temporal artery will have to be compressed to obtain the desired abnormal response in the left affected supraorbital-ophthalmic system, as demonstrated in Figure 8–14D.

References

1. Brokenbough EC. Periorbital velocity evaluation of carotid obstruction. *In* Bernstein EF (ed). Noninvasive diagnostic techniques in vascular disease. St Louis, CV Mosby, 1978:212–220.
2. Spencer MP. Technique of Doppler examination. *In* Spencer MP, Reid JM (eds): Cerebrovascular evaluation with Doppler ultrasound. The Hague, Martinus Nijhoff, 1981:77–80.
3. Zwiebel WJ, Crummy AB. Sources of error in Doppler diagnosis of carotid occlusive disease. AJR 1981; 137:231–242.
4. Barnes RW, Russell HE, Bone GE, et al. Doppler cerebrovascular examination: improved results with refinements in technique. Stroke 1977; 8:468–471.

9 • Anatomical Variations of the Carotid Bifurcation Vessels

Introduction

Anatomical variations of the extracranial carotid arteries present challenging technical problems in the vascular laboratory. Despite this fact, little is known about the true incidence of these variations. It is the purpose of this section, then, to review some of these variations and to give their incidence when possible. Angiograms are used to illustrate the vessel anatomy encountered on B-mode imaging of the carotid bifurcation vessels.

Aberrant External Carotid Artery

It is generally assumed that the external carotid artery (ECA) is the vessel imaged anterior to the internal carotid artery (ICA) at the bifurcation, as shown in Figure 9–1A. This assumption may be wrong at least 5 to 17% of the time because of the presence of an aberrant ECA.[1] An aberrant ECA is defined as any major variation from the usual position of the ECA, which is anterior and medial to the ICA, as seen on the lateral view of the carotid bifurcation (Fig. 9–1A). The most common location of an aberrant ECA is posterior and lateral to the ICA, as shown in Fig. 9–1B.[2] An ECA located posterior and medial to the ICA is the next most common form of an aberrant ECA (Fig. 9–1C). Both vessels may lie side by side on the lateral view of the carotid bifurcation with the ECA arising either medial (Fig. 9–1C) or lateral (Fig. 9–1E) to the ICA.

Equally perplexing is the fact that an aberrant ECA may be found on one side, whereas a carotid bifurcation with its usual anatomical configuration is present on the other side. This situation is illustrated in Figure 9–2. No carotid bifurcation is seen on the lateral angiogram of the right carotid vessels because the ECA and ICA are lying side by side (Fig. 9–2A). A carotid bifurcation is seen on the anteroposterior angiogram of these vessels with an aberrant ECA arising lateral to the ICA (Fig. 9–2B). The ECA is in its usual position anterior and medial to the ICA on the angiograms of the left carotid vessels in Figure 9–2C and D. This case illustrates that the carotid bifurcation vessels may not be symmetrical in the same patient because of the existence of an aberrant ECA.

Dolichocarotid Arteries

The dolichocarotid artery is discussed in this section on anatomical variations of the carotid bifurcation vessels because its etiology is unknown and it does not fit into any specific disease category. The numerous anatomical variations of dolichocarotid arteries have inspired a constellation of graphic labels: looped, coiled, tortuous, kinked, *sigma*-shaped, S-shaped, Z-shaped, U-shaped, and so forth. Admittedly, these adjectives furnish descriptive mental images, but they overlook the basic abnormality of the affected vessel, which is elongation. Dolichocarotid is the preferred term for this entity because it properly shifts the emphasis to the primary abnormality of increased length rather than the secondary shape distortions that are commonly caused by this condition. Three secondary shape distortions are the (1) tortuous, (2) coiled, and (3) kinked carotid artery. Although these are most commonly found in the dolicho-internal carotid artery, they may also exist in the dolicho-common carotid artery.

A tortuous dolicho-internal carotid artery is shown in Figure 9–3. It is defined as an S-shaped or C-shaped arterial configuration. Coiling occurs when an arterial segment forms a complete circle from its longitudinal axis (Fig. 9–4). A kink denotes a sharp angulation of 90° or less associated with a distinct stenosis in the affected arte-

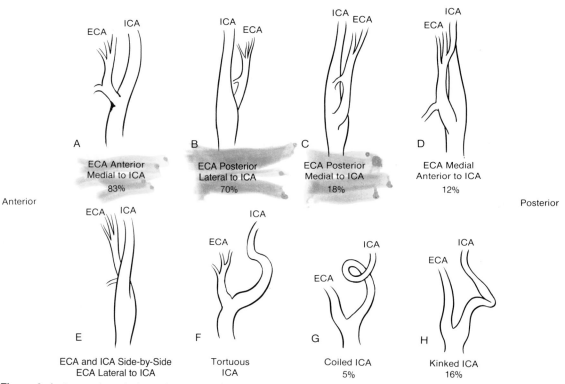

Figure 9–1. Anatomic variations of right carotid bifurcation, lateral view. *A,* Usual positions of external carotid artery (ECA) and internal carotid artery (ICA). *B–E,* Positions of aberrant ECA. *F–H,* Secondary shape distortions caused by dolicho-internal carotid artery.

rial segment (Fig. 9–5). The most important difference between a kinked ICA and a tortuous or coiled is that the kinked ICA is most often associated with symptoms of cerebral ischemia.[3]

Etiology

Theories concerning the etiology of the dolichocarotid artery include (1) congenital or developmental aberrations and (2) acquired mechanisms.

Congenital or Developmental Aberrations. The brachiocephalic vessels are normally coiled and kinked in the embryo. Straightening of these vessels occurs when the fetal heart and brachiocephalic vessels descend into the mediastinum. If this theory is correct, the brachiocephalic vessels should remain coiled and kinked when this descent is incomplete. The angiogram in Figure 9–6 shows an aortic arch that is in an unusually high cephalad position and is associated with the tortuosity of the right CCA and coiling of the vertebral arteries bilaterally, which tends to support this theory. However, there is no evidence for incomplete descent of the heart and brachiocephalic vessels into the mediastinum in the vast

majority of people with dolichocarotid arteries. Vascular dysplasias have also been implicated in causing elongation of the carotid arteries. Gass reported the association of ICA kinking in a 2-year-old patient with elastic tissue dysplasia.[4]

Acquired Mechanisms. Atherosclerotic degeneration, arterial hypertension, dorsal kyphoscoliosis, and obesity have been suggested as the acquired mechanisms for the development of elongated carotid arteries. The elongated, tortuous ICA in Figure 9–3 is characteristic of those found in patients with long-standing hypertension. Ultimately, however, the true etiology of this condition remains unknown.

Incidence

The true incidence of dolichocarotid vessels is also unknown. It has been reported to occur in the general population with an incidence ranging from 10 to 43%.[3] Tortuosity is the most common anatomical variation occurring in dolichocarotid arteries, whereas kinking is present with an incidence of 5 to 18%. Kinks usually are located 2 to 4 cm above the carotid bifurcation and are bilateral in 50% of patients. Dolichocarotid ar-

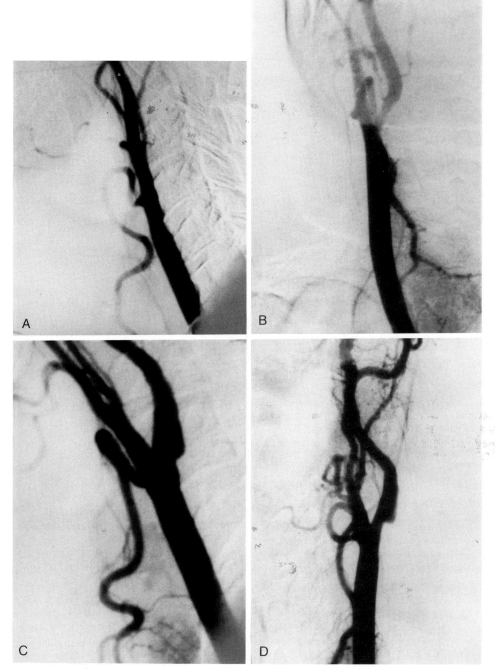

Figure 9–2. Aberrant right ECA with left ECA in its usual anatomical location. *A,* Right carotid bifurcation angiogram, lateral projection. No bifurcation is seen because the ECA and ICA are superimposed. *B,* Right carotid bifurcation angiogram, anteroposterior projection. Aberrant ECA arises lateral to ICA. *C,* Left carotid bifurcation angiogram, lateral projection, with ECA in its usual position anterior to ICA. *D,* Left carotid bifurcation angiogram, anteroposterior projection, with ECA in its usual position medial to ICA.

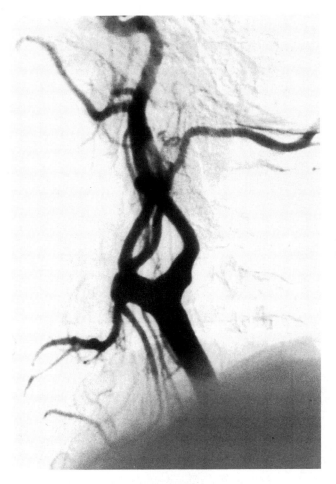

Figure 9–3. Tortuous dolicho-internal carotid artery on lateral angiogram of patient with long-standing hypertension.

teries have been found in people of all ages, including fetuses. The average age of incidence is 55 years.

The Kinked Vessel Segment

Stenosis occurring in a kinked vessel segment may cause cerebrovascular insufficiency either by interfering with cerebral perfusion or by being the source of emboli to the brain. Most often the kink is associated with cerebrovascular insufficiency that is brought about when the head is rotated in certain directions.[5, 6] These maneuvers further accentuate the stenosis caused by the kink and further reduce cerebral perfusion. Stanton and associates used oculoplethysmography to study this phenomenon in 16 patients with cerebral ischemic symptoms who were treated surgically for ICA kinks.[7] Oculoplethysmography was used to measure eye pulse arrival time and the time delay of one eye against the other in order to determine the degree of stenosis in the ICA. Oculoplethysmographs were made with the head of the patient rotated both to the right and left and to the hyperextended and flexed positions. This procedure was then repeated 4 to 7 days after surgical correction of the ICA kink. A preoperative oculoplethysmographic examination showed positive results in 14 of the 16 patients in this series when the head was placed in a rotated position. It was normal in the remaining two patients, regardless of the position of the head. All 14 patients were found at surgery to have a reduction in ICA blood flow as measured by an electromagnetic flow meter. The two patients who did not have preoperative abnormalities on oculoplethysmography were found to have no positional flow reduction during intraoperative electromagnetic flow meter testing. Postoperative oculoplethysmographic positional testing was normal in all 16 patients.

The results of this investigation are important because they demonstrate that flow reduction may occur in the kinked ICA during rotation of the head. The investigation also shows that the kinked ICA may cause cerebral ischemic symp-

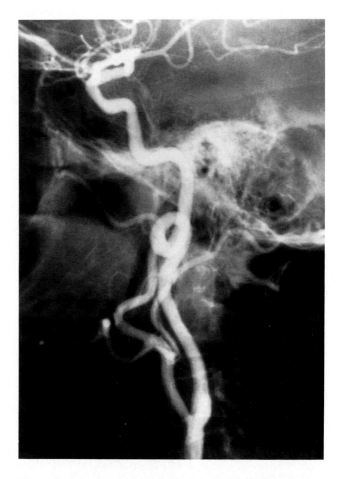

Figure 9–4. Coiled dolicho-internal carotid artery on lateral angiogram.

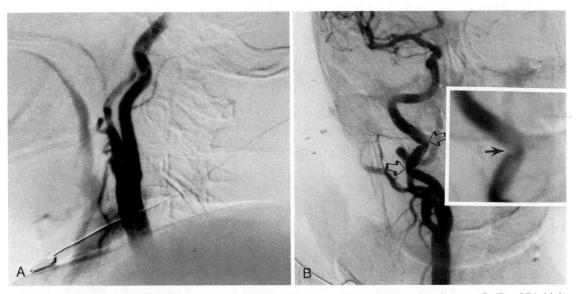

Figure 9–5. Kinked dolicho-internal carotid artery. *A,* Kinked ICA not seen on lateral angiogram. *B,* Two ICA kinks (open arrows) are readily seen on anteroposterior angiogram. Inset shows stenosis (arrow).

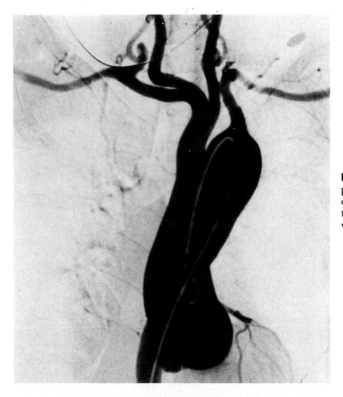

Figure 9–6. Thoracic aortogram, anteroposterior projection. The unusually high cephalad position of the aortic arch is associated with tortuosity of the right common carotid artery and coiling of the vertebral arteries bilaterally.

toms that were present preoperatively in all of the 16 patients reported in this series.[7] All 16 patients became asymptomatic following surgical correction of the ICA kink. In contrast, in two of the 16 patients with angiographic evidence of ICA kinking, oculoplethysmographic findings were normal prior to operation and ICA blood flow reduction was absent during intraoperative electromagnetic flow meter measurements. Derrick and Smith have also reported on intraoperative pressure studies in patients with ICA kinking and observed a definite pressure decrease across the kink when the head is in a rotated position.[8]

Vollmar and associates suggested that dilated, kinked carotid arteries are an important source of cerebral and retinal emboli.[9] They cite 173 patients with carotid artery reconstructions; emboli arose from kinked arteries in 66 cases. The turbulence from the jet of blood flowing through the stenosis in the kinked ICA segment may foster the formation of bland microthrombi of fibrin and platelet aggregates that shoot off into the cerebrovascular circulation.[10] The endothelium is smooth in the majority of dolichocarotid vessels unless there is superimposed atherosclerotic disease. Vannix and colleagues reported that it is not uncommon to find ulcerated atheromas within the lumen of dolichocarotid vessels

opened at surgery.[11] Atheromas are most likely to be the source of emboli in patients with dolichocarotid vessels. However, children without atherosclerosis but in whom ICA loops are present have been reported to have neurologic manifestations of microemboli,[10] indicating that emboli can arise from ICA loops in which there is no superimposed atherosclerotic disease.

Problems Associated with Duplex Sonography of Carotid Artery Variants

One of the most common errors made with duplex sonography is mistaking the ECA for the ICA. Because of the possible existence of an aberrant ECA, the usual anteromedial location of the ECA to the ICA cannot be relied upon to distinguish these two vessels from each other on the B-mode scan. The sound spectral analysis of the blood flow in these vessels is helpful in making this distinction because the ECA is characterized by a distinct high-resistance waveform pattern that is quite different from the low-resistance waveform pattern that characterizes the ICA. Unfortunately, disease may change the configurations of both the ECA and ICA waveform patterns. The ECA waveform can then mimic the ICA waveform and vice versa. Neither the B-mode image nor the sound spectral analysis can be used to distinguish the ECA from the ICA under these circumstances. A method of avoiding this problem is to search for branch vessels arising from the ECA. These can be used to identify the vessel under investigation as the ECA because there are no branch vessels that arise from the cervical ICA.

The Doppler frequency shift measurements are also affected by anatomical variations of the carotid bifurcation vessels. These are dependent on the angle of incidence of the sound beam with the plane of blood flow in the lumen of the vessel being examined. As a result, the Doppler frequency measurements will give misleading results if the vessel is angled one way or the other in relation to the direction of the sound beam. An example of this type of false information is shown in Figure 9–7.

In Figure 9–7, the sound spectral analysis waveform correctly identified the turbulent blood flow in the kinked dolicho-internal carotid artery containing atherosclerotic plaque disease. However, it also indicated that a tight stenosis was also present in the ICA. This was not found on angiography (Fig. 9–7). The abnormally high systolic peak Doppler frequency shift of 7.5 kHz was probably caused by the angled kink deformity, which resulted in a decreased angle of incidence between the sound beam and the plane of blood flow in the ICA. In this case, head rotation maneuvers failed to produce any abnormalities on the periorbital Doppler examination.

Ramirez has found that kinks give abnormal spectral analysis waveforms with loss of the systolic window and some elevation of the systolic peak Doppler frequency shifts.[12] To differentiate this spectral analysis waveform from one caused by an isolated atherosclerotic plaque stenosis requires identification of the kinked arterial segment by duplex sonography. This is not an easy task because the kinked arterial segments are often located above the angle of the mandible where they cannot be seen on B-mode imaging. Also, atherosclerotic plaque stenoses may occur in the kinked carotid artery, as shown in Figure 9–8. The plaque stenosis was diagnosed in this case, but the kink was too high to be seen on the B-mode image.

Because coils and kinks are so difficult to identify by noninvasive vascular techniques, the major role of these techniques centers around the hemodynamic evaluation of these variants once they are diagnosed by angiography. This type of information is extremely important because the coils and kinks often do not limit the cerebral blood flow and, therefore, may not be the true cause of the patient's symptoms. Angiography can show the anatomy of these variants but cannot determine their hemodynamic significance unless the blood flow through them decreases or completely stops during head rotation maneuvers. The dilemma at angiography is to decide in which position to rotate the head in order to document a decrease in blood flow through the involved arterial segment. Often this dilemma results in multiple contrast media injec-

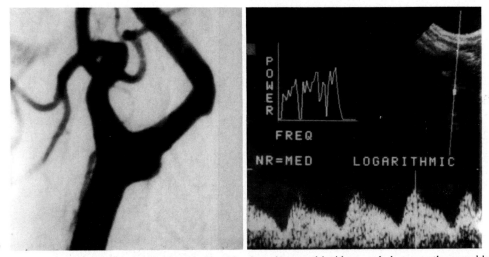

Figure 9–7. Kinked dolicho-internal carotid artery resulting in a decreased incident angle between the sound beam and the plane of blood flow in the ICA. Sound spectral analysis shows turbulence either from kink or atherosclerotic plaque or from both. Systolic peak frequency measured 7.5 kHz, but no significant stenosis is seen on the angiogram.

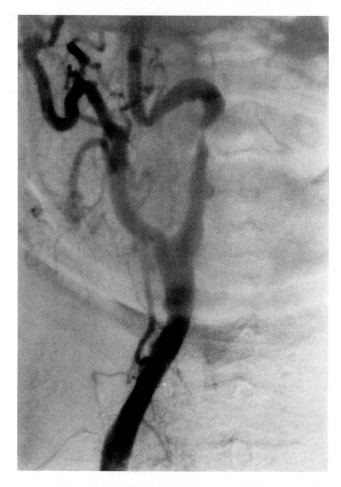

Figure 9–8. Atherosclerotic plaque stenosis in kinked dolicho-internal carotid artery.

Figure 9–9. Kinked dolicho-internal carotid artery, which does not appear to limit cerebral blood flow on the angiogram during head rotation maneuvers.

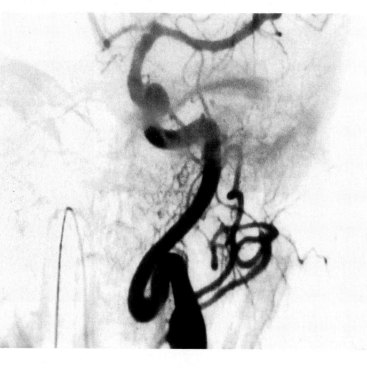

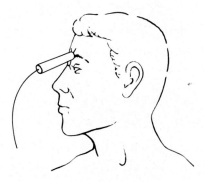
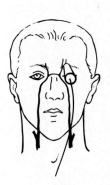
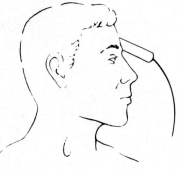

HEAD TURNED RIGHT   HEAD IN NEUTRAL POSITION   HEAD TURNED LEFT

Figure 9–10. Periorbital Doppler examination with blood flow reversal in the supraorbital-ophthalmic arterial system when the head is rotated to the left.

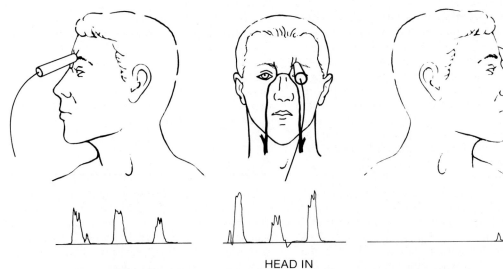

HEAD TURNED RIGHT   HEAD IN NEUTRAL POSITION   HEAD TURNED LEFT

Figure 9–11. Periorbital Doppler examination with partial blood flow reversal and damping of velocity waveforms. Obtained from the supraorbital artery of the patient whose angiogram is shown in Figure 9–5.

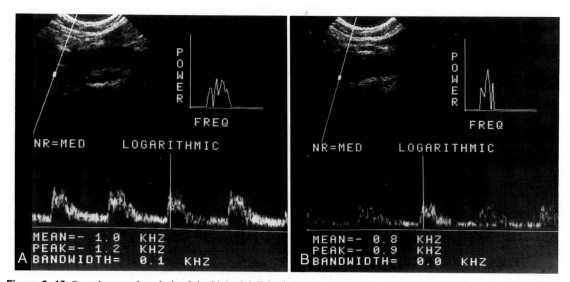

Figure 9–12. Sound spectral analysis of the kinked dolicho-internal carotid artery shown in Figure 9–5. Waveforms were obtained from the ICA at the carotid bifurcation below the level of the kinks.

A, ICA waveforms with patient's head slightly rotated to the left show mild, early diastolic spectral broadening and a systolic peak frequency of 1.2 kHz. The CCA resistivity index (RI) was 0.58.

B, ICA waveforms with patient's head further rotated to the left show depression of the diastolic frequency, shifts towards the zero baseline, and a systolic peak frequency of 0.9 kHz. The CCA resistivity index was 0.77.

tions that fail to demonstrate any limitation of blood flow through the involved segment. An example is shown in Figure 9–9 in which head rotation maneuvers failed to demonstrate any decrease in ICA blood flow through the kinked segment on angiography. A subsequent periorbital Doppler examination did show a reversal of blood flow in the left supraorbital-ophthalmic arterial system when the head was rotated to the left, as illustrated in Figure 9–10. This type of information offers evidence that a significant hemodynamic obstruction exists somewhere in the ICA circulation. It is this type of information along with the patient's symptoms that determines whether or not an isolated coil or kink uncomplicated by atherosclerosis is to be surgically corrected.

Figure 9–11 illustrates another example of a periorbital Doppler examination with abnormal results. It is from the patient whose angiogram is shown in Figure 9–5. A partial reversal of the blood flow in the supraorbital-ophthalmic arterial system was noted when the patient's head was rotated to the left. Spectral analysis was used to study the effect of the head rotation maneuvers on the blood flow in the ICA below the level of the kinks. When the patient's head was slightly rotated to the left, mild early diastolic spectral broadening with a systolic peak frequency of 1.2 kHz was seen by spectral analysis, which was

otherwise normal (Fig. 9–12A). A CCA resistivity index of 0.58 was obtained with the head in this position. Further rotation of the head to the left produced some damping of the waveforms with depression of the diastolic frequency shifts towards the zero baseline level and a decrease in the systolic peak frequency shifts from 1.2 to 0.98 kHz (Fig. 9–12B). The CCA resistivity index increased to 0.77. The progressive damping of the ICA waveforms and an increase in the CCA resistivity index yielded further information concerning the hemodynamic significance of the ICA kinks in this patient.

Summary

The anatomical variations that have been described in this chapter are important because of the limitations they place on obtaining the correct diagnosis of carotid artery disease by Duplex sonography. It is well recognized that high carotid bifurcations located deep in the neck above the angle of the mandible are difficult, if not impossible, to completely evaluate by this technique. The aberrant ECA may make it difficult to distinguish the ECA from the ICA in some cases. Anatomical variations of tortuous, coiled, and kinked dolichocarotid arteries are elusive on B-mode imaging, but the hemodynamic significance of these abnormalities is readily detected by spectral analysis and the periorbital Doppler examination.

References

1. Teal JS, Rumbaugh CL, Bergeron RT, et al. Lateral position of the external carotid artery: A rare anomaly? Radiology 1973; 108:77.
2. Faller A. Zur kenntnis der gesabverhaltnisse der carotisteilungsstelle. Schweiz Med Wochenschr 1946; 45:1156.
3. Schechter DC. Dolichocarotid syndrome. Cerebral ischemia related to cervical carotid artery redundancy with kinking: Part I. NY State J Med 1979; 79:1391–1397.
4. Gass HH. Kinks and coils of the cervical carotid artery. Surg Forum 1958; 9:721.
5. Bauer R, Sheehan S, Meyer JS. Arteriographic study of cerebrovascular disease. II. Cerebral symptoms due to kinking, tortuosity, and compression of carotid and vertebral arteries in the neck. Arch Neurol 1961; 4:119.
6. Weibel J, Fields WS. Tortuosity, coiling and kinking of the internal carotid artery. II. Relationship of morphological variation to cerebrovascular insufficiency. Neurology 1965; 15:462.
7. Stanton PE Jr, McCluskey DA Jr, Lamis PA. Hemodynamic assessment and surgical correction of kinking of the internal carotid artery. Surgery 1978; 84:793–802.
8. Derrick JR, Smith T. Carotid kinking as a cause of cerebral insufficiency. Circulation 1962; 9:721.
9. Vollmar J, Nadjafi AS, Stalker CG. Surgical treatment of kinked internal carotid arteries. Br J Surg 1976; 63:847.
10. Sarkari NB, Holmes JM, Bickerstaff ER. Neurologic manifestations associated with internal carotid loops and kinks in children. J Neurol Neurosurg Psychiatry 1970; 33:194.
11. Vannix RS, Joergenson EJ, Carter R. Kinking of the internal carotid artery. Clinical significance and surgical management. Am J Surg 1959; 134:82.
12. Henrikson J. The carotid kink. Bruit 1983; 8:33–37.

10 • Doppler Evaluation of Superficial Temporal Artery–Middle Cerebral Artery (ECA–ICA) Bypass Surgery

Introduction

The superficial temporal artery (STA)–middle cerebral artery (MCA) bypass (Fig. 10–1) provides blood flow to the intracranial circulation and alleviates cerebral ischemia. The technique was first described independently by Yasargil and Donaghy in 1967.[1] Since then, this procedure has technically improved because of the development of microscopic surgery. The main goal of the procedure is to bypass the occlusive lesion of the internal carotid artery (ICA) and/or MCA by furnishing collaterals. The small vessels of the external carotid artery (ECA)—branches of the STA—are anastomosed with the cortical opercular branch of the MCA because ischemia most commonly occurs in the distribution of the latter artery. The occipital branch of the external carotid artery is anastomosed with a branch of the posterior circulation to provide blood flow throughout the distribution of the basilar artery in the event of posterior cerebral vascular insult.

Collateral Routes in the Cerebrovascular System

The collateral routes are presented as follows.[2]
Intracranial collaterals
    Circle of Willis (Fig. 10–2)
    Persistent trigeminal artery (Fig. 10–3)
    Persistent hypoglossal artery
Extracranial-intracranial collaterals
    Ophthalmic artery
    Occipital artery
    Spinal anastomosis
    Meningeal branches from carotid siphon
    Corticotympanic artery

The cerebral circulation consists of anterior and posterior circulation. The internal carotid arteries and their branches form the anterior circulation. The two vertebral arteries unite to form the basilar artery, which in turn establishes the posterior circulation. The circle of Willis (Fig. 10–2) provides anastomoses between the anterior and posterior circulation. The anterior portion of the circle consists of a pair of internal carotid arteries, the A-1 (first or horizontal) segment of both anterior cerebral arteries, and the anterior communicating artery. Two posterior communicating arteries and the P-1 (first or horizontal) segment of both posterior cerebral arteries form the posterior portion. The posterior communicating artery joins the anterior portion of the circle of Willis to the ipsilateral posterior portion.

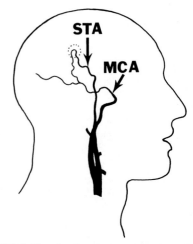

Figure 10–1. Line drawing shows an anastomosis between the superficial temporal artery (STA) and middle cerebral artery (MCA).

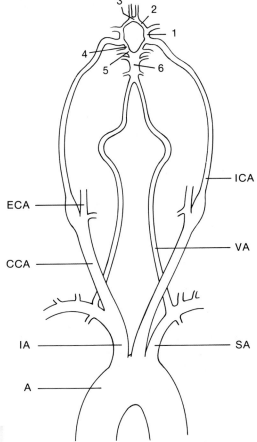

Figure 10–2. Line drawing demonstrates the circle of Willis and cerebral blood supply. *1*, Internal carotid artery. *2*, A-1 segment of the anterior cerebral artery. *3*, Anterior communicating artery. *4*, Posterior communicating artery. *5*, P-1 segment of the posterior cerebral artery. *6*, Basilar artery. ECA = External carotid artery; ICA = internal carotid artery; VA = vertebral artery; CCA = common carotid artery; IA = innominate artery; SA = subclavian artery; A = aorta.

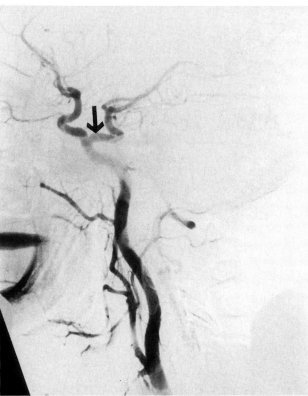

Figure 10–3. Arteriogram showing persistent trigeminal artery (arrow) providing collateral flow.

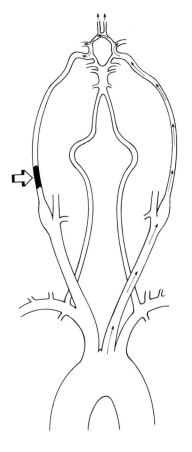

Figure 10–4. Line drawing shows the right internal carotid artery occlusion (open arrow). Arrows indicate the blood supply to the right cerebral hemisphere from the left carotid system via the anterior portion of the circle of Willis.

Figure 10–5. Line drawing demonstrates the right internal carotid artery occlusion (open arrow). Arrows indicate the blood supply to the right cerebral hemisphere via the posterior portion of the circle of Willis.

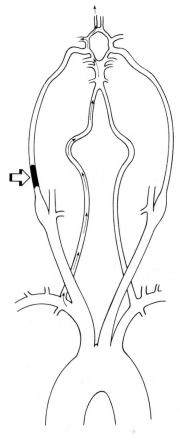

When the internal carotid artery is completely occluded or severely stenosed, the circle of Willis provides collateral supply. The cerebral hemisphere on the diseased side may receive blood from the contralateral carotid artery via the anterior cerebral and anterior communicating arteries (Fig. 10–4) or from the basilar artery via the posterior cerebral and the posterior communicating arteries (Fig. 10–5).[3, 4]

The circle of Willis was found to be normal in 52% of cases. In the remaining cases (48%), one or two of the arteries of the circle of Willis were hypoplastic.[5] Because of this normal variation (hypoplastic or absent A-1 segment of the anterior cerebral artery or anterior communicating artery; hypoplastic or absent P-1 segment of the posterior cerebral artery, or posterior communicating artery), the circle of Willis may not provide sufficient collateral flow in all cases (Fig. 10–6). Under these circumstances, the external carotid artery and its branches play an essential role in reconstituting the major collaterals. These collateral vessels are often small, but they gradually enlarge to render more blood flow to the obstructed side. The collateral flow is provided by the branches of the superficial temporal and facial arteries, which anastomose with the supraorbital branches of the ophthalmic artery (Fig. 10–7). The blood flows in a retrograde manner in the ophthalmic artery to the internal carotid artery on the side of the occlusion.

Collateral flow also occurs between leptomeningeal and cerebral vessels on the surface of the brain (Fig. 10–8).

Indications for Bypass

Cerebral revascularization by STA–MCA bypass is designed to augment the blood flow to the symptomatic or potentially symptomatic area. The primary function of the bypass is to alleviate ischemia by improving the blood flow. It is indicated in the following circumstances:[4]

1. Patients who experience multiple transient ischemic attack (TIA) episodes or patients with cerebral infarction with reversible ischemic deficits and angiographic evidence of advanced disease of the ICA or MCA that is not amenable to conventional therapy.

2. Patients with bilateral carotid occlusive disease with components of the generalized, low-perfusion syndrome (impaired mentation, syncopal episodes, ataxia, and transient or progressive visual loss).

3. Patients with moyamoya, carotid-cavernous fistula, intracranial aneurysm, or neoplastic disease may require occlusion of the ICA or MCA for therapeutic purposes or may experience occlusion secondary to the primary disease process.

However, each case should be individualized for ECA–ICA bypass.

Doppler Ultrasound

Arteriography has been the diagnostic procedure of choice for assessing the cerebral circulation prior and subsequent to the STA–MCA bypass. Arteriography not only appraises the patency of the bypass but also evaluates the results and complications of the procedure with a high degree of accuracy.[5-7] Because arteriography is invasive, it cannot be utilized frequently for follow-up examinations.

The plain film of the skull and the arteriogram for *Case I* are shown in Figure 10–9. *Case I* is a 50-year-old man who presented with multiple TIA episodes with bitemporal hemianopsia. The preoperative arteriogram demonstrates stenosis

Figure 10–6. Normal variations of the circle of Willis. *A,* Normal. *B,* Hypoplasia of A-1 segment of the anterior cerebral artery (arrow). *C,* Hypoplasia of the anterior communicating artery (arrow). *D,* Hypoplasia of the P-1 segment of the posterior cerebral artery (arrow). *E,* Hypoplasia of the posterior communicating artery (arrow). (From O'Connor RAJ. The anatomy and pathophysiology of extracranial atherosclerotic cerebrovascular disease. *In* Hershey FB, Barnes RW, Sumner DS (eds). Noninvasive diagnosis of vascular disease. Pasadena, Calif. Appleton-Davies, Inc, 1984: 158–176, with permission.)

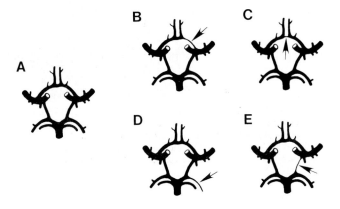

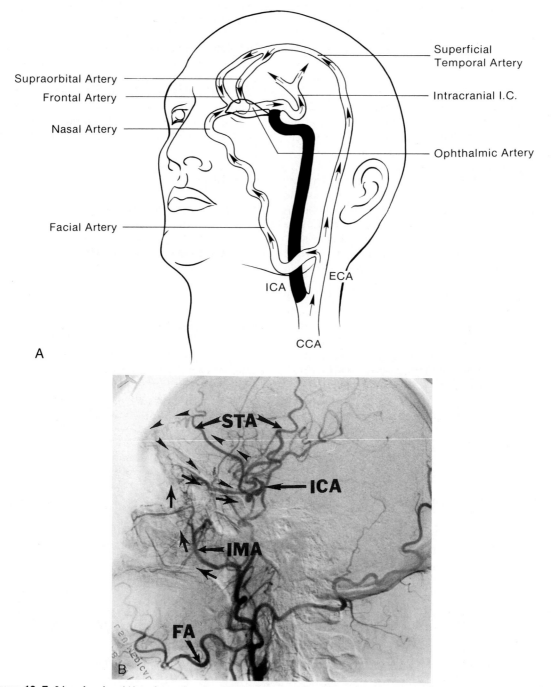

Figure 10–7. Line drawing *(A)* and arteriogram *(B)* of collateral circulation between the internal carotid artery (ICA) and external carotid artery (ECA). *A,* Line drawing shows occlusion of the left ICA with collateral flow through superficial temporal and facial arteries (branches of ECA). CCA = Common carotid artery. *B,* Arteriogram showing filling of ICA via superficial temporal (STA) and internal maxillary (IMA) arteries. Collateral flow via the STA as shown by arrowheads; collateral flow via the IMA is demonstrated by arrows. FA = facial artery.

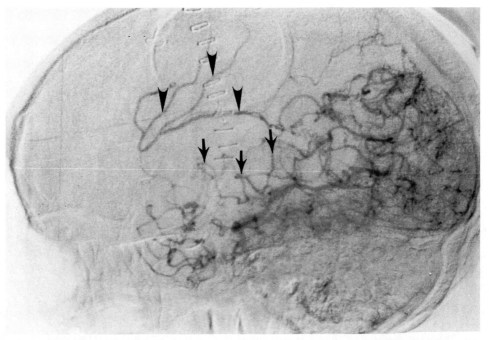

Figure 10–8. Arteriogram showing filling of anterior cerebral artery branches (arrowheads) and middle cerebral artery branches (arrows) via collaterals between leptomeningeal vessels (arrowheads) and cerebral vessels over the surface of the brain.

of both middle cerebral arteries (Fig. 10–9A and B). The plain film of the skull (Fig. 10–9C) reveals the craniotomy defect. The post-bypass arteriogram demonstrates patency of the STA–MCA bypass (Fig. 10–9D).

Doppler ultrasound provides an alternative method for making this determination. The technique is simple, rapid, reproducible, and noninvasive. It is as accurate as arteriography in determining the patency of the anastomotic site.[6–11] Because ultrasound is atraumatic, frequent follow-up evaluations can be performed without risk.

Although the superficial temporal artery can be detected without difficulty, the exact site of the anastomosis is not easy to locate with the Doppler probe. This problem can be solved by utilizing real-time ultrasonography with a 5 or 7.5 MHz frequency transducer. Figure 10–10 shows the lateral ventricles delineated by real-time ultrasonography. Normally, the intracranial structures are not visualized by sonography because the sound beam is attenuated by bone. When the bone is removed, sonography is capable of demonstrating intracranial contents.

With the use of sonography, the outline of the craniotomy site is demarcated on the scalp, as shown in Figure 10–11. The branch of the superficial temporal artery that enters the craniotomy

site is then located by means of a 4 or 8 MHz bi-directional Doppler probe. This technique allows the examination of the precise anastomotic branch and enhances the accuracy of the Doppler ultrasound.

When the 4 MHz bi-directional Doppler probe is placed over the extracranial portion of the superficial temporal artery and the probe is angled towards the direction of the blood flow, a positive signal is obtained (Fig. 10–12A). As the probe is moved in the direction of the craniotomy site and reaches the extracranial-intracranial anastomotic site, a negative signal will be obtained if the bypass is patent (Fig. 10–12B). This change in signal is due to the superficial temporal artery branch coursing away from the tip of the angled Doppler probe.

The following criteria indicate the success of the STA–MCA bypass as determined by Doppler examination:[10]

1. The STA shows significant increase in the blood flow on the side of the anastomosis when compared with the contralateral side.

2. There is significant improvement in the volume of the blood flow in the STA postoperatively.

3. The blood flow pattern in the STA changes from an external carotid to an internal carotid type.

Text continued on page 146

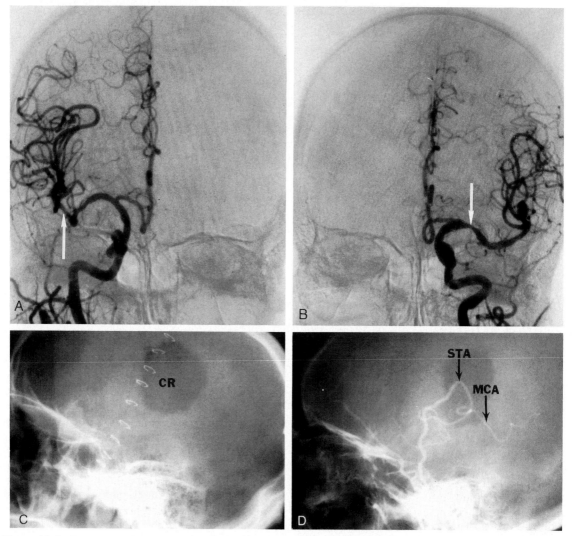

Figure 10–9. *Case 1. A* and *B*, right *(A)* and left *(B)* preoperative cerebral arteriogram showing stenosis (arrow) of the middle cerebral artery bilaterally. *C*, Plain film of the skull showing a craniotomy site (CR). *D*, Post bypass cerebral arteriogram showing patent anastomosis between superficial temporal artery (STA) and a branch of the middle cerebral artery (MCA).

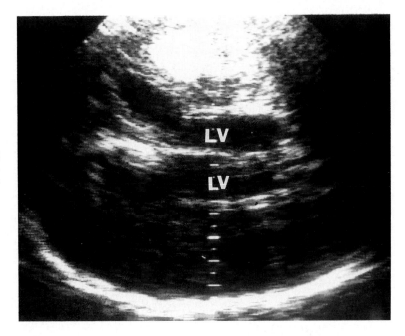

Figure 10–10. Real-time ultrasound of intracranial structures; lateral ventricles (LV) as seen through the craniotomy site.

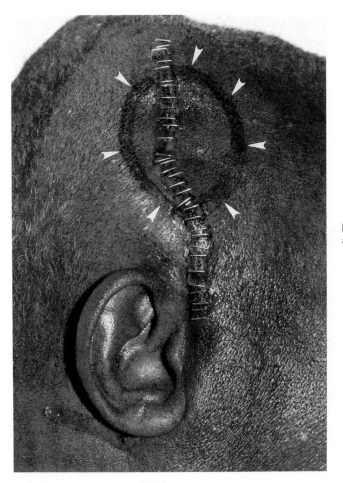

Figure 10–11. A photograph of the patient showing a craniotomy site marked by pen (arrowheads).

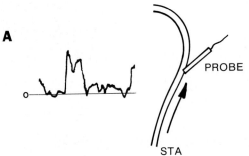

A

PROBE

STA

B

PROBE

STA

Figure 10–12. Doppler ultrasound. *A*, Doppler ultrasound demonstrating positive signal acquired from extracranial portion of the superficial temporal artery. *B*, Doppler ultrasound showing negative signal obtained from superficial temporal artery at the anastomosis site. STA = superficial temporal artery.

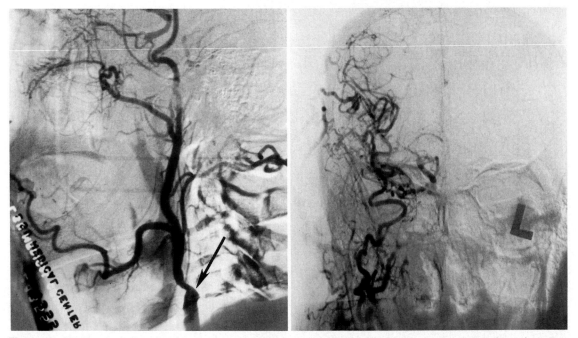

Figure 10–13. *Case 2. A*, Preoperative arteriogram demonstrates right internal carotid artery occlusion (arrow). *B*, Post right superficial temporal artery–middle cerebral artery (STA–MCA) bypass arteriogram showing patency.

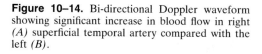

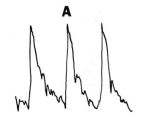

Figure 10–14. Bi-directional Doppler waveform showing significant increase in blood flow in right *(A)* superficial temporal artery compared with the left *(B)*.

4 khz   3 khz

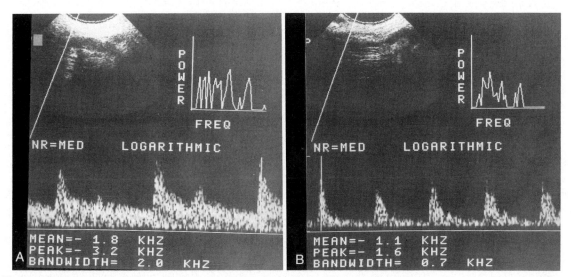

Figure 10–15. *Case 2. A,* Spectrum analysis showing internal carotid artery blood flow pattern in the right superficial temporal artery–middle cerebral artery (right STA–MCA bypass). *B,* Spectrum analysis showing external carotid artery blood flow pattern in the left superficial temporal artery.

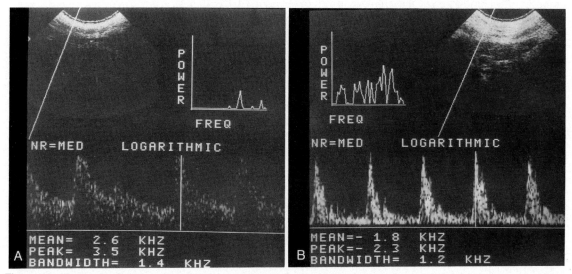

Figure 10–16. Spectrum analysis from the external carotid artery showing the internal carotid artery pattern on the right side *(A)* and the external carotid artery pattern on the left side *(B)*.

These findings are demonstrated in *Case II* and Figures 13 through 15.

Case II is a 60-year-old man who presented with a stroke along with a component of low perfusion syndrome. The preoperative arteriogram revealed occlusion of the right internal carotid artery (Fig. 10–13*A*). The postoperative right STA–MCA bypass arteriogram demonstrated the patency of the bypass (Fig. 10–13*B*). The postoperative Doppler examination of the bypass revealed a significant increase in the blood flow in the right STA compared with the left STA (Fig. 10–14). Spectral analysis of the right STA showed an internal carotid artery blood flow pattern with a significant diastolic component (Fig. 10–15*A*), whereas the left STA showed an external carotid blood flow pattern (Fig. 10–15*B*). Also, spectral analysis of the right ECA showed an ICA pattern whereas analysis of the left ECA demonstrated an ECA pattern (Fig. 10–16).

When blood flow is absent at the anastomotic site, an occlusion is suspected. The bypass is not functioning properly if the blood flow on the same side does not show improvement.[10] A properly functioning bypass is suggested when all three criteria are met.

Summary

Doppler ultrasonography is valuable for assessing the ECA–ICA bypass. Initially, this technique should be utilized to evaluate the patency and the function of the bypass. Arteriography should be reserved for those situations in which Doppler ultrasonography suggests occlusion or poor function. Doppler ultrasonography should be complemented by using real-time sonography to localize the anastomotic site and, hence, to increase its accuracy.

References

1. Yasargil MG. Microsurgery applied to neurosurgery. *In* Stuttgart Verlag GR (ed). Extracranial-intracranial anastomoses. New York and London, Academic Press, 1969:95–119.
2. O'Connor RAJ. The anatomy and pathophysiology of extracranial atherosclerotic cerebrovascular disease. *In* Hershey FB, Barnes RW, Sumner DS (eds). Noninvasive diagnosis of vascular disease. Pasadena, Calif, Appleton-Davies, Inc, 1984:158–176.
3. Osborn AG. The external carotid artery. *In* Osborn AG (ed). Introduction to cerebral angiography. 10th ed. Philadelphia, Harper & Row, 1980:49–86.
4. Sherman RL, Reichman OH. Superficial temporal artery to middle cerebral artery (STA–MCA) bypass. Bruit 1983; 7:50–53.
5. Alpers BJ, Berry RG. Circle of Willis in cerebral vascular disorders: the anatomical structure. Arch Neurol 1963; 8:398–402.
6. Anderson RE, Reichman OH, Davis DO. Radiological evaluation of temporal artery–middle cerebral artery anastomosis. Neuroradiology 1974; 113:73–79.
7. Deruty R, Duguesnel J, Lecuire J, Dechaume JP, Bret P. The extra-intracranial anastomosis: Radiological and clinical correlations. Neurochirurgia 1976; 22:469–476.
8. Handa H, Niimi H, Moritake K, Okumura A, Matsuda I, Hayashi K. Analysis of sound spectrographic pattern for assessment of vascular occlusive disorders by continuous wave ultrasonic Doppler flowmeter. Arch Jpn Chir 1977; 46:214–225.
9. Terwey B, Gahbauer H. A simple ultrasonographic method for evaluating the patency of an extra-intracranial bypass. Radiology 1982; 144:185.
10. Moritake K, Handa H, Yonekawa Y,, Nagata I. Ultrasonic Doppler assessment of hemodynamics in superficial temporal artery–middle cerebral artery anastomosis. Surg Neurol 1980; 13:249–257.
11. Hopman H, Gratzl O, Schmiedek P, et al. Doppler–Sonographie bei mikrovaskularem Bypass. Neurochirurgia 1976; 19:190–196.

11 • Carotid Endarterectomy

Introduction

This chapter will begin by describing some of the basic maneuvers used in performing a carotid endarterectomy. These are of interest because the abnormal findings seen with duplex sonography often result from some of the problems associated with this procedure. The areas where these problems may arise will be emphasized so that they can be thoroughly examined by duplex scanning. Figures 11–1 through 11–4 illustrate the basic surgical maneuvers involved in performing a carotid endarterectomy.

As shown in Figure 11–1A, a longitudinal incision is made at the carotid bifurcation to expose the outer surface of the diseased intima containing the plaque. Stay sutures are used to retract the edges of the incision. No attempt is made to cut into the plaque. Instead, a dissection plane is made around the plaque, as shown in Figure 11–1B. The optimum plane of dissection lies between the diseased intima containing the plaque and the circular fibers of the arterial media. Failure to enter this dissection plane is one of the first problems that may arise in this procedure. This problem will be addressed later.

Once the diseased intima is dissected free, it is incised at its junction with the normal intimal tissue in the common carotid artery (Fig. 11–1C). Blunt dissection is used to separate it from the normal intima of the internal and external carotid arteries. Removing the diseased intima containing the plaque in this manner constitutes the endarterectomy portion of the procedure. What remains behind to be examined by duplex scanning is the enlarged chamber at the carotid bifurcation, created by removing the diseased intima and the remaining tapered edges of the normal intima located in the common, internal, and external carotid arteries (Fig. 11–2A and B).

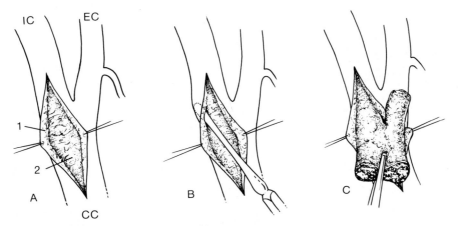

Figure 11–1. Surgical maneuvers for exposure and removal of diseased intima containing plaque.

A, Longitudinal incision through adventitia exposing outer diseased intimal plaque surface. *1*, Circular fibers of arterial media. *2*, Diseased intima containing plaque. CC = Common carotid artery; IC = internal carotid artery; EC = external carotid artery.

B, Blunt probe dissection of diseased intima from surrounding circular fibers of arterial media.

C, Circumferentially cored-out, diseased intima is removed from carotid bifurcation with forceps.

147

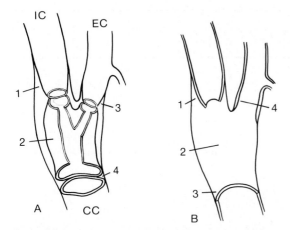

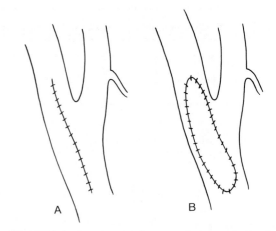

Figure 11–2. Illustration showing removal of diseased intima, which leaves behind an enlarged carotid bifurcation chamber and normal intimal margins in the common, internal, and external carotid arteries.

A, Diseased intima cut open and lying in carotid bifurcation. Its proximal end is excised from the normal intima of the common carotid artery (CC); its distal ends are torn away from the normal intima of the internal carotid (IC) and external carotid (EC) arteries by blunt dissection. Potential space between remaining normal intima and adventitia may produce intimal flap formations. *1, 3*, and *4*, Potential space between intima and adventitia. *2*, Diseased intima.

B, Diseased intima removed, showing enlarged carotid bifurcation chamber and potential remaining normal intimal edge abnormalities. *1*, Flap. *2*, Enlarged carotid bifurcation chamber. *3*, Step-off. *4*, Smooth tapering.

If the dissection plane is between the diseased intima and the circular fibers of arterial media, these edges should have smooth tapering, as shown in Figure 11–2*B*. Obtaining smooth taper-

Figure 11–4. Arteriotomy closure techniques. *A*, Continuous suture line. *B*, Patch graft.

ing of the remaining normal intimal edges may be more difficult when the dissection plane is between the arterial media and adventitia. This difficulty is caused by the increased thickness between the normal intimal tissue and the termination of the dissection separation points, as shown in Figure 11–2*A* and *B*.

Figure 11–2*A* shows the diseased intima dissected free and lying in the carotid bifurcation. The ends of the intima are separated from the normal intimal tissue remaining in the common, internal, and external carotid arteries. This figure shows the intimal thickness and potential spaces that may exist between the remaining edges of the normal intima and the adventitia.

The diseased intima has been completely removed in Figure 11–2*B*, leaving behind the enlarged carotid bifurcation chamber and the margins of the normal intima. These margins may be smoothly tapered or may contain flaps or step-offs between the margins and the arterial media and adventitia. It is important, therefore, to try to identify these intimal margins when examining the post-endarterectomized vessel with duplex scanning.

Other potential sources of intimal defects are shown in Figure 11–3. These may be caused by clamps and tapes placed on the vessels for hemostasis and wound exposure. Shunts used to bypass blood flow around the endarterectomy surgical site may also produce intimal dissections and abnormalities.

Intimal flaps occurring at the incised and dissected margins of the normal remaining intima are usually recognized and corrected during surgery. During surgery, the area of the carotid bifurcation dissection is irrigated generously with saline and any loose bits of debris or tiny intimal strips are carefully removed. Large, free intimal

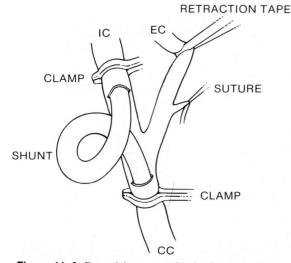

Figure 11–3. Potential sources of intimal defects. IC = Internal carotid artery; EC = external carotid artery; CC = common carotid artery.

edges or flaps are sutured to the vessel wall under direct vision. However, intimal defects caused by clamp and shunt tube placements may not be recognized because they are remote from the incision site and cannot be inspected by direct vision. It is helpful, therefore, to know where the clamps were placed and whether a shunt was used during surgery when these vessels are examined by duplex scanning.

Once the endarterectomy is complete, the arteriotomy is sutured closed, as shown in Figure 11–4. Fine bites are taken with each suture to prevent narrowing of the vessel lumen. A satisfactory closure can be achieved in most patients by the single-suture technique shown in Figure 11–4A. When it appears that such a closure will constrict the vessel lumen, the patch graft technique may be used, as shown in Figure 11–4B. The purpose of the patch graft is to allow the vessel to be closed without constricting its lumen. Generally, the patch graft is made from one of the arm veins, but it may also be constructed from an oblong piece of prosthetic material. Because these materials can produce artifacts during scanning, it is helpful to know whether or not this type of graft was used when these vessels are examined by duplex sonography.

Duplex Examination

Duplex examination of the postoperative carotid endarterectomy is performed primarily to determine the patency of the vessels and to evaluate the surgical correction of hemodynamically significant stenoses. Careful assessment of the surgical site and corresponding vessels (internal, external, and common carotid arteries) will identify any post-surgical changes, flaps, or residual tissue. The post-surgical examination is usually difficult for both the patient and the examiner because of the surgical staples overlying the vessels and the swollen edematous tissue. Hematomas may also be present, requiring additional transducer penetration in order to visualize the underlying vessels (Fig. 11–5).

The duplex carotid examination is performed using a 7.5 MHz transducer with integrated, pulsed Doppler. The higher frequencies often do not provide adequate penetration, whereas frequencies lower than 7.5 MHz cannot provide adequate resolution to identify surgical complications. A small scanning head is preferred because it provides easy manipulation and better visualization of the distal carotid vessels. The patient's head can be positioned in a true antero-posterior position with the transducer placed in a lateral plane, or the patient's head can be placed in a lateral position with the transducer placed in a 90° plane. Both positions are acceptable and avoid direct contact with the surgical staples, thereby reducing wound infection and eliminating skin artifacts.

Real-time imaging combined with spectral analysis is used to evaluate the vessel lumen and to demonstrate patency of the vessels. The post-

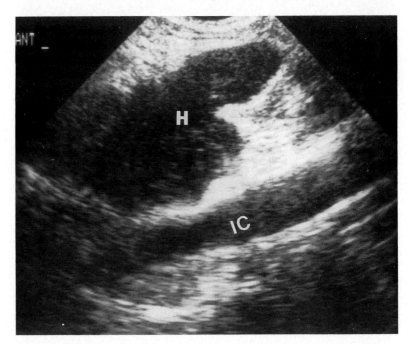

Figure 11–5. Real-time sonography shows hematomas (H) that do not occlude the internal carotid artery (IC).

surgical vessels usually appear slightly dilated, especially in the bulb and bifurcating arteries (Figs. 11–6 through 11–10). Any residual tissue, hemorrhage, calcium deposits, or intimal thickening is identified, and the site is evaluated with spectral analysis to identify post-stenotic areas (Fig. 11–11). During examination, special emphasis is placed on the surgical site in order to demonstrate post-surgical flaps (Fig. 11–12A, B, and C). These flaps are usually seen as small, discrete membranes moving in unison with the vessel wall. The spectral analysis at the flap will show a mild turbulent flow pattern. Usually, the post-endarterectomy vessel exhibits slightly increased frequencies with mild spectral broadening (Fig. 11–8). However, careful analysis should be made in order to demonstrate high-frequency areas where spectral broadening indicates post-stenotic zones and in order to re-evaluate the pre-stenotic areas for correction and return of a normal frequency range.

A good example of the pre-surgical and post-surgical examination is seen in Figures 11–13 and 11–14. In the patient shown in this figure, the internal carotid artery (ICA) was totally occluded and a high-grade stenosis of the external carotid artery (ECA) was present (Fig. 11–13A, B, and C). An external carotid endarterectomy was per-formed to correct the ECA stenosis prior to an ICA–ECA bypass. The ECA spectral analysis and duplex evaluation was obtained before the bypass was initiated. The post-surgical spectral analysis demonstrated a decrease in frequency resulting from the correction of the stenotic zone (Fig. 11–14A), which was confirmed by arteri-ography (Fig. 11–14B).

A baseline duplex examination is performed in the immediate postoperative period. The patient is usually re-examined at six months and then on a yearly basis unless clinical manifestations appear. The duplex examination is an excellent method for monitoring post-surgical endarterectomy patients.

Vessel Occlusion

One of the first priorities of noninvasive testing after carotid endarterectomy is to determine patency of the vessels. This can be done intraoperatively with the use of a continuous-wave Doppler probe. The importance of making this determination intraoperatively is illustrated by the arteriogram in Figure 11–15. The arteriogram was not obtained at the time of surgery. Instead, it was obtained several days after the surgery and

Text continued on page 155

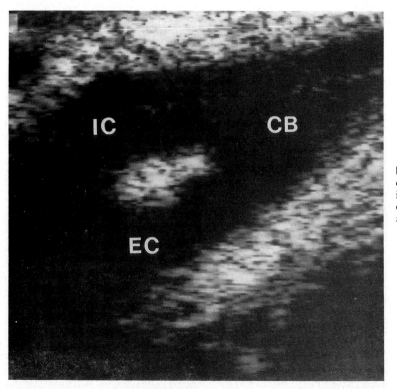

Figure 11–6. Real-time sonography of post carotid endarterectomy showing patent and mildly dilated internal carotid artery (IC), external carotid artery (EC), and carotid bulb (CB).

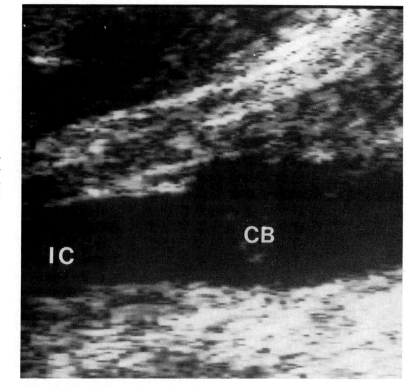

Figure 11–7. Real-time sonography of post carotid endarterectomy demonstrating patent, mildly dilated carotid bulb (CB) and internal carotid artery (IC).

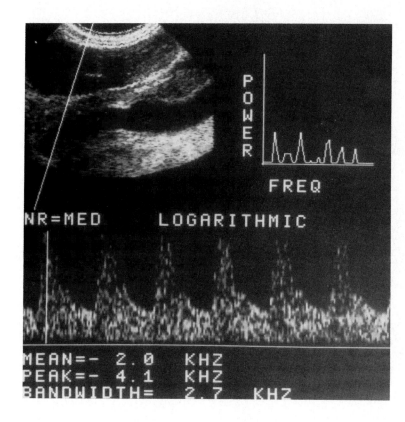

Figure 11–8. Continuous-wave Doppler examination showing mild elevation of Doppler frequency (normal <3.0 kHz).

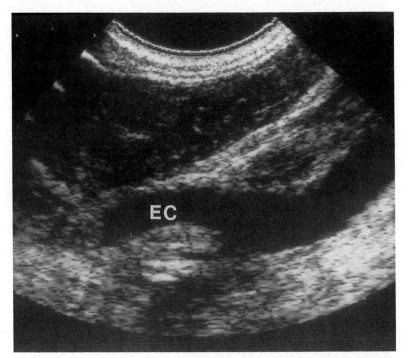

Figure 11–9. Real-time sonography of post carotid endarterectomy exhibiting patent external carotid artery (EC).

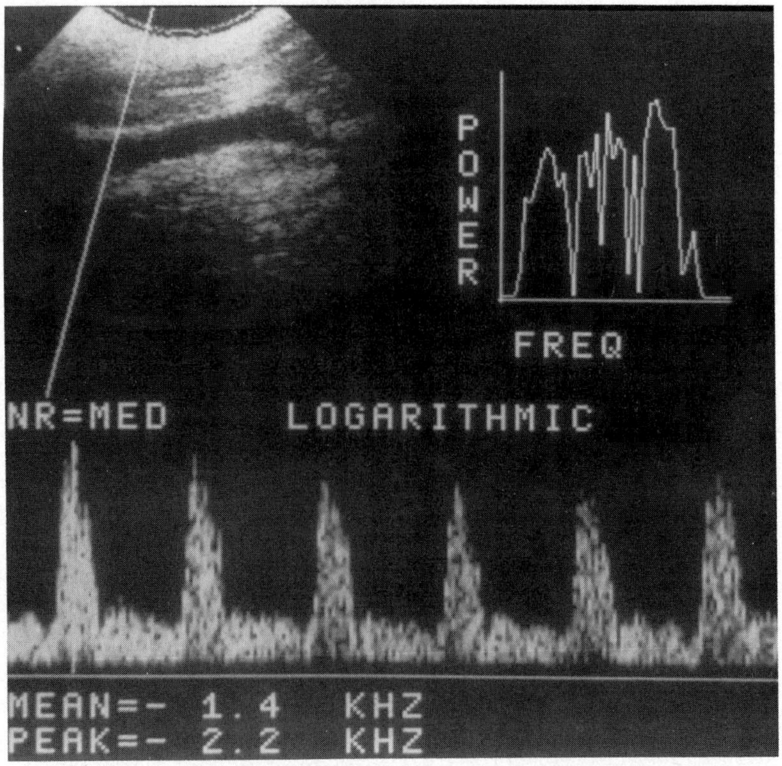

Figure 11–10. Spectral analysis showing normal external carotid artery waveforms.

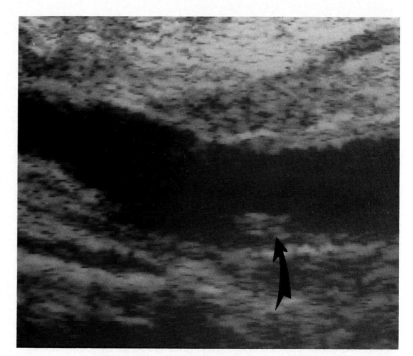

Figure 11–11. Real-time sonography of post carotid endarterectomy demonstrating residual tissue changes (arrow) in the carotid bulb.

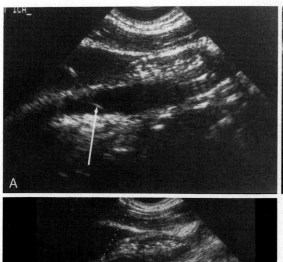

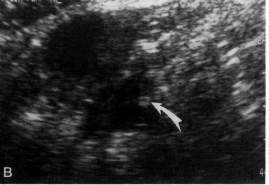

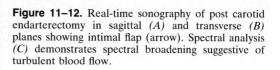

Figure 11–12. Real-time sonography of post carotid endarterectomy in sagittal *(A)* and transverse *(B)* planes showing intimal flap (arrow). Spectral analysis *(C)* demonstrates spectral broadening suggestive of turbulent blood flow.

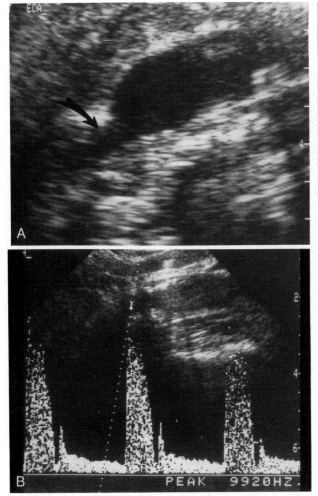

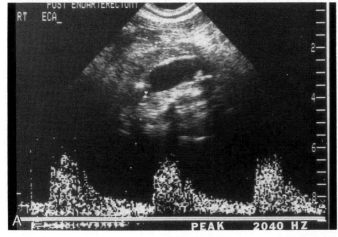

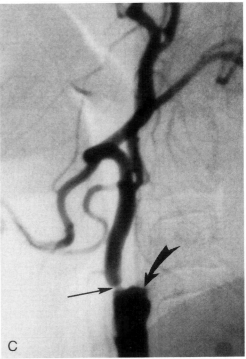

Figure 11–13. Pre-operative and postoperative examination for carotid endarterectomy. *A*, Pre-operative real-time sonogram showing stenosis (arrow). *B*, Pre-operative spectral analysis demonstrating markedly elevated Doppler frequency. *C*, Arteriogram in lateral view showing total occlusion of the right internal carotid artery (large arrow) and stenosis of external carotid artery (small arrows).

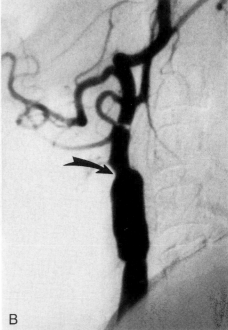

Figure 11–14. Pre-operative and postoperative examination for carotid endarterectomy. *A*, Pre-operative spectral analysis exhibiting return of Doppler frequency to normal. *B*, Arteriogram demonstrates improvement in stenotic zone (arrow).

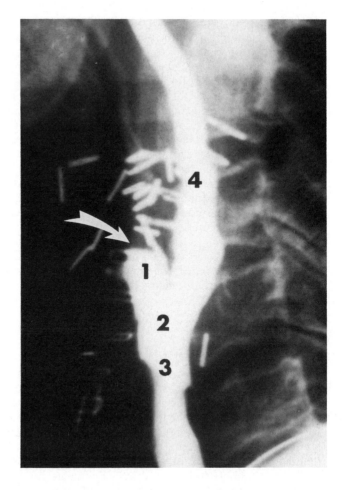

Figure 11–15. External carotid artery (ECA) occlusion (arrow) following post carotid endarterectomy. *1*, Occluded ECA. *2*, Enlarged carotid bifurcation chamber and internal carotid artery (ICA). *3*, Common carotid artery step-off. *4*, ICA step-off.

shows occlusion of the external carotid artery. If this occlusion was present at the time of surgery and had been detected by the Doppler probe examination, it could have been repaired while the operative wound was still open. This would have eliminated taking the patient back to surgery and re-opening the incision site to repair a lesion of this type.

Because the patient in Figure 11–15 remained asymptomatic, the external carotid artery was not surgically explored and the true cause of the occlusion remains unknown. From the arteriogram it can be speculated that the occlusion occurred at the site of the remaining normal intimal margin in the external carotid artery.

As illustrated in Figure 11–1B, blunt dissection is used to separate the diseased intima in the carotid bifurcation from the normal intima of the external and internal carotid arteries. During the dissection, the diseased intima is noted to become quite thin as it melts into the normal intima of the external and internal carotid arteries. This usually causes the diseased intima to dissect free and separate cleanly from the normal intima in

these vessels. The normal intima and media remain adherent to the adventitia of the distal endarterectomy sites in the external and internal carotid arteries. As a result, the remaining normal intima has a smooth tapered margin, as shown in the external carotid artery of Figure 11–2B.

When the diseased intima does not separate cleanly from the normal intima, an intimal flap may be created, as shown in the internal carotid artery of Figure 11–2B. This may occur when the plane of dissection is between the arterial media and adventitia instead of between the diseased intima and the circular fibers of the arterial media. Obtaining smooth tapering of the remaining normal intimal edges may be difficult under these circumstances. Instead, the increased thickness of the remaining normal intima may result in step-off or flap abnormalities at the termination of the dissection separation points, as shown in Figure 11–2A and B. An intimal flap may occlude the vessel, and the increased intimal thickness may produce the step-off abnormalities seen between the normal remaining intima and the termination of the dissection; separation points can be appreciated in both the common and internal carotid arteries in Figure 11–15.

The arteriogram in Figure 11–15 shows the enlargement of the carotid bifurcation chamber and internal carotid artery lumen that occurs when the diseased intima containing the atherosclerotic plaque is removed, as illustrated in Figure 11–2A and B. Figure 11–15 also shows the multiple vascular clips used for achieving hemostasis and for closing the incision site. These clips may make it difficult to evaluate the vessels with noninvasive techniques during the immediate postoperative period. They are of no concern intraoperatively beause the Doppler probe can be placed directly on the surface of the vessels to be examined. Should the Doppler assessment reveal an occluded vessel, an intraoperative arteriogram may be used to define the anatomy of the lesion prior to its repair.

Vessel Stenosis

An example of an internal carotid artery stenosis following a carotid endarterectomy is given in Figure 11–16. Again, the stenosis is present at the distal dissection site of the endarterectomy. It is caused by a thick margin of the remaining normal intima in the internal carotid artery. Note that the internal carotid artery lumen is enlarged in the region where the diseased intima containing the atherosclerotic plaque was removed. The stenosis occurs at the junction between the enlarged post-surgical carotid endarterectomy segment and the more normal-appearing lumen of the distal internal carotid artery. This is the point where the diseased intima of the proximal internal carotid artery is dissected and separated from the normal intima of the distal internal carotid artery.

Duplex scanning of the stenosis will show the narrow internal carotid artery lumen on the B-mode image and will show increased systolic peak Doppler shift frequencies with spectral broadening on the spectral analysis (Fig. 11–17A and B). Another example of post-surgical common carotid artery stenosis is shown in Figure 11–18A and B.

Complications

The patient is potentially subject to problems during four different periods. Optimally, nonin-

vasive vascular testing should be readily available during each of these periods.

Interoperatively. A continuous-wave Doppler probe may be used to detect either total occlusions or stenoses of the vessels after the carotid endarterectomy incision is closed. Should a total occlusion or stenosis be present, it may be explored and corrected immediately with or without the use of an intraoperative arteriogram. Duplex scanning, although more difficult to use intraoperatively, offers an opportunity to detect intraluminal filling defects, such as loose intimal edges, by means of its B-mode imaging capability. The pulsed Doppler probe capability is also used to detect vessel occlusions and stenoses. Detection of these abnormalities intraoperatively allows them to be corrected immediately without having to reopen and re-explore the operative site at a later date.

Immediately after Operation. Noninvasive testing may be used immediately after the operation for monitoring the patency of the vessels while the patient is in the recovery room. Immediate surgical re-exploration is generally performed for a patient found to be experiencing neurological deficits upon recovery from anesthesia. Because the surgery must be performed as quickly as possible, there may be no time for noninvasive testing under these circumstances.

Several Days after Operation. A neurologically threatening event occurring several days postoperatively while the patient is in the hospital room may necessitate immediate noninvasive testing, preferably with a duplex scanner. If this reveals an occluded vessel, nothing more may be done (Fig. 11–19A and B). However, if a stenosis is found, surgical procedures may be used to explore and correct the lesion causing the stenosis. Deciding whether or not to re-explore a patient under these conditions requires an analysis of many factors, such as the patient's symptoms and the ability of the patient to sustain another operative procedure. Duplex scanning and arteriography are important in this decision-making process because they can aid in evaluating the severity, site, and cause of the vessel abnormality. Because duplex scanning is noninvasive, it is often used prior to arteriography to determine whether or not an abnormality exists in the vessels. Once an abnormality is revealed by duplex scanning, arteriography is used to further define the anatomy of the abnormality as well as to evaluate the status of the intracranial vessels.

Follow-up. After discharge from the hospital, the carotid endarterectomy patient is followed

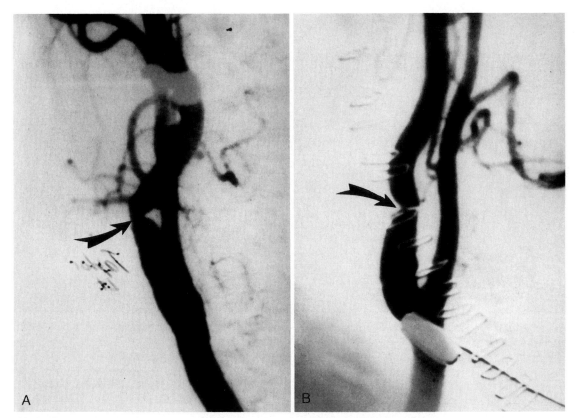

Figure 11–16. Internal carotid artery (ICA) stenosis following carotid endarterectomy. Arteriogram in both lateral *(A)* and anteroposterior *(B)* views. Arrow = ICA stenosis.

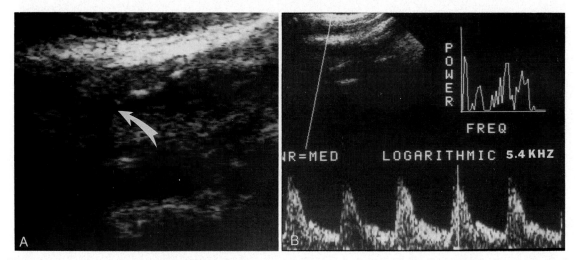

Figure 11–17. Post carotid endarterectomy examination. *A*, Real-time sonogram showing internal carotid artery stenosis (arrow). *B*, Spectral analysis showing elevated Doppler frequency.

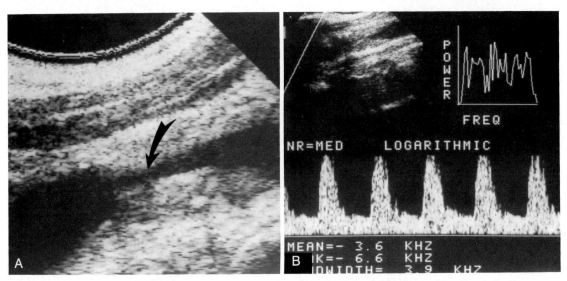

Figure 11–18. Post carotid endarterectomy examination. *A*, Real-time sonogram demonstrating stenosis in the common carotid artery (arrow) by fibrous plaque. *B*, Spectral analysis showing elevated Doppler frequency.

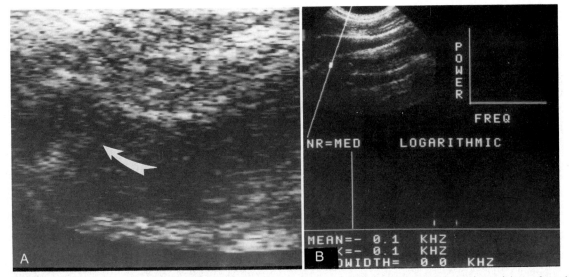

Figure 11–19. Real-time sonogram *(A)* demonstrating total occlusion of the internal carotid artery (arrow) is confirmed by absence of the Doppler signal *(B)*.

up in either the outpatient clinic or office. Duplex scaning can play a major role in these follow-up evaluations because it can detect areas of recurrent stenosis in the region of the endarterectomy site. Duplex scanning may also be used to monitor the status of any atherosclerotic disease that may be developing in the contralateral carotid artery bifurcation. Stenoses occurring at the site of a previous carotid endarterectomy may be caused by either myointimal hyperplasia or atherosclerosis. Early re-stenoses occurring within the first 18 months after endarterectomy are usually caused by myointimal hyperplasia. Late stenoses occurring more than two years after endarterectomy are commonly associated with the development of recurrent atherosclerosis.

Part III • Noninvasive Assessment of Venous Disease

12 • Hemodynamic Anatomy of the Lower Extremity Veins

Introduction

The lower extremity veins possess both a unique function and a complex anatomy. These must be understood before any attempt is made to examine them by noninvasive methods. Much of what is known about the functions and anatomy of these veins has been acquired through the use of contrast venography in the diagnosis of venous pathology. Unlike line drawing illustrations and the dissection of cadaver specimens, the venogram offers the opportunity to study both the anatomy and the function of these veins in vivo. The venogram, therefore, represents a method by which the information about hemodynamic anatomy is used to diagnose venous pathology. Venography is so accurate in defining this hemodynamic anatomy that its results are the "gold standard" for the diagnosis of venous disease. For these reasons, the venogram will be used throughout this section as the model for illustrating the hemodynamic anatomy of the lower extremity veins.

Superficial Veins

The major superficial veins seen on the venogram are the greater and lesser saphenous veins. The greater saphenous vein arises from the medial end of the dorsal venous arch at the foot and ascends in the ankle in front of the medial malleolus of the tibia. It spirals around the medial aspect of the leg posteriorly to cross behind the medial condyle of the femur at the knee (Figures 12–1 and 12–2). Extending up the medial aspect of the thigh (Fig. 12–3), it passes through the saphenous opening to drain into the femoral vein at about 3.7 cm below the inguinal ligament. In its course through the leg and thigh, the greater saphenous vein receives numerous cutaneous tributaries. Normally, the diameter of this vein is 2 to 3 mm in the calf and 6 mm in the thigh, as seen on the venogram.[1] Valves can be seen in the greater saphenous vein on the venogram; these range in number from zero to four in the lower leg and up to six in the thigh.[1]

The lesser saphenous vein begins at the lateral end of the venous arch on the dorsum of the foot

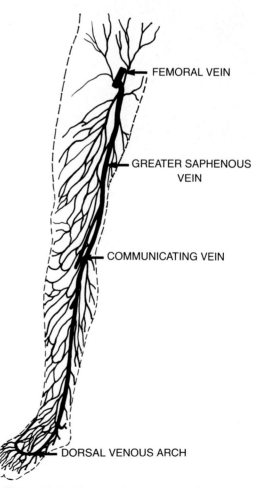

Figure 12–1. Diagram of greater saphenous vein.

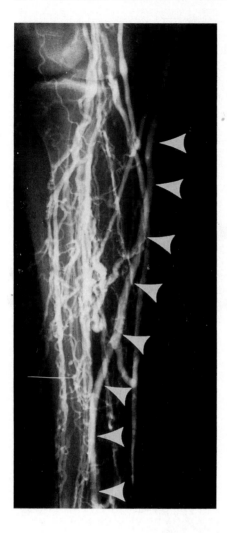

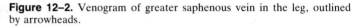

Figure 12–2. Venogram of greater saphenous vein in the leg, outlined by arrowheads.

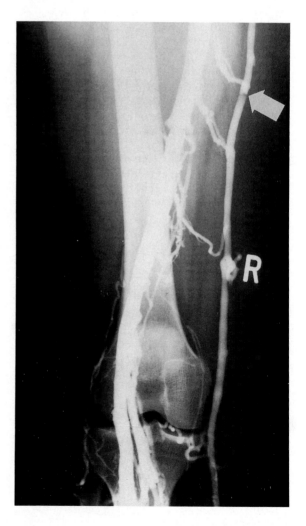

Figure 12–3. Venogram of greater saphenous vein extending up the medial aspect of thigh. Arrow points to the valve in the greater saphenous vein.

and ascends in the ankle behind the lateral malleolus of the fibula (Fig. 12–4). Extending up the back of the calf to the lower part of the popliteal fossa, the lesser saphenous vein perforates the deep fascia, passes between the two heads of the gastrocnemius muscle, and drains into the popliteal vein (Fig. 12–5). As this vein passes along the calf between the superficial and deep fascia, it receives numerous cutaneous veins from the heel and back of the leg. The greater and lesser saphenous veins can communicate through the femoropopliteal vein, which runs superficially over the popliteal fossa and lower thigh. Venographically, the diameter of the lesser saphenous vein normally measures up to 7 mm and possesses two to 12 valves.[1]

Because these veins lie in subcutaneous tissue and are superficial to the deep fascia, they can be occluded easily by the application of a tourniquet.

Deep Veins

The three principal deep veins of the lower leg are shown in Figure 12–6.

1. The *anterior tibial veins* begin in the dorsal venous rete and accompany the anterior tibial artery up the leg. Their origin in the dorsal venous rete is important because it is through this network that the anterior tibial veins comunicate with the superficial veins of the leg. The anterior tibial veins pass backward from the anterior compartment of the leg to go through the interosseous membrane and between the tibia and fibula to unite with the popliteal vein.

2. The *posterior tibial veins* arise from and drain the plantar venous arch and superficial venous rete of the foot. They follow the posterior tibial artery through the leg and receive the peroneal veins. The posterior and anterior tibial

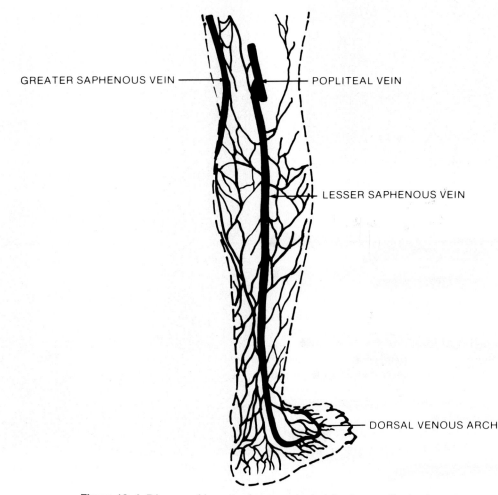

GREATER SAPHENOUS VEIN

POPLITEAL VEIN

LESSER SAPHENOUS VEIN

DORSAL VENOUS ARCH

Figure 12–4. Diagram of lesser saphenous vein draining into popliteal vein.

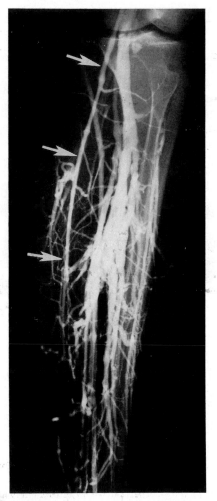

Figure 12–5. Venogram of lesser saphenous vein (arrows) extending up into the posterior aspect of the calf to drain into the popliteal vein.

veins unite at the distal border of the popliteus muscle to form the popliteal vein.

3. The *peroneal vein* arises medial to the lateral malleolus of the ankle. In the lower two thirds of the leg the peroneal vein follows the medial surface of the fibula; in the upper third it turns medially to join the posterior tibial vein.

All deep veins contain at least ten valves, are usually paired, and communicate by means of the communicating or perforating veins with the superficial venous system. On venography, the deep veins are spindle-shaped and measure up to 8 mm in diameter.

It is important to realize that these deep veins of the leg are surrounded by fascia and by the muscular mass of the leg. Any edema or swelling of the soft tissue or muscles of the leg can compress these veins. When this compression

occurs, no radiographic contrast media can enter these deep veins and the veins cannot be seen on the venogram.

These deep veins also function as the primary anatomical structures that form the deep venous pump.

Popliteal Vein

The popliteal vein is formed from the posterior tibial and anterior tibial veins at the knee. From the knee, it extends upward to the medial aspect of the femur, where it passes through the adductor hiatus to become the superficial femoral vein. The popliteal vein lies 1 to 2 cm from the posterior surface of the distal femur. The close

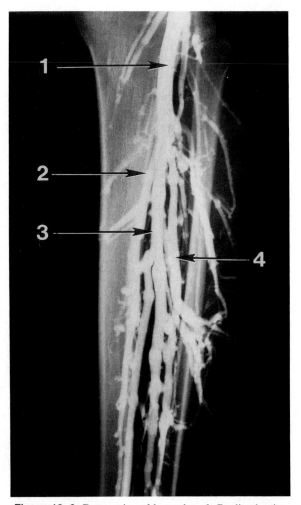

Figure 12–6. Deep veins of lower leg. *1*, Popliteal vein. *2*, Posterior tibial vein. *3*, Peroneal vein. *4*, Anterior tibial vein.

relationship of the popliteal vein to the femoral condyles has been implicated as a cause of the pseudo-obstruction of the popliteal vein seen on venography.[2] It is thought that when the leg is fully extended, the popliteal vein is stretched over the femoral condyle and is compressed by the plantaris muscle. In order to avoid this compression, the popliteal vein should be studied with the knee slightly flexed.

The normal diameter of the popliteal vein is 9 to 15 mm when measured on anteroposterior radiographs at a point 8 cm above the knee joint. In the popliteal vein, up to two valves may be present. This vein may be single (55.85%), double (39.15%), double with two femoral veins (2.78%), or triple (2.22%).[3] These variations in the popliteal vein may produce islet formations (Fig. 12–7). These are the result of small dupli-

cations of the popliteal vein and should not be mistaken for thrombus formation. The popliteal vein accompanies the popliteal artery, lying posterior and superficial to it throughout its course. A fascial sheath encircles both the popliteal artery and vein. At the lower part of the popliteal fossa, the vein is slightly medial to the artery; however, as the vein ascends, it crosses the artery to lie lateral to it in the proximal part of the fossa.

Superficial Femoral Vein and Profunda Femoris Vein

The superficial femoral vein (Fig. 12–8) is a continuation of the popliteal vein. It courses up the medial aspect of the thigh along with the superficial femoral artery to the inguinal ligament to form the common femoral vein. The superficial femoral vein measures 0.9 to 1.0 cm in diameter and usually contains two to five valves. May and Nissl have described four variations of the superficial vein.[4] These consist of (1) a normal single vein (62.34%); (2) duplication of the lower segment, sequentially uniting to form one single vein in the midthigh (21.16%); (3) multiple veins (13.72%); and (4) duplication of the entire superficial femoral vein (2.78%). Duplications of the superficial femoral vein are shown in Figures 12–8 and 12–9.

The deep femoral vein or profunda femoris vein (Fig. 12–8) arises from the venae comitantes corresponding to the perforating branches of the profunda artery. This vein drains into the lateral aspect of the superficial femoral vein.

Communicating (Perforating) Veins

The communicating veins connect the superficial venous system with the deep venous system throughout the leg and thigh. Their number and arrangement are presented here according to Limborgh's description.[5] The posterior group of communicating veins can be seen in the lateral venogram of the leg (Fig. 12–10A). These connect the lesser saphenous vein with the veins of the gastrocnemius muscle and the gastrocnemius plexus. In the anteroposterior radiographic projection, the communicating veins can be divided into two groups. These consist of the medial and lateral groups (Fig. 12–10B). The medial group is composed of those veins that connect the great saphenous vein with the posterior tibial veins.

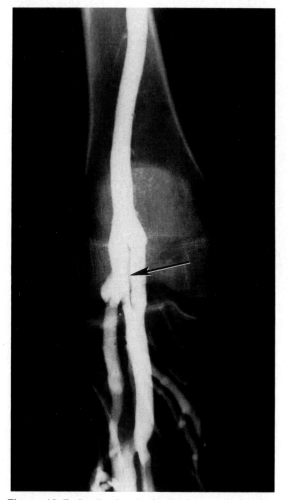

Figure 12–7. Popliteal vein duplication producing islet formation (arrow).

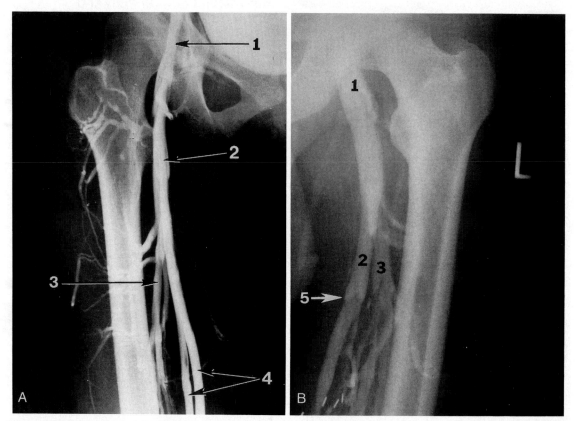

Figure 12–8. Deep veins of the thigh *(A)* and inguinal region *(B)*. *1,* Common femoral vein. *2,* Superficial femoral vein. *3,* Profunda femoris vein. *4,* Duplication of the lower segment superficial femoral vein uniting to form one single vein in midthigh. *5,* Valve in superficial femoral vein.

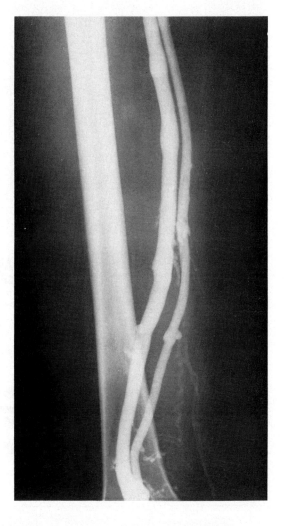

Figure 12–9. Duplication of the entire superficial femoral vein.

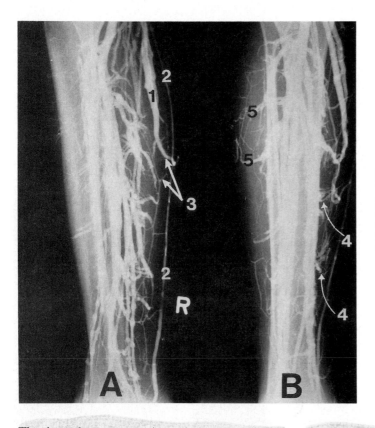

Figure 12–10. Communicating (perforating) veins of the leg. *A*, Leg venogram, lateral projection. *1*, Gastrocnemius venous plexus. *2*, Lesser saphenous vein. *3*, Posterior communicating veins. *B*, Leg venogram, anteroposterior projection. *4*, Medial communicating veins. *5*, Lateral communicating veins.

The lateral group consists of those veins that connect the greater saphenous vein with the anterior tibial and peroneal veins. On the venograms, one to 12 veins of the medial group are seen, whereas up to seven veins of the lateral group are seen and one to five veins of the posterior group are seen. The diameter of the communicating veins when measured at a point near their junction with the superficial veins is 0.5 to 4 mm. There are one to six communicating veins medially in the thigh. These connect the superficial femoral vein with the greater saphenous vein (Fig. 12–11). These communicating veins normally measure 2 to 5 mm in diameter.

Muscle Plexus Veins

The two muscle plexus veins that can be seen by venography are the soleus and gastrocnemius. The gastrocnemius plexus drains the blood from the gastrocnemius muscle and empties into the popliteal vein. These are seen as saccular venous structures in the medial calf region when viewed on the anteroposterior venographic projection (Fig. 12–12). While draining the soleus muscle, the soleus plexus veins empty into the posterior tibial vein. They are seen as saccular venous structures in the posterior calf region when viewed on the lateral venographic projection (Fig. 12–13). Visualization of the soleus plexus veins is important because deep vein thrombi may originate in these veins.[6, 7] An example of thrombi in the soleus muscular plexus veins is shown in Figure 12–14.

Deep Vein Muscular Pump

The vast venous anatomy of the lower extremity, as shown in the venograms of this section, is capable of containing a large volume of blood. In fact, as much as 15 to 20% of the body's total blood volume may be pooled in the lower extremity veins within 15 minutes of standing absolutely still. This accounts for the well-known example of soldiers fainting after standing at absolute attention for extended periods of time. While a person is standing still, the veins simply collect blood from the capillaries and passively transport it up the lower extremity to the heart. The energy for this transport is supplied totally through contraction of the left ventricle. Obviously, this is insufficient because a large amount of blood is allowed to pool in the lower extremity veins at rest. A mechanism that helps to com-

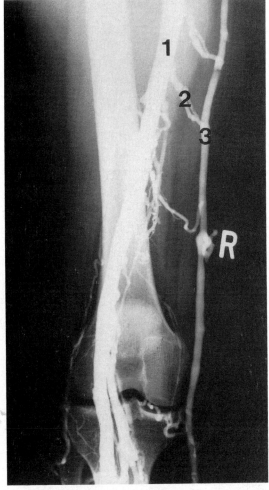

Figure 12–11. Communicating (perforating) veins of the thigh. *1,* Superficial femoral vein. *2,* Communicating veins. *3,* Greater saphenous vein.

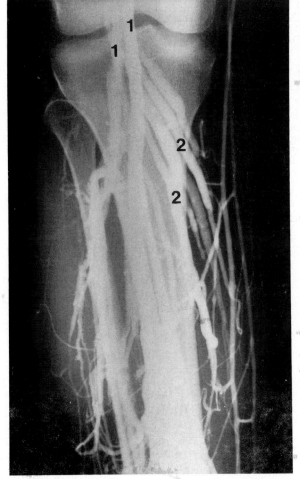

Figure 12–12. Venogram of muscle plexus veins, anteroposterior projection. *1,* Duplication of popliteal vein. *2,* Gastrocnemius muscle plexus veins, which drain blood into the popliteal vein.

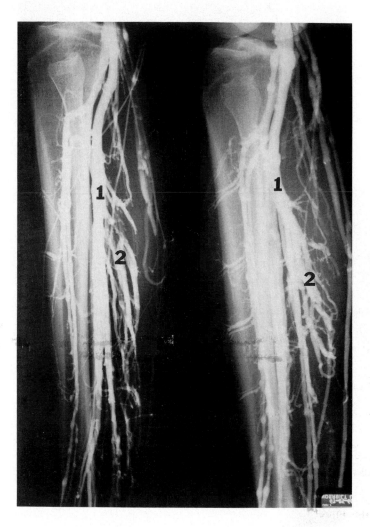

Figure 12–13. Venogram of muscle plexus veins, lateral projection. *1,* Posterior tibial vein. *2,* Soleus muscle plexus.

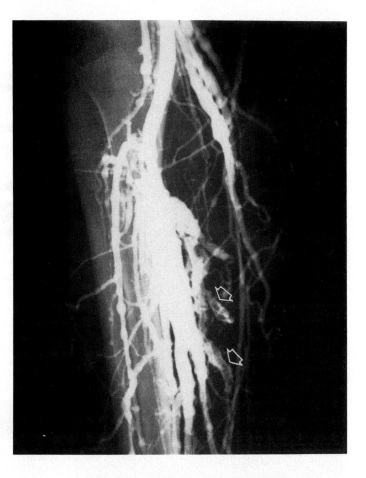

Figure 12–14. Thrombi in soleus muscle plexus veins (arrows).

pensate for this insufficiency is the deep vein muscular pump. Every time one moves the legs or even tenses the leg muscles, a certain amount of blood is propelled towards the heart because of this mechanism.

Another important function of the deep vein muscular pump is controlling the pressure in the lower extremity veins. Because of the hydrostatic pressure created by a column of blood extending from the feet to the heart in the standing individual, the venous pressure in the feet would always be around +90 mm Hg. However, the deep vein muscular pump acts to keep the pressure low in the leg veins by continually pumping the blood out of them. This allows the venous pressure in the feet of a walking adult to remain lower than 25 mm Hg.

Failure of the deep vein muscular pump to pump blood out of the leg veins results in both increased volume of blood and pressure in these veins. This failure causes the veins to distend, producing varicose veins. The increase in venous pressure also causes an increase in the pressure of the capillary bed, leading to a leakage of fluid

and red blood cells from the capillary blood into the tissues and resulting in edema and hyperpigmentation of the affected extremity. The edema in turn prevents adequate diffusion of nutritional materials from the capillaries to the muscle and skin cells so that the muscles become painful and the skin ulcerates. These pathological changes are most marked in those tissues that are subjected to the highest pressure. This includes the ankle region, where the pressures developed by calf muscle contractions are transmitted directly to the skin surface via incompetent perforating veins. An example of chronic venous insufficiency of the leg from failure of the deep vein muscular pump is shown in Figure 12–15. This example emphasizes just how important this mechanism is in returning blood from the leg to the heart and maintaining a low pressure in the veins.

The anatomy and function of the deep vein muscular pump has been described extensively by Almen and Nylander.[8] Their study was accomplished by the use of serial venograms of the lower extremity during contraction and relaxa-

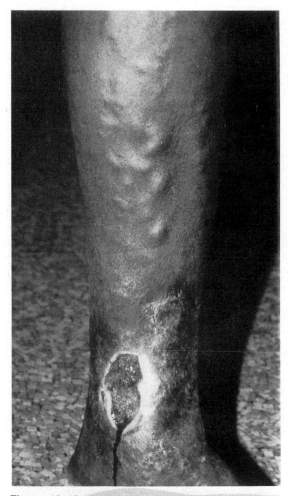

Figure 12–15. Chronic venous insufficiency owing to failure of the deep vein muscular pump, causing varicose veins, edema, hyperpigmentation, and a large ulcer over the medial ankle region.

tion of the leg muscles. These authors—by using this technique—were able to observe the method by which blood is pumped from the leg veins up into the thigh veins The movement of blood up the veins of the lower extremity is a complex function of the leg muscles and valves in the venous system. To simplify these functions, the actions of the leg muscles and valves of the venous system will be described as they occur during walking. With each step taken during walking, there are periods in which the leg muscles are relaxed and contracted. The flow of venous blood during these periods is outlined in Table 12–1.

Venography allows the function of the deep vein muscular pump to be observed in vivo. Figure 12–17A shows the veins filled with blood

opacified by contrast medium. This figure is analogous to the line drawing shown in Figure 12–16B. The muscles of the deep venous pump are relaxed, allowing the blood to flow into the deep veins from the superficial veins. This occurs because the pressure in the deep veins is lower than that of the superficial veins. The blood begins to flow from the deep leg veins up into the deep thigh veins as the leg muscles begin to contract and activate the deep vein muscular pump (Fig. 12–17B). Valves in the deep leg veins prevent the flow of blood towards the feet, and valves in the communicating veins prevent the flow of blood backward from the deep veins into the superficial veins during muscle contraction. As a result, all of the blood in the leg is pumped up into the thigh veins by the deep vein pump mechanism during contraction of the calf muscles (Fig. 12–17C and D). Figure 12–17D shows the post-exercise venographic appearance of a normal leg with competent valves in both the superficial and deep venous systems. The valves in the communicating veins are also competent.

Table 12–1. Deep Vein Muscular Pump

Beginning of Muscle Relaxation (Fig. 12–16A)
1. Leg muscles relax and no longer compress the leg veins.
2. The deep veins and muscle veins of the leg are empty of blood because the blood has been pumped into the thigh veins by the previous muscle contraction.
3. Valves in the popliteal vein close so that the blood in the thigh cannot reflux back down into the leg.
4. Pressure in the deep veins is low because the deep veins are empty of blood.
5. The superficial veins fill with blood, and the pressure in the superficial venous system increases. This increase in pressure causes the valves in the communicating veins to open.
6. Blood flows from the high pressure in the superficial veins to the low pressure in the deep veins through the communicating veins.

End of Muscle Relaxation (Fig. 12–16B)
1. The deep veins become filled with blood.
2. The muscle plexus veins become filled with blood.

End of Muscle Contraction (Fig. 12–16C)
1. The leg muscles have contracted, forcing the blood out of the deep veins and muscle veins of the leg and up into the thigh veins.
2. Valves in the communicating veins close so that blood cannot reflux back into the superficial venous system.
3. Once the blood is pumped into the thigh veins by the contraction of the leg muscles, it is held there by the closed valve in the popliteal vein.
4. The leg muscles begin to relax (Fig. 12–16A), and the deep veins and muscle veins again become filled with blood, as shown in Figure 12–16B.

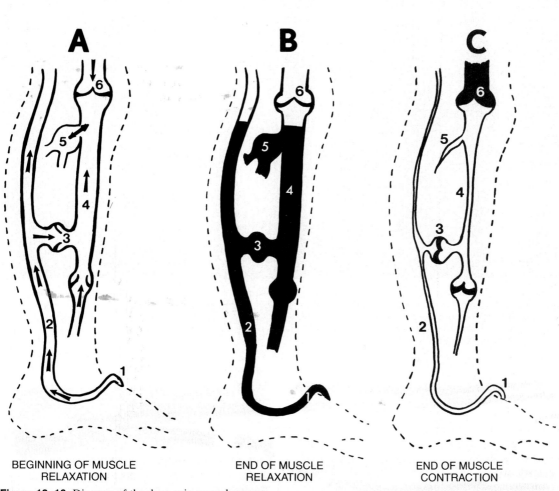

Figure 12–16. Diagram of the deep vein muscular pump.

A, Leg veins following muscular contraction and at the beginning of muscular relaxation showing the empty leg veins beginning to fill with blood. Arrows show direction of blood flow from the superficial veins through the communicating veins into the deep veins. *1*, Dorsal venous rete. *2*, Superficial venous system. *3*, Valve in the perforator vein. *4*, Deep venous system. *5*, Muscle plexus veins. *6*, Valve in the popliteal vein.

B, Leg veins are completely filled with blood as noted by the dark shading of the veins.

C, The muscle contraction forces the blood out of the leg veins into the popliteal vein. Here it cannot flow in a retrograde direction because of closure of the valve in the popliteal vein. Note the dark shading of the popliteal vein, showing this vein filled with blood.

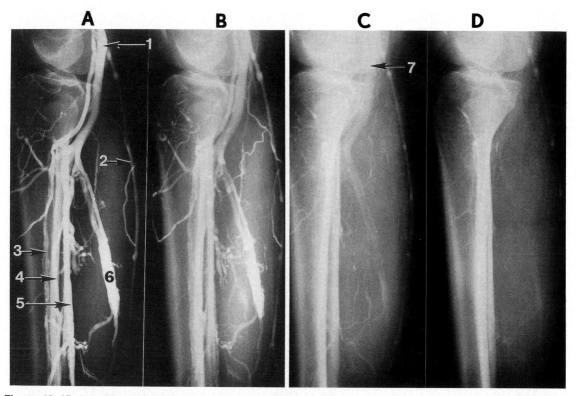

Figure 12–17. Function of deep vein muscular pump demonstrated by venography. *A*, Deep leg veins filled with opacified blood at the end of muscle relaxation. *1*, Popliteal vein. *2*, Lesser saphenous vein. *3*, Anterior tibial vein. *4*, Peroneal vein. *5*, Posterior tibial vein. *6*, Soleus muscle plexus. *B*, Veins are less opacified as blood begins to flow out of them during early muscle contraction. *C* and *D*, Contraction of the leg muscles pumps the opacified blood out of the leg veins up into the popliteal vein *(7)*.

Incompetence of the deep vein valves results in failure of the deep vein muscular pump mechanism. The blood in the deep leg veins cannot be transported successfully into the deep thigh veins once the deep vein muscular pump fails. Instead, the blood refluxes up and down in the deep leg veins with each contraction and relaxation of the deep vein muscular pump. An example of a deep vein muscular pump that has failed is shown in Figure 12–18.

The status of the deep vein valves is an important factor in determining the prognosis of patients with varicose veins and chronic venous insufficiency. The objective of the evaluation of patients with varicose veins is to define whether or not the varicosities are the only venous abnormality present. Varicose veins with incompetent superficial vein valves and competent deep vein valves are termed primary varicose veins. Those varicose veins with incompetent valves in both the superficial and deep veins are termed secondary varicose veins. This diagnostic distinction is of the utmost importance in planning therapy and assessing the patient's prognosis.

Patients with primary varicose veins improve after excision and ligation of the varicosities. Patients with secondary varicose veins, however, have a chronic venous problem that is rarely cured or significantly improved by surgical intervention on the superficial varicosities alone.

The pre-exercise and post-exercise venograms of a patient with primary varicose veins are shown in Figure 12–19. Opacified blood remains in the superficial veins after exercise (Fig. 12–19B), indicating that the valves are incompetent in these veins. It empties out of the deep leg veins, indicating competency of the valves in these veins. A post-exercise venogram of a patient with secondary varicose veins is shown in Figure 12–20. Here the opacified blood remains present in both the superficial and deep veins because all of these veins have incompetent valves.

The valves in the deep veins of the inguinal region and thigh may also become incompetent. Incompetent valves allow the blood in the thigh to reflux down the lower extremity into the deep leg veins. Contrast medium injected through a catheter placed in the external iliac vein in the

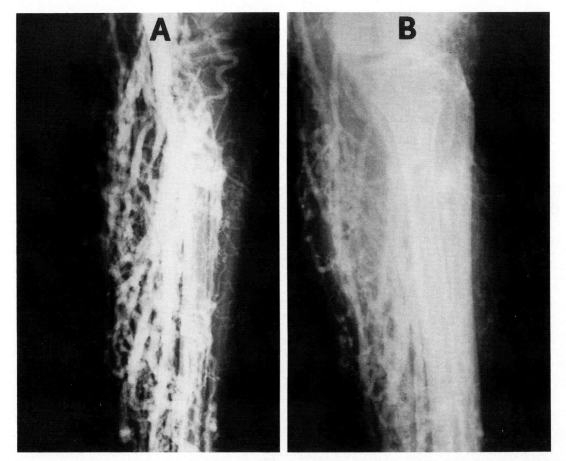

Figure 12–18. Venographic demonstration of an incompetent deep vein muscular pump. *A*, Leg muscles relaxed with deep veins filled with opacified blood. *B*, Leg muscles contracted; opacified blood remains in the deep veins because the deep vein muscular pump has failed.

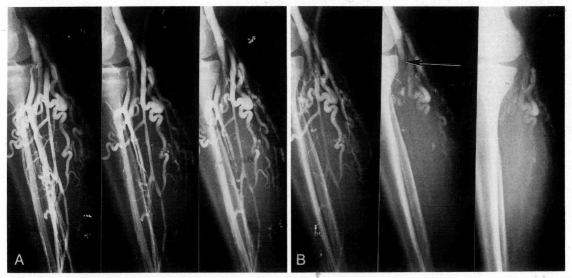

Figure 12–19. Venogram of competent deep vein muscular pump in a patient with primary varicose veins. *A*, Leg muscles relaxed; both superficial and deep veins are filled with opacified blood. *B*, Leg muscles contracted; deep veins are empty, indicating competent valves. Blood cannot reflux back down into deep leg veins because of competent popliteal vein valve (arrow). Opacified blood remains in the lesser saphenous vein, indicating incompetency of its valves.

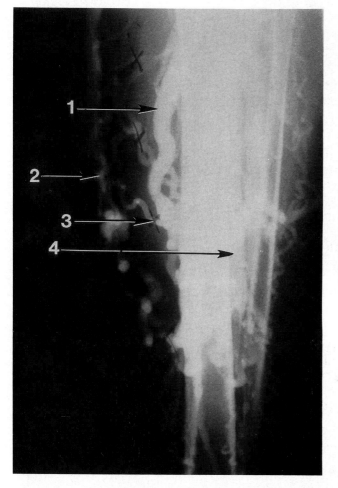

Figure 12–20. Post-exercise venogram of a patient with secondary varicose veins. The opacified blood remains in the deep veins and refluxes past the incompetent communicating vein valves into the dilated superficial veins. *1,* Dilated lesser saphenous vein. *2,* Dilated greater saphenous vein. *3,* Incompetent communicating vein. *4,* Opacified blood in deep leg veins.

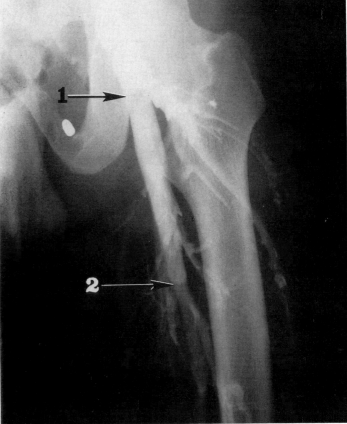

Figure 12–21. Venogram of incompetent iliofemoral *(1)* and superficial femoral *(2)* valves (arrows). These incompetent valves allowed contrast media injected into the external iliac vein to reflux down the thigh veins into the deep leg veins.

standing individual may be used to test the competency of the iliofemoral, superficial femoral, and popliteal vein valves. Competent valves will prevent the retrograde flow of the injected contrast medium down the thigh into the deep leg veins. Incompetent valves allow the contrast medium injected into the external iliac vein to reflux down the deep veins into the deep leg veins (Fig. 12–21).

References

1. Greitz T. Phlebography of the normal leg. Acta Radiol 1955; 44:1–20.
2. Arkoff RS, Gilfillan RS, Burhenne HJ. Pseudo-obstruction of the popliteal vein. Radiology 1968; 90:66–69.
3. DeWeese JA, Rogoff SM. Functional ascending phlebography of the lower extremity by serial long film technique: Evaluation of anatomic and functional detail in 62 extremities. AJR 1959; 81:851–854.
4. May R, Nissl R. Phlebographische studien zur anatomie der beinvenen. ROFO 1966; 104:171.
5. Linton RR. The communicating veins of the lower leg and the operative technique for their ligation. Ann Surg 1938; 107:582.
6. Nicholaides AN, Kakkar VV, Renney JTG. The soleal sinuses: origin of deep-vein thrombosis. Br J Surg 1968; 55:742.
7. Nicholaides AN, Kakkar VV, Field ES, Renney JTG. The origin of deep vein thrombosis: a venographic study. Br J Surg 1971; 44:653–663.
8. Almen T, Nylander G. Serial phlebography of the normal lower leg during muscular contraction and relaxation. Acta Radiol 1962; 57:264–272.

13 • Peripheral Venous Examination of the Lower Extremities

Introduction

The use of noninvasive vascular examinations of the peripheral venous system has gained popularity during the last few years. Although contrast venography remains the "gold standard," extraordinary efforts are being made to replace the venogram because of the expense, patient discomfort, and risks associated with the procedure. These efforts began as early as the 1960s with the Doppler principle[1] and continued with the development of indirect testing methods, such as strain gauge plethysmography (SPG) and photoplethysmography (PPG). More recently, duplex venous imaging has been utilized to evaluate the venous system. This new, direct assessment of the venous system offers anatomical detail along with hemodynamic data that enhances diagnostic accuracy.

Each laboratory employs various methods for appraising the venous system, depending upon the availability of the equipment and the expertise of the examiner. Figure 13–1 illustrates a typical venous protocol for complete evaluation of the venous system. This protocol includes duplex venous evaluation, which has been included in our laboratory.

Noninvasive Procedures

We routinely use the following noninvasive testing procedures.

1. Strain gauge plethysmography for determining vein patency and for ruling out deep vein thrombosis (DVT).

2. Photoplethysmography for evaluating the venous valves, determining reflux (incompetency), and localizing incompetency in the superficial or deep venous system.

3. Doppler techniques for ruling out DVT and determining incompetency of the deep and superficial venous systems.

4. Duplex imaging for verifying the findings of other noninvasive tests and for visualizing the venous system.

In a situation in which there are technical or patient limitations, not all of the tests can be performed. However, we try to combine the indirect tests (SPG, PPG) with at least one or both of the direct tests (Doppler, real-time imaging). By using multiple diagnostic tests procedures, we can increase the sensitivity of our findings and avoid certain pitfalls inherent in some of the noninvasive examinations.

Certain groups of patients derive the greatest benefit from noninvasive examinations, and, in some instances these examinations become the procedures of choice. These groups include:
• patients allergic to contrast media
• patients with poor renal function
• pregnant patients
• pediatric patients
• patients with a technically limited venogram
• patients in traction or casts
• post-surgical patients

Patient History and Physical Evaluation

A detailed patient medical history and a thorough physical examination are required in all vascular examinations. The clinical history can often aid in the diagnosis and can ensure that the correct examinations are performed. The clinical history of patients with peripheral vascular disease varies according to the cause and the site of involvement. It is important to determine any previous injury to the extremities, the presence of hypertension, any major disease (e.g., diabetes mellitus, heart disease), or any history of thrombophlebitis or varicose veins.[2]

Visual inspection of the extremities should be made to identify any physical signs of disease. This would include edema, swelling, inflamma-

VENOUS EVALUATION

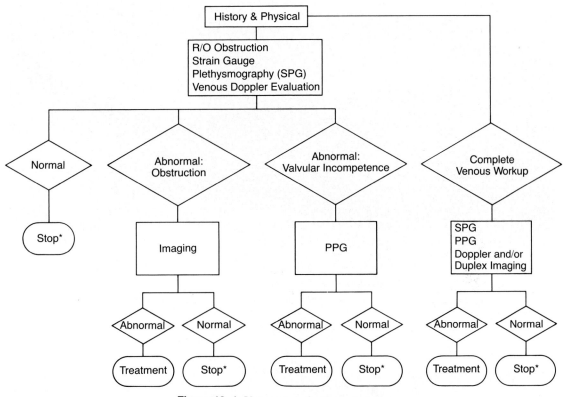

Figure 13–1. Venous examination protocol.

tory conditions, skin changes, ulcerations, varicose veins, and leg tenderness. Figure 13–2 demonstrates a classic example of unilateral swelling associated with deep vein thrombosis. The patient with DVT may present with severe pain, massive edema, coldness, cyanosis, or severe ischemia. In contrast, there may be no local symptoms or signs other than slight edema.[3] The classic signs and symptoms are nonspecific and cannot be depended upon to diagnose or rule out deep vein thrombosis. The overall accuracy for clinical diagnosis is only 50%.[4] Hence, there is a need for a more objective testing methodology.

The examiner performing the noninvasive examination utilizes any clinical findings along with the patient's history to determine the examination to be performed and to provide the clinician with the necessary information for treatment.

of reference, we have included Figure 13–3A and B. Additional anatomical diagrams with the respective clinical presentation are presented in Chapter 12. The examiner should have a thorough understanding of the venous system for anatomical localization and physiological function. The initial learning experience should include performance of all the basic venous examinations (SPG, PPG, Doppler, and duplex imaging) on both abnormal and normal patients. These examinations should be correlated with venography to enable the examiner to establish baselines, to determine normal values for noninvasive testing, to assess abnormal conditions, and to understand the function of the venous system. As examiners gain experience and perfect their knowledge of the venous system, a high degree of reliability will be achieved. Then the protocol may be varied for specific examinations.

Peripheral Venous Anatomy

The venous anatomy and physiology have been presented in detail in Chapter 12. For the sake

Strain Gauge Plethysmography

Strain gauge plethysmography, a method of assessing the patency of the venous system, was

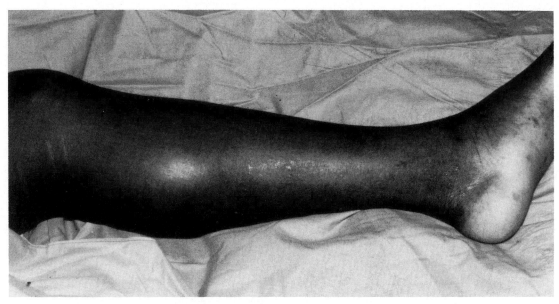

Figure 13–2. Deep vein thrombosis with unilateral swelling, edema, and leg tenderness.

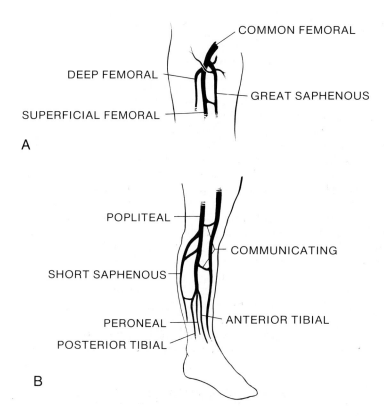

Figure 13–3. Anatomical diagrams of *(A)* the deep venous system in the thigh and *(B)* the deep venous system in the lower leg.

first described by Whitney in 1950. Initial studies were followed by the work done in the 1960s by Barnes who used SPG in the diagnosis of deep vein thrombosis above the knee. Cramer, using SPG and the outflow/capacitance discriminant line for the detection of deep vein thrombosis, provided the most recent innovation. This method provided a consistent, repeatable measuring interval for calculating the venous outflow.[5, 6] There are several other plethysmographic methods (air, water, and electricity) that are used in the assessment of venous patency. However, our laboratory utilizes the SPG method combined with the venous outflow/venous capacitance (VO/VC) discriminant line, which has proved to be simple, inexpensive, and reliable.

Strain gauge plethysmography measures volume changes in the limb, and these changes are indicated by the limb circumference. A fine elastic silicone rubber tube filled with an electrically conductive alloy (strain gauge) is gently stretched around the limb so that changes in the circumference are indicated by length changes of the tube. Because the electrical resistance of the alloy is proportional to both its length and area, the measurement of gauge resistance can be used to follow changes in the limb circumference. In fact, it can be shown that the change in resistance is directly proportional to the changes in volume, as seen in the equation in Figure 13–4.[7] By using the equation and observing the relationship between volume and resistance, we can obtain the volume changes and respective measurements.

Examination Techniques

To perform the SPG examination, the examiner places the patient in a supine position with all clothing removed from the lower extremities. A large sponge is placed under the feet to elevate the lower extremities at least 12 inches above the bed. The hips are rotated slightly lateral, with the knees flexed outward, which places the pa-

$$\frac{\Delta V}{V} = \frac{\Delta R}{R}$$

WHERE ΔV IS THE CHANGE IN LIMB VOLUME

WHERE V IS THE INITIAL LIMB VOLUME

WHERE ΔR IS THE CHANGE IN GAUGE RESISTANCE

WHERE R IS THE INITIAL RESISTANCE

Figure 13–4. Equation illustrating resistance and volume relationship.

tient in a semi-frogleg position. Small triangular sponges are placed under the upper thigh for support. Of prime importance is the relaxation state of the extremities. The patient must relax the extremities and be in a comfortable position throughout the test. This not only ensures a smooth curve but also allows for ease of flow in the vessels for proper recording and accuracy (Fig. 13–5).

A wide pneumatic cuff attached to an automated inflation system is placed around the upper thighs while the strain gauges are gently placed around the calf at the maximum circumference. Strain gauges come in various sizes; however, we use 24 and 34 cm sizes, depending upon the calf size. The cuff should be lightly (just touching the skin surface) wrapped around the calf circumference, with the gauge covering approximately 80% of the calf diameter. The SPG unit is coupled to a strip chart recorder and calibrated so that 1% capacitance is equal to a 10 mm deflection, allowing for computer calculation of the venous capacitance and outflow. An example is shown in Figure 13–6. The chart speed is set at 1 mm/sec, and the pneumatic thigh cuffs are inflated to 55 mm Hg to occlude the venous system. This prevents the outflow of venous blood but still allows the arterial inflow, thereby enlarging the venous vessels in the limb. Repeating the inflation (which is called *toning*) several times increases the capacitance and improves the outflow. The venous pressure rises until equilibrium and stability is achieved, which is 55 mm Hg on the cuff inflator.

During the final test, the cuff is rapidly deflated and the venous outflow is calculated and recorded by computer (Fig. 13–6). The maximum increase in the calf volume during venous occlusion is termed the *venous capacitance* (VC), which is normally at least 2% or 20 mm above the baseline during venous occlusion. The *maximum venous outflow* (MVO) is obtained by measuring the outflow between 0.5 and 2 seconds after the release of the venous occlusion cuff.[6] Following the release of the cuffs, the venous outflow should result in a decrease of the calf circumference. The normal venous outflow is at least 50% of the incremental volume within the first three seconds.[8] Based on the Cramer study and the standardization of the VO/VC curve, we use the computer calculation with a >25%/min normal value and a 5% equivocal zone.[5, 6] The VC and VO are both computed in the microprocessor, and the final values are plotted on the VO/VC discriminant curve (Fig. 13–7). The VO/VC discriminant line accurately defines normal and ab-

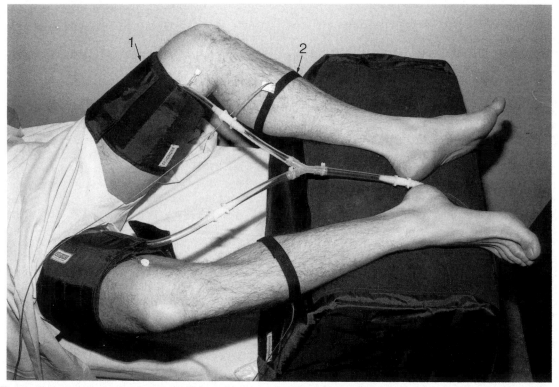

Figure 13–5. Venous strain gauge plethysmography: patient position and procedure setup. *1* = Wide pneumatic inflation cuff. *2* = Strain gauge.

normal patients when we employ SPG and calculate the outflow using the Cramer method. A standardization study of the VO/VC discriminant line curve indicated a 95% sensitivity and a 99% specificity.

In the presence of DVT, the venous capacitance will be reduced because the veins will be already partially distended. One of the most accurate indications of the SPG is the MVO, which will also be diminished in the presence of DVT (Fig. 13–8). When the results are equivocal or abnormal, the test is performed at least two more times with the patient's position checked and technical factors reviewed.

Abnormal Findings

There are various technical conditions that can produce artifacts and alter the values, producing abnormal results.

1. Kinking of the air inflation hoses produces ineffectual occlusion, resulting in diminished capacitance and outflow (Fig. 13–9).

2. A strain gauge of improper size or placed too tightly around the calf may result in diminished capacitance and outflow (Fig. 13–10).

3. Patient movement or sitting during examination causes fluctuations in the curve. However, the outflow calculations will be correct (Fig. 13–

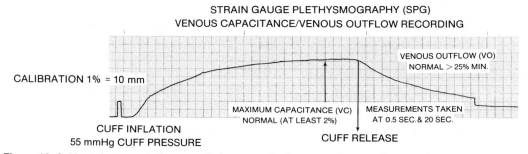

STRAIN GAUGE PLETHYSMOGRAPHY (SPG)
VENOUS CAPACITANCE/VENOUS OUTFLOW RECORDING

CALIBRATION 1% = 10 mm

VENOUS OUTFLOW (VO)
NORMAL > 25% MIN.

MAXIMUM CAPACITANCE (VC)
NORMAL (AT LEAST 2%)

MEASUREMENTS TAKEN
AT 0.5 SEC. & 20 SEC.

CUFF INFLATION
55 mmHg CUFF PRESSURE

CUFF RELEASE

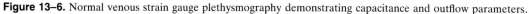

Figure 13–6. Normal venous strain gauge plethysmography demonstrating capacitance and outflow parameters.

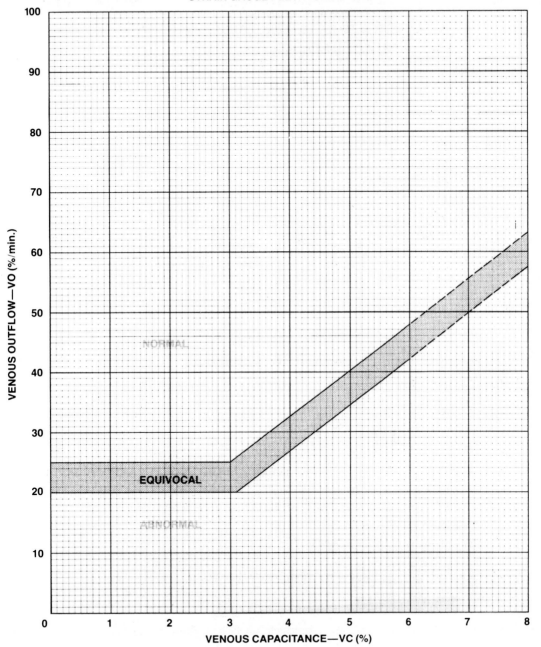

Figure 13–7. Venous outflow/venous capacitance (VO/VC) discriminant line chart based on Cramer's study; used for venous strain gauge plethysmography.

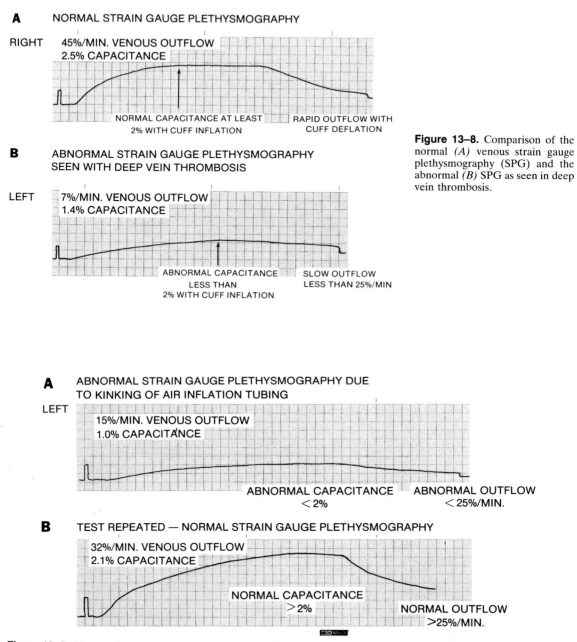

Figure 13–8. Comparison of the normal *(A)* venous strain gauge plethysmography (SPG) and the abnormal *(B)* SPG as seen in deep vein thrombosis.

Figure 13–9. Abnormal venous strain gauge plethysmography resulting from tube kinking *(A)* and the normal repeated study *(B)*.

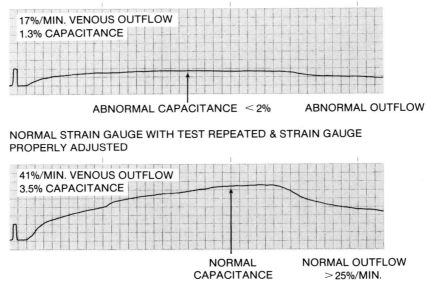

A ABNORMAL STRAIN GAUGE DUE TO TIGHT STRAIN GAUGE

17%/MIN. VENOUS OUTFLOW
1.3% CAPACITANCE

ABNORMAL CAPACITANCE < 2%   ABNORMAL OUTFLOW

B NORMAL STRAIN GAUGE WITH TEST REPEATED & STRAIN GAUGE
PROPERLY ADJUSTED

41%/MIN. VENOUS OUTFLOW
3.5% CAPACITANCE

NORMAL   NORMAL OUTFLOW
CAPACITANCE   > 25%/MIN.
>2%

Figure 13–10. Abnormal venous strain gauge plethysmography resulting from a tight strain gauge *(A)* and the normal repeated study with the strain gauge properly adjusted *(B)*.

11). Capacitance values will be normal with movement artifacts but will be greatly increased if the patient sits.

4. Patient placing the extremity in a stretched position produces tautness and compression of the venous vessels, resulting in diminished capacitance and outflow (Fig. 13–12*A* and *B*).

5. Placement of the strain gauge over an artery, resulting in a pulsating curve (Fig. 13–13).

Strain gauge plethysmography can be performed only on a patient who can assume the correct position and maintain a relaxed state for the duration of the examination, which usually requires 15 to 20 minutes.

In addition to the technical limitations, there are other limiting factors that should be considered, with appropriate corrective measures taken.

In patients with recurring DVT or chronic venous disease, the SPG will often produce equivocal results (Fig. 13–14). As mentioned earlier, we routinely back up the indirect noninvasive testing procedures with a direct noninvasive testing procedure. In this case, the Doppler examination was performed, which clearly demonstrated a patent deep venous system with secondary venous incompetency. Doppler or duplex scanning will provide a good assessment of chronic venous disorders and verify the SPG results.

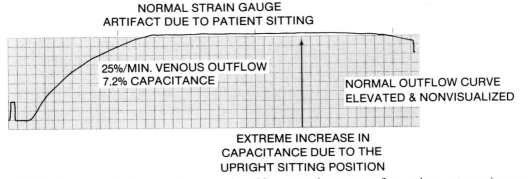

NORMAL STRAIN GAUGE
ARTIFACT DUE TO PATIENT SITTING

25%/MIN. VENOUS OUTFLOW
7.2% CAPACITANCE

NORMAL OUTFLOW CURVE
ELEVATED & NONVISUALIZED

EXTREME INCREASE IN
CAPACITANCE DUE TO THE
UPRIGHT SITTING POSITION

Figure 13–11. Venous strain gauge plethysmography with a normal venous outflow and an extreme increase in capacitance caused by the patient sitting up.

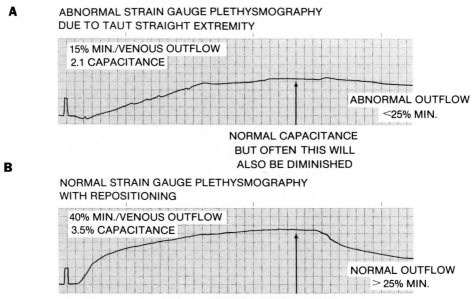

Figure 13–12. Abnormal venous strain gauge plethysmography resulting from a straight taut extremity and compression of the veins *(A)*. Repeated examination is normal after repositioning *(B)*.

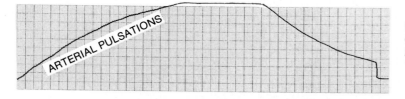

NORMAL STRAIN GAUGE PLETHYSMOGRAPHY

Figure 13–13. Arterial pulsations demonstrated by placing the strain gauge over an artery.

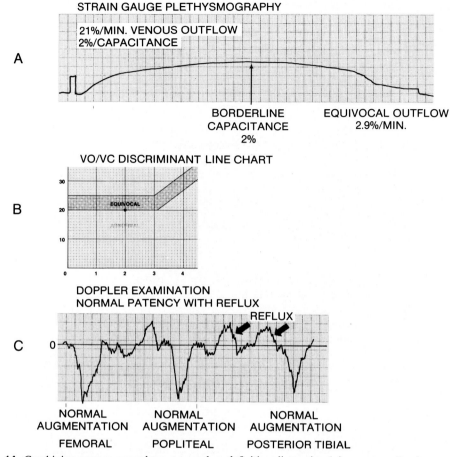

Figure 13–14. Combining venous procedures to reach a definitive diagnosis. *A* is an example of an equivocal strain gauge examination using the venous outflow/venous capacitance (VO/VC) discriminant line chart *(B)*. The Doppler examination *(C)* demonstrates patency with normal augmentation and reflux resulting from chronic venous disease.

Nonocclusive thrombi are not always defined by SPG when the venous system is patent. Depending upon the re-canalization and collateral flow patterns, the SPG may fall in an equivocal or normal pattern. Combining SPG with other noninvasive procedures will provide a more definitive diagnosis. Some venous examinations will be more complex because of problems with the patient (e.g., obesity, inability to maintain position) or because of chronic disease or equipment-related problems. Figure 13–15A illustrates a normal SPG of both the right and left lower extremities. Doppler correlation (Fig. 13–15B) demonstrated DVT of the left femoral vein; duplex scanning illustrated left femoral obstruction with extensive collateral flow, which produced the equivocal results (Figs. 13–16 and 13–17).

External compression of the venous system can also produce a false-positive result. This external compression may be due to tumors, hematomas, Baker's cysts, or lymph nodes. The SPG will reflect equivocal or abnormal results because of compression of the veins restricting the venous flow. However, the direct testing procedures (Doppler or duplex scanning) will confirm the patency. Duplex scanning is preferred because the compression structures can be visualized. Figures 13–18 through 13–20 demonstrate SPG and duplex scanning of lymph node compression of the venous system. The lymph nodes were visualized, and normal flow was documented in the compressed veins.

Strain gauge plethysmography is very accurate in determining patency of the venous system in the major veins, which include the iliac, femoral, and popliteal, and provides a safe, reliable method of screening patients for DVT. However, its limitations must be considered in patients with chronic venous disease and during the more

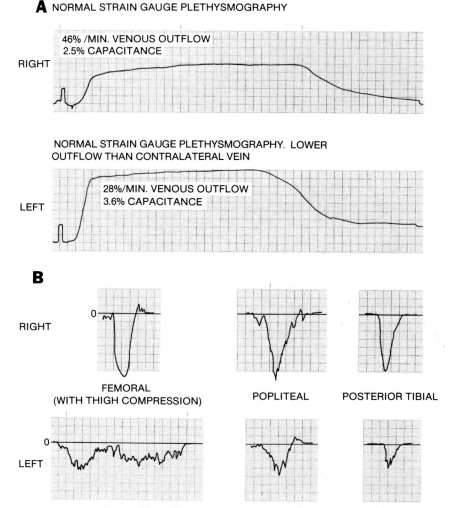

A NORMAL STRAIN GAUGE PLETHYSMOGRAPHY

46% /MIN. VENOUS OUTFLOW
2.5% CAPACITANCE

RIGHT

NORMAL STRAIN GAUGE PLETHYSMOGRAPHY. LOWER
OUTFLOW THAN CONTRALATERAL VEIN

28%/MIN. VENOUS OUTFLOW
3.6% CAPACITANCE

LEFT

B

RIGHT

0

FEMORAL
(WITH THIGH COMPRESSION)   POPLITEAL   POSTERIOR TIBIAL

0

LEFT

Figure 13–15. An example of a normal strain gauge plethysmography, *(A)* produced by extensive collateralization. The Doppler venous examination *(B)* provided the definitive diagnosis of left deep vein thrombosis resulting from the lack of venous flow and augmentation.

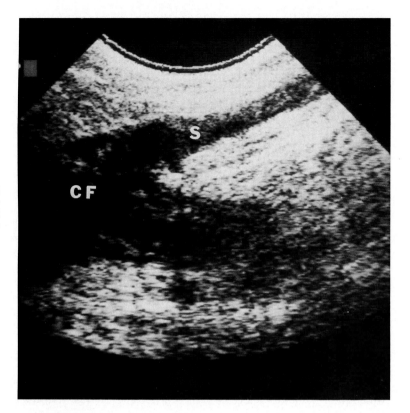

Figure 13–16. Real-time longitudinal view of the femoral veins demonstrating low-level echoes that represent deep vein thrombosis. CF = Common femoral; S = saphenous.

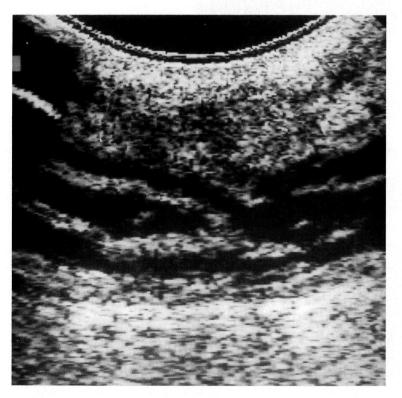

Figure 13–17. Real-time longitudinal view of the collateral vessels.

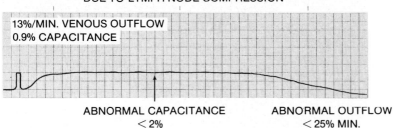

ABNORMAL STRAIN GAUGE PLETHYSMOGRAPHY
DUE TO LYMPH NODE COMPRESSION

13%/MIN. VENOUS OUTFLOW
0.9% CAPACITANCE

ABNORMAL CAPACITANCE
< 2%

ABNORMAL OUTFLOW
< 25% MIN.

Figure 13–18. Abnormal venous strain gauge plethysmography resulting from lymph node compression.

complex examinations. We recommend using multiple noninvasive procedures for a thorough assessment and a more definitive diagnosis.

Doppler Techniques

Some of the most important uses of the Doppler ultrasound blood flow detector were pioneered at the University of Washington by Dr. Eugene Strandness and his coworkers.[9] Doppler ultrasonography detects the motion of particles (red blood cells) in such a way that the pitch of the signals is related to the velocity of motion, which can then be heard and recorded. The

examination can be performed in the vascular laboratory or at the patient's bedside. Because of portability and ease of operation, the Doppler examination is an ideal technique for use in specialized areas such as surgery, recovery, intensive care, or angiographic suites.

A continuous, bi-directional unit with an analog strip chart recorder is used for demonstrating patency of the venous system. A bi-directional unit is not necessary for demonstrating patency of the venous system; this can be done with a simple hand-held unidirectional unit. However, to assess the venous system and venous reflux completely, the bi-directional unit is a necessity. The transducer is a small hand-held device hous-

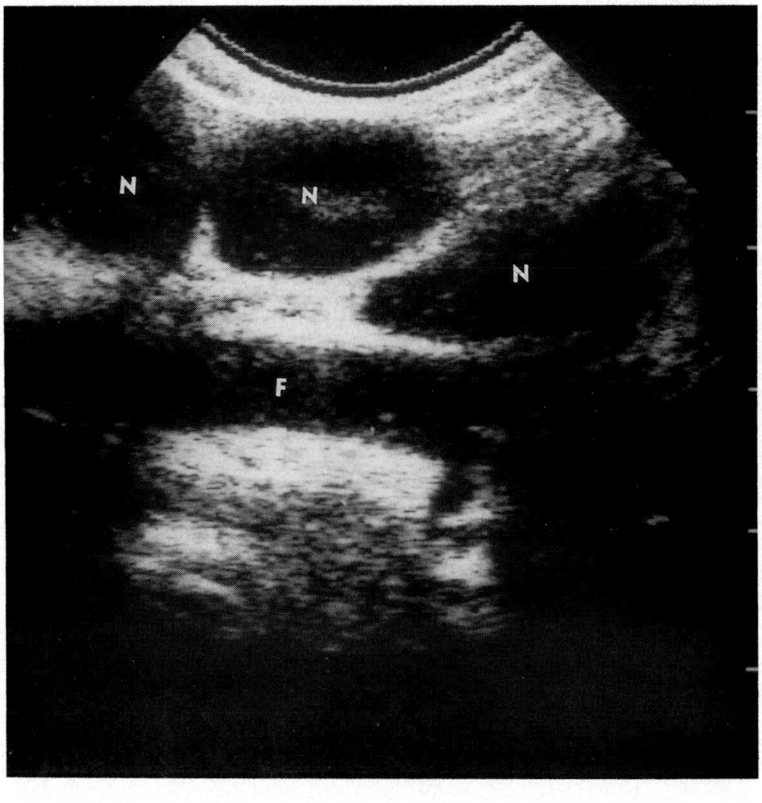

Figure 13–19. Real-time longitudinal view of the femoral vein (F) with lymph node (N) compression. Patency of the femoral vein was confirmed with the duplex scan shown in Figure 13–20.

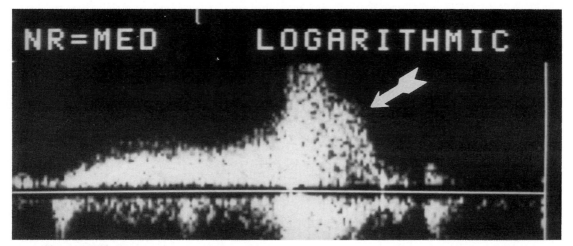

Figure 13–20. Duplex spectral analysis demonstrates a normal venous flow with augmentation (arrow).

ing two piezoelectric crystals: one for sending soundwaves and one for receiving soundwaves. Frequencies usually range from 5 to 10 MHz, with higher frequencies used for examination of the superficial vessels and lower frequencies for the deeper vessels. The strip chart recorder is calibrated with a 1 kHz negative deflection (Fig. 13–21). This calibration allows for quantitative measurement of the venous augmentation flow. The baseline is set at approximately 20 to 30 mm below the top margin of the recording paper to allow for positive reflux and negative venous deflections.

Examination Techniques

The patient is placed in a recumbent position with the torso elevated, thus allowing pooling of the venous blood in the lower extremities and enhancing the performance of the examination. The patient is turned slightly to the side being examined, and the knee is flexed. It is important that the leg be relaxed for ease of blood flow.

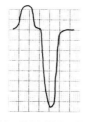

1 kHz CALIBRATION

Figure 13–21. Calibration of the strip chart recorder denoting a 1 kHz negative deflection.

The transducer is placed at a 45° angle to the vessel and towards the heart, producing a negative deflection. Because the angle cannot be visualized, it is determined by the sound pitch. The maximum pitch will indicate the correct angle. The examiner should lightly place the transducer on the skin surface because any excessive pressure can alter the flow. The sites of examination for the deep venous system include the posterior tibial, popliteal, superficial femoral, and common femoral veins. The superficial venous sites include the greater saphenous and the perforating veins.

Venous Qualities

Each examination site is examined for five venous qualities, which are illustrated in Figure 13–22.

1. **Spontaneity.** The venous sound is automatically elicited at the proper location. This holds true for all of the examination sites except the posterior tibial vein, which may be in a vasoconstricted state. Slight distal compressions may be necessary to localize the vein.

2. **Phasity.** The venous flow varies in pitch with respiration. In deep inhalation, the venous sounds discontinue but augment with expiration.

3. **Augmentation.** Compression maneuvers augment or increase the venous flow, which indicates the patency of the vein.

4. **Competency.** Proximal compression or a Valsalva maneuver will demonstrate the competency of the venous valves. Normal valves will demonstrate a negative deflection, whereas an incompetent vein will have both positive and negative deflections because of reflux.

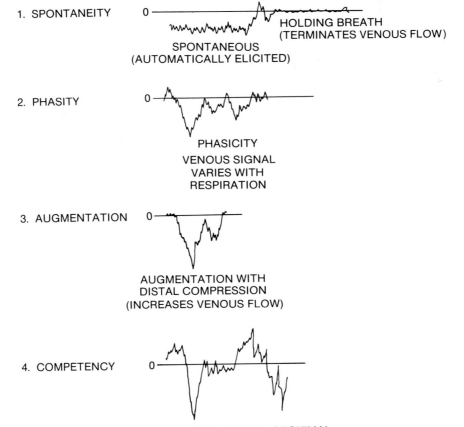

Figure 13–22. Diagrammatic illustration of the five venous qualities.

5. **Pulsatility.** Normally, there is no pulsatility with venous sounds. This occurs only with arterial sounds. In cases of venous hypertension or chronic heart failure and excessive fluid, pulsatility of the veins will occur.

It is important that the examiner become thoroughly familiar with the venous sounds and understand the nature of the signals. It is equally important that the sounds be recorded and available for inspection and interpretation. The veins exhibit a low-pitched, roaring, phasic sound, which varies with respiration and ceases with a deep breath-holding maneuver.

Figure 13–23 demonstrates the Doppler examination of the lower extremity venous system. Each vessel site is examined for the five venous qualities and documented. The veins are evalu-ated bilaterally for comparison values—the primary objective being demonstration of patency and competency.

Abnormal Findings

Normally, the venous flow is in one direction (towards the heart). However, when venous incompetency (reflux) is present, the venous flow will be heard in a forward and backward motion with proximal compression maneuvers (Figs. 13–24 and 13–25). Incompetency should be assessed in the deep and superficial systems to determine whether the condition is primary or secondary. The perforators can also be examined for competency by placing a tourniquet just below the knee to occlude the superficial system. The ex-

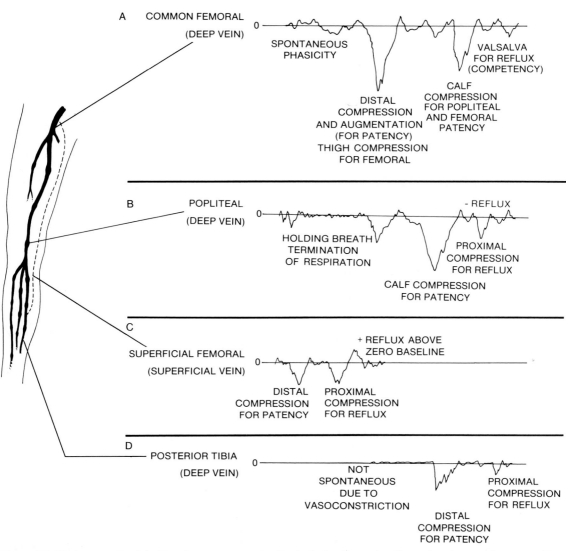

Figure 13–23. An example of the Doppler venous examination including the probe sites and analog waveform recordings using the venous qualities (A–D).

Figure 13–24. A normal Doppler venous study with negative augmentations (arrows).

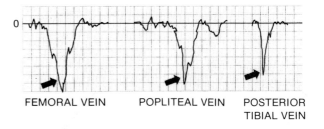

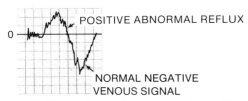

Figure 13–25. An abnormal venous waveform with positive deflection that is due to reflux.

aminer listens with the Doppler probe at the medial aspect of the lower leg while distal compressions are performed. There should be no sounds of reflux.

In patients with deep vein thrombosis, the venous flow will be greatly reduced or absent (Fig. 13–26). The signal below an obstructed vein will become continuous with a high-pitched "windstorm" effect that cannot be augmented (Fig. 13–27). This characteristic is a common finding and reflects the extent of venous hypertension that exists. When the vein is partially occluded by thrombus, this windstorm effect may be difficult to determine in some instances. Careful comparison with the contralateral side for augmentation values will verify any decrease in value. There may be some augmentation; however, it is usually harder to elicit, and the augmentation deflection will be decreased in comparison with the contralateral vein (Fig. 13–26). Duplex scanning can further identify this condition and should be used in any instance in which equivocal results or difficulties are encountered.

Another phenomenon associated with obstruction is collateralization. The collateral routes may vary and may be minimal or extensive, depending upon the type and degree of obstruction. The collateral routes may be confusing for the examiner and may be mistaken for a patent vessel. The collateral vessels usually are more continuous in nature, abnormally located, and difficult to compress. Figures 13–28 through 13–30 illustrate various collateral routes. They are much easier to document with duplex scanning. Figure

13–31 illustrates a duplex scan of the collateral vessels distal to the occlusion, and Figure 13–32 demonstrates a spectral analyzer recording of the continuous-waveform pattern with no augmentation and no respiratory motion.

Doppler techniques in our laboratory are combined with the indirect testing methods to evaluate the venous system. In patients evaluated for DVT, the Doppler is combined with the SPG examination. For venous incompetency, the Doppler techniques are combined with the photoplethysmography examination. The examinations are then compared for accuracy and diagnostic definition. If they do not correlate or if there are equivocal results, duplex scanning is required. The recordings and documentation are placed on a worksheet for interpretation and reporting. The venous worksheet is illustrated in Figure 13–33.

Photoplethysmography

Photoplethysmography provides a qualitative measurement of the venous refilling time after exercise. Early studies using the PPG to measure the venous recovery time and assess the veins for competency were performed by Barnes.[10] The accuracy of the PPG was later validated against direct venous pressure measurements in a study by Abramowitz and colleagues.[11] Photoplethysmography is now an accepted method of assessing venous refilling time and incompetency.

Photoplethysmography does not measure volume changes as does strain gauge plethysmography. Photoplethysmography records the flow in the cutaneous region by means of a photoelectric cell. The photoelectric cell emits an infrared light from a light-emitting diode into the subcutaneous tissue. In turn, the backscattered light is received by the photoelectric detector. Both PPG and SPG can be used to record venous refilling time; however, we use PPG because of its simplicity.

A ABNORMAL DECREASED AUGMENTATION DUE TO OBSTRUCTION

B

NORMAL

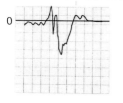

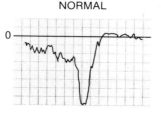

Figure 13–26. An example of deep vein thrombosis with decreased augmentation (A) and the normal augmentation for comparison (B).

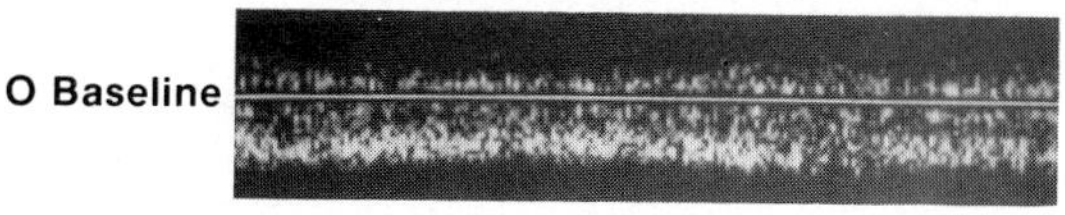

Figure 13–27. Spectral analysis of a continuous, high-pitched venous signal.

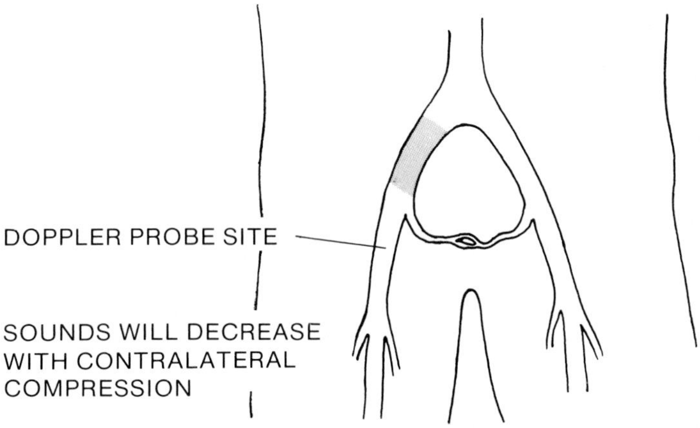

O Baseline

DOPPLER PROBE SITE

SOUNDS WILL DECREASE
WITH CONTRALATERAL
COMPRESSION

Figure 13–28. Iliac vein occlusion with a crossover collateral vessel. Occlusion indicated by shaded area.

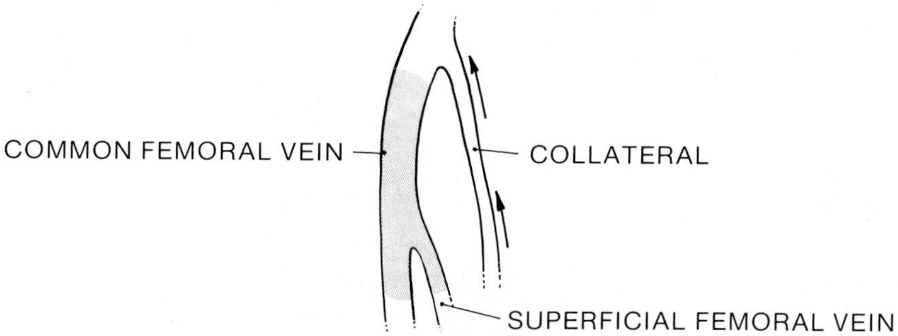

COMMON FEMORAL VEIN

COLLATERAL

SUPERFICIAL FEMORAL VEIN

Figure 13–29. Common femoral vein occlusion with a large accessory collateral vessel. There will be no sounds elicited at the site of obstruction (shaded area). The venous sounds will be located in an abnormal location. They will have a continuous, high-pitched sound that does not augment easily and is not phasic with respiration.

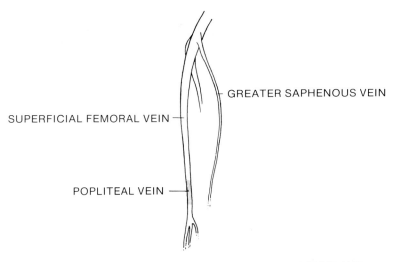

SUPERFICIAL FEMORAL VEIN —|

GREATER SAPHENOUS VEIN

POPLITEAL VEIN —|

Figure 13–30. Popliteal vein occlusion with a greater saphenous vein as collateral. Occlusion indicated by shaded area.

POPLITEAL VENOUS SOUNDS WILL BE ABSENT AND
VENOUS FLOW WILL BE FOUND MORE
LATERAL THAN NORMAL. THE SOUND WILL
BE HIGHER IN PITCH WITH NO PHASITY
AND MAY ALSO BE CONTINUOUS.

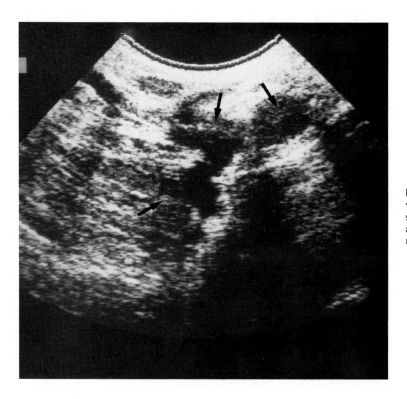

Figure 13–31. Real-time longitudinal view of the collateral vessels demonstrating multiple irregular anechoic areas in an abnormal location (arrows).

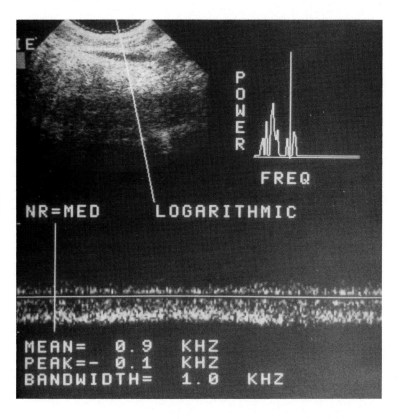

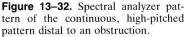

Figure 13–32. Spectral analyzer pattern of the continuous, high-pitched pattern distal to an obstruction.

Examination Techniques

The patient is placed in a sitting position with the lower extremities hanging unencumbered at a 90° angle. The PPG photoelectric cell sensor is attached bilaterally to the skin surface of the medial lower leg (Figs. 13–34 and 13–35). The sensor is placed approximately 6 cm above the malleolus. The position is not critical and may need to be altered if ulcerations are present. The photoplethysmograph is set on the direct current venous mode with the dual strip chart recorder running at 5 mm/sec. The recorder is centered 10 mm below the top margin. The patient is instructed to exercise the lower extremities by dorsiflexing the feet five times. If the patient is unable to exercise the feet and empty the veins sufficiently, the examiner can squeeze the calf muscles. The patient relaxes after the exercise maneuver to allow venous refilling, which is expressed in the refilling curve as seen in Figure 13–36. The recovery time from the end of the exercise to the leveling of the refill time is calculated. In normal patients, the venous refilling time is 20 seconds or greater. If the venous refilling time is less than 20 seconds, this is considered abnormal, indicating valvular incompetency (Fig. 13–37). The procedure is repeated

with a tourniquet placed just below the knees to occlude the superficial venous system. The application of the tourniquet will determine whether the incompetency is primary (superficial system) or secondary (deep venous system). If the venous refilling time becomes normal (20 seconds or more) after application of the tourniquet, superficial incompetency (Fig. 13–38) is indicated. If the venous refilling time remains abnormal, the deep venous system is incompetent (Fig. 13–39). This determination will aid in deciding the course of treatment and whether surgical procedures are indicated.

Photoplethysmography is a simple, reliable method of assessing valve patency and venous refilling time. However, caution should be exercised to avoid artifacts and to ensure the quality of the examination. Artifacts can occur with improper exercising, misplacement of the photoelectric cell, and tense muscles or undefined curves. A few examples are illustrated in Figures 13–40 and 13–41.

In our laboratory, PPG is routinely correlated with Doppler ultrasound to enhance the diagnostic accuracy. Currently, studies are being conducted using the duplex scanner to document valvular status. For the Doppler examination, the patient is placed in a supine position with the

Text continued on page 204

PERIPHERAL VENOUS EXAMINATION

Hospital No. _____

Patient's Name _____

Date _____

Strain Gauge Plethysmography

Duplex Imaging

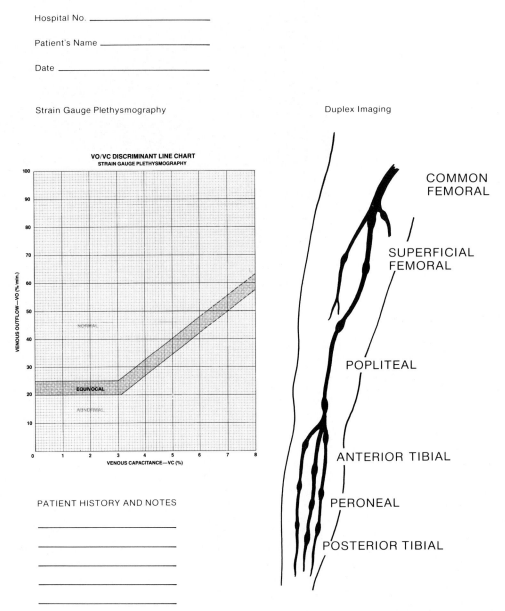

VO/VC DISCRIMINANT LINE CHART
STRAIN GAUGE PLETHYSMOGRAPHY

VENOUS OUTFLOW—VO (%/min.)

VENOUS CAPACITANCE—VC (%)

NORMAL

EQUIVOCAL

ABNORMAL

COMMON FEMORAL

SUPERFICIAL FEMORAL

POPLITEAL

ANTERIOR TIBIAL

PERONEAL

POSTERIOR TIBIAL

PATIENT HISTORY AND NOTES

_____
_____
_____
_____
_____

Figure 13–33. An example of the venous worksheet. The waveform recordings are attached to the back.

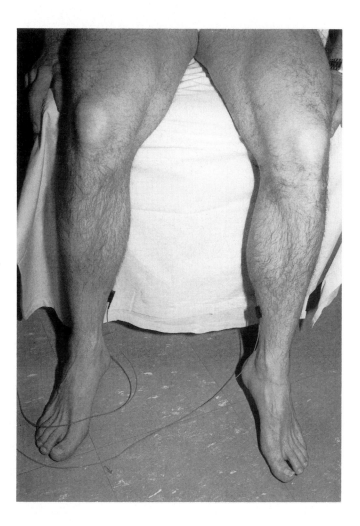

Figure 13–34. Bilateral placement of the photoplethysmography photocells.

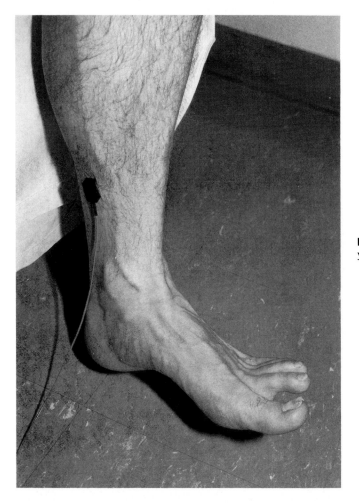

Figure 13–35. Enlarged view of the photoplethysmography photocell placement.

Figure 13–36. Normal bilateral photoplethysmography examination.

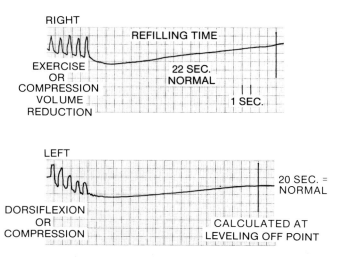

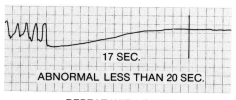

Figure 13–37. An abnormal photoplethysmograph indicating venous incompetency.

PHOTOPLETHYSMOGRAPHY DEMONSTRATION OF SUPERFICIAL
VENOUS INCOMPETENCY

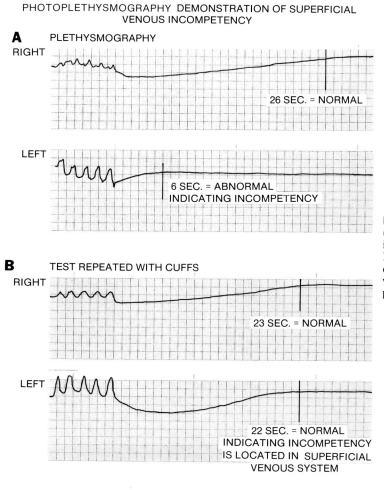

A PLETHYSMOGRAPHY
RIGHT

26 SEC. = NORMAL

LEFT

6 SEC. = ABNORMAL
INDICATING INCOMPETENCY

B TEST REPEATED WITH CUFFS
RIGHT

23 SEC. = NORMAL

LEFT

22 SEC. = NORMAL
INDICATING INCOMPETENCY
IS LOCATED IN SUPERFICIAL
VENOUS SYSTEM

Figure 13–38. Photoplethysmography (PPG) without cuffs *(A)* demonstrates incompetency in the left venous system. Repeat PPG examination with a tourniquet *(B)* indicates a normal refilling time, which verifies superficial venous incompetency.

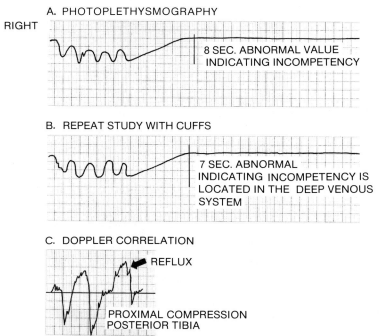

A. PHOTOPLETHYSMOGRAPHY

RIGHT

8 SEC. ABNORMAL VALUE INDICATING INCOMPETENCY

B. REPEAT STUDY WITH CUFFS

7 SEC. ABNORMAL INDICATING INCOMPETENCY IS LOCATED IN THE DEEP VENOUS SYSTEM

C. DOPPLER CORRELATION

REFLUX

PROXIMAL COMPRESSION POSTERIOR TIBIA

Figure 13–39. Deep venous incompetency. *A,* The photoplethysmography examination demonstrates abnormal refilling time, suggesting venous incompetency. *B,* The repeat examination with a tourniquet remains abnormal, indicating deep vein incompetency. *C,* The Doppler study further verifies the deep venous incompetency.

torso elevated so that the blood will pool in the lower extremities. Examination sites include the common femoral, superficial femoral, popliteal, greater saphenous, perforator, and posterior tibial veins. These sites are used to evaluate the superficial and deep systems.

To determine incompetency (reflux), the transducer probe is placed 45° cephalad to the vessel. Proximal compression maneuvers are performed at each of the vessel sites except the common femoral site, where the Valsalva maneuver is used. Normally, venous flow will be heard as a single sound in one direction towards the heart

and expressed on the analog waveform as a negative deflection. In abnormal veins with reflux, there will be two sounds heard: one as the compression forces the blood backward through the incompetent valve and another as the compression is released and blood flows normally.

The reflux is also documented on the chart strip recording as a positive deflection, whereas the normal venous flow is documented as a negative deflection. Because arterial flow is also recorded as a positive deflection, reflux should be labeled on the paper recording. Absence of

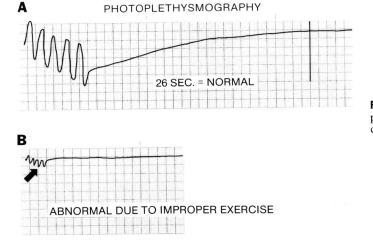

A   PHOTOPLETHYSMOGRAPHY

26 SEC. = NORMAL

B

ABNORMAL DUE TO IMPROPER EXERCISE

Figure 13–40. Normal photoplethysmography *(A)* compared with abnormal findings caused by improper exercise *(B).*

PHOTOPLETHYSMOGRAPHY

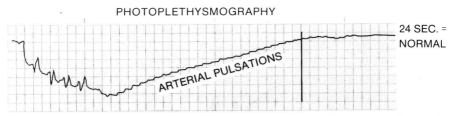

24 SEC. = NORMAL

ARTERIAL PULSATIONS

Figure 13–41. Photoplethysmography examination with photocell placed over the artery, causing arterial pulsations.

reflux should also be noted for the convenience of the interpreter. Examples of reflux are seen in Figures 13–42 and 13–43 using PPG and Doppler correlation.

Duplex Venous Imaging

Venous imaging using a duplex system is quickly becoming the state of the art for venous evaluations. Duplex scanning provides a direct assessment of the veins by combining anatomical information with hemodynamic data. The first successful attempt to visualize the venous system using real-time imaging was reported by Talbot in 1982. This was followed by studies using the duplex scanner and, even more recently, the color-coded duplex scan systems.

The traditional gold standards for evaluating the venous system are contrast venography and venous pressure measurements; however, be-

cause of the expense and discomfort to the patient, noninvasive methods have evolved. The traditional methods of noninvasive examinations include strain gauge plethysmography, photoplethysmography, and Doppler techniques. These are still in use and provide rapid, simple assessment of the venous system. However, artifacts and the limitations of the examinations must be borne in mind, and, in order to correct discrepancies, the duplex system can be a valuable tool. As previously mentioned, we use at least two of the noninvasive venous procedures, often combining the indirect tests (SPG and PPG) with the direct methods of testing (Doppler and duplex).

Duplex imaging utilizes a high-resolution imaging system combined with Doppler techniques. It is preferable to have continuous and pulse-gated capabilities incorporated into one scanhead. The continuous mode can search for ve-

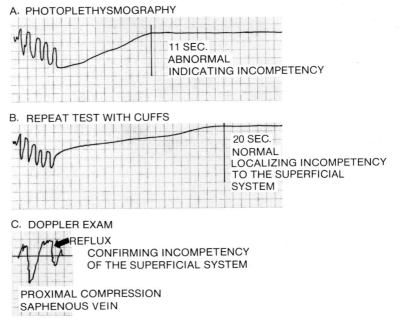

Figure 13–42. Superficial venous incompetency. *A*, Photoplethysmography (PPG) demonstrating incompetency. *B*, Repeated PPG with a tourniquet becomes normal, indicating superficial venous incompetency. *C*, Doppler examination further verifies the diagnosis by demonstrating the positive reflux (arrow) in the superficial veins.

A. PHOTOPLETHYSMOGRAPHY

11 SEC. ABNORMAL INDICATING INCOMPETENCY

B. REPEAT TEST WITH CUFFS

20 SEC. NORMAL LOCALIZING INCOMPETENCY TO THE SUPERFICIAL SYSTEM

C. DOPPLER EXAM

REFLUX CONFIRMING INCOMPETENCY OF THE SUPERFICIAL SYSTEM

PROXIMAL COMPRESSION SAPHENOUS VEIN

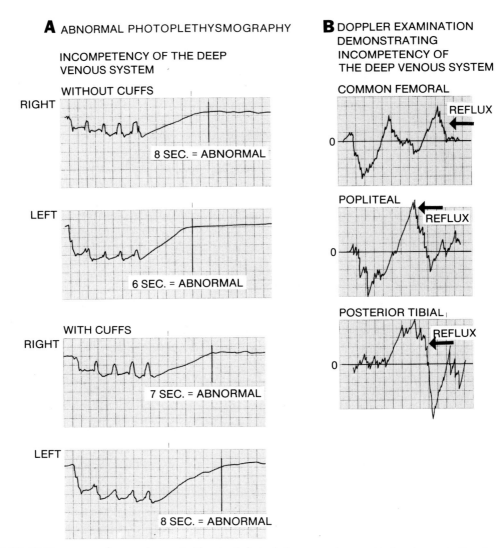

Figure 13–43. Deep venous incompetency. *A*, Abnormal photoplethysmography examination demonstrating deep venous incompetency. *B*, The Doppler examination confirms the diagnosis with positive reflux in the deep veins (arrows).

nous sounds by using Doppler techniques; the gated sample volume can be used to discriminate between the arterial and venous vessels. The identification and localization of specific veins often constitute a problem in venous imaging because the vessels frequently overlap.

Examination Techniques

Either 7.5 or 10 MHz frequency is used for imaging, whereas either 4.5 or 5 MHz is used for detecting blood flow. The 10 MHz frequency provides excellent detail and resolution; however, difficulties arise in visualizing deeper vessels with the short focal length of the 10 MHz frequency. We recommend using a 7.5 MHz fre-

quency for deeper structures to provide adequate penetration. The time-gain compensation curves, along with the power controls, are adjusted to identify the veins as sonolucent vessels with fine echogenic particles moving in a cephalad direction. The normal flow should always be labeled on the film so that it will not be confused with a thrombus-filled lumen, as could easily happen when viewing still photography (Figs. 13–44 and 13–45). The valves will be seen as thin, membranous structures rapidly opening and closing. Adjustments in the near field curve may have to be made to demonstrate the fine echogenic structure properly (Fig. 13–46). In cases of fresh thrombus, power gains will have to be altered during the examination because thrombi may appear either

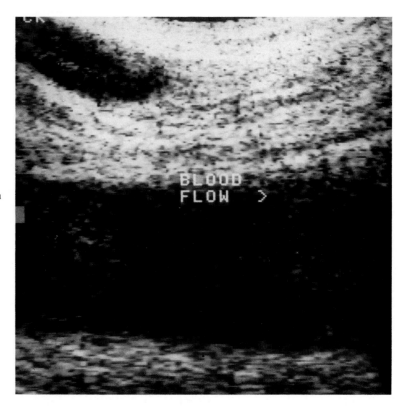

Figure 13–44. Real-time sonogram of the vein with blood flow.

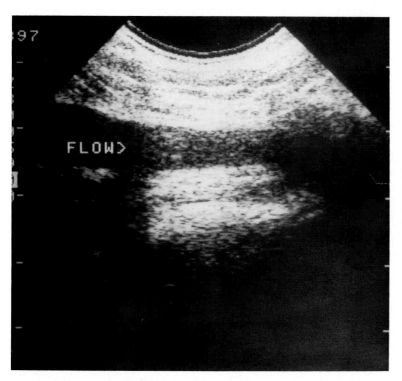

Figure 13–45. Real-time sonogram of the deep vein with increased power levels enhancing the flow pattern. The blood flow is labeled because this could mimic a thrombus-filled lumen.

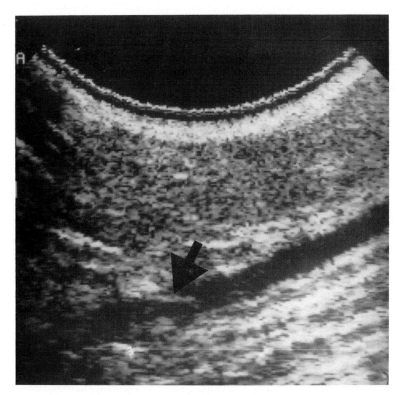

Figure 13–46. Real-time sonogram of the venous valve (arrow).

sonolucent or may contain low-level echoes. The Doppler mode with spectral analysis is set to hear the venous flow profiles adequately and to display the venous flow in a negative deflection (Fig. 13–47).

Various techniques and positions have been described for visualization of the venous system. These include examining the patient in a supine, sitting, or standing position. We prefer to image the veins with the patient in a supine, recumbent position. If the calf veins are difficult to visualize, a sitting position is required and a tourniquet may be applied, thus making visualization easier.

To begin the examination, the patient is placed in the supine position with the hip slightly externally rotated. The knee is slightly flexed to relax the leg and to ease muscle tension. The examination begins at the common femoral vein in a transverse position. Scanning is performed in a normal, relaxed state with light compression techniques. Compression is achieved by applying light transducer pressure on the vein while scanning, which normally will decrease the diameter substantially and verify patency of the vessel (Figs. 13–48 and 13–49).

Just inferior to the common femoral vein, the saphenous femoral junction can be visualized, identifying the superficial femoral, the deep fem-

oral, and the saphenous veins (Figs. 13–50 and 13–51). The superficial vein can be followed down the extremity in a transverse projection using normal pressures and compression maneuvers to verify patency (Fig. 13–52). The popliteal vein is then visualized transversely in the popliteal fossa either from the posterior surface while the knee is flexed or in a prone position with the foot slightly elevated (Figs 13–53 and 13–54). From the popliteal vein, we continue transverse to the lower leg, identifying the trifurcation, which includes the anterior tibial (AT), posterior tibial (PT), and the peroneal veins (PV) (Figs. 13–55 and 13–56). The peroneal vein and posterior tibial vein are seen from the medial side in the calf area inferior to the saphenous vein. The anterior tibial vein is seen from the anterior side between the tibia and fibula (Figs. 13–57 and 13–58).

The superficial system can also be demonstrated by following the greater saphenous vein inferiorly (Fig. 13–59). The saphenous vein lies superficially, approximately 1.2 cm below the skin surface in the medial portion of the leg. This vein is often utilized in coronary bypass procedures and is routinely evaluated by noninvasive methods for patency. The perforators are not routinely visualized but can be assessed by apply-

Text continued on page 214

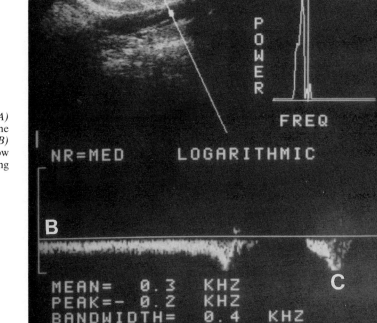

Figure 13–47. Duplex image *(A)* with the pulsed Doppler gated in the vein lumen. The spectral analyzer *(B)* demonstrates the normal venous flow with a negative projection increasing with augmentation *(C)*.

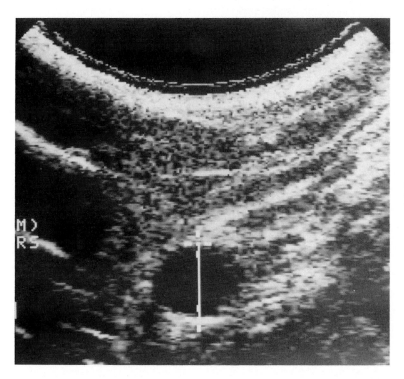

Figure 13–48. Transverse view of the deep femoral vein with cursor measuring the anteroposterior diameter.

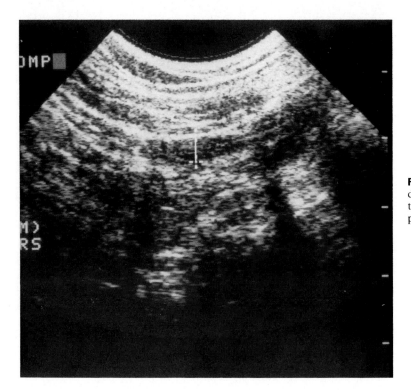

Figure 13–49. Transverse view of the deep femoral vein using compression to decrease the diameter and verify patency.

Figure 13–50. Anatomical cross-sectional diagram of the saphenous femoral junction.

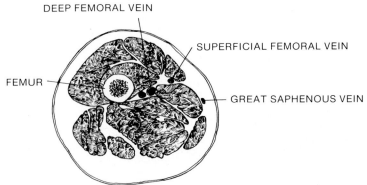

DEEP FEMORAL VEIN

SUPERFICIAL FEMORAL VEIN

FEMUR

GREAT SAPHENOUS VEIN

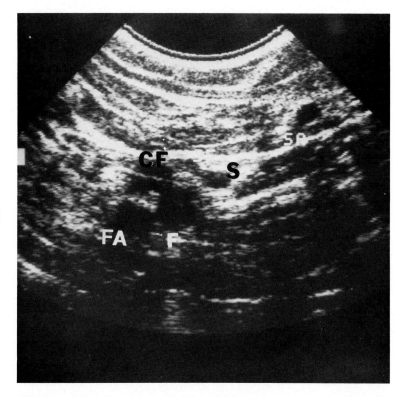

Figure 13–51. Cross-sectional image of the saphenous femoral junction. CF = Common femoral vein; FA = femoral artery; F = deep femoral vein; S = superficial femoral vein; SP = saphenous vein.

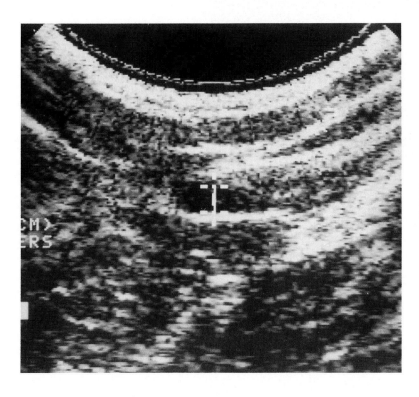

Figure 13–52. Cross-sectional view of the superficial femoral vein in the midthigh.

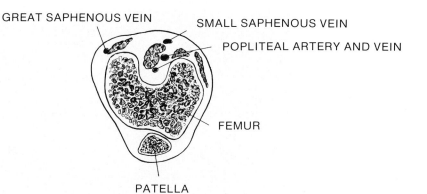

Figure 13–53. Cross-sectional anatomical diagram of the popliteal vein.

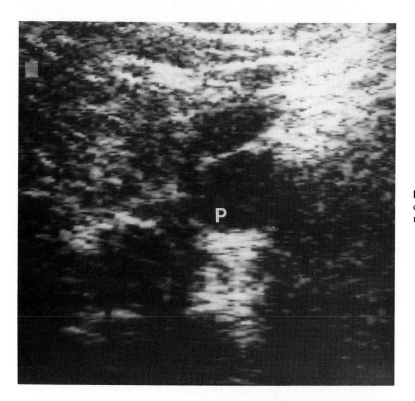

Figure 13–54. Cross-sectional view of the popliteal *(P)* vein in a normal, relaxed state.

Figure 13–55. Cross-sectional anatomical diagram of the lower leg identifying the posterior tibial and peroneal veins.

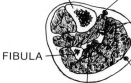

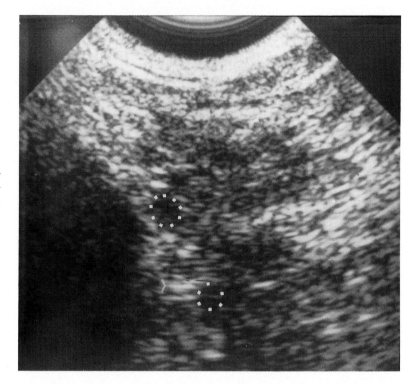

Figure 13–56. Cross-sectional view of the lower leg identifying the posterior tibial and the peroneal veins.

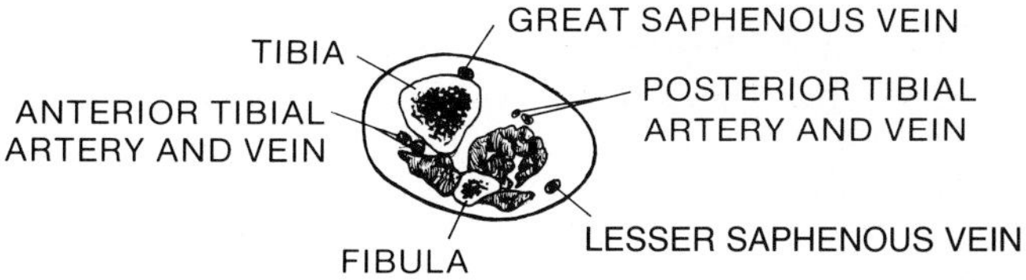

TIBIA

GREAT SAPHENOUS VEIN

ANTERIOR TIBIAL
ARTERY AND VEIN

POSTERIOR TIBIAL
ARTERY AND VEIN

FIBULA

LESSER SAPHENOUS VEIN

Figure 13–57. Cross-sectional anatomical diagram of the lower leg demonstrating the anterior tibial vein.

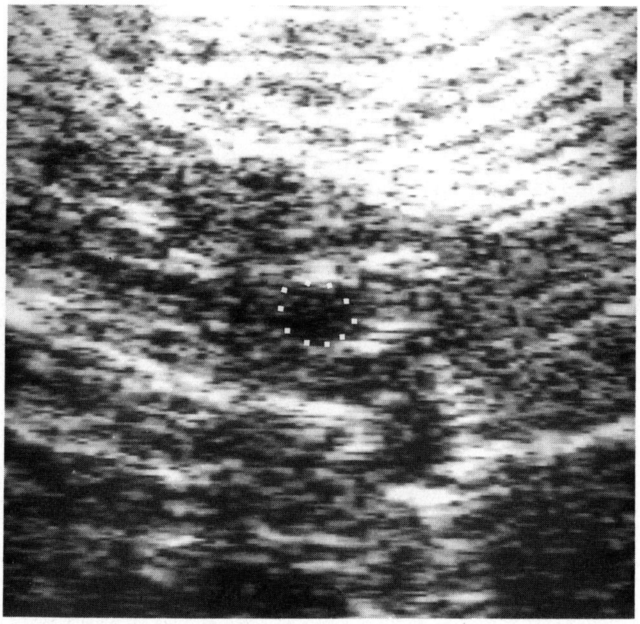

Figure 13–58. Cross-sectional view of the lower leg identifying the anterior tibial vein.

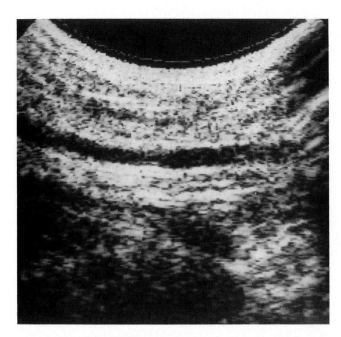

Figure 13–59. Real-time sonogram of the greater saphenous vein.

ing a tourniquet just below the knee and scanning the medial portion of the calf. Collateral flow patterns indicating disease states are easily identified because of their irregularity and location. In patients with obstruction, if collaterals have developed, the collateral system and its pattern of flow should be identified. Examples of various collateral patterns were given in the section on Doppler techniques. Duplex imaging is especially valuable because collateral flow can be mistaken for a patent vessel with Doppler examination alone. Figure 13–60 demonstrates collateral vessels that have developed secondary to deep vein thrombosis. Figure 13–61 depicts the superficial vein, which has become a collateral route secondary to deep vein thrombosis.

Longitudinal views may be obtained at primary sites. These primary sites include the following.

1. The common femoral vein and superficial femoral vein, including the bifurcation (Fig. 13–62).

2. The popliteal vein and its trifurcation (Fig. 13–63).

3. The saphenous vein (Fig. 13–64).

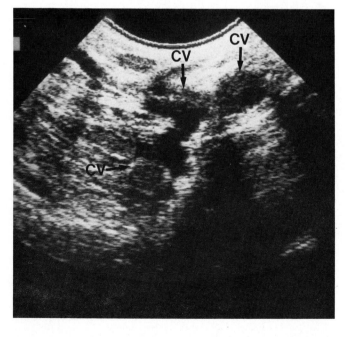

Figure 13–60. Real-time sonogram illustrating collateral vessels (CV), which were irregular in shape and located abnormally.

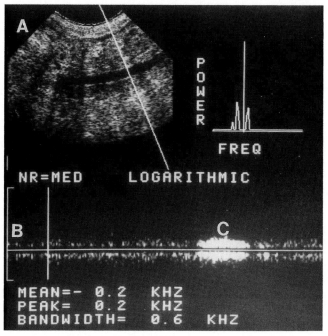

Figure 13–61. Duplex imaging *(A)* and Doppler spectral analysis *(B)* of the superficial vein, which has become a collateral vessel. The flow is a continuous, high-pitched sound with no augmentation *(C)*.

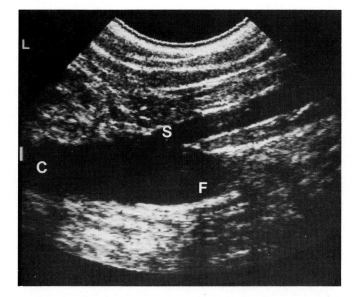

Figure 13–62. Real-time sonogram of the common femoral vein bifurcation. C = Common femoral vein; F = deep femoral vein; S = superficial femoral vein.

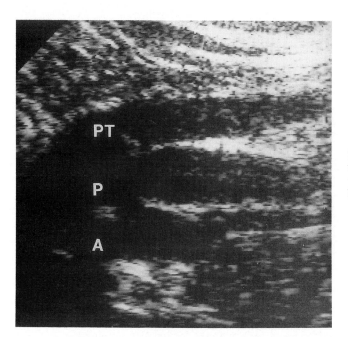

Figure 13–63. Real-time view of the venous trifurcation just inferior to the popliteal vein. A = Anterior tibial vein; P = peroneal vein; PT = posterior tibial vein.

Each site evaluation includes:

1. Visualization of the sonolucent vessel, with slightly echogenic blood flow profiles.

2. Doppler assessment of the flow profile for the routine qualities and augmentation maneuvers in order to determine patency.

3. Compression maneuvers with measurements in the normal and compressed states.

4. Observation of the general area to identify any masses, enlarged lymph nodes, or collateral vessels.

Normally, the veins demonstrate a patent vessel with a spontaneous flow pattern that is phasic with respiration. The veins are easily compressed, which further identifies patency (Fig. 13–65). The flow can be augmented by distal compression maneuvers, thus ruling out deep vein thrombosis. Valves can be identified as thin, echogenic mem-

Figure 13–64. Real-time sonogram of the greater saphenous vein.

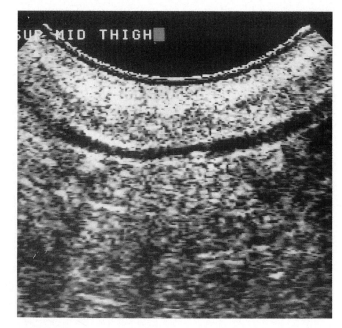

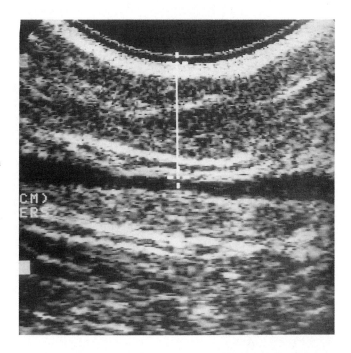

Figure 13–65. Real-time sonogram of a vein with compression.

branes rapidly opening and closing, as was seen in Figure 13–46. The valves are located predominantly in the lower part of the extremity, and the veins will be slightly bulbous at their locations.

Abnormal Findings

Deep vein thrombosis in a totally occluded state will present as an echogenic, filled lumen, usually complex in nature, which does not compress and has no Doppler venous sounds (Figs. 13–66 through 13–68). Figures 13–69 through 13–71 demonstrate occlusion of the deep femoral vein with patency of the common femoral and superficial femoral veins. The thrombus in the initial stage or "fresh clot" is somewhat sonolucent and an increase in gain is required for identification. The age of the clot is determined by the echogenicity, which increases with age. In

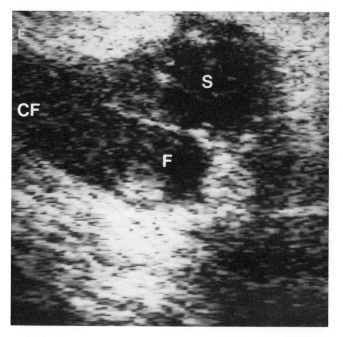

Figure 13–66. Real-time sonogram of the common femoral (CF), deep femoral (F), and superficial femoral (S) veins with total occlusion.

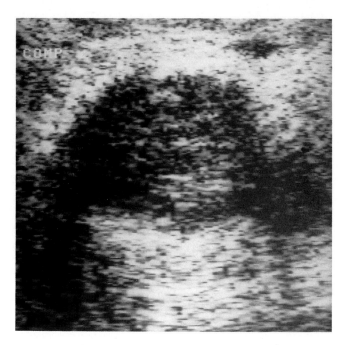

Figure 13–67. Transverse view of the common femoral vein thrombosis: A lumen filled with medium-level echoes that does not compress.

Figure 13–68. Spectral analysis of the femoral vein with absence of venous sounds.

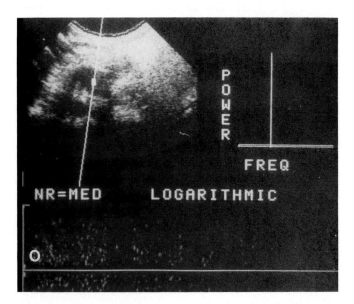

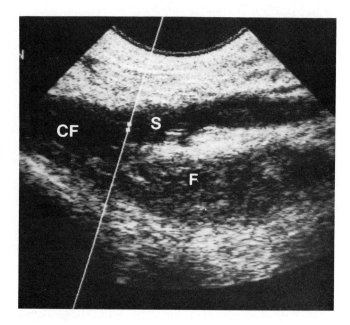

Figure 13–69. Real-time sonogram of the thrombus-filled femoral vein (F) and the patent superficial (S) and common femoral (CF) veins.

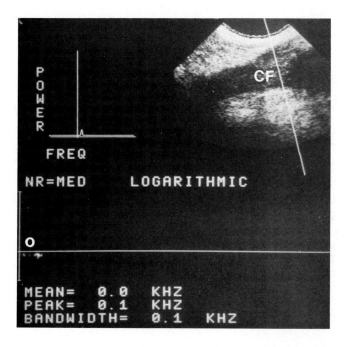

Figure 13–70. Spectral analysis of the femoral vein demonstrates no flow (0). CF = Common femoral vein.

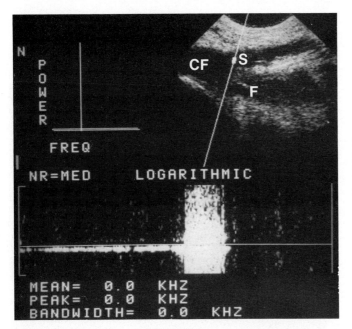

Figure 13–71. Duplex examination of the superficial (S) and common (CF) femoral veins identifies the venous flow and augmentation with compression maneuvers. F = Deep femoral vein.

the acute stage, the clot may be free-floating with a "tail" effect; the older clot is more echogenic or complex with collateral channels.

Partial obstruction will present as a partially fixed lumen that is very hard to compress, with limited closure and flow patterns around the thrombi (Figs. 13–72 and 13–73). When the partial obstruction is difficult to identify by SPG or Doppler, duplex scanning becomes the method of choice because it can visualize the partially occluded vessel and identify the flow patterns.

Collateral flow associated with occlusive states is marked by multiple irregular vessels that exhibit a continuous sound and do not augment. The collateral system may be a single vessel (e.g., superficial vein) or may be very extensive, depending upon the occlusive nature and the amount of time the collateral has had to develop. Careful scanning and observation should be made to determine these collateral routes.

The post-phlebitic state can also be determined by duplex scanning. Resolution of the clot can

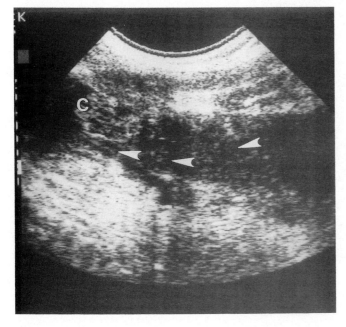

Figure 13–72. Real-time sonogram of the deep femoral vein, demonstrating partial clot formation (C) with a limited flow (arrows).

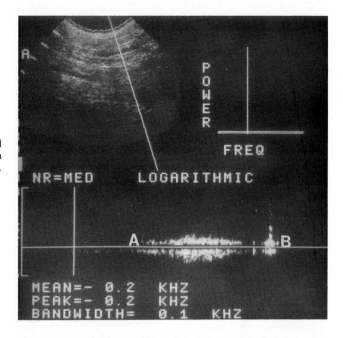

Figure 13–73. Spectral analysis of the deep femoral vein in the area of restricted flow demonstrates a minimal flow *(A)* with decreased augmentation *(B)*.

be followed and flow profiles demonstrated as patency of the vessel returns. In turn, the valves can be observed in order to demonstrate competency or incompetency following DVT episodes.

Compression of the venous system by external pressure from the lymph nodes, Baker's cysts, tumors, or hematomas often produces equivocal results on other noninvasive procedures by compressing the vessel and compromising the flow. This pathologic condition is easily demonstrated

by duplex scanning (Figs. 13–74, 13–75, and 13–76).

Primarily, duplex imaging of the venous system has been used for evaluation of DVT. Other uses include postoperative assessment of veins and in situ venous mapping of the veins for grafting and venous incompetency. Future trends will probably focus on more extensive evaluation of the entire venous system, especially in surgical patients, and evaluation of chronic venous disease.

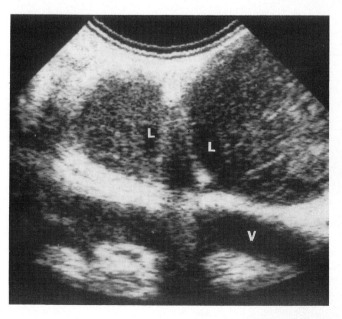

Figure 13–74. Real-time sonogram of enlarged lymph nodes (L) compressing the veins (V) and producing equivocal results on the strain gauge plethysmograph.

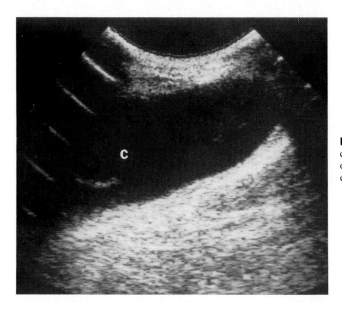

Figure 13–75. Real-time sonogram of a Baker's cyst (C), which can also produce abnormal results on the strain gauge plethysmographic and Doppler examinations.

Figure 13–76. Real-time sonogram of a hematoma (H), which causes compression of the vessels.

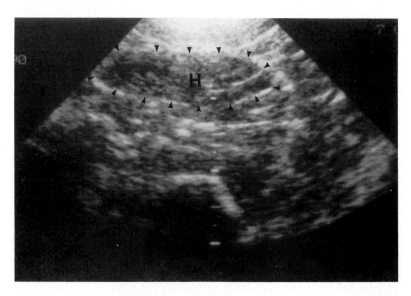

References

1. Bernstein E. Introduction. *In* Bernstein E (ed). Noninvasive diagnostic techniques: vascular disease. 3rd ed. St Louis, CV Mosby, 1985:1.
2. Yamada EM. Disorders of the peripheral vascular system. *In* Beyers M, Dudor S (eds). The clinical practice of medical surgical nursing. 2nd ed. Boston, Little, Brown & Co, 1984:590.
3. Horwitz O, Casey MP, Maslock MM. Venous thrombosis: pulmonary embolus complex. *In* McCombs RB (ed). Diseases of blood vessels. Philadelphia, Lea & Febiger, 1985:264.
4. Sufian S. Noninvasive vascular laboratory diagnosis of deep venous thrombosis. Am Surg 1981; 47:254.
5. Shaw L, Holland R, Englebrecht L, et al. Standardization of VO/VC curve using strain gauge plethysmography with vacuum deflation. Mountain View, Calif, MedaSonics (9-070584 DW).
6. Cramer MBS. The detection of proximal deep vein thrombosis by strain gauge plethysmography through the use of outflow/capacitance discriminant line. Bruit, vol. 7, December 1983.
7. Hokanson DE, Sumner DS, Strandness DE. An electrically calibrated plethysmograph for direct measurement of limb blood flow. Trans Biomed Eng 1975; 22:25–29.
8. Barnes RW. Noninvasive diagnostic techniques in peripheral vascular disease. Medical College of Virginia 1980; 4:140.
9. Strandness DE Jr, Sumner DS. Ultrasonic velocity detector in the diagnosis of thrombophlebitis. Arch Surg 1972; 104:180–183.
10. Barnes RW, Garrett WV, Hummel BA, et al. Photoplethysmographic assessment of altered cutaneous circulation in the postphlebitic syndrome. Technology in diagnosis and therapy. AAMI 13th Annual Meeting, 1978; 25.
11. Abramowitz HB, Queral LA, Flinn WR, et al. The use of PPG in the assessment of venous insufficiency: a comparison to venous measurements. Surgery 1979; 86:434.

14 • Lower Extremity Deep Vein Thrombosis

Introduction

Deep vein thrombosis (DVT) should be diagnosed and treated early to prevent the complications of pulmonary embolism and the sequelae of chronic venous insufficiency. Unfortunately, this is often difficult because the clinical symptoms and signs of DVT cannot be relied upon for determining the diagnosis. [1-6] Significant intraluminal thrombosis may be present in a patient with no physical symptoms, [7] and even unilateral limb swelling is an unreliable finding. [2] Studies have shown that not only are there no clinical signs or symptoms referable to the lower extremities in 50% of the patients with extensive thrombosis but in 33 to 55% of symptomatic patients there is also no venographic evidence of DVT. [1-3] An exception is the patient with phlegmasia cerulea dolens in whom the diagnosis of massive iliofemoral thrombosis is clinically obvious. However, this syndrome affects less than 1% of patients with symptomatic venous thrombosis.

It must be emphasized that patients with relatively minor symptoms and signs may have extensive DVT, whereas those with florid symptoms and signs suggesting extensive DVT frequently are shown to be free of this disorder upon objective testing. The nonspecificity of the clinical diagnosis makes it essential that the diagnosis of DVT be confirmed by other methods before starting treatment. Currently, the method used is *contrast venography*.

Contrast venography is highly accurate, but it has some severe limitations. These center around the invasiveness of the procedure. The placement of the needle in the foot vein can cause considerable patient discomfort, and there are situations in which this cannot be accomplished at all. For instance, given the patient with a swollen lower extremity, it may be most difficult, if not impossible, to find a suitable vein. Concern also exists about infection from the venipuncture and

chemical phlebitis from the injected contrast media. Although clinical studies have demonstrated an incidence of chemical phlebitis of only 2.3%, [8] radioactive fibrinogen uptake tests have indicated that it may be as high as 33%. [9]

Other less common complications include hypersensitivity reactions to the contrast media and local skin and tissue necrosis caused by extravasation of the contrast media at the injection site. Radiation exposure to the fetus precludes the routine use of contrast venography in pregnant patients. [10] Some patients are confined in intensive care units and cannot be taken to the radiology department for the examination. Others are outpatients who need to be screened for DVT. Logistically, it may be difficult to perform contrast venography on these patients in some centers. Consequently, patients with suspected DVT may be hospitalized and treated with heparin until venography can be done.

Because of these problems, there is considerable interest in the development of a noninvasive modality that can be used to diagnose DVT. As a result, a wide variety of these procedures have emerged over the past three decades. The following procedures will be discussed in this chapter.

• plethysmography
• Doppler ultrasonography
• real-time B-mode ultrasound imaging
• duplex scanning

The results obtained with each of these techniques have varied widely, and none has been conclusively shown to have sufficient accuracy to completely replace contrast venography in all instances. Contrast venography remains the gold standard to which other modalities must be compared because of its ability to consistently demonstrate a clear image of the offending thrombus. [11, 12] However, it should be noted that a 10% rate of error has been reported when the same venograms are reviewed by independent and equally experienced observers. [13]

Pathology

Detection of venous thrombosis is the primary goal of all these diagnostic modalities. A venous thrombus or phlebothrombosis consists of a total coagulation of blood in some predisposed segment of a vein. The thrombus that forms is much like that which occurs from the clotting of blood in a test tube. Venous thrombi are almost always occlusive and often form a quite accurate cast of the veins in which they arise. Plethysmography and Doppler ultrasonography rely on the venous obstruction for the diagnosis of thrombi; real-time B-mode ultrasonography relies on the image of the venous cast for the diagnosis. Duplex sonography uses both the obstruction and the cast formed by the thrombus in the diagnosis of DVT. Phlebothrombosis is found predominantly in the veins of the lower extremities. Ninety percent of the cases of phlebothrombosis occur in the leg veins in approximately the following order of frequency: deep calf, femoral, popliteal, and iliac veins. Venous thrombi appear to begin in the sinuses, behind the cusps of venous valves. Exactly why venous thrombi occur remains unknown. Some theories leading to phlebothrombosis include the presence of endothelial damage, blood flow stasis with eddy current formation, and the presence of a hypercoaguable state. A high risk of venous thrombosis is known to be associated with congestive heart failure, varicosities of the lower legs, severe burns, other forms of trauma, postoperative and postpartum states and disseminated cancer.

The evolution of a thrombus goes through three main phases regardless of its origin. These consist of (1) *inflammation*, (2) *organization*, and (3) *canalization*.

When a thrombus is formed, it acts as a foreign body and excites an inflammatory process in the underlying vein wall. The *inflammatory reaction* is followed by the invasion of fibroblasts and capillary buds into the thrombus. Eventually, the thrombus becomes converted into a mass of vascularized connective tissue referred to as an *organized thrombus*. As the capillaries progress, they anastomose to form channels that carry blood through the thrombus. The fibrous tissue contracts in the course of weeks to months until the thrombus is virtually incorporated within the vein wall as a fibrous lump or thickening. If a valve cusp is in the region of fibrous tissue contraction, it will be incorporated into the vein wall also and rendered incompetent. The *canalization phase* then leaves the vein as a valveless conduit through which blood can flow.

Plethysmography

Before real-time ultrasound, B-mode imaging, and duplex scanning were available, plethysmography was the principal method for objectively obtaining data on venous disease of the lower extremities. Plethysmography works by detecting volume changes in the calf of the lower extremity, which increase when blood is pooled in the deep leg veins and decrease as the blood is allowed to empty out of the deep leg veins. These volume changes can be evaluated by measuring the changes either in the calf circumference with a strain gauge or in the resistive impedance of the calf with electrodes.

Types of Plethysmography

Strain Gauge Plethysmography

Strain gauge plethysmography (SPG) is used to measure the changes in leg circumference by means of a small cuff-like device wrapped around the calf. This device is made from a fine-bore silicone rubber tube that is filled with mercury or a liquid metal alloy to form the strain gauge cuff, which can be placed around the calf to measure changes in its circumference. Because the electrical resistance of the liquid or mercury in this gauge is proportional to its length, a greater resistance is obtained when the strain gauge is elongated and a lesser value is obtained when it is shortened. These changes in the resistance of the gauge are then recorded for interpretation on a strip chart recorder.

Initially, the strain gauge is placed around the calf, as shown in Figure 14–1*A*, and the plethysmographic curve is calibrated to the baseline level. Next, blood is pooled in the calf veins by the inflation of a pneumatic cuff placed above the knee and around the thigh, as shown in Figure 14–1*B*. With the strip chart recorder running, the thigh cuff is quickly inflated to 50 mm Hg. The resultant venous pooling expands the calf veins and increases the calf volume, which elongates the strain gauge. As the strain gauge elongates, its resistance increases, as shown by the upslope of the curve of the plethysmograph in Figure 14–1*B*.

The curve reaches a plateau when the venous pressure exceeds the cuff occlusion pressure and the calf veins cease to be filled by blood pumped into them from the arterial circulation. This segment of the curve is also termed the *venous capacitance* (VC), indicating the point at which full expansion of the calf veins with pooled blood is achieved. It is measured on the plethysmo-

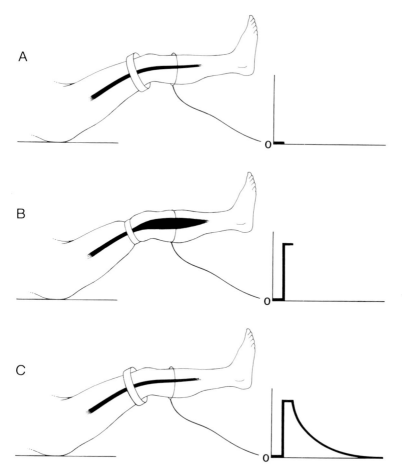

Figure 14–1. Line drawing of strain gauge plethysmographic method of detecting calf volume changes.

A, Strain gauge placed around calf and pressure cuff placed around thigh. Strip chart recorder calibrated to baseline level.

B, Thigh cuff inflated, pooling blood in the expanding calf veins. Calf volume increases, elongating strain gauge and causing a curve upslope that levels off in a plateau of maximum venous filling or venous capacitance (VC).

C, Thigh cuff released; blood in the calf veins flows out into popliteal and femoral veins, decreasing the calf volume. The strain gauge shortens, causing the curve to slope downward to the baseline level during the venous outflow (VO) phase.

graph as the height in millimeters from the initial baseline to the plateau two minutes after the thigh cuff is inflated. Generally, this is compared with an electrical standard, with each 10 mm rise in the curve representing a 1% volume increase in the calf size. A 2 to 3% volume increase or an elevation in the height of the plateau 20 to 30 mm above the baseline level is considered within the normal range.

Once the plateau of venous capacitance is reached, the cuff is released and the blood pooled in the expanded calf veins is allowed to flow out into the popliteal and femoral veins. The emptying of the leg veins then decreases the calf volume and circumference, which shortens the strain gauge length and decreases its resistance. This emptying causes the curve in Figure 14–1C to slope downward to the baseline level during the *venous outflow* (VO) phase of the plethysmographic examination. The venous outflow is generally expressed in terms of decrease in calf volume per unit time after the cuff is released or the percentage of decrease in volume per minute

(%/min). A decrease in calf volume of >20%/min is considered normal.

The diagrammatic illustration in Figure 14–1 is used to show that the normal unobstructed deep calf veins are capable of large increases in blood volumes. Normally, intraluminal pressures in the deep calf veins are low and the vein walls are in a semi-collapsed state, allowing increases in blood volume when the thigh cuff is inflated. This ability is lost when an outflow venous obstruction exists in the popliteal, femoral, or pelvic veins. The obstruction causes the intraluminal pressure in the deep calf veins to increase, and their walls become stiff and distended. Because these veins are already distended with blood, their further expansion in response to inflation of thigh cuff is limited, as illustrated in Figure 14–2, which shows a thrombus in the femoral-popliteal system. The deep calf veins in Figure 14–2A are already distended and filled with blood before the plethysmographic examination begins because of the outflow obstruction in the femoral-popliteal system. Therefore, the extent to which the calf is able to expand in response to the thigh cuff inflation is reduced, as shown by the decreased height of the curve in Figure 14–2B. The plateau is flat and close to the baseline because the venous capacitance is low. Venous outflow from the calf is decreased by the femoral-popliteal vein obstruction also, as shown in Figure 14–2C. In general, venous outflow decreases as the distended volume or venous capacitance of the calf veins decreases and vice versa. For this reason, both venous capacitance and outflow are used in the interpretation of the results of the plethysmographic examination.

Impedance Plethysmography

Impedance plethysmography (IPG) can also be used to obtain curves similar to the one shown in Figures 14–1 and 14–2. Impedance is a measure of the opposition to the flow of electric current. The electrical impedance of the tissues in the calf is changed by the varying amounts of blood the tissues contain. Because blood is more conductive than tissue, the presence of a slightly increased amount of blood reduces the impedance of the tissue. Therefore, changes in the impedance of the calf can be used to measure changes in its blood volume. This measurement is accomplished by placing a series of four circumferential electrodes on the calf and recording the impedance changes on a chart strip recorder during the inflation and deflation of a pressure cuff placed above the knee on the thigh. Inflation of the cuff causes the blood to pool in the calf, increasing blood volume and lowering impedance. This cuff inflation is recorded as an upswing on the curve similar to the one shown in Figure 14–1B. A plateau is reached when the calf veins become filled with blood and reach the point of maximum expansion. This plateau represents the same venous capacitance that was obtained with strain gauge plethysmography. Releasing the thigh cuff allows the blood pooled in the calf to flow out into the popliteal and femoral veins, decreasing blood volume in the calf and increasing impedance. Release of the thigh cuff is recorded as a downswing of the curve towards the baseline level and represents the same venous

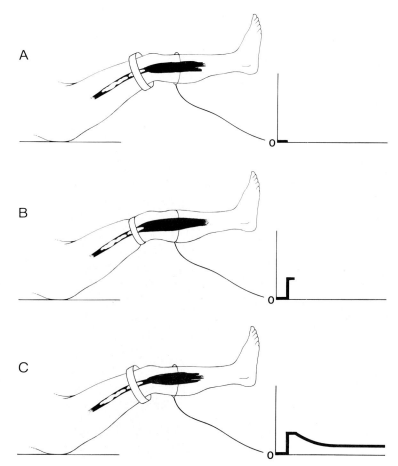

Figure 14–2. Line drawing illustrating how strain gauge plethysmography is used to detect outflow obstruction in the popliteal and femoral veins.

A, Strain gauge is placed around calf, and the strip chart recorder is calibrated to the baseline level. Note thrombi obstructing the popliteal and superficial femoral veins, causing the calf veins to be already distended with blood.

B, Inflating thigh cuff results in little curve upslope and a decreased flat plateau (venous capacitance) close to baseline level because calf veins are already filled with blood and cannot distend further.

C, Prolonged downslope curve to baseline after cuff release is due to poor venous emptying caused by venous outflow obstructive disease. Note that deep calf veins remain expanded and filled with blood after cuff is deflated.

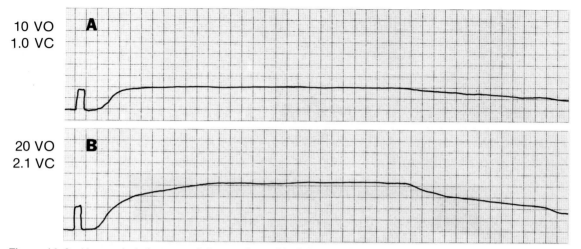

Figure 14–3. Abnormal plethysmograph in a patient with deep vein thrombosis of the left popliteal and superficial femoral veins. Normal plethysmographic examination of the right lower extremity is included for comparison.

A, Abnormal left plethysmograph shows flat venous capacitance (VC) plateau of 10 mm above the zero baseline and a prolonged venous outflow (VO) (<10%/min).

B, Normal right plethysmograph shows venous capacitance (VC) 20 mm above the zero baseline with a good venous outflow curve which slopes downward towards the baseline (VO of 20%/min).

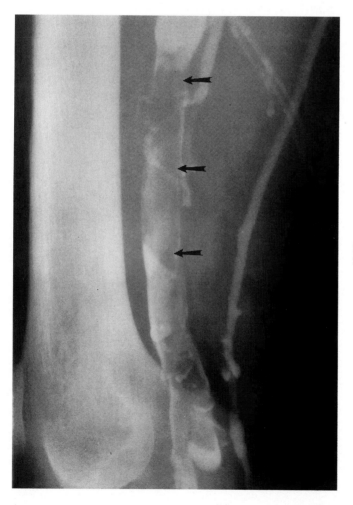

Figure 14–4. Venogram of popliteal and superficial femoral vein thrombosis (arrows).

outflow phase of the examination as shown in the strain gauge plethysmograph in Figure 14–1.

An example of a normal and abnormal plethysmographic examination is shown in Figure 14–3. It is from a patient with DVT of the left popliteal and superficial femoral veins. There is no evidence of venous obstructive disease in the right lower extremity. The contrast venogram in Figure 14–4 shows popliteal vein thrombosis.

Accuracy of Plethysmography

A composite analysis of the reported data in which occlusive impedance plethysmography has been compared with 2,561 contrast venograms reveals an overall sensitivity of 93% and a specificity of 94%.[14] However, it must be realized that strain gauge and impedance plethysmography are indirect tests and do not give the same primary evidence of DVT as contrast venography because they cannot present an image of the thrombus. Instead, these tests depend on the changes in the hemodynamics of the calf veins caused by outflow obstructions in the popliteal, femoral, or iliac veins for indicating the diagnosis of DVT. Therefore, they are sensitive and specific for thrombosis of these proximal veins and relatively insensitive to calf vein thrombosis. A plethysmographic examination with negative results does not exclude DVT of the calf as a possible cause of the symptoms in a patient with calf pain and swelling. Plethysmographic findings may also be negative when proximal vein thrombosis is associated with well-developed collaterals.

False-positive results are caused by the fact that plethysmography cannot distinguish between thrombotic and nonthrombotic obstructions of the venous outflow from the calf veins. This inability can result in the false-positive diagnosis of DVT being made when the patient is positioned incorrectly and the popliteal vein is compressed by pillows or when the deep calf veins are compressed by tense contracted leg muscles. The proximal veins may also be compressed by extrinsic masses. This compression can occur from hemorrhage into the thigh following trauma or pseudoaneurysm rupture, pelvic or groin lymphadenopathy, dissecting posterior synovial cyst, or Baker's cysts. Examples of false-positive plethysmographic examinations for DVT are shown in Figures 14–5 through 14–8. A false-positive result was caused by compression of the external iliac vein by lymph nodes, as shown by the venogram in Figure 14–8. The B-mode ultrasound scan in Figure 14–6 was most helpful in demonstrating the enlarged lymph nodes in the inguinal region. This modality combined with the duplex scan findings in Figure 14–7, was used to exclude DVT of the common femoral vein. No intraluminal echoes of thrombus formation were seen on the B-mode images (Figs. 14–6 and 14–7), and good blood flow was noted by the augmented velocity waveform shown on the duplex scan in Figure 14–7. This waveform was obtained with the probe placed over the common femoral vein during compression of the thigh. This augmentation maneuver squeezes the blood out of the thigh veins into the common femoral vein, where it passes beneath the probe face. Because

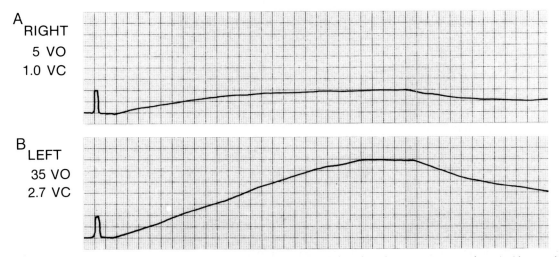

Figure 14–5. Abnormal strain gauge plethysmograph caused by extrinsic lymph node venous compression. *A*, Abnormal right side venous capacitance (VC) is <2% and the venus outflow (VO) is < 20%/min. *B*, Normal left side for comparison.

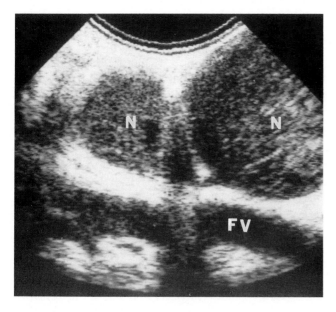

Figure 14–6. B-mode ultrasound image of enlarged inguinal lymph nodes (N) and noncompressed superficial femoral vein (FV).

the probe over this vein is angled towards the heart, the flow of blood is directed away from the probe face, resulting in a waveform that is deflected downward below the zero baseline level, as shown in Figure 14–7.

Another cause for false-positive examinations is an increase in the central venous pressure, which may prevent the outflow of blood from the calf veins into femoral and pelvic veins. Reduced arterial inflow into the lower limb can also cause

a reduced outflow of blood from the calf veins and thus produce a false-positive result.

Significance of Calf Vein Thrombosis

The fact that plethysmography cannot be relied upon to detect thrombosis confined to the calf veins is well recognized.[15–17] This fact also raises the following question. Are thrombi in the deep calf veins below the knee significant? The an-

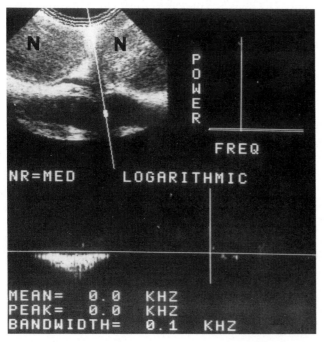

Figure 14–7. Duplex scan of common femoral vein blood flow and B-mode image without internal echoes of thrombus formation. The augmented velocity waveform was obtained by compression of the thigh. It is below the baseline because the blood flow direction is away from the probe face. N = Lymph nodes.

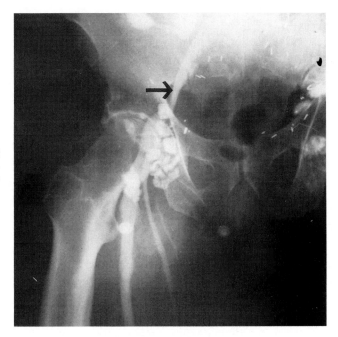

Figure 14–8. Venogram showing compression of external iliac vein (arrow) by lymph nodes containing contrast media from a previous lymphangiogram. There is no associated deep vein thrombosis.

swers to this question center around two schools of thought. Although it is agreed that the vast majority of clinically significant pulmonary emboli arise from clots in the major veins of the thigh or pelvis, there is disagreement concerning the significance of thrombi in the deep calf veins.

Thrombi Are Not Significant

One group of authors considers calf vein thrombi to be of no significance because they are too small to cause clinically significant pulmonary emboli. This group does not believe that thrombi arising in the deep calf vein propagate up into the veins of the thigh and pelvis. Also, because deep calf veins are not thought to be significant, the complications of treating with anticoagulation may be greater than the risk of not detecting and treating them at all.

Benedict reported on a study conducted by Wheeler and Patwardhan in which the clinical records of 400 patients with normal impedance plethysmographs were reviewed for a follow-up of possible DVT.[17] Their patient population consisted mainly of postoperative patients and those bedridden as a result of major medical diseases. The review disclosed that 114 of the 400 patients were already receiving heparin because of the clinical impression of DVT. Seven of these sustained a major hemorrhagic complication. Of the 286 patients who were not taking anticoagulants, only one developed a clinically documented pulmonary embolism (lung scan with positive find-

ings). That patient did well when placed on anticoagulant therapy. The results of this study are included here because they suggest that the complications of treating deep calf vein clot may be greater than the risk of not detecting it with impedance plethysmography.

Thrombi Are Significant

The second group of authors considers calf vein thrombi to be highly significant because, if left undiagnosed and untreated, they may extend up into the larger proximal veins of the thigh and pelvis where they can become enlarged, possibly producing clinically significant pulmonary emboli. This group of authors also believes that whenever and wherever DVT exists it poses a potentially serious threat to the patient and should be treated aggressively. This approach is used to prevent not only the complication of pulmonary emboli but also the destruction of the valves in the deep venous pump mechanism of the calf. Destruction of these valves may lead to the complications of chronic venous insufficiency, an entity that cannot be effectively treated at this time.

Conclusion

Controversy exists concerning the significance of calf vein thrombosis because there is evidence that supports both sides. Concerning the origin of thrombi, Kakkar and colleagues[18] and Secker-

Walker and Potchen[19] report that thrombi almost always arise in the calf veins and propagate up into the popliteal-femoral vein segments. Mahaffy and coworkers,[20] on the other hand, counter with their data, which show that most iliofemoral clots arise de novo in this segment. The postmortem findings of Sevitt and Gallagher support a multicentric origin for lower extremity clot.[21]

Whether or not only proximal vein thrombi are significant remains to be clarified by randomized clinical trials.

Doppler Ultrasonography

Venous Examinations

The Doppler ultrasound examination consists of obtaining a blood flow velocity waveform signal from a bi-directional Doppler probe placed directly over the vein being studied, as illustrated in Figure 14–9. The Doppler probe in this figure is placed over the superficial femoral vein with the probe face angled towards the heart. The velocity waveform obtained with the probe in this position should be phasic during quiet respiration, as shown in Figure 14–9A. In this figure, the blood flow towards the probe face causes a positive deflection above the zero baseline level; blood flow away from the probe face causes a negative deflection below the baseline. The probe face is always directed towards the heart for peripheral vascular examinations in our laboratory.

The small deflections in the waveform above and below the zero baseline level shown in Figure 14–9A are phasic because of the changes in respiration. During inspiration, the intra-abdominal pressure increases as the diaphragm descends down into the abdomen, causing the blood in the lower extremity veins to stop flowing or to flow away from the heart towards the probe face for a short distance. This results in a small wave being deflected above the zero baseline. On expiration, the blood flow in the lower extremity veins is towards the heart and away from the probe face. This results in the small wave below the zero baseline level occuring during expiration, as shown in Figure 14–9A. Normally, the small phasic waveform in Figure 14–9A taken during quiet breathing can be augmented by calf compression, as shown in Figure 14–9B. Compressing the calf region squeezes the blood out of the deep calf veins, causing blood to rush up into the superficial femoral vein and to flow away from the probe face. This augmentation maneuver is recorded as an increase in the height of the negative wave below the zero baseline, as shown in Figure 14–9B.

In DVT, both the respiratory phasic and aug-

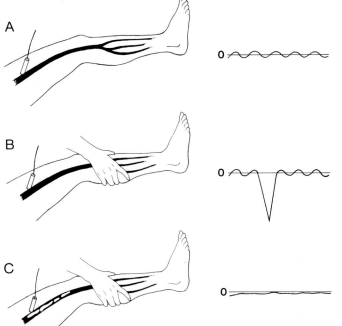

Figure 14–9. Line drawing illustrating Doppler ultrasound method of detecting venous obstructive disease.

A, Phasic waveform of quiet-breathing patient obtained from probe placed over the superficial femoral vein. Waveform above the zero baseline occurs during expiration, and waveform below zero baseline occurs during inspiration.

B, Phasic waveform of quiet-breathing patient augmented by calf compression maneuver because no obstruction exists between the point of calf compression and the site of the Doppler probe.

C, Phasic waveform of quiet-breathing patient is absent and not augmented by calf compression because thrombus in popliteal and superficial femoral veins obstructs blood flow between the point of calf compression and the Doppler probe site.

mented waveforms may be absent, indicating absence of blood flow in the obstructed venous segment, as shown in Figure 14–9C. This figure illustrates that when the calf region is compressed, blood cannot flow past the probe face placed over the superficial femoral vein because this vein is obstructed with thrombus.

An example of how the Doppler ultrasound examination is used to detect an obstructing thrombus in the common femoral vein is shown in Figure 14–10. The waveforms in this figure were obtained with the Doppler probe placed over the common femoral veins with its face angled towards the heart during augmentation compression maneuvers of the thighs. A good augmentation waveform is obtained from the left common femoral vein shown in Figure 14–10B.

This waveform indicates that no point of obstruction exists in the venous system between the point of thigh compression and the Doppler probe site over the left common femoral vein. As shown in Figure 14–10A, the augmented waveform is diminished over the right common femoral vein, indicating that an obstruction does exist in the venous system between the point of thigh compression and site of the Doppler probe over the common femoral vein. The obstruction was caused by a thrombus in the right common femoral and superficial femoral veins, as shown on the venogram in Figure 14–11. An example of a popliteal vein obstruction is given in Figure 14–12. In this example, the Doppler probe is placed over the popliteal vein during manual compression of the deep calf veins. There is good

A

RIGHT

B

LEFT

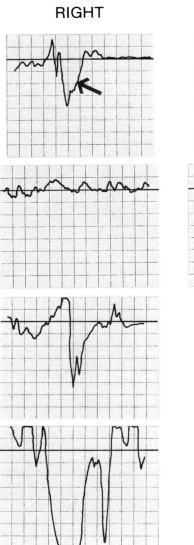
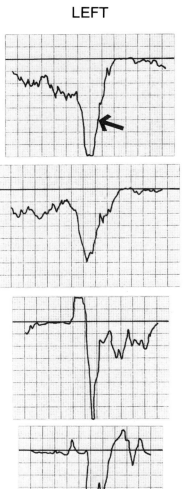

Figure 14–10. Doppler ultrasound of right common femoral vein obstruction. Normal left common femoral vein is shown for comparison.

A, Diminished augmented velocity waveform (arrow) over right common femoral vein, indicating that an obstruction is present between the point of thigh compression and the site of the Doppler probe.

B, Normal augmented velocity waveform (arrow) from left common femoral vein, indicating that no obstruction exists between point of thigh compression and site of Doppler probe.

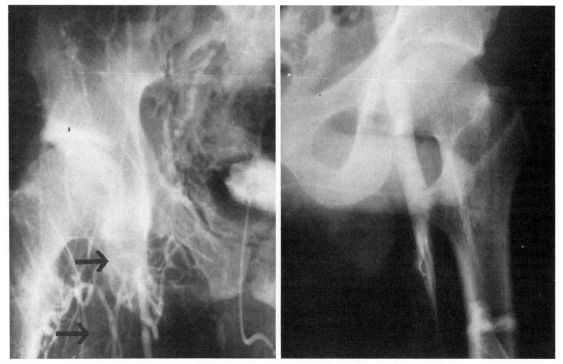

Figure 14–11. Venogram shows thrombus obstructing right common femoral and superficial femoral veins (arrows). Venogram of left side is normal.

augmentation of the waveform from the right popliteal vein (Fig. 14–12*A*), whereas a greatly diminished augmented waveform (Fig. 14–12*B*) is obtained from the left popliteal vein. These findings indicate an obstructive process affecting the blood flow, in the left popliteal vein. This obstruction was found to be caused by a thrombus, as demonstrated on the venogram in Figure 14–13.

A technique for obtaining augmented velocity waveforms from the greater saphenous vein and deep calf veins is given in Figure 14–14. Gener-

ally, this technique consists of manually compressing the foot veins while recording the velocity waveforms from the greater saphenous vein or the deep calf veins. As shown in Figure 14–14*A*, a cuff placed around the leg below the knee can be used to pool blood in the superficial and deep leg veins. Releasing the cuff causes the blood pooled in the calf veins to rush up into the thigh veins, increasing blood velocity, as shown in Figure 14–14*B*. A clot occluding these veins results in an absence of the augmented waveform (Fig. 14–14*C*).

A

RIGHT POPLITEAL

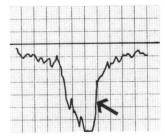

B

LEFT POPLITEAL

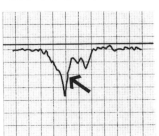

Figure 14–12. Doppler ultrasound of left popliteal vein obstruction. Normal right popliteal vein included for comparison.

A, Normal augmented velocity waveform (arrow) from right popliteal vein, indicating that no obstruction exists between point of calf compression and site of Doppler probe.

B, Abnormal diminished augmented velocity waveform (arrow) from left popliteal vein, indicating that an obstruction exists between the point of calf compression and site of Doppler probe.

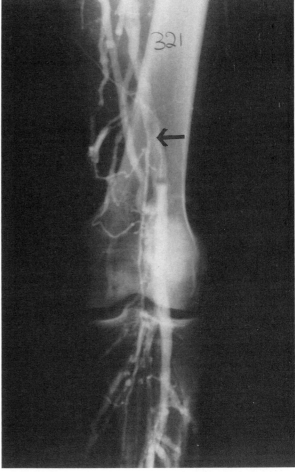

Figure 14–13. Venogram showing thrombus in popliteal vein (arrow).

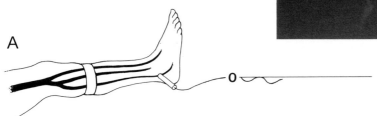

CLOT

Figure 14–14. Occlusion cuff method of obtaining augmented velocity waveforms from greater saphenous and deep calf veins.

A, Inflated cuff pools blood in superficial and deep leg veins. Doppler probe over deep calf vein shows no waveform because blood flow in these veins ceases during cuff inflation.

B, Deflated cuff releases blood pooled in calf veins, which rushes out of greater saphenous and deep calf veins, augmenting velocity waveform.

C, Obstructing clot in deep calf vein causes absence of augmented velocity waveform.

Accuracy of Doppler Ultrasonography

In experienced hands, the Doppler bi-directional blood flow velocity probe offers an accurate, versatile, simple, and rapid method of detecting DVT. Several reports have suggested that the sensitivity of the venous Doppler examination may exceed 95% in detecting major calf vein thrombosis and deep vein thrombosis at or above the level of the knee.[22–25] Like plethysmography, Doppler ultrasonography is not capable of detecting thrombi that do not significantly obstruct venous blood flow. It is also not specific for DVT, inasmuch as any condition that may extrinsically compress the venous system can result in a false-positive diagnosis of DVT. False-negative findings occur when the Doppler sounds or velocity waveforms coming from a collateral vein going around an obstructing thrombus are mistaken for patency of the main vein under investigation.

Real-Time B-Mode Ultrasonography

Real-time ultrasonography uses a 7.5 or 10 MHz transducer to obtain an image of the vein lumen in both the longitudinal and transverse planes.

Examination Sites

All of the primary locations in the lower extremity where thrombi occur can be examined by real-time B-mode imaging. These locations are as follows:
1. The iliac veins.
2. The common femoral veins.
3. The superficial femoral and popliteal veins near the adductor ring.
4. The posterior tibial vein.
5. The soleus muscular plexus veins.[26]
The greater and lesser saphenous veins of the superficial venous system can also be examined by this method.

Ultrasonographic Findings

The ultrasonographic findings in DVT include:
1. Thrombus-producing intraluminal echoes.[27–29]
2. No change of vessel size with the Valsalva maneuver.[27, 28]
3. Nonvisualization of flowing blood and valve leaflet motion.[27]
4. Noncompressibility of the vein lumen.[27, 30]

The vein is considered free of thrombus when the vein walls touch on compression of the vein with the transducer and no intraluminal echogenic material is seen.

Intraluminal Echoes

Thrombus is considered present when echogenic material is seen within the vein lumen on both the longitudinal and transverse scans, as shown in Figures 14–15 and 14–16. Characterization of the thrombus may be used to determine whether it is acute or chronic. As a general rule, acute clot, like that seen in Figure 14–16A, is less echogenic than chronic clot, and very fresh clot may not be echogenic at all. An example of a chronic thrombus is shown in Figure 14–17. The texture of an acute thrombus is generally homogeneous and exhibits a smooth surface, whereas a chronic thrombus is more heterogeneous and many times has a rough or irregular surface. Acute thrombus is soft and may be compressed to a certain extent; chronic thrombus is not compressible to any extent. Adherence to the vessel wall occurs within 2 weeks and indicates the presence of a chronic thrombus. A free-floating clot, in contrast, is usually indicative of an acute thrombus.

Valsalva Maneuver

A forced expiration against a closed glottis or the Valsalva maneuver causes the intrathoracic pressure to rise. This rise in intrathoracic pressure impedes the venous drainage from the lower extremities, causing expansion and pressure increases in the peripheral veins. During periods in which the patient is breathing quietly, the pressure in the common femoral vein is low, causing it to be partially collapsed and narrow in the anteroposterior diameter (Fig. 14–18A).

The Valsalva maneuver or abdominal compression promptly expands the common femoral vein, causing it to increase in size and assume a circular configuration, as shown in Figure 14–18B. In fact, its diameter may double during these maneuvers as compared with its size in the resting state.[28] Immediately on release of the Valsalva maneuver or expiration, the common femoral vein collapses and becomes even more narrow in the anteroposterior diameter than when the patient is breathing quietly (Fig. 14–18C). These responses are not as pronounced in veins below the level of the common femoral vein, such as the popliteal vein. Both the common femoral and popliteal veins also change in size with postural changes (e.g., diameter increases with upright position).

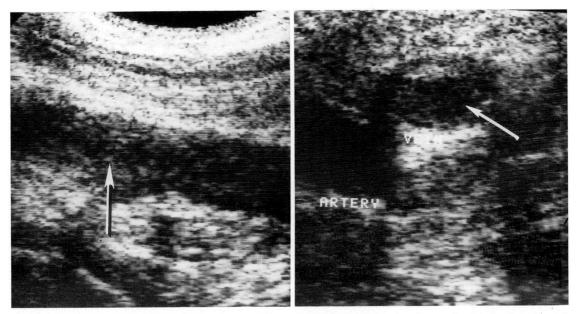

Figure 14–15. Freeze frame images from real-time B-mode ultrasonography showing popliteal vein thrombus. *A*, Thrombus on sagittal projection (arrow). *B*, Thrombus on transverse projection (arrow).

When the iliofemoral system is obstructed by thrombus, the common femoral vein becomes fixed in its expanded, circular configuration, as shown in Figure 14–19, and there is no change in this configuration during inspiration, the Valsalva maneuver, quiet breathing, or expiration. When the veins below the common femoral vein are thrombosed while the iliac and common femoral veins remain patent, the size of the common femoral vein may change its configuration from collapsed to circular with respiratory movements; however, these changes are slow and damped. Total occlusion of the iliac veins or ligation of the inferior vena cava results in no change in the common femoral vein during the Valsalva maneuver or deep inspiration. More importantly, the common femoral vein never collapses to its normal configuration because of the persistent, elevated intraluminal pressure caused by the iliac vein or inferior vena cava occlusion.

Blood Flow Visualization

Blood flow within the entire vein lumen is seen inconsistently but, when present, is a definite indicator that clot is not present. An example of intraluminal echoes originating from blood flow is seen in Figure 14–20. Flow can be seen around acute or chronic thrombi and can be helpful in outlining the size of the thrombus.

Valve Leaflet Motion

Clot can form in the sinuses behind the valve leaflets and cause their dysfunction in acute thrombosis. The total absence of any valve leaflets can be found as a result of chronic DVT.

Compressibility of Vein Lumen

Compressibility of the vein lumen is defined as the ability to coapt the vessel walls with slight pressure on the probe and is indicative of a normal vein that does not contain clot. The example in Figure 14–21 shows complete collapse of the vein lumen so that one wall touches the other. It is important to realize that if the transducer is allowed to rest on the skin surface, its weight alone is usually enough to collapse the vein, resulting in nonvisualization of the vein lumen. This is especially true of veins that lie close to the skin surface, such as the common femoral, superficial femoral, and popliteal veins. Therefore, it is essential that the transducer probe be held gently against the skin surface to achieve clear visualization of the vein.

Noncompressibility of a vein is a good indicator that its lumen contains a thrombus. Raghavendra and colleagues reported an inability to compress the vein lumen in all their cases of thrombus occurring in either the common femoral or popliteal vein.[29] Cronan and coworkers also noted

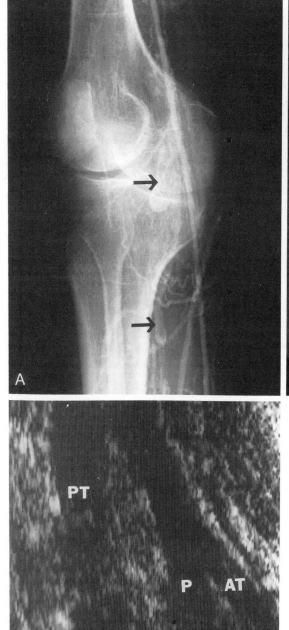

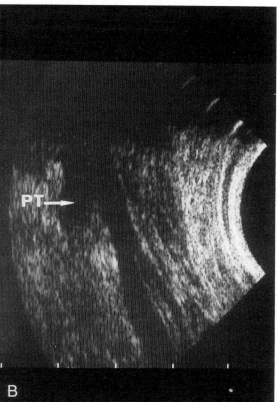

Figure 14–16. Ultrasound of acute vein thrombosis correlated with venogram. *A*, Venogram of popliteal and tibial vein clots (arrows). *B*, Noncompressibility of posterior tibial veins (PT) on ultrasound. *C*, Close-up view of low-level echoes in anterior tibial (AT), posterior tibial (PT), and peroneal (P) veins.

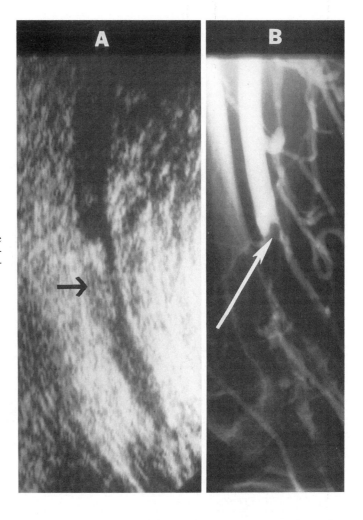

Figure 14–17. Chronic thrombus on B-mode ultrasound containing dense echoes. *A*, Echogenic thrombus (arrow). *B*, Thrombus in popliteal vein on venogram (arrow).

noncompressibility of the veins in their patients with DVT.[32] These investigators found this finding so reliable that they reported that it obviates the need to search for the intraluminal echoes of the thrombus, hence avoiding false-positive results generated by poorly established gain settings and false-negative results from anechoic fresh clot.

There are, however, some veins that cannot be completely compressed normally. The veins that are normally difficult to compress are the profunda femoral vein, the superficial femoral vein at the adductor canal region, and the posterior tibial vein at the medial malleolus.[31] Inability to compress these veins at these locations should be approached with caution in diagnosing DVT. It is also important to consider, when the pregnant patient is examined (especially during the third trimester), that the fetal head can compress the inferior vena cava and iliac veins, resulting in venous obstruction. This may lead to

noncompressibility of the lower extremity veins and to a false-positive diagnosis of DVT.[33] Placing the patient on his or her side relieves the pressure on the veins exerted by the uterus and helps to eliminate this problem.

Accuracy of Real-Time B-Mode Ultrasound

Hannan and colleagues correlated the real-time B-mode venous scans with contrast venograms for 68 cases. All were performed within 48 hours of each other. They found the overall specificity to be 89%, the sensitivity 95%, the positive predictive value 93%, and the negative predictive value 92%.[31]

Cronan and associates also correlated real-time B-mode venous scans with contrast venograms performed within 24 hours of each other in 51 patients.[32] Deep vein thrombosis was seen on 28 venograms; ultrasonographic findings were true-

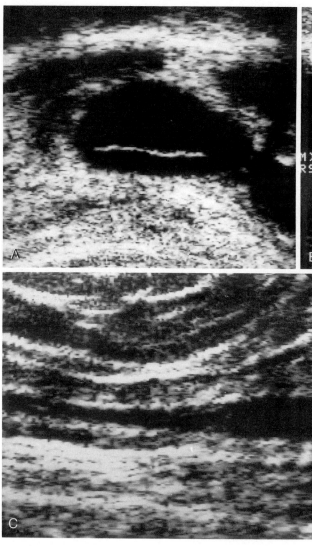

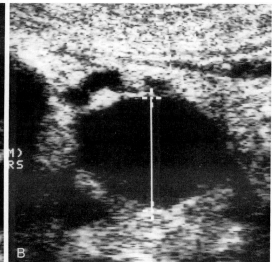

Figure 14–18. Transverse B-mode ultrasound of common femoral vein showing effects of Valsalva maneuver. *A*, Femoral vein partially collapsed during quiet breathing. *B*, Femoral vein round and expanded during Valsalva maneuver. *C*, Femoral vein collapses during expiration.

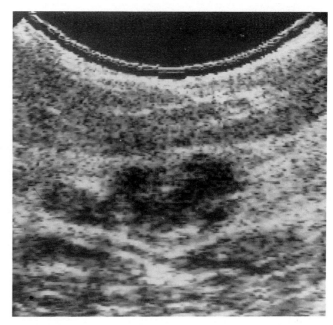

Figure 14–19. Transverse B-mode ultrasound of common femoral vein fixed in circular configuration because of deep vein thrombosis.

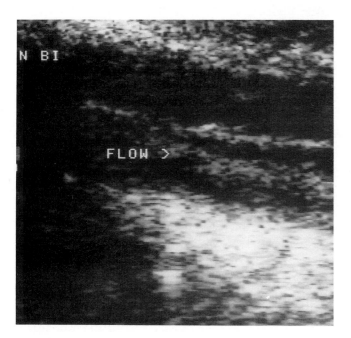

Figure 14–20. Intraluminal echoes from venous blood flow.

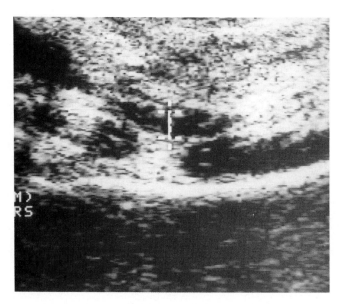

Figure 14–21. Normal vein lumen collapsed by slight pressure on the probe.

positive in 25 patients and false-negative in three patients. The three false-negative ultrasound examinations were the result of:

1. Clot limited only to the anterior tibial vein on the venogram, not seen by ultrasonography.

2. Clot isolated to a single valve leaflet in the proximal popliteal vein on the venogram, not seen by ultrasonography.

3. The profunda femoral vein being misinterpreted as a patent superficial femoral vein by ultrasonography and the superficial femoral vein being found to be occluded on the venogram.

All 23 patients in this series with negative venograms also had negative ultrasound findings. Accuracy measurements from this series of 51 patients showed sensitivity to be 89% and specificity to be 100%. The positive predictive value of the ultrasound examination was 100%, and the overall accuracy was 95%.

Real-time B-mode ultrasonography is different from plethysmography and Doppler ultrasonography because it produces an image of the thrombus and is not affected by masses causing extrinsic venous compression. Its ability to image structures outside of the vein lumen provides information that cannot be obtained by contrast venography. For example, it is possible with ultrasonography to make a diagnosis that accounts for the patient's symptoms (such as Baker's cyst or calf muscle hemorrhage) even when the venous ultrasound examination is normal.

Duplex Sonography

Duplex sonography essentially combines real-time B-mode imaging and Doppler ultrasonog-

raphy, allowing both the anatomy and blood flow characteristics of veins to be studied simultaneously. Normal veins are characterized by applying light pressure with the probe, resulting in compression of the vein with coaptation of its walls and no evidence of internal intraluminal echoes. When seen, blood flow and valve motion also reflect a normal vein. Phasic and velocity waveform augmentation are evaluated with spectral analysis of the pulsed Doppler signal.

Venous Examinations

The duplex sonographic criteria for a normal venous examination includes:
- compressibility
- anechoic lumen
- blood flow with normal valve motion
- normal Doppler signals

Abnormal veins caused by DVT are distended, are incompressible with probe pressure, contain internal echoes, and have absent Doppler signals when thrombus totally occludes the vein lumen. The duplex scan in Figures 14–22 and 14–23 is an example of these abnormalities. The scan shows noncompressibility of the common femoral vein lumen, which is filled with echogenic thrombus. The Doppler velocity waveform in Figure 14–23 is from a collateral vein bypassing the thrombus-filled common femoral vein. This finding reveals a collateral vein because its waveform cannot be augmented by either the Valsalva or the thigh compression maneuvers. A normal Doppler waveform of the common femoral vein is shown in Figure 14–24. This waveform shows how the velocity waveform of quiet breathing can be damped by the Valsalva maneuver. Dur-

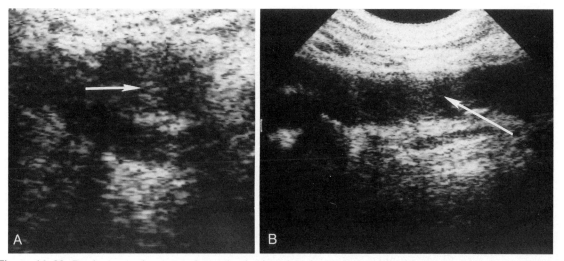

Figure 14–22. Duplex scan of common femoral vein thrombus. *A*, Transverse B-mode image of circular, expanded, noncompressible vein lumen filled with echogenic thrombus (arrow). *B*, Sagittal B-mode image of thrombus (arrow).

ing the Valsalva maneuver, the increased intra-abdominal pressure decreases the velocity of the venous blood flow from the lower extremities. Cessation of the Valsalva maneuver causes the blood flow velocity to return to quiet breathing levels, indicating that no obstruction exists in the common femoral vein.

Figures 14–25 and 14–26 illustrate how duplex sonography may be used to follow-up the results of fibrinolytic therapy for DVT. The treated popliteal vein thrombus is shown on the venogram and B-mode scan in Figure 14–25. Doppler examination of the popliteal fossa revealed collateral venous blood flow around the thrombus-filled popliteal vein, as demonstrated in Figure

14–26*A*. Again, blood flow in this collateral pathway is continuous and cannot be augmented by respiratory or compression maneuvers (Fig. 14–26*A*). Three days after streptokinase therapy, the popliteal vein velocity waveform is readily augmented by calf compression, as shown in Figure 14–26*B*. Six days after therapy the waveform is easily augmented by the Valsalva maneuver (Fig. 14–26*C*), indicating continued patency of the popliteal vein and a good response to therapy

Accuracy of Duplex Sonography

Oliver used duplex sonography correlated with contrast venography to evaluate its accuracy in

Figure 14–23. Doppler waveform of collateral blood flow around thrombus-filled common femoral vein. Blood flow velocity not changed by Valsalva maneuver.

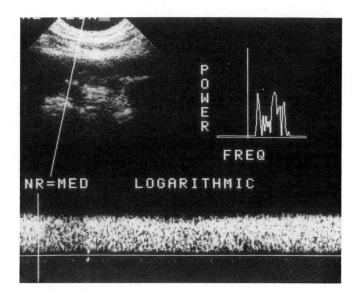

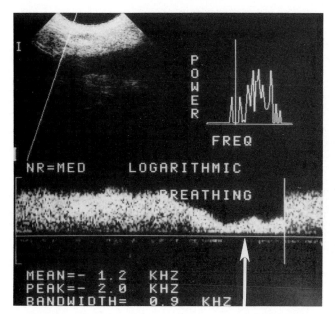

Figure 14–24. Doppler waveform of normal common femoral vein. Blood flow velocity decreased by Valsalva maneuver (arrow).

30 limbs (two upper, 28 lower).[34] All venograms were done within 48 hours of the duplex scan examination; the overall sensitivity of this technique was found to be 90%[9, 10], and the specificity was found to be 95%. The one false-negative finding was a peroneal thrombus that could not be visualized, and the one false-positive finding was in a patient with a very narrow popliteal vein, which led to a false interpretation of the duplex scan results.

Summary

Various noninvasive procedures are available to the clinician who must evaluate and treat patients with suspected DVT. The continuing need for these procedures arises from the recognized fallibility of the clinical diagnosis of DVT and the time, discomfort, expense, and potential risk of contrast venography. Plethysmography and Doppler ultrasonography are particularly

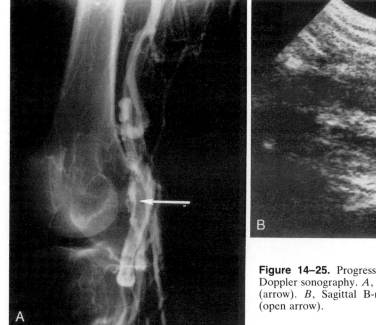
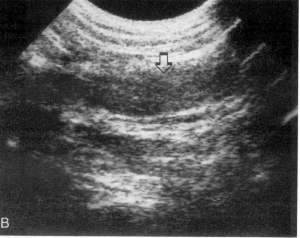

Figure 14–25. Progress of fibrinolytic therapy followed by Doppler sonography. *A*, Venogram of popliteal vein thrombus (arrow). *B*, Sagittal B-mode image of echogenic thrombus (open arrow).

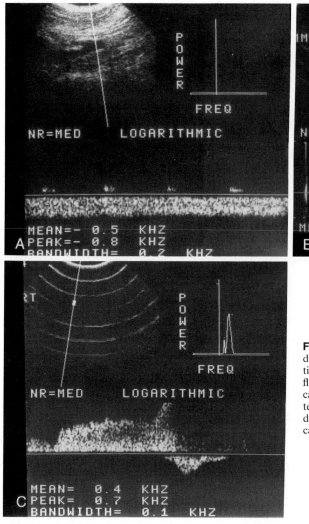

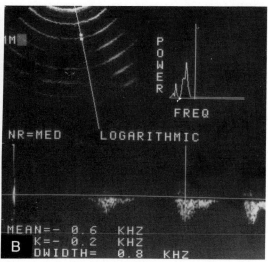

Figure 14–26. Doppler velocity waveform changes during fibrinolytic therapy. *A*, Pre-streptokinase continuous, non-augmented waveform of collateral blood flow around thrombus. *B*, Post-streptokinase (3 days) calf compression-augmented waveform, indicating patency of popliteal vein lumen. *C*, Post-streptokinase (6 days) Valsalva maneuver-augmented waveform, indicating patency of popliteal vein lumen.

suited to screen patients suspected of having major DVT at or above the level of the knee. Real-time B-mode ultrasonography and duplex sonography may be even more useful because, like contrast venography, these modalities also produce an image of the offending thrombus and can be used to examine the deep calf veins below the knee. There may be no need to use contrast venography when the thrombi are seen by either real-time B-mode ultrasonography or duplex sonography. If the clot or thrombus cannot be identified by either real-time B-mode ultrasonography or duplex sonography, contrast venography may be required to make the diagnosis, and one should not hesitate to use this method.

References

1. Evans DS. The early diagnosis of deep vein thrombosis by ultrasound. Br J Surg 1970; 57:726–731.
2. Haeger K. Problems of acute venous thrombosis. Angiology 1969; 20:219–223.
3. Nicholas GN, Miller FJ, Demuth WE, Waldhausen JA. Clinical vascular laboratory diagnosis of deep vein thrombosis. Ann Surg 1977; 186:213–216.
4. Cranley JJ, Canos AJ, Sull WF. The diagnosis of deep venous thrombosis: Fallibility of clinical symptoms and signs. Arch Surg 1976; 111:34–36.
5. McLachlin JT, Richards T, Paterson JC. An evaluation of clinical signs in the diagnosis of venous thrombosis. Arch Surg 1962; 85:738–740.
6. Barnes RW, Hoak JC. The fallibility of the clinical diagnosis of venous thrombosis. JAMA 1975; 234:605–608.
7. Lambie JM, Mchaffy RG, Barber DC, Karmody AM, Scott MM, Matheson NA. Diagnostic accuracy in venous thrombosis. Br Med J 1970; 2:142–143.
8. Athanasoulis CA. Phlebography for the diagnosis of deep vein thrombosis. *In* Fratantoni J, Wessler S (eds). Prophylactic therapy of deep vein thrombosis and pulmonary embolism. Bethesda, NIH, 1975:62–76.
9. Albrechtsson J, Olsen CG. Thrombotic side effects of lower limb phlebography. Lancet 1976; 1:723–734.
10. Bonnar J. Venous thromboembolism and pregnancy. Clin Obstet Gynecol 1981; 8:455–473.
11. Lea TM. Phlebography. Arch Surg 1972; 104:145–151.
12. Rabinov K, Paulin S. Roentgen diagnosis of venous thrombosis in the leg. Arch Surg 1972; 104:134–144.
13. Sauerbrei E, Thomson JG, McLachlan MS, Musial J. Observer variation in lower limb venography. J Can Assoc Radiol 1981; 32:28–29.
14. Wheeler HB, Anderson FA Jr. Can noninvasive tests be used as the basis for treatment of deep vein thrombosis? *In* Bernstein EF (ed). Noninvasive diagnostic techniques in vascular disease. 2nd ed. St Louis, CV Mosby, 1982:545–559.
15. Hull R, Hirsh J, Sackett DL, Stoddart G. Cost effectiveness of clinical diagnosis, venography, and noninvasive testing in patients with symptomatic deep-vein thrombosis. N Engl J Med 1981; 304:1561–1567.
16. Hull R, Van Aken WG, Hiesh J. Impedance plethysmography using the occlusive cuff technique in the diagnosis of venous thrombosis. Circulation 1976; 53:696.
17. Benedict KT Jr, Wheeler HB, Patwardhan NA. Impedance plethysmography correlated with contrast venography. Radiology 1977; 125:695–699.
18. Kakkar VV, Howe CT, Flanc C, et al. Natural history of postoperative deep vein thrombosis. Lancet 1969; 2:230–232.
19. Secker-Walker R, Potchen EJ. Radiology of venous thrombosis—Current status. Radiology 1971; 101:499–452.
20. Mahaffy RG, Mavor GE, Galloway JMG. Iliofemoral phlebography in pulmonary embolism. Br J Radiol 1971; 44:172–183.
21. Sevitt S, Gallagher NG. Venous thrombosis and pulmonary embolism. Br J Surg 1961; 48:475–489.
22. Sumner DS, Baker DW, Strandness DE Jr. The ultrasonic velocity detector in a clinical study of venous disease. Arch Surg 1968; 97:75–80.
23. Siegel B, Popky GL, Wagner DK, et al. Comparison of clinical and Doppler ultrasound evaluation of confirmed lower extremity venous disease. Surgery 1968; 64:332–338.
24. Yao ST, Gourmos C, Hobbs JR. Detection of proximal vein thrombosis by the Doppler ultrasound flow detection method. Lancet 1972; 1:4.
25. Strandness DE Jr, Sumner DS. Ultrasonic velocity detector in the diagnosis of thrombophlebitis. Arch Surg 1972; 104:180–183.
26. Sevitt S. Venous thrombosis and pulmonary embolism. Am J Med 1962; 33:703–704.
27. Sullivan ED, Peter DJ, Cranley JJ. Real-time B-mode venous ultrasound. J Vasc Surg 1984; 1:456–571.
28. Effeney DJ, Friedman MB, Gooding GAW. Iliofemoral venous thrombosis real-time ultrasound diagnosis, normal criteria, and clinical application. Radiology 1984; 150:787–792.
29. Raghavendra BN, Rosen RJ, Lam S, Riles T, Horii SC. Deep venous thrombosis: detection by high-resolution real-time ultrasonography. Radiology 1984; 152:789–793.
30. Raghavendra BN, Horii SC, Hilton S, Subramanyam BR, Rosen RJ, Lam S. Deep vein thrombosis: detection by probe compression of veins. J Ultrasound Med 1986; 5:89–95.
31. Hannan LJ, Stedje MJ, Skorcz MJ, Karkow WS, Flanagan LD, Cranley JJ. Venous imaging of the extremities: our first twenty-five hundred cases. Bruit 1986; 10:29–32.
32. Cronan JJ, Dorfman GS, Scola FH, Schepps B, Alexander J. Deep venous thrombosis: US assessment using vein compression. Radiology 1987; 162:191–194.
33. Langsfeld M, Hurley JJ, Thorpe LE, Hershey FB. Real-time venous imaging in pregnancy: a case report illustrating the potential pitfalls in diagnosing deep vein thrombosis. Bruit 1986; 10:244–247.
34. Oliver MA. Duplex scanning in venous disease. Bruit 1985; 10:206–209.

15 • Venous Insufficiency

Chronic Venous Insufficiency

Normally, contraction of the calf muscles, competent venous valves, and muscular compression of the leg veins are responsible for venous return to the heart. This mechanism is known as the *peripheral venous pump*.[1] While a person is at rest, the normal venous system blood flows in a cephalad direction through both the superficial and deep veins because of the pressure difference between the right atrium and left ventricle (Fig. 15–1A). While one is walking or standing, the calf muscles contract and push the blood towards the heart via both the superficial and deep systems. The reflux of blood is prevented by valves in the distal veins and perforators (Fig. 15–1B). With relaxation of the calf muscles, the pressure is reduced in the deep veins and the valves open in the perforators; this allows the blood to enter from the superficial system to the deep venous system and on to the heart (Fig. 15–1C). This mechanism decreases the ambulatory venous pressure and, hence, prevents venous stasis.

Failure of the peripheral venous pump mechanism from various causes results in venous stasis, which then leads to *chronic venous insufficiency*. Chronic venous insufficiency is caused by various entities, including varicose veins, post-thrombotic syndrome, and chronic recurrent thrombosis.[2] This process is characterized clinically by chronic swelling of the leg, malleolar ulceration, cutaneous hyperpigmentation, varicose veins, and leg pain (Fig. 15–2).[2]

Varicose Veins

Varicose veins represent dilated, tortuous, and elongated superficial veins. A varicose vein may be *primary* or *secondary*.[3]

Primary Varicose Veins

Primary varicose veins usually affect the superficial venous system (greater saphenous vein, lesser saphenous vein, and their tributaries). The deep veins remain normal. Occasionally, primary varicose veins may also involve the perforating veins. The exact cause is unknown; however, the development of varicose veins is hereditary. Abnormal wall weakness, increased distending force, and multiple, small arteriovenous fistulas have been suggested as possible contributing factors.[4–6] The condition is associated with venous valvular incompetency. The valves in the greater saphenous vein, in the iliac vein, and at the saphenofemoral junction are often absent or incompetent.[3]

The process initially occurs in the proximal portion of the saphenous vein and gradually descends to affect the distal part of the vein and its perforators. Figure 15–3 demonstrates the venous dynamics in a patient with primary varicose veins. At rest and during exercise or walking, blood flows in both the superficial and deep veins towards the heart (Fig. 15–3A and B). Unlike the normal venous system, however, when the muscles relax following exercise, the blood flows in a retrograde manner in the superficial veins to re-enter the deep veins through the perforating veins (Fig. 15–3C). The resulting venous stasis maintains a high venous pressure in the superficial veins, which, along with the inefficient circular motion of a portion of the blood, leads to varicose vein formation.

Secondary Varicose Veins

Secondary varicose veins involve the deep and communicating veins. The most common etiologic factor is previous deep vein thrombosis. Arteriovenous fistula, (congenital or acquired), and Klippel-Trenaunay syndrome (deep vein hypoplasia or aplasia) are other causes of secondary varicose veins. Deep vein obstruction may or may not be present.

Both chronic venous thrombosis and post-phlebitic syndrome are associated with venous out-

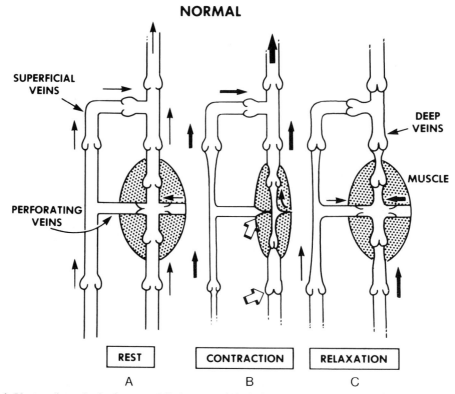

Figure 15–1. Venous dynamics in the normal limb at rest *(A)*, during exercise *(B)*, and after exercise *(C)*.

A, Blood flows to the heart through both superficial and deep venous systems in the direction of the arrows.

B, Blood flows to the heart via both superficial and deep venous systems in the direction of the arrows. Closed valves (open arrow) in the perforating and deep veins prevent retrograde flow.

C, Blood flows from the superficial system to enter the deep system via open valves in the perforators and then flows to the heart (arrows).

(From Sumner D. Venous dynamics—varicosities. Clin Obstet Gynecol 1981; 24:751, by permission.)

flow obstruction and/or venous valvular insufficiency. Previous deep vein thrombosis is also responsible for these conditions.[7] Some thrombi may gradually resolve with time by the action of thrombolysin; others may undergo the process of recanalization. Venous valves are destroyed by these thrombi, resulting in venous valvular incompetency. This event is followed by progressive dilatation of collateral veins, which results in secondary varicose veins. The venous dynamics associated with secondary varicose veins are illustrated in Figure 15–4.

In a patient with secondary varicose veins and chronic recurrent deep vein thrombosis, the blood flows from the deep veins to the superficial veins, even while one is at rest. When the muscles relax after exercise, the blood flows in a retrograde manner into both the superficial and deep veins at all times. This increased pressure results in exudation of fluid and red blood cells into the subcutaneous tissue. The exudated fluid organ-

izes, causing induration of the tissue, which then leads to ulceration.

Evaluation Methods

Chronic venous insufficiency can be evaluated by the following tests:
- photoplethysmography
- Doppler ultrasonography
- descending contrast venography
- ascending contrast venography
- ambulatory venous pressure

Photoplethysmography

Photoplethysmography (PPG) is a simple, rapid, nontraumatic, and noninvasive method of assessing chronic venous insufficiency. The technique was first described by Barnes and associates.[8] They noticed that it took a longer time for cutaneous blood to refill following exercise in a normal limb compared with one with chronic venous insufficiency. The condition is associated with abnormal blood content in the cutaneous tissue of the lower extremities, which then can be detected by photoplethysmography.

Technique

A photoelectric transducer is placed just above the medial malleolus (Fig. 15–5), which is a common site of ulcer formation in chronic venous insufficiency. The transducer has two components: an infrared light-emitting diode and a photodetector that is attached to an amplifier and a strip chart recorder in the direct current (DC) mode. The patient is examined while sitting down, with the legs in a dependent, non–weight-bearing position.

The patient is asked to plantarflex and dorsiflex the foot five times to contract the calf muscles and then to relax the lower extremity completely. The recording on the strip chart recorder continues before exercise, during exercise, and there-

after until a stable point is achieved and maintained. Details of the technique, instrumentation, and precautions are described in the chapter on venous techniques (see Chapter 13, "Peripheral Venous Examination of the Lower Extremities.")

Venous Refilling Time

After cessation of exercise, the time required for the PPG curve to attain and sustain a stable end point for a period of five or more seconds is called the *venous refilling time* (VRT). One must be sure that the time is determined from the end of exercise rather than from the beginning of exercise. *Cases I* and *II* (Figs. 15–6 and 15–7) demonstrate the importance of calculating the proper venous refilling time.

Case I

The accurate refilling time in the patient in Figure 15–6 is 27 seconds, which is calculated from the end of the exercise. If one calculates from the beginning of exercise, the venous refilling time is 32 seconds, which is inaccurate. In this patient, the diagnosis did not

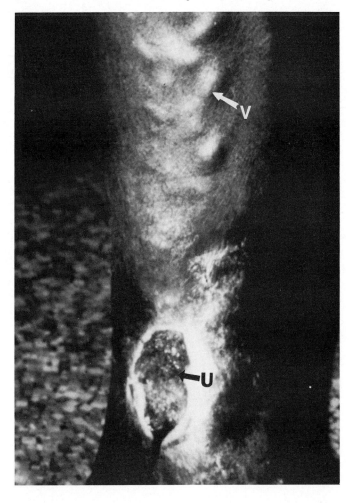

Figure 15–2. A photograph of a patient with chronic venous insufficiency showing ulceration (U) and varicose veins (V). (By permission, Travis J. Phifer, M.D., Department of Surgery, Louisiana State University Medical Center, Shreveport, Louisiana.)

PRIMARY VARICOSE VEINS

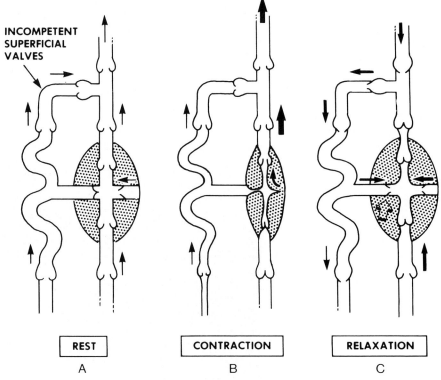

Figure 15–3. Venous dynamics in the limb with primary varicose veins at rest *(A)*, during exercise *(B)*, and after exercise *(C)*.

A, Blood flows to the heart through both superficial and deep venous systems in the direction of the arrows.

B, Blood flows to the heart via superficial and deep venous systems in the direction of the arrows.

C, Blood flows in a retrograde fashion in the superficial venous system and enters the deep system via open valves (open arrow) in the perforating veins.

(From Sumner D. Venous dynamics—varicosities. Clin Obstet Gynecol 1981; 24:752, by permission.)

CHRONIC VENOUS INSUFFICIENCY
INCOMPETENT PERFORATING VEINS, SECONDARY VARICOSE VEINS

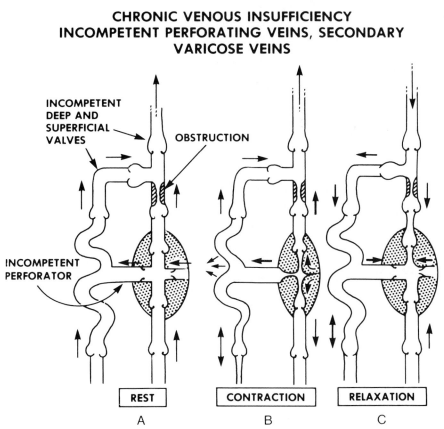

Figure 15–4. Venous dynamics in a limb with chronic venous insufficiency at rest *(A)*, during exercise *(B)*, and after exercise *(C)*.

A, Blood flows in the superficial and deep veins in the direction of the arrows.

B, Blood flows in an antegrade as well as retrograde manner in the deep and superficial venous system.

C, Blood flows in an antegrade as well as a retrograde manner in the deep and superficial venous systems.

(From Sumner D. Venous dynamics—varicosities. Clin Obstet Gynecol 1981; 24:753, by permission.)

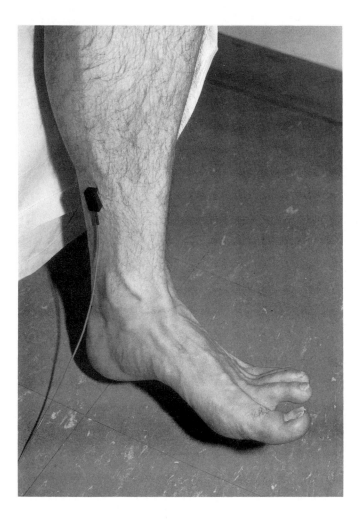

Figure 15–5. A photograph showing a plethysmographic photo sensor placed above the medial malleolus.

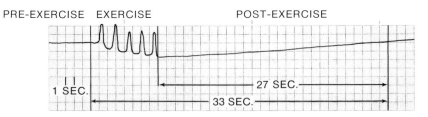

Figure 15–6. Photoplethysmographic tracing calculating accurate and inaccurate venous refilling time (VRT). Accurate VRT = 27 seconds; inaccurate VRT = 33 seconds.

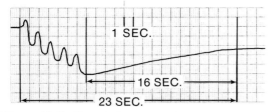

Figure 15–7. Photoplethysmographic tracing calculating accurate and inaccurate venous refilling time (VRT). Accurate VRT = 16 seconds; inaccurate VRT = 23 seconds.

differ because both venous refilling times are within the normal range.

Case II

The accurate venous refilling time at the end of exercise for the patient in Figure 15–7 is 16 seconds, which is abnormal. However, if one calculates from the beginning of exercise, the venous refilling time is 23 seconds, which is within the normal range. In this patient, the diagnoses did differ, and the erroneous diagnosis would have altered the patient's management.

Normal Venous Refilling Time

The normal venous refilling time is 20 seconds or greater (Fig. 15–8).[8] Usually, following leg muscle exercise, there is almost complete emptying of the venous system, which results in a rapid decline in the venous pressure and volume. The venous refilling then occurs via the arterial system because the competent venous valves prevent the retrograde flow of blood. Therefore, it takes a longer time for normal veins to fill with blood.

Chronic Venous Insufficiency

Chronic venous insufficiency is associated with valvular incompetency with or without venous obstruction. Following exercise, there is no significant decrease in venous volume and pressure in these patients because outlet obstruction prevents complete emptying of the veins and incompetent valves allow retrograde flow of blood to refill the venous system. This state results in

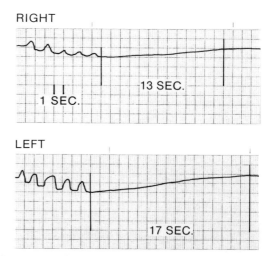

Figure 15–9. Chronic venous insufficiency. Photoplethysmographic tracing with abnormal venous refilling time, suggesting chronic venous insufficiency. Right = 13 seconds; left = 17 seconds.

shortening of the venous refilling time to less than 20 seconds, the value depending upon the severity of the condition (Fig. 15–9). In a patient with severe venous insufficiency, particularly when the deep veins and perforators are involved, the refilling time may be reduced even further and may be less than 10 seconds (Fig. 15–10).

Primary Venous Insufficiency

The venous refilling time is also abnormal in a limb with primary venous insufficiency. The ambulatory venous pressure after exercise is low, but not as low as seen in a limb with a normal venous system. A tourniquet, or pressure cuff, is utilized to differentiate primary from secondary venous insufficiency. The tourniquet is placed above the knee to occlude the superficial venous system but not the deep venous system. The test is repeated again as previously described. If the venous refilling time returns to normal (>20 seconds), the superficial venous system is responsible for the insufficiency. This is illustrated in *Case III* and Figure 15–11.

Figure 15–8. Normal photoplethysmography. Photoplethysmographic tracing with normal venous refilling time of 22 seconds.

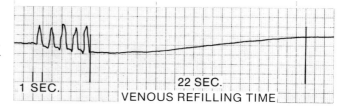

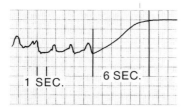

Figure 15–10. Severe chronic venous insufficiency. Photoplethysmographic tracing with markedly abnormal venous refilling time of 6 seconds, suggesting severe chronic venous insufficiency.

Case III

A 34-year-old woman presented with signs and symptoms of chronic venous insufficiency. The PPG showed a VRT of 7 seconds (Fig. 15–11*A*), which improved to 21 seconds after the application of a tourniquet (Fig. 15–11*B*). These findings suggested the presence of primary venous insufficiency.

Secondary Venous Insufficiency

In chronic venous insufficiency the pressure remains elevated in both the superficial and deep systems all of the time. Unlike that in the normal venous system, the ambulatory venous pressure does not fall following exercise. Therefore, the VRT remains abnormal, even after the application of a tourniquet. This is shown in *Case IV* and Figure 15–12.

Case IV

A 43-year-old man presented with chronic leg pain. The PPG demonstrated a short VRT of 8 seconds (Fig. 15–12*A*). The VRT remained abnormal after the ap-

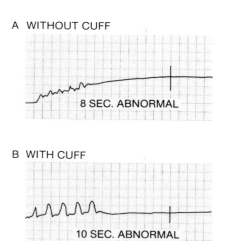

Figure 15–12. Secondary venous insufficiency. Photoplethysmographic (PPG) tracing of secondary venous insufficiency without pressure cuff *(A)* and with pressure cuff *(B)*. *A*, PPG tracing with an abnormal venous refilling time (VRT) of 8 seconds. *B*, PPG with VRT (10 seconds) remained abnormal after tourniquet application.

plication of a tourniquet (Fig. 15–12*B*). These findings indicated venous insufficiency of the deep system.

Uses of Photoplethysmography

Photoplethysmography is used for the following purposes:

1. To confirm the clinical diagnosis of chronic venous insufficiency.

2. To differentiate primary from secondary venous insufficiency and, thus, to predict the success of varicose vein stripping. If the VRT returns to normal after the application of the

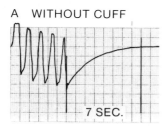

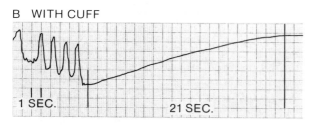

Figure 15–11. Primary venous insufficiency. Photoplethysmographic (PPG) tracing of primary venous insufficiency without pressure cuff *(A)* and with pressure cuff *(B)*. *A*, An abnormal venous refilling time (VRT) of 7 seconds. *B*, PPG tracing with VRT returning to normal (21 seconds) after tourniquet application, suggesting primary venous insufficiency.

tourniquet, surgery may help the patient and vice versa.

3. To follow the results of reconstructive surgery.

Limitations

Like the venous pressure measurement, photoplethysmography is not reliable in the presence of arterial obstructive disease. The plethysmographic examination cannot be calibrated accurately to measure blood flow.

Doppler Ultrasonography

Doppler ultrasonography is another noninvasive technique for evaluating venous insufficiency. It can aid in detecting both venous valvular incompetency and venous outlet obstruction secondary to thrombosis in the superficial as well as the deep venous system.

The test consists of a bi-directional Doppler probe (5 to 10 MHz frequency) containing two crystals, one that sends and one that receives the sound. The probe is connected to the amplifier and strip chart recorder. The veins that are accessible to the Doppler probe are the common femoral, superficial femoral, popliteal, posterior tibial, anterior tibial, lesser and greater saphenous, and the perforators.

The examination is performed with the patient in the supine position. Superficial veins should be examined without any pressure applied on the skin surface; deep veins can be examined with slight pressure applied on the skin. Each vein should be examined separately for patency and valvular incompetency. Details of this technique have been described in Chapter 13.

Two methods are used to assess valvular incompetency: (1) *proximal limb compression* and (2) *Valsalva maneuvers*.

The first method consists of compression of the limb proximal to the Doppler probe (Fig. 15–13). This method impedes the venous blood flow,

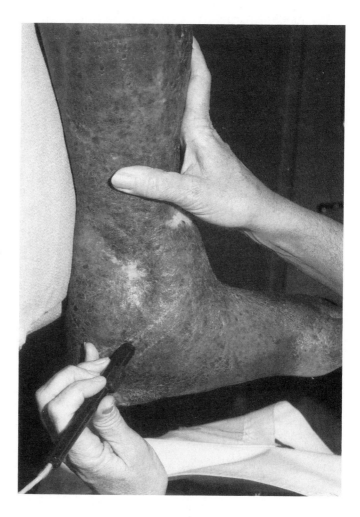

Figure 15–13. A photograph showing compression of the limb proximal to Doppler probe.

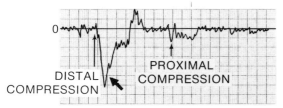

Figure 15–14. Doppler ultrasound showing normal response to compression of the limb distal and proximal to Doppler probe. Note the augmentation of flow following distal compression (large arrow) and decrease in flow following proximal compression (small arrow).

which is seen as a change in the Doppler velocity (Fig. 15–14). The competent valves between the probe and point of compression prevent retrograde flow of blood. This situation can be visualized as absence of the positive waveform deflections, indicating absence of reflux. When valves are incompetent, retrograde flow will be detected as positive waveform deflection (Fig. 15–15). This technique is usually used for distal veins.

The proximal compression technique cannot be used in proximal veins such as the common femoral vein. The Valsalva maneuver will be helpful in this situation. Valsalva maneuvers (deep breathing, coughing) increase the intraabdominal pressure and, hence, impede venous return from the lower extremity (Fig. 15–16). Competent valves in the common femoral vein prevent retrograde flow of blood from the inferior vena cava and iliac veins. If the femoral vein valve is incompetent, reflux can be documented in the femoral vein by this method. Reflux in distal veins can also be detected using this method.

After release of compression of the limb distal to the probe, the examiner must be careful not to mistake the positive deflection for an indication of reflux (Fig. 15–17).[9] This confusing finding is sometimes seen, and it occurs because the blood, which is pushed superiorly by distal compression of the limb, tries to flow in a retro-

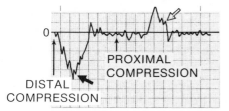

Figure 15–15. Doppler ultrasound showing positive deflection (open arrow), indicating reflux during compression of the limb proximal to probe. Augmentation (solid arrow) indicates absence of outlet obstruction.

grade manner to occupy the empty vein upon release of compression.

Chronic venous insufficiency from secondary varicose veins and post-thrombotic syndrome is usually due to previous thrombophlebitis. The affected vein may undergo recanalization, and numerous collateral venous channels may also be present. Therefore, obstruction may or may not be present with chronic venous insufficiency. Hence, Doppler ultrasonography may or may not be able to detect outflow obstruction in spite of the diseased veins; however, Doppler ultrasonography can aid in differentiating primary varicose veins from secondary varicose veins by demonstrating reflux. In the primary condition, reflux will be demonstrated in the superficial venous system of the lower extremity greater and lesser saphenous veins. It is illustrated in *Case V* and Figure 15–18.

Case V
A 40-year-old man presented with signs and symptoms of chronic venous insufficiency. Doppler ultrasound (Fig. 15–18) and strain gauge plethysmography (SPG) (Fig. 15–19) showed no venous outlet obstruction. The venous flow was phasic with good augmentation. The proximal compression and Valsalva maneuvers revealed reflux in the saphenous vein without deep system involvement (Fig. 15–18). This finding suggested a diagnosis of primary varicose vein or superficial venous insufficiency. The Doppler finding was also confirmed by PPG. The VRT without the cuff was 11 seconds (Fig. 15–20A). The VRT returned to normal (20 seconds) when the test was repeated with a tourniquet (Fig. 15–20B). The patient also was examined by means of ascending venography, which showed normal superficial femoral, popliteal, and deep veins in the extremity (Fig. 15–21). Venography demonstrated varices of the superficial veins and incompetent perforators (Fig. 15–22). Contrast material was retained in the superficial venous system and emptied out of the deep system following exercise (Fig. 15–23). The use of venography established the diagnosis of superficial venous insufficiency with normal deep venous pump, as had been suggested by the noninvasive tests.

In some cases of primary varicosity, reflux may be present in the common femoral vein because the iliofemoral valve is often incompetent in primary varicose veins (Fig. 15–24). However, reflux should not be present in the other deep veins, such as the popliteal and posterior tibial veins. This example of reflux is demonstrated in *Case VI* and Figure 15–24.

Case VI
A middle-aged woman presented with chronic pain in the left leg. Doppler ultrasonography demonstrated reflux in the common femoral and saphenous veins

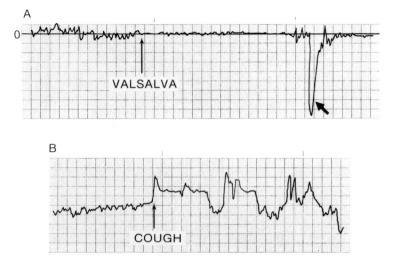

Figure 15–16. Doppler ultrasound during Valsalva maneuver *(A)* and coughing *(B)* showing change in velocity without reflux. Augmentation of flow shown by large arrow.

(Fig. 15–24). There was no evidence of associated obstructive venous disease. Photoplethysmogrpahy confirmed the diagnosis of superficial venous insufficiency. The shortened VRT of 16 seconds improved to 26 seconds when the pressure cuff was applied (Fig. 15–25). Ascending venography showed engorgement and tortuosity of the great saphenous vein (Fig. 15–26). There was no associated deep vein thrombosis, and both the superficial and deep venous systems were empty of contrast media on the post-exercise radiograph (Fig. 15–27).

With deep venous incompetency, reflux may be present in both the deep and superficial veins. An example of deep venous incompetency is discussed in *Case VII.*

Case VII

A 34-year-old man presented with ulceration and pain in both lower extremities. Doppler ultrasonography exhibited a phasic pattern with good augmentation, suggesting absence of venous outlet obstruction (Fig. 15–28). Reflux was seen as a positive deflection waveform for both deep and superficial venous systems, indicating deep venous insufficiency. The SPG was equivocal bilaterally (Fig. 15–29). Pre-exercise ascending venography displayed irregularities of the

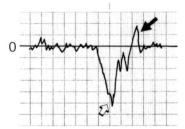

Figure 15–17. Doppler ultrasound showing positive deflection (solid arrow) following release of distal compression. Augmentation is demonstrated by open arrow.

deep veins secondary to previous thrombophlebitis (Fig. 15–30). Varices of the superficial venous system and incompetent communicating veins were also identified on contrast venography. Post-exercise venography showed retention of the contrast within the superficial as well as the deep venous system (Fig. 15–31), suggesting the diagnosis of chronic venous insufficiency with valvular incompetency. Photoplethysmography demonstrated shortening of the VRT with no improvement following the application of the pressure cuff (Fig. 15–32).

Descending Venography

Venous valves play a very essential role in venous physiology. The most important pathogenesis in the development of chronic venous insufficiency is the absence of valves or the presence of incompetent venous valves, particularly in saphenofemoral and femoropopliteal veins.[10–12] Primary varicose veins are associated with hypoplastic-to-absent proximal valves, whereas secondary venous insufficiency results from incompetency of valves damaged most commonly by thrombophlebitis. More recently, attention has been paid to the function of venous valves because of the improvement of surgical techniques for correcting chronic venous insufficiency.

Noninvasive techniques cannot quantitatively assess venous insufficiency. Although ascending venography can be used to exhibit varicose veins, recanalized post-phlebitic veins, and collaterals, it cannot appraise the function of the proximal valves in the lower extremity. Descending venography, by directly visualizing venous valves, offers the capability of assessing valvular function.

Text continued on page 267

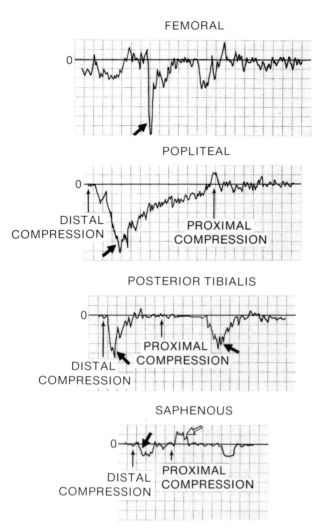

FEMORAL

POPLITEAL

DISTAL
COMPRESSION

PROXIMAL
COMPRESSION

POSTERIOR TIBIALIS

PROXIMAL
COMPRESSION

DISTAL
COMPRESSION

SAPHENOUS

DISTAL
COMPRESSION

PROXIMAL
COMPRESSION

Figure 15–18. *Case V.* Primary venous insufficiency. Doppler ultrasound showing phasic respiration with augmentation (solid arrows) in femoral, popliteal, posterior tibial, and saphenous veins, indicating no venous outlet obstruction. Reflux (open arrow) is seen in the saphenous vein.

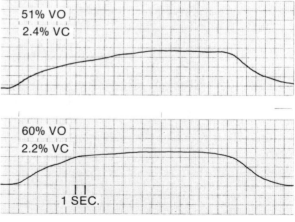

51% VO
2.4% VC

60% VO
2.2% VC

1 SEC.

Figure 15–19. *Case V.* Primary venous insufficiency. Strain gauge plethysmography showing normal venous capacitance (VC) and venous outflow (VO).

A WITHOUT CUFF

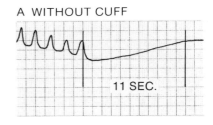

11 SEC.

Figure 15–20. *Case V.* Primary venous insufficiency. Photoplethysmographic (PPG) tracing without pressure cuff *(A)* and with cuff *(B)*. *A*, PPG without cuff showing short venous refilling time (VRT) of 11 seconds. *B*, PPG with cuff showing VRT returning to normal (20 seconds).

B WITH CUFF

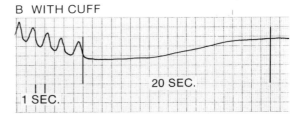

1 SEC.   20 SEC.

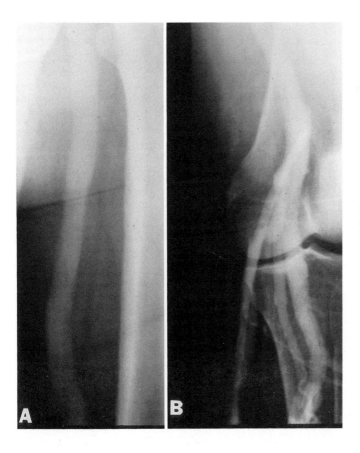

Figure 15–21. *Case V.* Primary venous insufficiency. Ascending venograms of thigh *(A)* and lower leg *(B)* showing normal superficial femoral, popliteal, and deep veins of the leg.

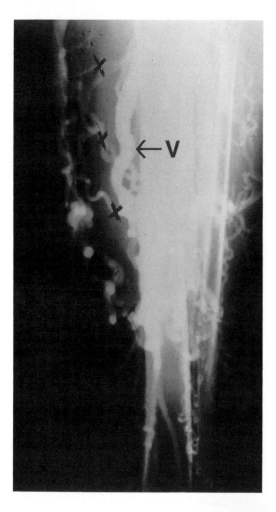

Figure 15–22. *Case V.* Primary venous insufficiency. Ascending venogram of leg showing superficial vein varices (V) and incompetent communicating veins (X).

Figure 15–23. *Case V.* Primary venous insufficiency. Post-exercise venography (*A*, *B*, and *C*) showing contrast media emptying out of normal deep veins of the leg and retained in the superficial veins.

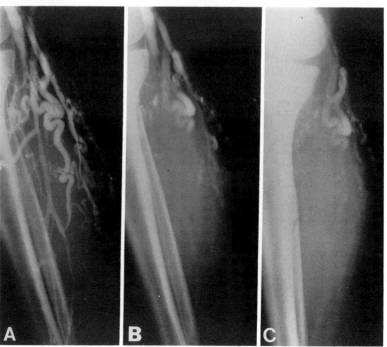

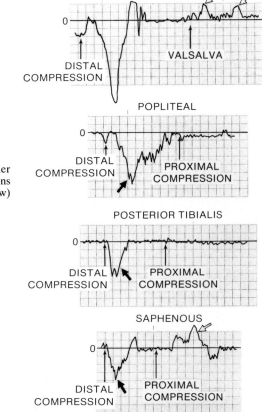

Figure 15–24. *Case VI.* Primary venous insufficiency. Doppler ultrasound showing reflux in the femoral and saphenous veins (open arrows). Phasic pattern with augmentation (closed arrow) indicating absence of venous outflow obstruction.

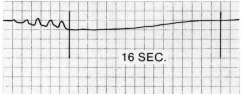

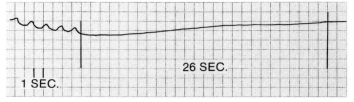

Figure 15–25. *Case VI.* Primary venous insufficiency. Photoplethysmographic tracing without *(A)* and with *(B)* pressure cuff. *A,* Shortened venous refilling time (VRT) of 16 seconds indicating venous insufficiency. *B,* Improved VRT of 26 seconds following cuff application, indicating superficial venous insufficiency.

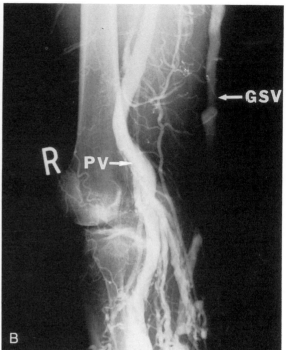

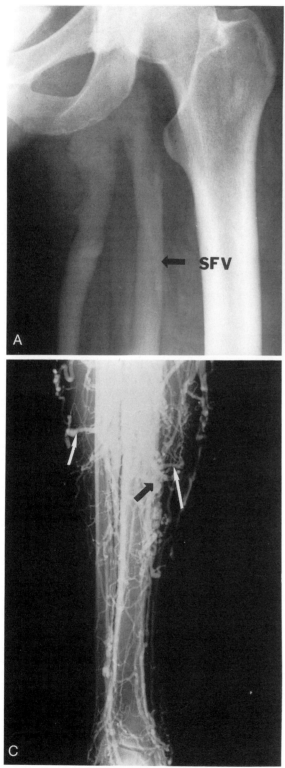

Figure 15–26. *Case VI.* Primary venous insufficiency. Ascending venography: thigh *(A)*, knee *(B)*, and lower leg *(C)*. *A*, Patent superficial femoral vein (SFV) without thrombosis. *B*, Patent popliteal vein (PV) without thrombosis. [Enlarged and tortuous saphenous vein (GSV).] *C*, Varices of the superficial veins (black arrow) with incompetent perforators (white arrows).

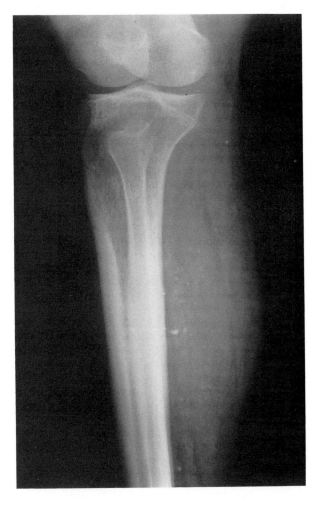

Figure 15–27. *Case VI.* Primary venous insufficiency. Post-exercise venogram showing almost complete emptying of the superficial and deep venous system.

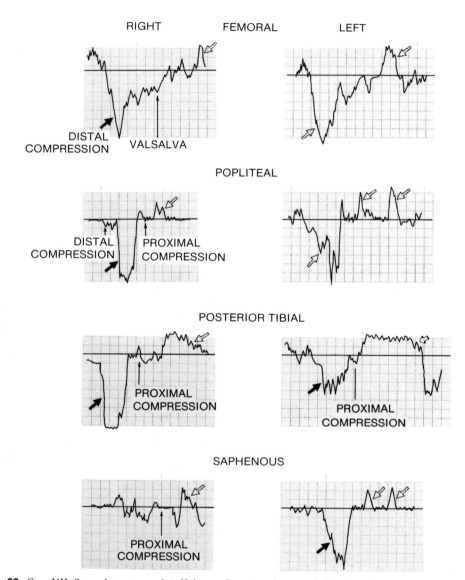

Figure 15–28. *Case VII.* Secondary venous insufficiency. Doppler ultrasound showing reflux in both the superficial and deep venous systems (open arrows), indicating deep venous insufficiency. Augmentation (closed arrows) suggests absence of obstruction.

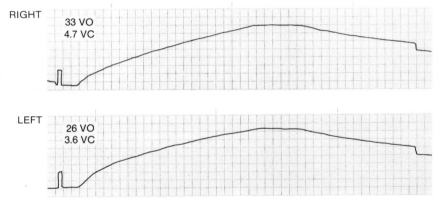

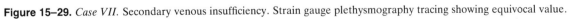

Figure 15–29. *Case VII.* Secondary venous insufficiency. Strain gauge plethysmography tracing showing equivocal value.

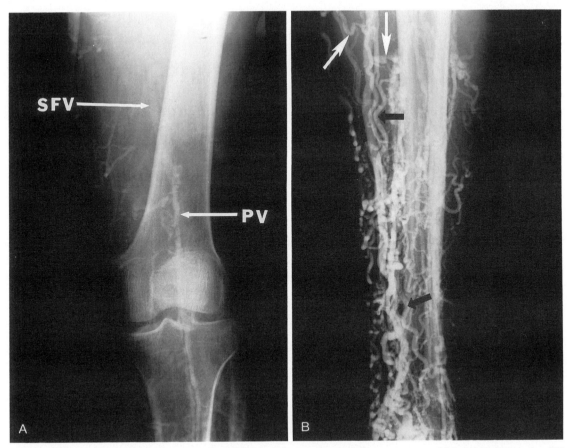

Figure 15–30. *Case VII.* Secondary venous insufficiency. Pre-exercise ascending venogram: thigh *(A)* and lower leg *(B)*. *A*, Irregularities of the popliteal (PV) and superficial femoral (SFV) veins suggest deep vein thrombosis. *B*, Varices of the superficial veins (black arrows) and incompetent perforators (white arrows).

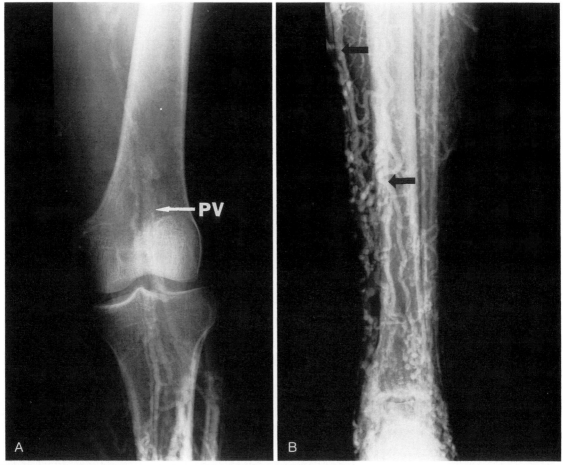

Figure 15–31. *Case VII.* Secondary venous insufficiency. Post-exercise venogram: thigh *(A)* and lower leg *(B)*. *A*, Retention of contrast material in the popliteal vein (PV). *B*, Retention of contrast material in the superficial venous system (arrows).

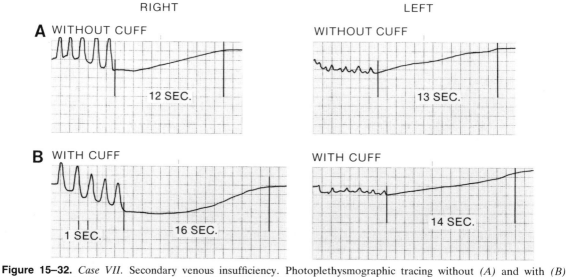

Figure 15–32. *Case VII.* Secondary venous insufficiency. Photoplethysmographic tracing without *(A)* and with *(B)* pressure cuff. *A*, Abnormal venous refilling time (VRT) of 12 seconds on the right and 13 seconds on the left. *B*, The VRT remained abnormal after the application of the cuff.

Technique

A No. 6 French end-hold catheter is placed into the common femoral vein percutaneously. The catheter is then moved superiorly to the level of the superior pubic rami. The patient is positioned 60° in a semi-upright position, and 15 ml of 60% meglumine diatrizoate is injected under fluoroscopic control. The patient is allowed to breathe during the examination. Spot films of the iliofemoral junction are acquired in multiple projections. Spot films of the thigh and lower leg are also taken at the same time. Radiographs of the thigh and leg are also acquired during the course of the injection while the patient performs the Valsalva maneuver.

Interpretation

Reflux of contrast material distally into the venous system is classified by Kistner[11] and is shown in Table 15–1. A reflux of Grade II or greater should be considered clinically valuable because minimal competency or less than Grade

Table 15–1. Grading of Venous Insufficiency

Grade 0	Competence. No reflux of contrast material beyond the upper aspect of the femoral vein.
Grade I	Minimal incompetence. Reflux of contrast material beyond the uppermost valve in the femoral vein but not beyond the proximal aspect of the thigh.
Grade II	Mild incompetence. Reflux into the femoral vein to the level of the knee.
Grade III	Moderate incompetence. Reflux to a level just below the knee.
Grade IV	Severe incompetence. Reflux into the paired calf veins to the level of the ankle.

Data from Kistner RL. Transvenous repair of the incompetent femoral vein valve. *In* Bergan JJ and Yao JST (eds). Venous Problems. Copyright © by Year Book Medical Publishers, Chicago. (Modified and reproduced with permission.)

II reflux has been found to occur in 40% of normal subjects.[10] Normal descending venography of a competent femoral valve is illustrated in Figure 15–33.

The level of valvular incompetency can be

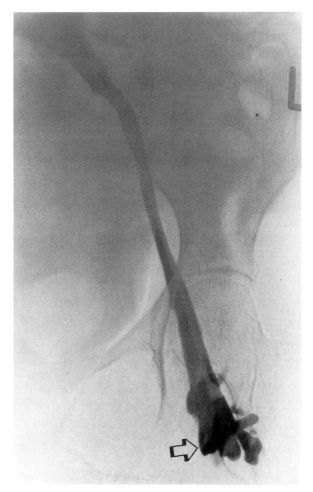

Figure 15–33. Normal descending venogram with competent valve (open arrow).

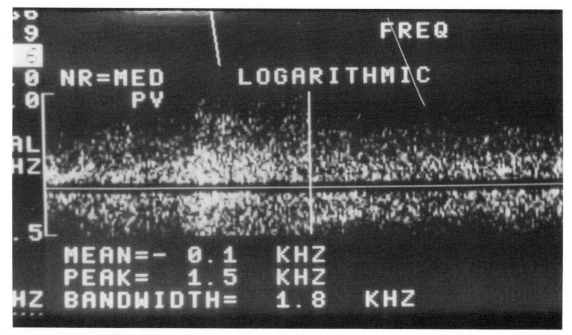

Figure 15–34. *Case VIII.* Spectral analysis shows bi-directional flow, indicating incompetency of the iliofemoral valves.

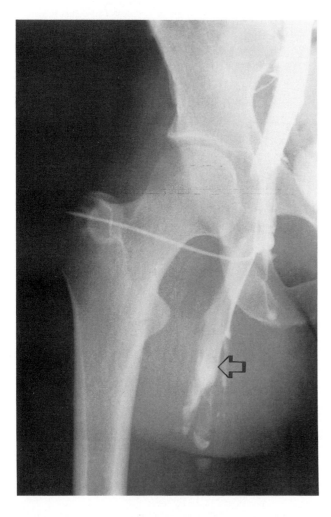

Figure 15–35. *Case VIII.* Descending venogram displaying reflux of the contrast material into the superficial femoral vein (open arrow), suggesting incompetent iliofemoral valves.

accurately determined by descending venography; this information cannot be provided by bi-directional ultrasonography, photoplethysmography, or radionuclide or contrast venography. However, findings should be correlated with those from ascending contrast venography to determine the cause of the patient's symptomatology, and other tests should be employed to assess chronic venous insufficiency. The following cases show descending venography used in collaboration with other invasive and noninvasive techniques to achieve the diagnosis of valvular insufficiency.

Case VIII

A 30-year-old woman presented with leg pain. Duplex ultrasonography showed bi-directional flow from the left femoral vein during the Valsalva maneuver, indicating incompetency of the iliofemoral valves (Fig. 15–34). The descending venogram exhibited reflux of the contrast material into the superficial femoral vein (Fig. 15–35), confirming the finding of the duplex examination. There was good correlation between the duplex examination and descending venography. The patient was symptomatic in spite of findings of Grade I reflux.

Case IX

A middle-aged man presented with left leg pain. The Doppler ultrasound examination demonstrated a positive deflection waveform from the femoral vein during the Valsalva maneuver and from the popliteal vein during proximal compression (Fig. 15–36). Photoplethysmography with and without the pressure cuff was abnormal, suggesting incompetency of the deep venous system (Fig. 15–37). The descending venogram exhibited reflux of the contrast material in the superficial femoral vein up to the knee level (Fig. 15–38). This finding indicates a Grade II reflux and shows good correlation between descending venography, Doppler ultrasonography, and PPG.

Case X

A 40-year-old man presented with signs and symptoms of chronic venous insufficiency. Doppler ultrasonography identified reflux in the femoral and popliteal veins (Fig. 15–39). The femoral vein was compressible and showed good augmentation on the real-time ultrasound examination, indicating patency (Fig. 15–40). Descending venography revealed incompetency of the iliofemoral valves, occlusion of the common iliac vein and collaterals (Fig. 15–41).

Descending venography can also be used to assess the results of surgical correction of valvular incompetency of the femoral vein.

Ascending Venography

Ascending contrast venography plays a major role in achieving the diagnosis of deep vein

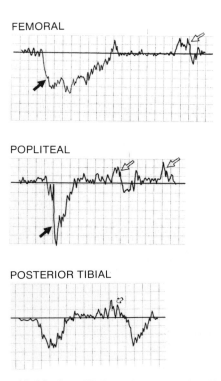

Figure 15–36. *Case IX.* Secondary venous insufficiency. Doppler ultrasound showing incompetency of the iliofemoral valves (open arrows). Phasic venous flow and augmentation (closed arrows), indicating a patent venous system.

thrombosis. However, it plays a secondary role in the assessment of chronic venous insufficiency because it does not have the capability of evaluating valvular function.[12] Ascending venography can aid in appraising the anatomical status of the

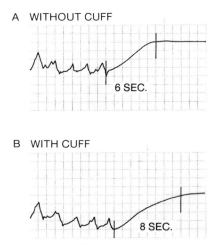

Figure 15–37. *Case IX.* Secondary venous insufficiency. Photoplethysmography without *(A)* and with *(B)* pressure cuff. *A,* Abnormal venous refilling time (VRT) of 6 seconds. *B,* The VRT remained abnormal after pressure cuff application, indicating deep venous insufficiency.

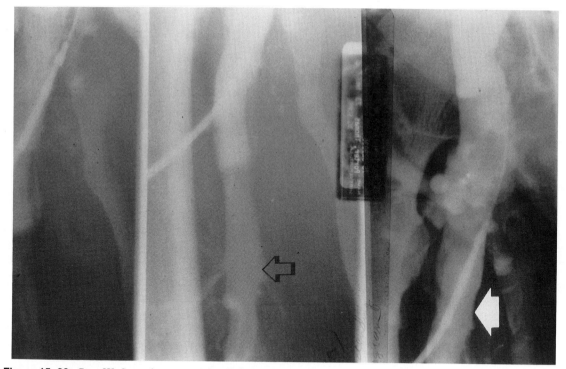

Figure 15–38. *Case IX.* Secondary venous insufficiency. Descending venogram showing reflux of contrast material into superficial femoral vein. Proximal = Closed white arrow; distal = open black arrow.

FEMORAL

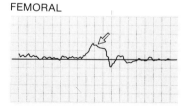

POPLITEAL

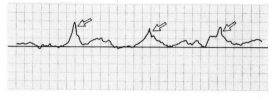

Figure 15–39. *Case X.* Secondary venous insufficiency. Doppler ultrasound showing incompetency of the femoral, popliteal, and posterior tibial veins (open arrows). Augmentation is shown by closed arrow.

POSTERIOR TIBIAL

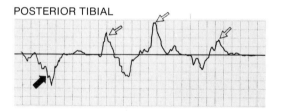

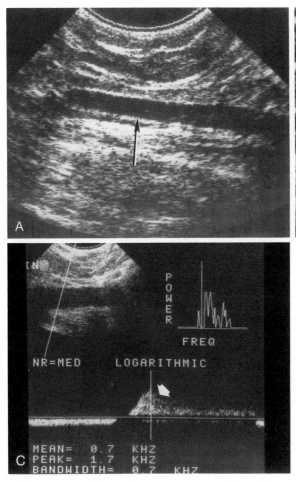

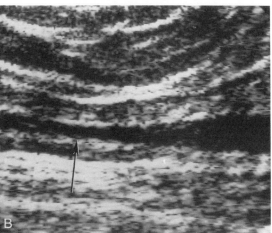

Figure 15–40. *Case X.* Secondary venous insufficiency. Real-time ultrasound without *(A)* and with *(B)* compression, and spectral analysis *(C)*. *A,* Patent femoral vein (arrow). *B,* Femoral vein compressed with slight pressure, indicating patency (arrow). *C,* Spectral analysis shows augmentation, suggesting patency (arrow).

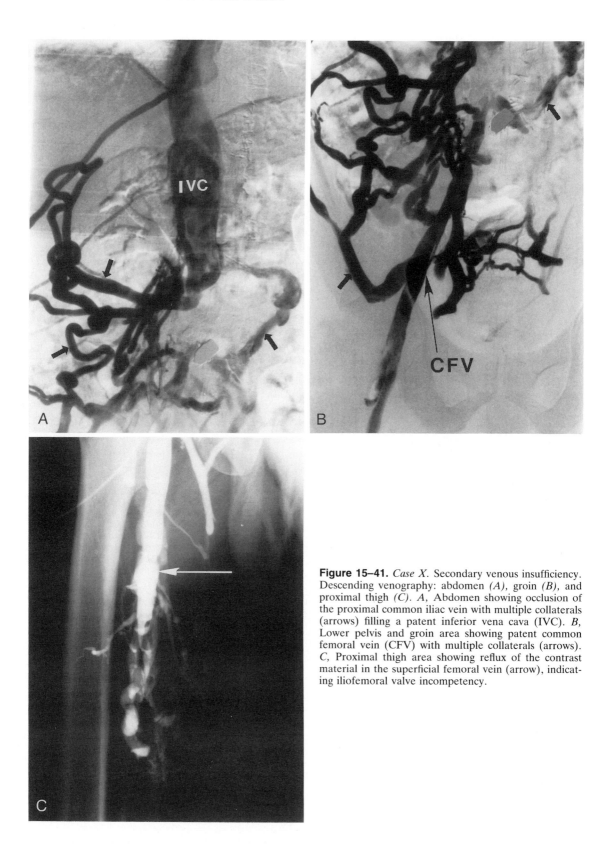

Figure 15–41. *Case X.* Secondary venous insufficiency. Descending venography: abdomen *(A)*, groin *(B)*, and proximal thigh *(C)*. *A,* Abdomen showing occlusion of the proximal common iliac vein with multiple collaterals (arrows) filling a patent inferior vena cava (IVC). *B,* Lower pelvis and groin area showing patent common femoral vein (CFV) with multiple collaterals (arrows). *C,* Proximal thigh area showing reflux of the contrast material in the superficial femoral vein (arrow), indicating iliofemoral valve incompetency.

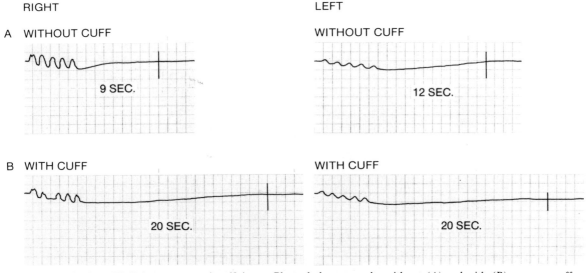

Figure 15–42. *Case XI.* Primary venous insufficiency. Photoplethysmography without *(A)* and with *(B)* pressure cuff. *A,* Abnormal venous refilling time (VRT) of 9 seconds on the right and 12 seconds on the left. *B,* VRT returned to normal after pressure cuff application.

deep and communicating veins and in detecting deep venous obstruction as well as a recanalized channel indicating previous thrombophlebitis. The absence or presence of the varicosity and the location of the incompetent perforator can also be documented by this technique.[15]

Post-exercise venography is helpful in differentiating primary from secondary varicose veins. In a patient with primary varicose veins, contrast material will remain in the superficial system and will empty from the deep veins following exercise (Fig. 15–23). In some patients with superficial venous insufficiency, contrast may empty from

both the superficial and deep systems. This is illustrated in *Case XI.*

Case XI
Photoplethysmography exhibits a shortened VRT of 9 seconds on the right and 12 seconds on the left. The VRT improved to 20 seconds on both sides when the pressure cuff was applied (Fig. 15–42). Doppler ultrasonography confirmed the presence of reflux in the superficial venous system (Fig. 15–43). The ascending venogram demonstrated varices of the superficial veins (Fig. 15–44). Films taken after exercise revealed complete emptying of both superficial and deep venous systems (Fig. 15–45).

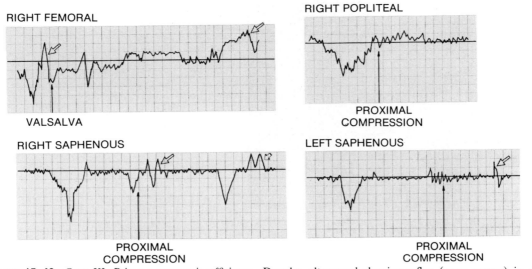

Figure 15–43. *Case XI.* Primary venous insufficiency. Doppler ultrasound showing reflux (open arrows) in right superficial femoral and superficial veins.

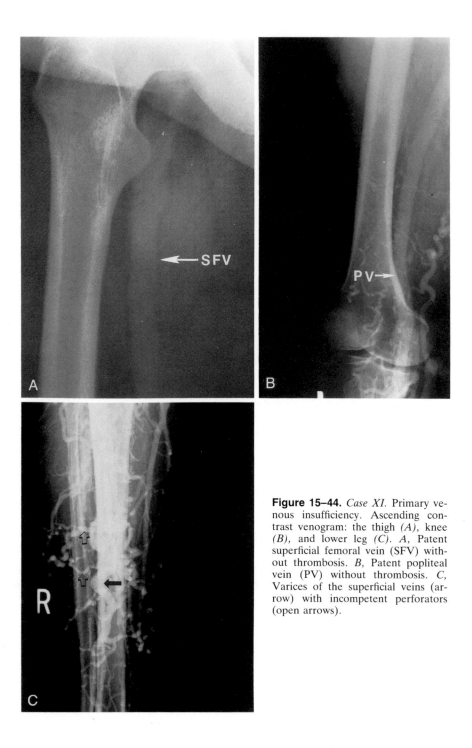

Figure 15–44. *Case XI.* Primary venous insufficiency. Ascending contrast venogram: the thigh *(A)*, knee *(B)*, and lower leg *(C)*. *A,* Patent superficial femoral vein (SFV) without thrombosis. *B,* Patent popliteal vein (PV) without thrombosis. *C,* Varices of the superficial veins (arrow) with incompetent perforators (open arrows).

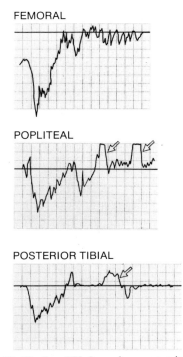

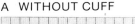

Figure 15–46. *Case XII.* Secondary venous insufficiency. Doppler ultrasound displaying reflux in the popliteal and posterior tibial veins (open arrows).

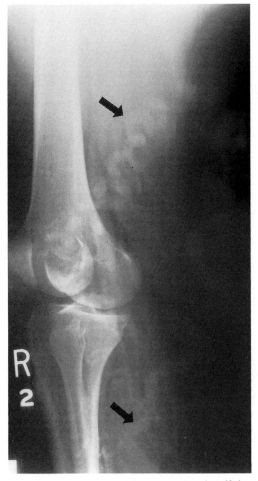

Figure 15–45. *Case XI.* Primary venous insufficiency. Post-exercise venogram showing retention of contrast in the collaterals (arrows), suggesting superficial venous insufficiency.

With deep venous insufficiency, contrast will be seen only in the deep venous system following exercise. This occurrence is illustrated in *Case XII.*

Case XII
The Doppler ultrasound examination in this case exhibited reflux without outlet obstruction in the deep venous system (Fig. 15–46). Photoplethysmography demonstrated an abnormal response to exercise with a shortened VRT that did not improve following application of the pressure cuff (Fig. 15–47). The presence of varices of the superficial veins with incompetent perforators was seen on the ascending contrast venogram (Fig. 15–48). After exercise, contrast was retained in the superficial as well as the deep venous system (Fig. 15–49), indicating deep venous insufficiency.

Ambulatory Venous Pressure

The measurement of venous pressure is an old diagnostic test for directly determining venous pressure. It is a quantitative test for assessing chronic venous insufficiency. The test not only confirms the clinical diagnosis but also differentiates primary from secondary chronic venous insufficiency.[14, 15] The diagnosis relies on determining the venous pressure before and after

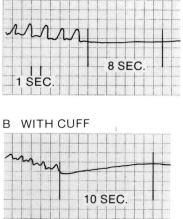

Figure 15–47. *Case XII.* Secondary venous insufficiency. Photoplethysmography without *(A)* and with *(B)* pressure cuff. *A,* Abnormal venous refilling time (VRT) of 8 seconds. *B,* VRT remains abnormal following pressure cuff application, indicating deep venous insufficiency.

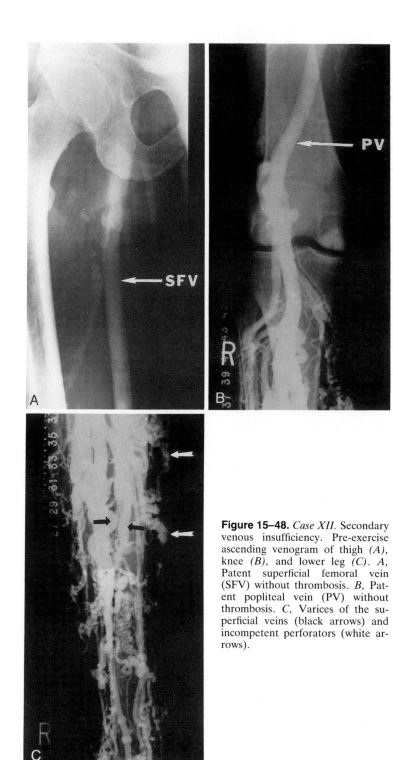

Figure 15–48. *Case XII.* Secondary venous insufficiency. Pre-exercise ascending venogram of thigh *(A)*, knee *(B)*, and lower leg *(C)*. *A*, Patent superficial femoral vein (SFV) without thrombosis. *B*, Patent popliteal vein (PV) without thrombosis. *C*, Varices of the superficial veins (black arrows) and incompetent perforators (white arrows).

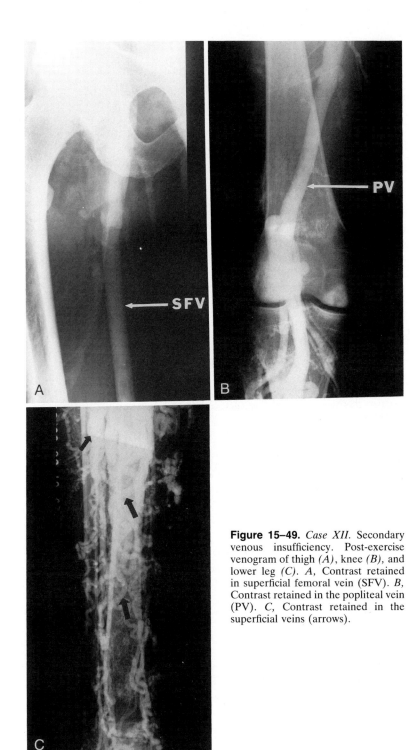

Figure 15–49. *Case XII.* Secondary venous insufficiency. Post-exercise venogram of thigh *(A)*, knee *(B)*, and lower leg *(C)*. *A,* Contrast retained in superficial femoral vein (SFV). *B,* Contrast retained in the popliteal vein (PV). *C,* Contrast retained in the superficial veins (arrows).

exercise. Normally, the venous pressure is reduced significantly after exercise, whereas it does not change significantly in the patient with chronic venous insufficiency.

Technique

A needle or catheter is placed into the vein on the dorsum of the foot or into the greater saphenous vein near the malleoli. The pressure in the superficial venous system is not significantly different from the pressure in the deep venous system. Therefore, pressure measurements from the superficial veins indirectly indicate the deep venous pressure. The catheter or needle is connected by fluid-filled tubing to the transducer, amplifier, and pen recorder.

Initially, venous pressure is acquired at rest in either a supine or a standing position. Then the patient is asked to exercise, either by rising on the toes or by bending the knees ten times in 15 seconds. The pressure is monitored continuously during and also after the cessation of the exercise until it either stabilizes or reaches the pre-exercise level.

Normal Values

The normal pressure in the superficial venous system at the ankle while the patient is in a standing position is approximately 80 to 90 mm Hg.[16] This value is equivalent to the hydrostatic pressure of the blood column between the foot and head. The height and position of the patient do affect the venous pressure. The venous pressure is essentially the same in both males and females.[17]

After exercise, the venous pressure falls to 50 to 80% of the pre-exercise level.[16] This means the pressure falls from 80 to 90 mm Hg to 20 to 40 mm Hg. After the patient stops exercising, the pressure returns to the pre-exercise level. After exercise, the time required for the venous pressure to return to the pre-exercise level is the *recovery time*, which is a function of the normal arterial inflow system, venous outflow system, and the venous valvular competency. The normal recovery time ranges from 10 to 60 seconds (Table 15–2).

Chronic Venous Insufficiency

There is no significant difference in the resting venous pressures of a normal extremity and an extremity with chronic venous insufficiency. However, the maximum pressure fall and the rate of fall as well as the recovery time are

Table 15–2. Venous Pressure Measurement

	Resting Venous Pressure (mm Hg)	Pressure Reduction During Exercise (%)	Recovery Time (sec)
Normal	80–90	60–80 (20–30 mm Hg absolute venous pressure)	10–60
Chronic venous insufficiency	80–90	<60	<10

different in a limb with chronic venous insufficiency when compared with a normal limb. All of these factors are often abnormal in a patient with chronic venous insufficiency.

Following exercise, there is a 20 to 30 mm Hg reduction in venous pressure in a patient with mild to moderate venous insufficiency. This means that venous pressure may drop from 80 to 90 mm Hg to only 50 to 60 mm Hg compared with a 20 to 30 mm Hg drop in a normal limb. In severe venous insufficiency, the post-exercise venous pressure either may remain unchanged or may increase when compared with the resting pressure. The recovery time is also very short (<10 seconds) in venous insufficiency (Table 15–2).

In patients with primary varicose veins, the post-exercise pressure is reduced significantly when a tourniquet is applied over the thigh. The recovery time is also prolonged in these patients after tourniquet application. However, in patients with secondary varicose veins, the post-exercise pressure remains elevated even after the tourniquet application over the thigh.

Limitations

The venous pressure measurement test cannot be used as a screening test or repeated frequently because it is time consuming and because it is invasive. Also, it is capable of assessing only the overall efficiency of the venous pump and is not useful in determining the individual abnormality in the presence of multiple abnormalities.

Because numerous noninvasive tests of high accuracy are currently available to evaluate venous insufficiency, the venous pressure test is now used only as a gold standard to compare the results of other tests.

Summary

Classically, venous insufficiency has been evaluated by means of contrast venography and direct venous pressure measurements. However, photoplethysmography and Doppler techniques have been used for years as noninvasive testing methods. There were certain technical limitations and pitfalls associated with these noninvasive methods that made them less reliable than the classical methods. With the addition of duplex scanning, the use of noninvasive procedures is becoming more popular. We are now able to visualize the venous system and combine the duplex examination with other noninvasive testing to obtain a more definitive diagnosis. This combination of tests will eliminate the technical and physiological limitations previously encountered and will provide an easier, less costly method for evaluating venous disease. In turn, these methods will allow for earlier detection, better management of chronic disease, and better surgical planning.

References

1. Sumner DS. Venous dynamics: varicosities. Clin Obstet Gynecol 1981; 24:743–760.
2. Barnes RW. Noninvasive techniques in chronic venous insufficiency. *In* Bernstein EF (ed). Noninvasive diagnostic techniques in vascular disease. 3rd ed. St Louis, CV Mosby, 1985.
3. Lofgren KA. Varicose veins: their symptoms, complications and management. Postgrad Med 1979; 65:131.
4. Cotton LT. Varicose veins: gross anatomy and development. Br J. Surg 1961; 48:589.
5. Edward EA. Varicose veins and venous stasis. Bol Asoc Med PR 1957; 49:49.
6. Alexander CJ. The theoretical basis of varicose vein formation. Med J Aust 1978; 1:258.
7. Linton RR. The post thrombotic ulceration of the lower extremity: its etiology and surgical treatment. Ann Surg 1953; 128:415.
8. Barnes RW, Garrett WV, Hummel BA, Slaymaker EE, Maixner W, Reinertson JE. Photoplethysmographic assessment of altered cutaneous circulation in the post-phlebitic syndrome. Proc Assoc Adv Med Instrum 1978; 13:25.
9. Sumner DS. Diagnosis of deep venous thrombosis by Doppler ultrasound. *In* Nicolaides A, Yao JST (eds). The investigation of vascular disorders. Edinburgh, Churchill Livingstone, 1981:736–802.
10. Herman RJ, Neiman HL, Yao JST, et al. Descending venography: a method of evaluating lower extremity venous valvular function. Radiology 1980; 137:63–69.
11. Kistner R. Transvenous repair of the incompetent femoral vein valve. *In* Bergan JJ, Yao JST (eds). Venous problems. Chicago, Year Book Medical Publishers, 1978: 145–251.
12. Queral LA, Whitehouse WM, Flinn WR, et al. Surgical correction of chronic venous insufficiency by valvular transposition. Surgery 1980; 87:688.
13. Thomas ML. Phlebography. Arch Surg 1972; 104:145.
14. DeCamp PT, Schramel RJ, Ray CJ, et al. Ambulatory venous pressure determination in postphlebitic and related syndromes. Surgery 1951; 29:44.
15. Warren R, White EA, Belcher CD. Venous pressures in the saphenous system in normal, varicose and postphlebitic extremities: alteration following femoral vein ligation. Surgery 1949; 26:435.
16. Browse NL. Venous pressure measurements. *In* Bernstein EF (ed). Noninvasive diagnostic techniques in vascular disease. 3rd ed. St Louis CV Mosby, 1985:834–838.
17. Kriessmann A. Ambulatory venous pressure measurements. *In* Nicolaides A, Yao JST (eds). The investigation of vascular disorders. Edinburgh, Churchill Livingstone, 1980:461–477.

Part IV • Noninvasive Assessment of the Lower Extremity Arterial System

16 • Hemodynamic Anatomy of the Lower Extremities

Introduction

Vascular disease that affects the blood flow in the lower extremity may be located in any or all of the vessels extending from the aorta to the distal arteries of the toes. Both the anatomy and function of this vast array of vessels may be understood by grouping them into three main systems. As shown in Figure 16–1, these are (1) the *aortoiliac inflow* (2) the *femoropopliteal outflow*, and (3) the *tibioperoneal run-off* systems. These three systems link together to form a chain of vessels that carries blood flow to and through the lower extremities. Any weak link or obstructive lesion in this vascular chain may cause the affected limb to become ischemic.

Noninvasive vascular tests are used to locate the weak link in this vascular chain. They do so by detecting changes in systolic segmental pressures and in velocity waveforms caused by the obstructive lesion. Understanding how these tests work requires a knowledge of how the pulse and velocity waveforms are propagated through each of the three systems in the vascular chain; this will be described in this chapter.

Anatomy

Gross Anatomy

Aortoiliac Inflow System

The aortoiliac inflow system begins at the level of the renal arteries and ends at the level of the inguinal ligaments. The angiographic anatomy of this system is shown in Figure 16–2. This system carries the blood pumped from the left ventricle into the arteries of the lower extremities. Obstructive lesions located in this system will limit the blood inflow into either one or both of the lower limbs. The common sites of obstructive lesions are shown in Figure 16–3. Total occlusions

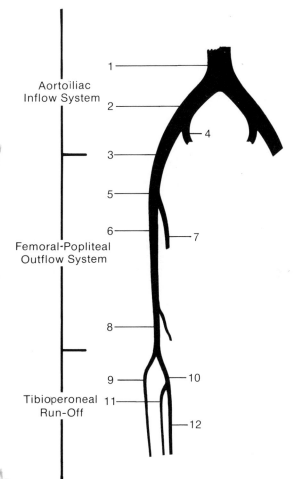

Aortoiliac
Inflow System

Femoral-Popliteal
Outflow System

Tibioperoneal
Run-Off

Figure 16–1. Vascular systems anatomy.
Aortoiliac inflow system: 1, Infrarenal abdominal aortic segment. *2,* Common iliac artery. *3,* External iliac artery. *4,* Internal iliac (hypogastric) artery.
Femoral-popliteal outflow system: 5, Common femoral artery. *6,* Superficial femoral artery. *7,* Profunda femoral artery. *8,* Popliteal artery.
Tibioperoneal run-off system: 9, Anterior tibial artery. *10,* Tibioperoneal trunk. *11,* Peroneal artery. *12,* Posterior tibial artery.

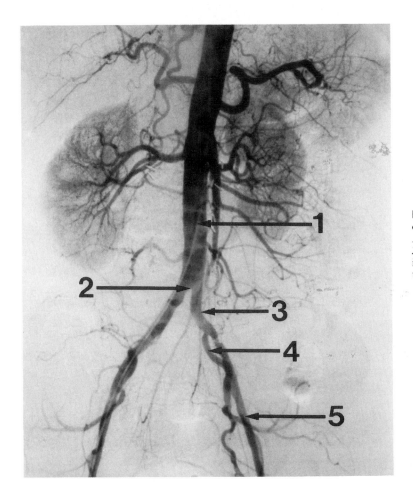

Figure 16–2. Angiographic anatomy of the aortoiliac inflow system. *1,* Infrarenal aortic segment. *2,* Aortic bifurcation. *3,* Common iliac artery. *4,* Internal iliac (hypogastric) artery. *5,* External iliac artery.

Figure 16–3. Sites of obstructive lesions in the aortoiliac inflow system. *1,* Infra-abdominal aortic segment. *2,* Common iliac artery. *3,* Internal iliac artery origin. *4,* External iliac artery.

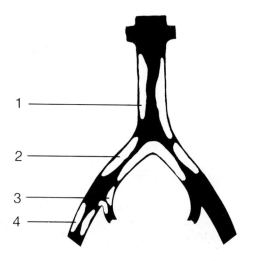

or severe stenoses of the infrarenal abdominal aortic segment, the aortic bifurcation, or the iliac arteries bilaterally will limit the inflow of blood into both of the lower extremities. Lesions of the infrarenal abdominal aortic segment usually extend from just below the level of the renal artery origins to the level of the aortic bifurcation. However, these lesions may involve both the renal artery origins and the aortic bifurcation. Such lesions may also be associated with abdominal aortic aneurysms.

The aortoiliac segment is the second most common site for atherosclerotic obstructive disease in the lower extremities. Isolated unilateral iliac artery obstructions will limit blood inflow into the affected lower limb, whereas the inflow into the unaffected lower limb remains entirely normal. Iliac obstructions range from short segmental stenoses located in either the common or the external iliac arteries to total occlusion of both of these vessels. Bilateral iliac artery obstructions will limit the blood inflow into both of the lower extremities. Isolated obstructions at the origins of the internal iliac arteries do not limit the blood inflow into the affected extremity. The internal iliac arteries do act as a valuable source of collateral blood inflow into the lower extremities when an obstruction exists in the aortoiliac system. Internal iliac artery obstructions will then severely limit the blood inflow into the affected lower extremities under these circumstances.

Femoropopliteal Outflow System

The femoropopliteal outflow system begins at the level of the inguinal ligament and ends at the trifurcation of the popliteal artery into the tibioperoneal vessels. The function of this system is to receive the outflow of blood from the aortoiliac system and carry it to the tibioperoneal run-off system. Obstructions in this system limit blood flow to one or both of the lower extremities by decreasing the blood outflow from the aortoiliac vessels. Common sites of obstructive lesions are shown in Figure 16–4.

The superficial femoral artery (SFA) is the most common site of atherosclerotic obstructive disease in the lower extremities. The SFA usually becomes obstructed either at its origin from the common femoral artery or in its distal segment, which lies within the adductor canal on the medial aspect of the thigh just above the knee. These SFA obstructions may not cause a marked decrease in the outflow of blood from the aortoiliac system when the profunda femoral artery

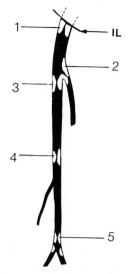

Figure 16–4. Sites of obstructive lesions in the femoral-popliteal outflow system. *1,* Common femoral artery. *2,* Profunda femoral artery origin. *3,* Superficial femoral artery origin. *4,* Superficial femoral artery (adductor canal). *5,* Popliteal artery. IL = Inguinal ligament.

(PFA) remains patent. This is because the PFA can act as a collateral pathway around the obstructions for carrying blood flow into the popliteal artery.

Atherosclerotic common femoral artery (CFA) obstructions are usually caused by disease that extends from the external iliac arteries to involve the CFA. An obstruction of one or both of these arteries severely limits the aortoiliac outflow of blood into the affected lower limb.

The angiographic anatomy of the CFA and its bifurcation branches is shown in Figure 16–5. Figure 16–5 shows that the profunda femoral artery is in a good position to receive the outflow of blood from the aortoiliac system when the SFA is obstructed. Also, note that a CFA obstruction would block the origins of both the superficial femoral and profunda femoral arteries and markedly decrease the outflow of blood into the lower extremity. The same results would occur if the origins of both the superficial femoral and profunda femoral arteries were obstructed.

The angiographic anatomy of the superficial and profunda femoral arteries is shown in Figure 16–6. The SFA descends superficially down the anteromedial aspect of the thigh, and the PFA sinks deeply into the thigh to lie posterolaterally to the SFA. The SFA continues down the thigh to form the popliteal artery; the PFA ends at the lower one third of the thigh to supply the hamstring muscles on the back of the thigh. During its course down the thigh, the SFA passes

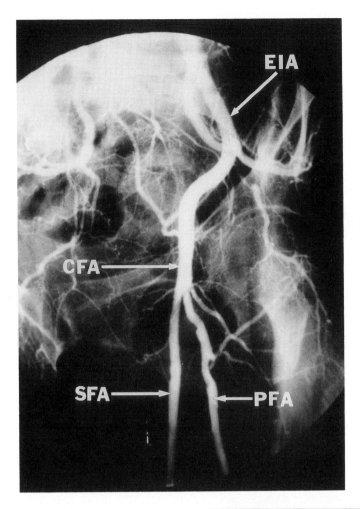

Figure 16–5. Angiographic anatomy of common femoral artery bifurcation vessels. EIA = External iliac artery; CFA = common femoral artery; SFA = superficial femoral artery; PFA = profunda femoral artery.

Figure 16–6. Angiographic anatomy of superficial femoral and profunda femoral arteries. SFA = Superficial femoral artery descending down the anteromedial aspect of the thigh to form the popliteal artery; PFA = profunda femoral artery, which ends at lower one-third of thigh.

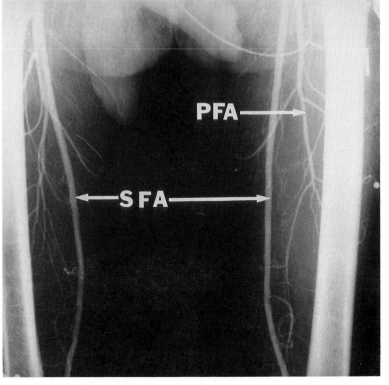

through the adductor canal. This canal is a fascial compartment surrounded by the thigh muscles and conducts both the superficial femoral artery and vein through the middle one third of the thigh. The canal ends at the tendinous insertion of the adductor magnus thigh muscle on the medial aspect of the femur (Fig. 16–7). This point marks the end of the superficial artery and vein and the beginning of the popliteal artery and vein. Both the popliteal artery and vein pass posteriorly to the femur to lie in the popliteal fossa behind the knee, where they end to form the tibioperoneal vessels.

The angiographic anatomy of the popliteal artery is shown in Figure 16–7. The popliteal artery begins at the termination of the adductor canal and ends at the level of the tibioperoneal vessels. Obstructive lesions located in either the distal SFA or the popliteal artery prevent the blood outflow of the aortoiliac system from passing into the tibioperoneal run-off system.

Tibioperoneal Run-Off System

The tibioperoneal run-off system begins at the termination of the popliteal artery in the popliteal fossa behind the knee and ends at the ankle. The system receives the blood run-off from both the aortoiliac and femoropopliteal systems. The blood flow in both of these systems is decreased when the tibioperoneal arteries are obstructed because the blood has no place to go.

As shown in Figure 16–8, the angiographic anatomy of the tibioperoneal run-off system in the leg is composed of the anterior tibial, posterior tibial, and peroneal arteries. The anterior tibial artery begins at the termination of the popliteal artery in the popliteal fossa behind the knee. The anterior tibial artery passes forward between the interosseous membrane of the tibia and fibula to descend down the anterior aspect of the leg, where it ends at the ankle to form the dorsalis pedis artery on the dorsum of the foot. Both the posterior tibial and peroneal arteries often arise from a common trunk at the termination of the popliteal artery. This is called the *posterior tibial peroneal trunk.* The posterior tibial artery extends from this trunk to descend down the posterior aspect of the leg, where it ends at the ankle to form the plantar arteries of the foot. Pulsations from the posterior tibial artery are readily obtained as it passes superficially behind the medial malleolus at the ankle.

The peroneal artery arises from the posterior tibial peroneal trunk and descends down the leg in the deep muscles located between the tibia

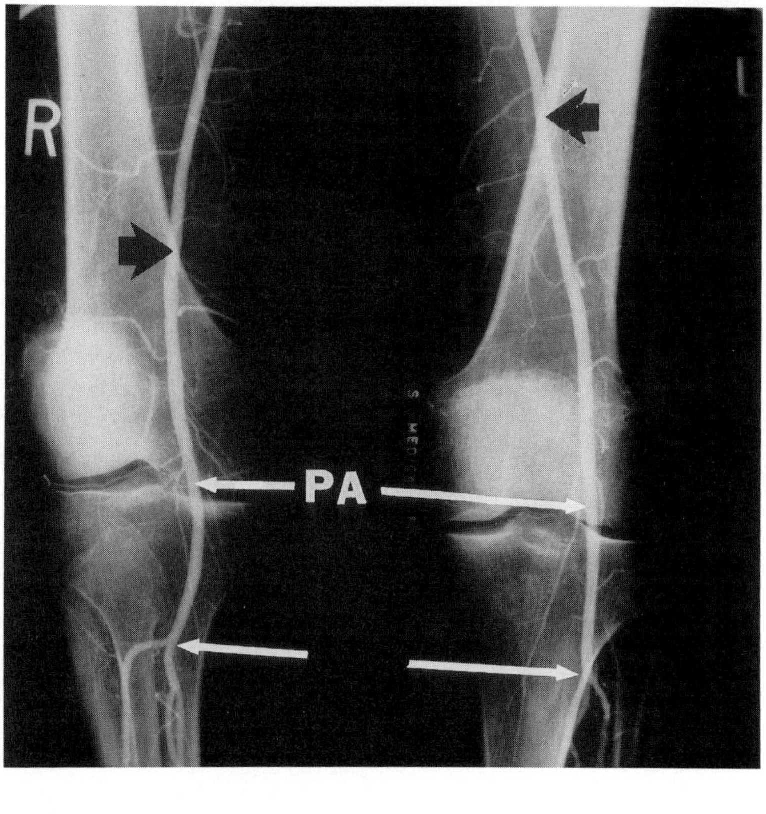

Figure 16–7. Angiographic anatomy of popliteal artery. Termination of adductor canal and beginning of popliteal artery (black arrows). Popliteal artery (PA) ends at tibioperoneal vessels (white arrows).

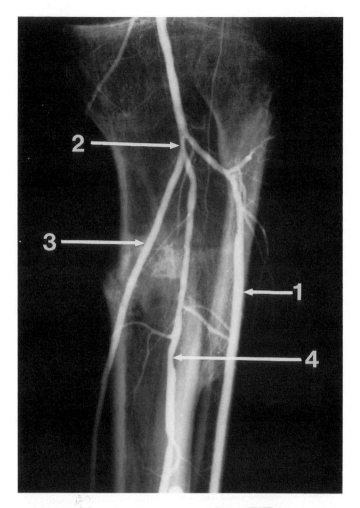

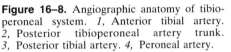

Figure 16–8. Angiographic anatomy of tibio-peroneal system. *1,* Anterior tibial artery. *2,* Posterior tibioperoneal artery trunk. *3,* Posterior tibial artery. *4,* Peroneal artery.

and fibula. The peroneal artery ends at the ankle, where it lies behind the tibiofibular syndesmosis. Here the artery gives off communicating branches to the anterior and posterior tibial arteries. These communicating branches act as a source of collateral blood flow to the tibial arteries when they are obstructed by atherosclerotic lesions. Because the peroneal artery ends at the ankle, it does not supply vessels to the foot.

Common sites of obstruction in the tibioperoneal run-off system are shown in Figure 16–9. These sites involve the proximal segments of one or more of the tibioperoneal arteries. A fair amount of blood flow run-off into the lower extremity may be maintained when only one of these vessels remains patent. This is possible because of the rich network of collateral vessels about the ankle. Because only the proximal portions of the tibial arteries may become occluded, their patent distal segments can be perfused through these collateral vessels as long as one of the arteries in this system remains open. In

extremely severe cases, all three of the arteries in this system are completely obstructed and only small collateral vessels remain to carry the run-off of blood flow into the leg, as shown in Figure 16–10.

Vascular Anatomy of the Foot

The angiographic anatomy of the foot is shown in Figures 16–11 through 16–14. These arteries are of particular interest because their pulsations are often evaluated during the course of noninvasive vascular testing of the lower extremities.

The dorsalis pedis artery, the continuation of the anterior tibial artery, is directed across the dorsum of the foot towards the base of the first toe (Fig. 16–11A). The major branches of the dorsal pedis artery are the tarsal and arcuate arteries. The tarsal artery passes superficially over the navicular bone to supply the extensor digitorum brevis muscle and tarsal articulations of the foot (Fig. 16–11A). The arcuate artery

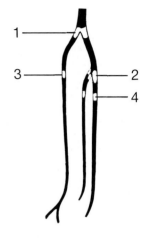

Figure 16–9. Sites of obstructive lesions in the tibioperoneal run-off system. *1,* Origin of anterior tibial artery and tibioperoneal trunk. *2,* Origin of posterior tibial and peroneal artery. *3,* Proximal anterior tibial artery. *4,* Proximal posterior tibial artery.

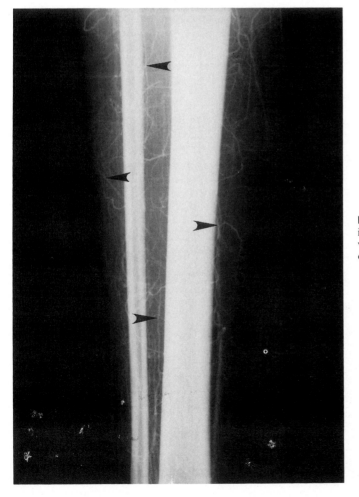

Figure 16–10. Obstruction of all three arteries in the tibioperoneal run-off system. Collateral vessels remain (arrowheads) to carry the run-off of blood flow into the leg.

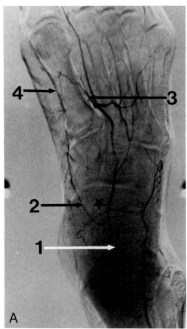

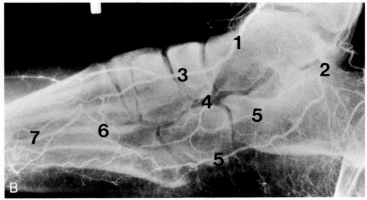

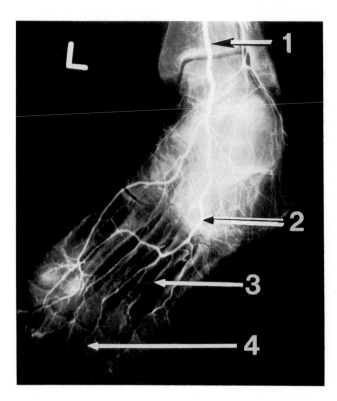

Figure 16–11. Angiographic anatomy of the foot. *A,* Anteroposterior projection. *1,* Dorsalis pedis artery directed over dorsum of foot towards first toe. *2,* Tarsal artery. Asterisk denotes navicular bone of the foot. *3,* Arcuate artery. *4,* Metatarsal artery (dorsal). *B,* Lateral projection. *1,* Anterior tibial artery. *2,* Posterior tibial artery. *3,* Dorsalis pedis artery. *4,* Tarsal artery. *5,* Plantar arteries. *6,* Arcuate artery. *7,* Metatarsal artery (dorsal).

Figure 16–12. Plantar metatarsal arteries arising from the plantar branches of the posterior tibial artery. *1,* Posterior tibial artery. *2,* Plantar artery. *3,* Plantar metatarsal artery. *4,* Digital artery.

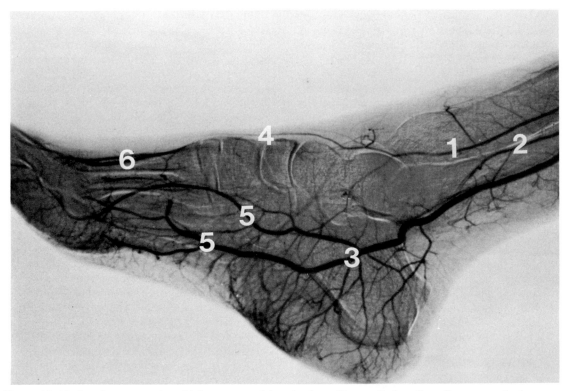

Figure 16–13. Dominant posterior tibial artery supplying the foot. The small dorsalis pedis artery pulsations were difficult to feel in this case. *1,* Anterior tibial artery. *2,* Peroneal artery. *3,* Posterior tibial artery. *4,* Dorsalis pedis artery. *5,* Plantar arteries. *6,* Metatarsal artery.

Figure 16–14. Posterior tibial artery occlusion. The foot is supplied with blood from the dorsalis pedis artery through the arcuate artery collateral pathway. *1,* Dorsalis pedis artery. *2,* Anterior tibial artery. *3,* Tarsal artery. *4,* Arcuate artery collateral pathway. *5,* Metatarsal artery.

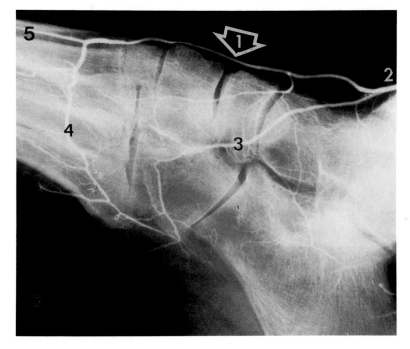

arises over the bases of the metatarsal bones and runs in a lateral direction across the dorsum of the foot to anastomose with the plantar arteries of the posterior tibial artery (Fig. 16–11B).

The plantar arteries are terminal branches of the posterior tibial artery and lie deep within the sole of the foot. Three dorsal metatarsal arteries arise from the arcuate artery and four plantar metatarsal arteries arise from the plantar artery. These metatarsal arteries branch into the digital arteries that supply the toes. Figure 16–12 shows the plantar metatarsal arteries arising from the plantar branches of the posterior tibial artery and ending in the digital arteries of the toes.

It is of particular interest to note that the posterior tibial and plantar arteries may normally be the dominant vessels supplying the foot. An example of this is shown in Figure 16–13. This figure shows large plantar branches arising from an enlarged posterior tibial artery and a small dorsalis pedis artery arising from a small anterior tibial artery. A variation of this type occurs in 5% of feet,[1] making the dorsalis pedis arterial pulse unobtainable or difficult to palpate. Failure to palpate pulses in the dorsalis pedis artery does not automatically indicate obstructive disease of the anterior tibial artery. Instead, it may mean that the dorsalis pedis artery is hypoplastic or small because of the presence of a dominant posterior tibial artery and its plantar branches.

When either the anterior or posterior tibial artery is obstructed, the foot receives its blood supply through the arcuate artery collateral pathway, as shown in Figure 16–14. The posterior tibial artery is occluded in this figure, and the metatarsal branches of the arcuate artery receive blood supply from the dorsalis pedis artery and its branches.

Hemodynamics

Lower Extremity Arterial Pressures

Intra-arterial catheters may be used in invasive techniques to obtain the two pressure waveforms shown in Figure 16–15. These waveforms were obtained by placing a catheter tip in both the aortic root segment above the aortic valve and the dorsalis pedis artery of the foot. These catheters are then connected to a pressure transducer for recording the pressure waveforms from both of these sites, as shown in Figure 16–15. The contours of these waveforms illustrate how the pressures in these vascular structures rise and fall during systolic contraction and diastolic relaxation of the left ventricle.

Investigations of this type are most helpful in explaining the following observations concerning the indirect pressure measurements used in the

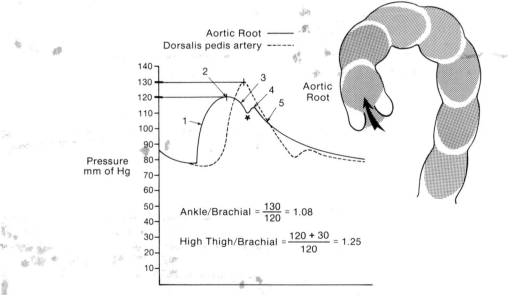

$$\text{Ankle/Brachial} = \frac{130}{120} = 1.08$$

$$\text{High Thigh/Brachial} = \frac{120 + 30}{120} = 1.25$$

Figure 16–15. Pressure waveforms. Aortic inset illustrates transmission of pulsatile, high-pressure aortic root (arrow) waveform to distal aortic segment. *1,* Pressure rises during systole. *2,* Systolic peak pressure. *3,* Pressure falls during early diastole (aortic valves open). *4,* Pressure rises as aortic valves snap shut. *5,* Pressure falls throughout late diastole. Asterisk = Incisura.

noninvasive vascular examination of the lower extremities.

Transmission of Pressure Pulse

The pumping action of the heart creates a pressure wave that is transmitted from the proximal aortic root towards the digital arteries of the toes. Because of the intermittent pumping action of the heart between systole and diastole, the pressure wave varies in a pulsatile manner. The left ventricle contracts during systole, pumping blood out of the heart into the proximal aortic root segment. Because the proximal aortic root segment is already filled with blood, the addition of more blood from the left ventricle causes the pressure of this root segment to rise and its walls to distend. A high-pressure wave is then created, which is transmitted down the aorta into the peripheral arteries of the lower extremities. The aortic inset in Figure 16–15 illustrates how a high-pressure wave, which began in the proximal aortic root segment, is transmitted down the aorta in a pulsatile manner. As the transmitted high-pressure wave travels out into the lower extremity arteries, the pressure increases in these vessels and the arterial walls also distend in a pulsatile manner. It is this transmitted high-pressure wave that forms the systolic pressure measurement used in the noninvasive vascular examination of the lower extremity. Any obstructive lesion in the pathway of this transmitted high-pressure wave may alter its configuration. For example, an obstructive lesion located in the popliteal artery will damp the high-pressure wave as it is transmitted through it. This causes the systolic pressure measurement to be lower below the level of the obstruction than above it.

Systolic Peak Pressure Delay

Figure 16–15 shows that the systolic peak pressure in the dorsalis pedis artery occurs after that in the proximal aortic root segment. This phenomenon occurs because the pressure rise in the aortic root caused by left ventricular systolic contraction is not transmitted immediately into the peripheral vessels of the lower extremities. Instead, it is transmitted in a pulsatile manner down the aorta towards these vessels, as illustrated by the aortic inset in Figure 16–15.

Systolic Pressure Values

A comparison of the two pressure waveforms in Figure 16–15 shows that the systolic pressure is higher in the dorsalis pedis artery than it is in the aortic root. This pressure difference occurs because the resistance to blood flow in the small-diameter arteries of the feet is greater than that of the large-diameter aortic root. As the primary high-pressure wave moves out from the aortic root, it meets the increased peripheral resistance of the foot vessels, which causes a secondary reflected pressure wave to bounce back up the lower extremity arteries towards the aortic root. It is the summation of both the primary and secondary pressure waves that constitutes the final systolic pressure measurement in the dorsalis pedis artery.

Intra-arterial direct pressure measurements show that femoral artery systolic pressure at the groin corresponds closely to the brachial artery systolic pressure in the arm.[2] These measurements also show that the systolic pressure increases distally in the lower limb, with the pressure in the dorsalis pedis artery of the foot being consistently greater than the femoral artery pressure at the groin.[3, 4]

The systolic pressure in the distal tibial arteries about the ankle is 10 to 20 mm Hg higher than systolic pressures in the brachial artery or the aortic root as a result of the reflected wave phenomenon. This phenomenon explains why the ankle/brachial index (ABI) is greater than 1.0 in the normal lower extremity. Because the brachial systolic pressure measured by an upper arm cuff is not affected by this rebound phenomenon, it closely approximates the aortic root pressure, assuming that no obstruction exists in the innominate, subclavian, or axillary arteries. The brachial systolic pressure can then be used to approximate the aortic root pressure, as shown in Figure 16–15. Dividing the higher dorsalis pedis systolic pressure by the lower brachial artery pressure results in the normal measurement, which is greater than 1.0 (Fig. 16–15). Systolic pressures are used because they are reduced by lesser degrees of stenosis than are the diastolic measurements.[5] For this reason, systolic pressures are used extensively for determining the segmental pressure of any vessel under investigation.

The systolic peak pressures in the digital arteries of the toes are less than these in either the tibial or the brachial arteries. Normal systolic toe pressure is no lower than 50 mm Hg or approximately 64% of the brachial artery systolic pressure.[6] The pressure in the digital arteries is not affected by the reflected pressure waves that increase the systolic pressure measurements in the lower segments of the tibial vessels about the ankle. The resistance in the toe vessels serves to bounce backward a pulse wave into the larger tibial vessels; however, they are located too far distally to be affected by this phenomenon.

Peripheral vasoconstriction, induced by body cooling, reduces the systolic pressure in digital arteries but increases it in the medium and small arteries of the lower limb.[7] Peripheral vasodilatation, induced by body heating, decreases the systolic pressure in the medium and small arteries of the lower limb but increases it in the digital arteries of the toes.[7] However, peripheral vasodilatation induced by either reactive hyperemia or exercise does not decrease the systolic pressure in the arteries of the lower limbs and toes. Instead, the systolic pressure in these arteries increases.

Factors Causing a Pressure Drop across a Stenosis

Figure 16–16 illustrates a popliteal artery stenosis. Normally, the pressure P^1 and the pressure P^2 approximate each other, and there is little change in the systolic peak pressure measurement from one end of the popliteal artery to the other end. When P^2 becomes lower than P^1, it indicates an obstruction between the two ends of the popliteal artery. Noninvasive vascular techniques are used to detect the differences between P^1 and P^2 and, therefore, to diagnose an obstructive lesion in the popliteal artery.

There are instances in which the obstruction does not cause a significant pressure difference. Why some obstructions cause a difference between P^1 and P^2 and others do not can be understood through an explanation of the factors regulating the amount of blood flowing through the popliteal artery stenosis in Figure 16–16. These factors include (1) the systolic aortic root pressure, (2) the diameter of the popliteal artery, and (3) the resistance to blood flow through the popliteal artery caused by the arterioles in the peripheral vascular bed. How each of these factors affects the blood flow across the popliteal artery stenosis in Figure 16–16 will be explained by the following concepts.

Flow-Limiting Concept

Tight stenoses or totally occlusive lesions decrease the diameter of the popliteal artery and limit the amount of blood flowing through it. The decrease in blood flow causes P^2 to become lower than P^1, creating a pressure drop across the obstructing lesion. These obstructions are readily diagnosed by the use of noninvasive vascular techniques and systolic pressure measurements.

Increased Blood Flow Concept

Moderate stenoses may not reduce the diameter of the popliteal artery enough to limit the blood flow through it to the extremity at rest. Under these circumstances, the blood flow remains the same throughout the popliteal artery and there is no difference between P^1 and P^2. Increasing the amount of blood flowing through the popliteal artery will intensify the effect of the stenosis, as shown by the equation in Figure 16–16. The equation indicates that if the blood flow (Q) is increased by a factor of 10, the resistance (R) of the stenosis also increases by a factor of 10. The increase in resistance caused by the increase in blood flow through the stenosis causes P^2 to be lower than P^1. For example, assume that Q = 10, R = 1, and P^1 = 120 mm Hg. The equation shows a 10 mm Hg pressure drop across the stenosis.

$$P^2 = P^1 - (Q \times R)$$
$$P^2 = 120 - 10$$
$$P^2 = 110$$
$$P^1 - P^2 = 120 - 110 = 10 \text{ mm Hg pressure drop across stenosis}$$

Next, increase the blood flow (Q) by a factor of 50. The equation shows a 50 mm Hg pressure drop across the stenosis.

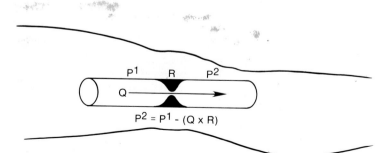

$$P^2 = P^1 - (Q \times R)$$

Figure 16–16. Factors causing a systolic peak pressure drop across a popliteal artery stenosis. P^1 = Pressure above stenosis; R = resistance caused by stenosis; P^2 = pressure below stenosis; Q = blood flow.

$$P^2 = P^1 - (Q \times R)$$
$$P^2 = 120 - 50$$
$$P^2 = 70$$
$$P^1 - P^2 = 120 - 70 = 50 \text{ mm Hg pressure drop across stenosis}$$

Note that the pressure drop across the stenosis is increased even though P^1 and R remain constant.

Increasing the blood flow through the popliteal artery is a way of diagnosing a moderate stenosis that might otherwise go undetected (Fig. 16–16). Various procedures are used to accomplish this by placing a demand on the popliteal artery for more blood to flow through it. This is done by dilating the arterioles in the peripheral vascular bed. This dilatation decreases the resistance in the peripheral vascular bed and allows an increased amount of blood to flow through the popliteal artery. The increase in blood flow enhances the significance of the stenosis, allowing it to be diagnosed by the use of noninvasive vascular procedures, and systolic pressure measurements.

The increased blood flow demand concept is used in the post-exercise segmental pressure examination of the lower extremities. After exercise, increased metabolic activity necessitates greater blood flow through the popliteal artery to the lower extremity muscles. *Reactive hyperemia* may also be used to increase the blood flow through the popliteal artery. When the blood supply to the lower extremities is blocked for 3 to 5 minutes and then is unblocked, the flow through the popliteal artery to the ischemic tissues may increase up to five times normal. This phenomenon may be used to unmask a popliteal stenosis (Fig. 16–16).

Understanding this concept explains why there may be no need to use exercise or reactive hyperemia in a patient with a significant pressure drop across a popliteal artery stenosis. The arterioles may already be fully dilated in response to the need for more blood to flow through the popliteal artery to supply the ischemic leg tissues. Fully dilated arterioles cannot respond either to exercise or to reactive hyperemia under these circumstances. There are instances in which no matter how much the arterioles dilate, they cannot cause more blood to flow through the popliteal artery because the flow is limited by the stenosis. These stenoses may not cause P^2 to be less than P^1 at rest because flow is maintained across the stenosis. However, when the arterioles are dilated by either exercise or reactive hyperemia and the flow cannot be maintained across

the stenosis, P^2 becomes less than P^1. Exercise testing and reactive hyperemia are then used to unmask stenoses that do not cause a difference between P^1 and P^2 in the lower extremities at rest. These procedures may also be used to further examine the significance of a known stenotic lesion.

The increased blood flow demand concept shows the importance of the peripheral vascular bed arterioles in the regulation of the blood flow through the arteries of the lower extremities. The blood flow through these arteries inceases when the arterioles are dilated and decreases when they are constricted. Of further practical importance is the fact that cool temperatures tend to constrict the arterioles and decrease the blood flow through the lower extremity arteries. This reduction in blood flow may mask an underlying stenosis in an extremity at rest. Exercise testing or reactive hyperemia would be necessary to unmask the stenosis in this case. Situations of this type exist when patients are exposed to cold weather or are allowed to lie in a cool, air-conditioned examining room environment with their bare feet exposed prior to the examination. A warm blanket placed over the lower extremities keeps the arterioles from constricting under these circumstances and ensures a more accurate measurement of the difference between P^1 and P^2 in the extremity at rest. This procedure may also eliminate the need for exercise or reactive hyperemia testing in a certain group of patients, although these procedures may still be required to further evaluate the severity of the obstructive lesions.

Decreased Aortic Root Pressure Concept

The increase in the aortic root systolic pressure caused by left ventricular contraction creates the force that drives the blood out of the aorta into the peripheral arteries, as shown in Figure 16–15. Any decrease in aortic root systolic pressure will subsequently decrease the pressure in the lower extremity arteries. The blood flow through the stenosis decreases as the aortic root systolic pressure drops. This concept is important because stenoses that do not limit blood flow under normal aortic root systolic pressure may do so when this pressure is decreased as a result of diminished cardiac output or hypovolemic shock.

Lower Extremity Velocity Waveforms

The Doppler velocity waveform is a graphic display of the pulsatile blood flow through an artery. An example of a velocity waveform from a normal peripheral artery is shown in Figure 16–17. To understand its components, the arterial tree should be considered as a liquid-filled elastic tube that is set into a pulsatile motion by each heart beat.

Systole

Each left ventricular contraction during systole ejects even more blood volume into the already blood-filled proximal aortic root segment. As the blood enters the proximal aortic root segment, it pushes the blood already present in this segment ahead of it in a forward direction down into the descending aorta and peripheral vessels of the lower extremities. As the red blood cells (RBCs) move forward, past a bi-directional Doppler probe placed over a peripheral artery segment, they produce a positive deflected velocity wave upward above the zero baseline level, as shown in Figure 16–17. This wave reaches its peak at the end of systole when the RBCs are moving at their maximum forward velocities through the peripheral vessels. A maximum peak systolic Doppler frequency shift, which is proportional to the maximum forward velocities of RBCs, is recorded by the probe at this point. The elastic arterial walls become distended as the increased blood volume enters the peripheral arteries during systole. This distention occurs because the increased blood volume entering the arteries cannot pass out immediately into the venous circulation because of the resistance of the peripheral arterioles.

Because the blood does not immediately flow out of these arteries, they become high-pressure storage reservoirs for the increased amount of blood volume pumped into them during systole. The velocity of the blood flow into these arteries begins to slow down at the end of systole and the beginning of early diastole as the pressure in these storage reservoirs rises. This deceleration of the RBC velocities marks the beginning of early diastole and is recorded as a decrease in their Doppler shift frequencies, which approach the zero baseline level, as illustrated in Figure 16–17.

Early Diastole

The walls of the arteries, which become distended in systole, begin to contract in a recoil manner during early diastole. This causes the blood to flow in a reversed direction away from the high-resistance, small-diameter arterioles of the peripheral vascular bed towards the low-resistance, large-diameter aorta. The increase in the velocities of the RBCs is now in a reversed direction as the blood flows away from the lower extremities towards the heart, marking the end of early diastole. A bi-directional Doppler probe placed over a peripheral vessel will record the velocity of this reversed blood flow as a negative wave deflected downward below the zero baseline level, as shown in Figure 16–17. This negative wave deflection is termed the *dicrotic notch*. It is not to be confused with the *incisura*.

The incisura begins to form before the aortic valve closes at the end of systole. When the left

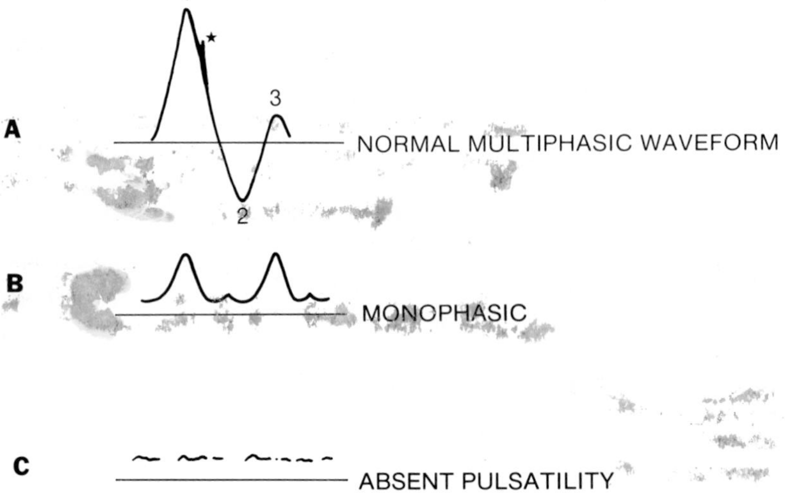

A — NORMAL MULTIPHASIC WAVEFORM

B — MONOPHASIC

C — ABSENT PULSATILITY

Figure 16–17. Velocity waveforms. *A,* Normal velocity waveform. *1,* Positive wave peak of systolic segment. *2,* Negative wave of early diastolic segment (dicrotic notch). *3,* Positive wave of late diastolic segment. Asterisk = Incisura. *B,* Velocity waveform below hemodynamically significant obstruction. *C,* Velocity waveform below severe obstruction.

ventricle relaxes at the end of systole, the decreased interventricular pressure allows the blood, which is under high pressure in the aortic root, to flow backward through the open aortic valve cusps. The flow reversal in the proximal aortic root segment causes the velocity of the forward blood flow in the peripheral arteries to slow down for a brief instant. A sudden decrease in the Doppler shift frequencies of the RBCs is recorded by the Doppler probe placed over a peripheral artery at this instant. The backward flow of blood from the aortic root into the left ventricle is then suddenly stopped as the aortic valve cusps snap shut. The blood, which is now under high pressure in the aortic roots, begins to flow in a forward direction again. This causes a brief acceleration of RBCs in the peripheral arteries, which is recorded by the Doppler probe as a sudden increase in their Doppler shift frequencies.

The incisura occurs immediately after systole or in early diastole as the aortic valves snap shut; the dicrotic notch occurs at the end of early diastole because of the recoil contraction of the distended peripheral arterial walls. Also, the incisura formation results in a velocity decrease of the forward blood flow in a peripheral vessel, whereas the dicrotic notch formation results in a velocity increase with blood flow reversal. Both the incisura and the dicrotic notch are more pronounced in the common femoral, superficial femoral, and popliteal arteries than they are in the tibial, dorsalis pedis, and digital arteries.

The magnitude of the dicrotic notch with flow reversal is directly proportional to the amount of resistance caused by arterioles in the peripheral vascular bed. High-resistance, constricted arterioles increase the magnitude of the dicrotic notch. Low-resistance, dilated arterioles decrease the magnitude of the dicrotic notch. A velocity waveform of an artery leading to a constricted arteriolar peripheral vascular bed will have a prominent dicrotic notch with marked reversed flow velocity and relatively little forward flow velocity. The velocity waveform of an artery leading to a dilated arteriolar peripheral vascular bed will have little or no dicrotic notch or flow reversal but will have good forward flow velocity throughout late diastole.

Late Diastole

Late diastole begins as the pressure in the distended, high-pressure artery reservoirs dissipates as a result of recoil contraction. Blood now begins to flow in a forward direction again. It passes out of the arteries through the arterioles and into the venous circulation. The Doppler probe records this forward blood flow as a positive wave deflected above the zero baseline level and composed of declining Doppler shift frequencies from the decelerating velocities of the RBCs. An increase in the peripheral resistance caused by a constriction of the arterioles will decrease the RBC velocities. The result is a decrease in Doppler shift frequencies that approach the zero baseline level. A decrease in the peripheral resistance caused by dilatation of the arterioles will increase the RBC velocities. The result is an increase in Doppler shift frequencies above the zero baseline level.

The Cardiac Cycle

Each of the three components of the cardiac cycle produces a distinct segment of the velocity waveform in a peripheral artery.

Systole produces a positive wave segment composed of ever-increasing Doppler shift frequencies as the RBCs are accelerated into and distend the peripheral arteries. It ends in the peak systolic Doppler frequency shift in which RBCs are accelerated to maximum velocities.

Early diastole produces a positive wave segment of declining Doppler shift frequencies as the velocities of the RBCs decelerate during filling of the arterial high-pressure reservoirs. Early diastole ends in a negative wave segment when the distended walls of these reservoirs undergo recoil contraction and force blood flow in a reversed direction towards the heart.

Late diastole produces a positive wave segment of declining Doppler shift frequencies as the continued, sustained contraction of the distended artery walls forces blood forward through the arterioles into the venous circulation.

All three components of the cardiac cycle combine to make the normal multiphasic or triphasic waveform shown in Figure 16–17. An arterial obstruction results in a damping of the multiphasic waveform below the site of the lesion. When the obstruction is hemodynamically significant (e.g., >50% diameter reduction), the systolic segment is decreased in height and the diastolic segments are absent. The velocity waveform becomes monophasic because only the systolic segment remains, as shown in Figure 16–17.

An extremely severe obstruction will reduce the systolic Doppler shift frequencies even more because the velocity of the blood flow below the lesion is further diminished or absent. The pulsatility of the velocity waveform is completely

EFFECT OF PROBE ANGLE ON DOPPLER WAVEFORM

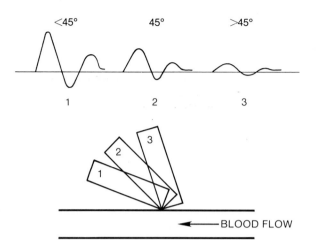

Figure 16–18. Effect of probe angle on Doppler velocity waveform. *1*, Probe angle <45° to plane of blood flow results in a normal velocity waveform. *2* and *3*, Probe angles 45° or greater result in a false-positive abnormal velocity waveform.

absent under these circumstances, as shown in Figure 16–17. It is important to realize that variations in the probe angle to the plane of blood flow in the artery under investigation can produce these same velocity waveform abnormalities. This is illustrated in Figure 16–18.

References

1. Huber JF. The arterial network supplying the dorsum of the foot. Anat Rec 1941; 80:373–376.
2. Pascarelli EF, Bertrand CR. Comparison of blood pressures in the arms and legs. N Engl J Med 1964; 270:693–695.
3. Carter SA. Effect of age, cardiovascular disease, and vasomotor changes on transmission of arterial pressure waves through the lower extremities. Angiology 1978; 29:601–604.
4. Lassen NA, Tonnesen KH, Holstein P. Distal blood pressure (editorial). Scand J Clin Lab Invest 1976; 36:705–706.
5. Carter SA, Clinical measurements of systolic pressures in limbs with arterial occlusive disease. JAMA 1969; 207:1869–1874.
6. Carter SA, Lezack JD. Digital systolic pressures in the lower limb in arterial disease. Circulation 1971; 43:905–908.
7. Carter SA. Hemodynamic considerations in peripheral and cerebrovascular disease. Semin Ultrasound 1981; 2:254–262.

17 • Noninvasive Vascular Examinations of the Lower Extremity Arteries

Introduction

Noninvasive vascular laboratories are rapidly being established throughout the United States. These laboratories specialize in a variety of vascular examinations, including cerebrovascular, peripheral arterial, and venous studies. Multiple methods of testing are usually required to define the disease process and to determine the severity of disease.

Peripheral arteries are assessed by several techniques, which include Doppler, plethysmography, and systolic pressure recordings. These combined techniques not only verify the presence of vascular disease but define the extent of disease. Noninvasive examinations can also indicate the most suitable form of therapy and suggest the predicted outcome.

Noninvasive vascular studies provide an excellent method of identifying those patients who require angiography and may be candidates for surgery.[1]

Indications for Examination

Indications for performing peripheral arterial examinations include:

1. Lower extremity pain (claudication and/or rest pain).
2. Traumatic injuries.
3. Tissue necrosis and ulceration.
4. Pre-operative evaluation.
5. Selection of surgical candidates.
6. Prediction of healing.
7. Determination of amputation levels.
8. Postoperative assessment for patency and function.
9. Long-term monitoring.
10. Follow-up for specialized radiological procedures (embolization, angioplasty).

The indication and patient history should be clearly stated on the requesting consultation form. This ensures that the correct examination is performed and that the patient's clinical problems have been evaluated. The request form shown in Figure 17–1 was designed for a large teaching institution. It provides a listing of all examinations for the clinician as a reference guide. Selection of the examination by checking the appropriate box also provides billing data. Space is available for the patient's history and any previous examinations. Upon completion of the examination, the interpretation is typed on the request form and forwarded to the referring physician.

Patient History

Prior to the noninvasive vascular examination, the patient's medical history and clinical symptoms are obtained from the request form and also from the patient. Pertinent information should include:

1. Any traumatic injury to the lower extremities that may alter the normal flow patterns or occlude the lower extremity vessels.
2. Any history of major diseases that may influence the peripheral vascular system (diabetes, hypertension, cardiac disease, or venous disease).
3. Previous vascular surgery, such as bypass, reconstruction, or shunts.
4. Previous noninvasive vascular examinations that may provide baseline data and follow-up guidelines.
5. Presence of numbness, unilateral coldness, tingling, or color changes that may signify vascular impairment.
6. Presence of any sores, ulcerations, or edematous areas. (Tissue necrosis and gangrene are seen in the most advanced stages of arterial

LOUISIANA STATE UNIVERSITY
MEDICAL CENTER - Shreveport
Ultrasound - Radiology

NON INVASIVE VASCULAR LABORATORY

☐ STAT ☐ ROUTINE PATIENT HISTORY	Name I.D. No. Billing No. Date
	Clinic or Ward
	Telephone and make appointments for all clinic patients and place appointment time in this space Date: Time:
List Patient's Previous Studies.	
	PHYSICIAN SIGNATURE

CHECK PROCEDURE REQUESTED

Duplex Deep Doppler

☐ Aorta
☐ Renal Arteries
☐ Portal Splenic
☐ Renal Transplant
☐ Misc_____

Extracranial Duplex/Doppler

☐ Carotid with Supraorbital
☐ Vertebral Arteries
☐ ECA-ICA By Pass Evaluation
☐ Subclavian Steal
  Upper Extremity
☐ Palmer Arch
☐ Thoracic Outlet Compression
☐ Upper Extremity Arterial
☐ Upper Extremity Venous
☐ Misc _____

Lower Extremity

☐ Peripheral Arterial (with exercise
  PPG, SBP, Doppler, Imaging)
☐ Limited Study
_____
☐ Post-Operative Evaluation
☐ Peripheral Venous
  (SPG, Doppler, Imaging)
☐ Limited Study

Misc._____

Exam Completed (DATE) _____ SONOGRAPHER_____

Figure 17–1. Vascular examination request form.

disease. These patients may require additional tests for predicting healing or determining amputation levels.)

7. Presence of trophic changes—hair loss, nail thickness, excessively dry skin, or tissue necrosis. These conditions may reflect arterial insufficiency.

8. Description of pain symptoms, including type, duration, location, and means of relief. Generally, there are two types described:

a. *Claudication*, produced by insufficient blood flow during exercise and usually relieved by short periods of rest. The ankle/brachial index (ABI), which is described later in this chapter, will usually range from 0.6 to 0.9. Exercise or hyperemia testing will demonstrate a greater decrease in the ABI as a result of primary vessels being unable to supply sufficient blood flow during stress or exercise.

b. *Rest pain,* presenting as a continuous aching in the lower extremity at rest that often becomes unbearable. The rest pain frequently occurs during the night and awakens the patient. These symptoms are suggestive of severe arterial disease and are associated with an ABI of 0.5 or less.

Preliminary Procedures

After the pertinent information is obtained, the patient is placed in a supine, recumbent position for at least 15 minutes prior to the examination. The extremities should be kept warm, either by maintaining correct room temperatures or by covering the extremities.

The extremities are then inspected for coldness, color changes, trophic changes, and tissue necrosis. This inspection is followed by palpation of the major peripheral arterial pulses (femoral, popliteal, and posterior tibial arteries). The pulse of each vessel, if present, should be evaluated for rate, rhythm, and amplitude and scored by one of the criteria listed in Table 17–1.[2, 3]

The Examination

The baseline peripheral arterial examination usually includes (1) segmental systolic blood pressures, (2) the ABI, and (3) Doppler waveform analysis. This combination of examinations will allow for the identification and localization of the area of disease and will indicate what additional tests are required. The exact protocol will vary for different laboratories, depending on the avail-

Table 17–1. Grading Systems

0 = Absent	0 = Absent
1 = Markedly impaired	
2 = Moderately impaired	+ = Reduced
3 = Almost normal or slightly impaired	
4 = Normal	+ + = Normal

ability of equipment and the expertise of the examiner. A protocol should be established and strictly adhered to for standardization and reproducibility of findings. A typical protocol provided by a commercial company is shown in Figure 17–2. Once the protocol has been established, the medical director should inform the clinicians of the availability and the sequence of testing to ensure the ordering of correct examinations and to provide a line of communication for patient follow-up.

Segmental Systolic Blood Pressure Recordings

The segmental (SBP) examination is a simple, noninvasive method for diagnosing and localizing arterial disease. This method was first introduced by Winsor in 1950[4] and still remains the most sensitive indicator of arterial disease. The SBP may be obtained using standard pneumatic cuffs with a hand-held aneroid manometer. However, considering the time involved for multiple measurements, it is advisable to use an automated, computerized system (Fig. 17–3). These systems have automated cuff inflators combined with microprocessors for memory storage, and they are preprogramed for specific testing procedures with predetermined limits. They also have remote controls for ease of operation and for multiple site recordings in sequence (Fig. 17–4). The automated system is less time-consuming and is more accurate than the manual hand-held system.

The brachial systolic pressure is the reference standard and is used to calculate the ABI. Systolic pressure recordings are obtained from both arms, and the higher value becomes the standard. A pneumatic cuff is placed on the upper arm, and the Doppler probe is placed over the brachial or radial artery. The pneumatic cuff is inflated above the systolic pressure, at which time the Doppler signal disappears. The cuff is then allowed to slowly deflate until the Doppler signal re-appears. When the Doppler signal re-appears, the systolic pressure is recorded. The return signal is audibly heard and is seen as an amplitude spike on the strip chart recording (Fig. 17–5).

ARTERIAL EVALUATION

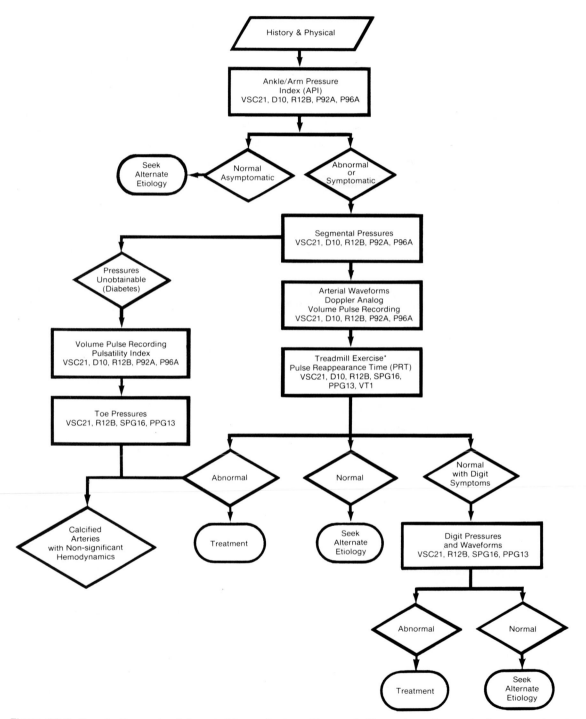

Figure 17–2. Examination protocol for arterial examinations. For treadmill exercise, take monitoring precautions in event of coronary artery involvement. (Courtesy of MedaSonics.)

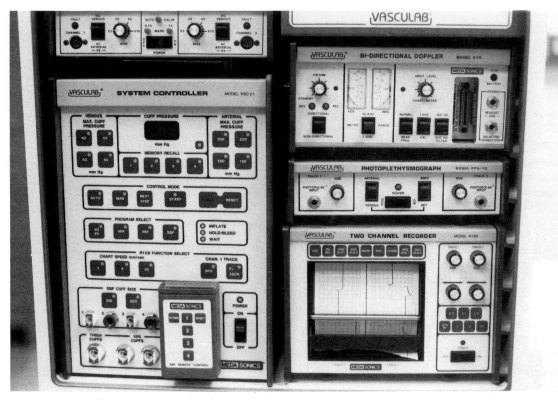

Figure 17–3. Automated computerized vascular unit. (Courtesy of MedaSonics.)

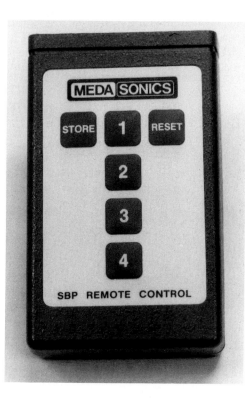

Figure 17–4. Segmental systolic blood pressure remote control unit with a four channel memory recording system. (Courtesy of MedaSonics.)

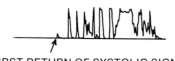

FIRST RETURN OF SYSTOLIC SIGNAL
(PULSE REAPPEARANCE)

Figure 17–5. Analog tracing of the systolic blood pressure recording.

There should be no more than 10 mm Hg difference in the brachial pressures. If the difference exceeds 10 mm Hg, the side with lower pressure indicates stenosis or occlusion of the ipsilateral innominate, subclavian, axillary, or proximal brachial artery. In this situation, vascular examination of the upper extremity is required.

After the brachial systolic pressures are taken, the lower extremity systolic pressures are obtained. A three-cuff or four-cuff method may be used. The blood pressure measurements are more accurate when the width of the cuff is 20% greater than the diameter of the limb. However, the cuff on the thigh would be so wide that only one cuff could be used (three-cuff method). The use of two thigh cuffs (four-cuff method) can be achieved by using narrower cuffs, resulting in an artificially high thigh pressure measurement.

The advantage of the four-cuff method is that it provides differentiation of aortoiliac disease from superficial femoral artery disease. This advantage outweighs the disadvantage of the artificially high pressure measurement obtained with the narrower cuffs.[5] With the four-cuff method, the pneumatic cuffs are placed at four levels: *ankle* (A), *below knee* (BK), *above knee* (AK),

and at the *upper* or *high thigh* (HT). Placement of the cuffs is shown in Figure 17–6. The Doppler probe is placed over the posterior tibial or dorsalis pedis artery, whichever has the best signal (Fig. 17–7). Note that the level of pressure measurement is determined at the site of pneumatic cuff inflation and not the site of the Doppler probe. Each cuff, beginning with the ankle and progressing upward, is inflated to a pressure above the systolic pressure. When the Doppler signal disappears, the cuff is slowly released and allowed to deflate. As the Doppler signal returns, the systolic pressure is recorded.

Once the baseline and bilateral systolic pressures are recorded, the values should be evaluated for any artifacts and to determine whether additional testing is required.

Artifacts

Artifacts may give erroneous measurements or limit the pressure recording. Typical examples of artifacts are listed as follows:

1. Pulsatile venous signals present in patients with congestive heart failure may be mistaken for arterial signals. These will give erroneous measurements, and values should be re-evaluated at other sites.

2. Collateral flow seen in severe occlusive states may be difficult to evaluate and may provide inadequate measurements. Re-evaluation using another Doppler probe site with stronger signals will ensure a correct measurement.

3. Absence of the Doppler signal because of extremely low flow states or occlusion may pre-

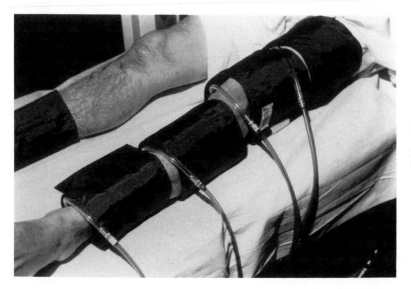

Figure 17–6. Pneumatic cuff placement for segmental systolic blood pressure recordings using the four-cuff method.

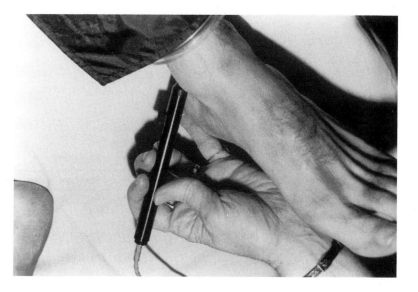

Figure 17–7. Doppler probe site over the posterior tibial artery.

vent measurements at certain levels. Alternate testing methods, such as toe pressures or pressures obtained at a higher level, may be used.

4. Calcified vessels (frequently seen in diabetic patients) restrict pressure recordings and give excessively high values because of the noncompressibility of the vessel and occlusion of the flow. Therefore, a correct measurement cannot be obtained. In these cases, plethysmographic techniques or toe pressures may be used.

5. Extreme obesity and large thighs may distort the pressure measurement. This is caused by the relationship of thigh cuff width and limb diameter. Emphasis is then placed on other values, such as the ABI and Doppler waveform recordings.

6. Multiple vessels located at or above the recording site may not be separated, making it impossible to distinguish the affected vessel. For instance, the high-thigh measurement includes the evaluation of the aortic, iliac, and common femoral arteries reflecting inflow disease but not specifying the vessel involved. If there is a stenotic lesion of the superficial femoral combined with the profunda femoris, the high-thigh pressure will also reflect a low pressure. This finding should be further tested by Doppler analog waveform and real-time imaging to specify the diseased vessel.

Normal Systolic Pressure Measurements

Interpretation of normal values (Table 17–2 and Fig. 17–8) may vary slightly, depending on the equipment standards, the size of the pneu-

matic cuffs, and the laboratory protocol. Once the values have been established, they should be evaluated using angiographic correlation to determine the accuracy and to define the limitations. In our laboratory, four (12.5 cm × 40 cm) cuffs are used. Our initial guidelines and standards were obtained from MedaSonics[6] but were modified as we gained further expertise.

Healing Prediction

The systolic pressure measurement can predict the healing of lesions of the lower calf and feet. Ankle pressures greater than 55 mm Hg in a nondiabetic patient indicate spontaneous healing of lesions; a pressure of 80 to 90 mm Hg in a diabetic patient indicates favorable healing.[7] Toe pressure (TP) measurement can provide an alternate testing procedure, but a systolic pressure of 30 mm Hg or higher is required to predict favorable healing of skin lesions.[7]

Ankle/Brachial Index

Included in the segmental pressure study of the lower extremities is the ankle/brachial index (ABI), often also termed the ankle/pressure index (API). The ABI is a simple, reliable index that is essentially free of technical artifacts and that defines the severity of arterial disease in the lower extremities. The ratio equation is shown in Figure 17–14. Each ankle pressure is divided by the highest brachial systolic pressure to obtain this ratio. The normal ABI value is 1 or slightly greater with the abnormal value being less than 1. There are two divisions in the abnormal

Text continued on page 310

Table 17–2. Normal Segmental Systolic Pressure Values

Cuff Location	Standard Value	Example
Brachial systolic pressure	Reference for procedures. Bilateral pressures are obtained and not to exceed 10 mm Hg difference. The highest of the two values is used. 1. Figure 17–9A illustrates normal brachial systolic pressures. 2. Figure 17–9B illustrates abnormal difference between systolic pressures, necessitating upper extremity evaluation.	150 mm Hg
High-thigh (HT) systolic pressure	20 to 30 mm Hg or more above the brachial pressure because of artifact from the narrow cuffs. 1. Low pressures indicate stenosis or occlusion of the aorta, iliac artery, or common femoral artery (aortoiliac inflow disease). 2. Superficial femoral artery disease combined with stenosis or occlusion of the profunda femoris artery may also present a low pressure.	181 mm Hg
Above-knee (AK) systolic pressure	Less than 20 to 30 mm Hg compared with high-thigh pressure. This level should be at least the value of the brachial pressure. An abnormal gradient between the proximal thigh and above the knee suggests stenosis or occlusion of the superficial femoral artery. Lower gradients indicate stenosis; larger gradients indicate occlusion.	171 mm Hg
Below-knee (BK) systolic pressure	All gradients not to exceed 20 to 30 mm Hg, decreasing in value from HT to A. An abnormal gradient between the AK and BK values suggests distal superficial femoral or popliteal artery obstruction.	163 mm Hg
Ankle (A) systolic pressure	Equal to or slightly greater than the brachial pressure. An abnormal gradient between the BK and A values suggests tibioperoneal (run-off) occlusive disease that usually involves two or three of the BK vessels. Each vessel (posterior tibial, dorsalis pedis, and anterior tibial arteries) can be evaluated with segmental pressures to determine individual status.	154 mm Hg
Toe systolic pressure	60% or greater of the ankle pressure. Toe pressures (TP) measure the cutaneous flow to the digit and are not usually affected by calcification. Toe pressures provide essential information when ankle pressures cannot be obtained.	97 mm Hg

[handwritten annotation: 1.2 is better →]
[handwritten annotation: Down to 1.0 – be reluctant to call this signif.]

Figures 17–10 through 17–13 illustrate the abnormal systolic pressure measurements for various levels of arterial disease.

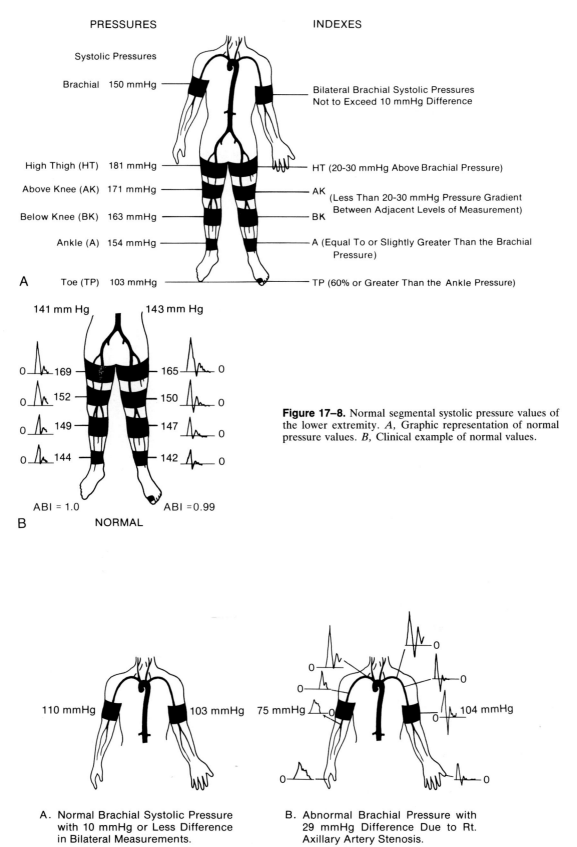

PRESSURES

INDEXES

Systolic Pressures

Brachial   150 mmHg

Bilateral Brachial Systolic Pressures
Not to Exceed 10 mmHg Difference

High Thigh (HT)   181 mmHg

HT (20-30 mmHg Above Brachial Pressure)

Above Knee (AK)   171 mmHg

AK

(Less Than 20-30 mmHg Pressure Gradient
Between Adjacent Levels of Measurement)

Below Knee (BK)   163 mmHg

BK

Ankle (A)   154 mmHg

A (Equal To or Slightly Greater Than the Brachial
Pressure)

A   Toe (TP)   103 mmHg

TP (60% or Greater Than the Ankle Pressure)

141 mm Hg   143 mm Hg

0 — 169   165 — 0

0 — 152   150 — 0

0 — 149   147 — 0

0 — 144   142 — 0

ABI = 1.0   ABI = 0.99

B   **NORMAL**

Figure 17–8. Normal segmental systolic pressure values of the lower extremity. *A*, Graphic representation of normal pressure values. *B*, Clinical example of normal values.

110 mmHg   103 mmHg   75 mmHg   104 mmHg

A. Normal Brachial Systolic Pressure
with 10 mmHg or Less Difference
in Bilateral Measurements.

B. Abnormal Brachial Pressure with
29 mmHg Difference Due to Rt.
Axillary Artery Stenosis.

Figure 17–9. Systolic pressure recordings. *A*, Normal pressure recording of the brachial artery. *B*, Abnormal pressure recording of the brachial artery with stenosis of the axillary artery.

307

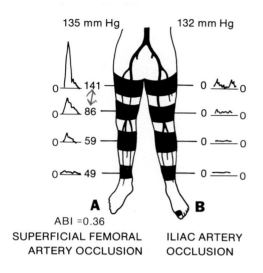

135 mm Hg   132 mm Hg

A

ABI =0.36

SUPERFICIAL FEMORAL
ARTERY OCCLUSION

B

ILIAC ARTERY
OCCLUSION

Figure 17–10. Lower extremity occlusion. *A*, Right superficial femoral artery occlusion. *B*, Left iliac artery occlusion.

Figure 17–11. Lower extremity stenosis and occlusion. *A*, Right profunda and superficial femoral artery occlusion. *B*, Left iliac stenosis combined with popliteal stenosis.

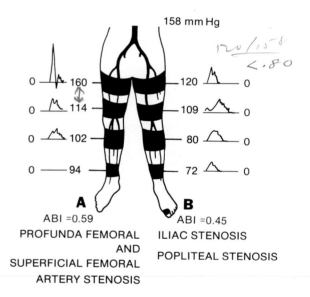

158 mm Hg

A

ABI =0.59

PROFUNDA FEMORAL
AND
SUPERFICIAL FEMORAL
ARTERY STENOSIS

B

ABI =0.45

ILIAC STENOSIS

POPLITEAL STENOSIS

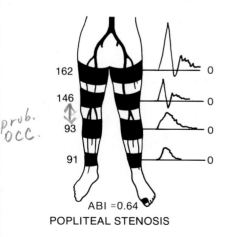

BRACHIAL 142 mm Hg

ABI =0.64

POPLITEAL STENOSIS

Figure 17–12. Popliteal stenosis.

BRACHIAL 140 mm Hg

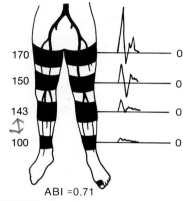

Figure 17–13. Tibioperoneal occlusive disease.

TIBIOPERONEAL OCCLUSIVE DISEASE

ANKLE BRACHIAL INDEX (ABI)

EXPRESSES ANKLE PRESSURE AND BRACHIAL
PRESSURE AS A RATIO.

1. THE BRACHIAL PRESSURE IS MEASURED IN BOTH
   ARMS WITH THE HIGHER MEASUREMENT BEING
   USED TO CALCULATE THE PRESSURE INDEX FOR
   BOTH THE RIGHT AND LEFT LEG.

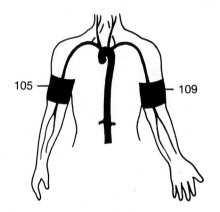

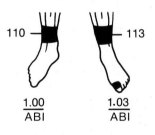

ANKLE PRESSURES

$$\frac{\text{ANKLE PRESSURE}}{\text{BRACHIAL PRESSURE}} = \text{ABI}$$

NORMAL VALUE   ABI = 1 OR SLIGHTLY GREATER

CLAUDICATION (MODERATE STENOSIS OR OCCLUSIVE STATES)   ABI = 0.6-0.9

REST PAIN (SEVERE OCCLUSIVE STATES)   ABI = 0.5 OR LESS

Figure 17–14. Ankle brachial index ratio equation.

ranges, classified according to patient symptoms and ABI value.

1. *Claudication (ABI 0.6 to 0.9)*. Claudication is seen in moderate stenosis and occlusive states. Claudication presents as intermittent pain associated with exercise. This condition is due to the inability of the collateral circulation to meet the needs of the exercising muscle. Thus, all patients whose ABI ranges from 0.6 to 0.9 should have systolic pressure measurements taken after exercise. Stress or exercise testing is also indicated in those patients who are symptomatic but in whom pressure measurements are borderline or normal under resting conditions. The ABI in these patients usually ranges from 0.9 to normal at rest.

2. *Severe occlusive states (ABI <0.5)*. If the ABI is 0.5 or less, there is no need for exercise testing. Doppler waveform analysis is performed to complete the examination and to correlate with the segmental pressures. The ABI defines the severity of the disease, whereas the segmental pressures localize the area of involvement.

Stress Testing

Stress testing (ST) is performed in all patients when the ABI indicates claudication. Stress testing is especially beneficial in patients with borderline pressure values at rest but who present with claudication symptoms. Vascular obstructive disease will be compensated through collateral flow and dilatation of the arteries in the resting state. However, with stress or exercise, the increased demands of the exercising muscle and the increased resistance of the distal extremity vessels will exceed the limit of arterial flow, thus causing a decrease in the pressure value.

Stress testing can be performed by having the patient walk or use a treadmill with a 12° grade moving at 2 miles per hour. Pneumatic cuffs are placed on the ankle above the malleoli and are left in place during the exercise period. The patient walks for 5 minutes or until pain symptoms occur. It is recommended that electrocardiogram monitoring be performed if treadmill testing is used. Immediately following the exercise period, sequential ankle pressures are obtained, initially at 30 second intervals for the first 4 minutes and then every minute until the pressure measurement returns to normal or to the pre-exercise level. In cases of severe occlusive disease, it may take 30 minutes or longer for pressures to return to normal; however, 10 to 15 minutes is sufficient recording time to evaluate vascular status.

In the normal response to exercise, there is usually no significant drop in pressure with increased flow. There may even be elevation in the pressure measurement. The abnormal response is a decrease in pressure. Any drop in pressure is an indicator of significant disease, and the degree of impairment will be reflected in the time it takes for the pressure to return to normal. Usually, when a single level of disease is present, the pressure will return to normal values within 2 to 6 minutes. With multiple levels of disease, it takes up to 12 minutes for pressures to return to normal. In a patient with a severe occlusive state, it may take up to 30 minutes or longer for pressures to return to normal. Figures 17–15 and 17–16 illustrate normal and abnormal responses to stress testing.

Reactive Hyperemia Testing

Patients who are disabled or unable to participate in conventional exercise testing can be evaluated by means of reactive hyperemia techniques. Wide pneumatic cuffs are placed on the upper thigh, and narrow cuffs are placed above the malleoli (Fig. 17–17). The upper thigh cuff is inflated to a pressure of 50 mm Hg above the thigh systolic pressure, which is maintained for 3 minutes to occlude the arterial flow. After 3 minutes, the cuff pressure is released, and ankle pressure measurements are obtained every 30 seconds for the first 4 minutes, then every minute for 4 to 10 minutes or until the pressure returns to normal or to the pre-exercise level. Hyperemia testing differs from routine exercise testing in that there will be a drop of pressure following the release of the cuff in all patients. However, the normal patient's ankle pressure will fall no more than 35% to the pre-ischemic level and will return to the baseline value within 1 minute. In contrast, the abnormal patient will show a pressure drop of more than 35%, and the ankle pressure will take more than 1 minute to return to the baseline. In severe occlusive disease involving multiple sites, there will be a greater than 50% pressure drop that will necessitate significant time for recovery.

Systolic Toe Pressure Measurement

Toe pressure measurement is an alternate method for determining the severity of arterial disease and assessing the circulatory status of the digits. This method of testing is used in severe occlusive states when lower extremity vessels

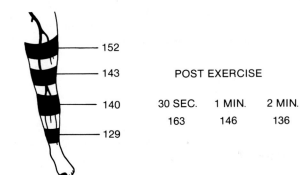

BRACHIAL 132 mm Hg

— 152

— 143   POST EXERCISE

— 140   30 SEC.   1 MIN.   2 MIN.

Figure 17–15. Normal response to stress testing.   163   146   136

— 129

ABI =0.9

Ankle Brachial Index indicates
borderline exercise testing
produced increase in pressures, a
normal response.

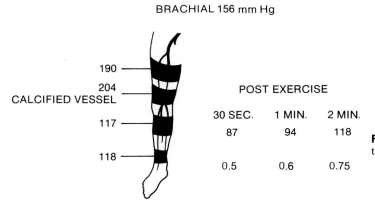

BRACHIAL 156 mm Hg

190 —

204 —

CALCIFIED VESSEL   POST EXERCISE

117 —   30 SEC.   1 MIN.   2 MIN.

               87   94   118   **Figure 17–16.** Abnormal response to stress
118 —   testing with a single-level stenosis.

               0.5   0.6   0.75

ABI = 0.76

Ankle Brachial Index indicates
claudication range. Exercise
testing indicates decrease in flow
returning to original state within 2
min. due to single level stenosis.

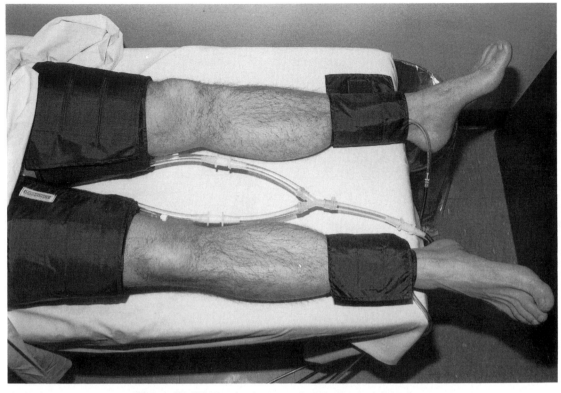

Figure 17–17. Examination procedure for hyperemia testing.

cannot be localized and the ABI cannot be obtained.

Toe pressure measurement utilizes photoplethysmography (PPG), which is used for detecting the cutaneous blood. A photoelectric cell consisting of an infrared light-emitting diode coupled with a phototransistor is placed in contact with the skin surface (Fig. 17–18). The infrared light emission is transmitted into the superficial tissues and reflected back to the phototransistor by the subcutaneous red blood cells. The acquired data are represented by a pulse waveform that is similar to the Doppler waveform. These pulse waveforms cannot be calibrated but present a distinct pulsatile configuration. The normal pulse waveform has a sharp systolic upsweep, rising rapidly to a peak and then dropping towards the baseline. The dicrotic notch will be seen on the downslope (Fig. 17–19).

To obtain the digit systolic pressure, place the

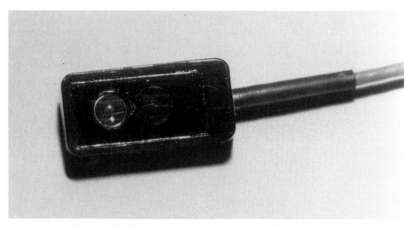

Figure 17–18. Photoplethysmography (PPG) photocell.

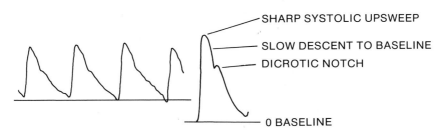

SHARP SYSTOLIC UPSWEEP
SLOW DESCENT TO BASELINE
DICROTIC NOTCH

0 BASELINE

Figure 17–19. Normal photoplethysmography digit pulse waveform.

digit pneumatic cuff around the proximal great toe, with the PPG photocell secured to the plantar surface of the toe (Fig. 17–20). Note the use of the 2.5 cm cuff. Always use the widest cuff possible to obtain the greatest sensitivity and to increase the accuracy of the pressure measurement. The alternating current (AC) electrical mode is normally used; however, in extremely low flow states the direct current (DC) mode may be used. The strip chart recorder is activated at a running speed of 5 mm/second, and the waveform is centered. The height of the waveform is usually set at 20 to 30 mm. The pneumatic cuff is inflated above the brachial systolic pressure or until the pulse disappears. The cuff is then slowly deflated until the pulse waveform reappears (pulse re-appearance time). The strip chart recorder is continuously running, and counter markings are made at specific intervals, usually every 10 mm Hg. The time of pulse reappearance represents the systolic toe pressure. Figure 17–21 demonstrates a recording of the toe pressure.

The normal toe systolic pressure is less than the systolic brachial pressure and is 60% or more of the ankle pressure.[8] In cases of severe occlusive disease with rest pain, the toe pressure may be less than 20 mm Hg. To obtain the systolic pressure recording in low flow states, the DC mode is used. The rise endpoint as blood enters the digit is recorded as the systolic pressure. An example is seen in Figure 17–22.

Reactive Hyperemia Toe Testing

Toe stress testing can be performed to demonstrate the functional severity of lower limb arterial disease. The PPG is set up for digit pressures, with the cuff pressure inflated and maintained for 5 minutes to occlude the arterial flow. The pressure cuff is then released, and the toe pulse re-appearance time (PRT) is demonstrated on the strip chart recording. The normal toe PRT is approximately 1 second. In cases of severe ischemic disease, the PRT will increase in direct proportion to the severity of the disease.[9]

Digit Pulse Waveform Recording with Photoplethysmography

Digit pulse waveforms (DPWs) are easily obtained using the PPG photocell. Digit pulse waveform recording is a simple method of verifying the pressure of arterial flow and of demonstrating

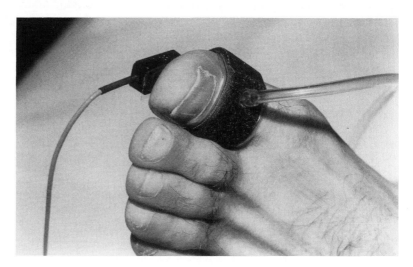

Figure 17–20. Placement of the photocell and the digit pneumatic cuff for toe pressure examination.

NORMAL BILATERAL TOE PRESSURES

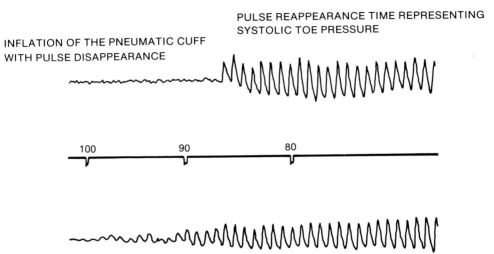

PULSE REAPPEARANCE TIME REPRESENTING
SYSTOLIC TOE PRESSURE

INFLATION OF THE PNEUMATIC CUFF
WITH PULSE DISAPPEARANCE

100   90   80

Figure 17–21. Normal toe pressure recording.

obstructing lesions. Although the DPW is not a quantitative waveform, it provides a good correlation with other testing procedures and can provide additional information in some circumstances.

Applications of the DPW include:

1. Assessment of blood flow in patients for whom no tibioperoneal vessels can be localized or in patients with severe obstruction.

2. Demonstration of blood flow in patients who have lower extremity ulcerations preventing routine pressure studies or Doppler waveform analysis.

3. Postoperative monitoring for patency and assessment of reconstructive procedures.

4. Monitoring and evaluation of radiological procedures, such as angioplasty and heart catheterization.

5. In ischemic states, the determination of the level of arterial flow at multiple levels. It should

be emphasized that segmental pressures and Doppler waveform analysis provide the most reliable quantitative data. However, in those patients who cannot be routinely assessed, the DPW provides an alternate form of verifying arterial flow.

6. Examination of the neonate and pediatric patient. The DPW recording is easy to use and rapidly demonstrates arterial flow.

The DPW is obtained by placing the PPG photocell on the digit or the area of interest. The chart strip recorder is activated at 25 mm/second, and the waveform is obtained. The height and baseline are adjusted by the examiner. It is recommended that the dial settings be recorded for each examination so that they become reproducible.

Examples of DPW waveform recordings include the following:

1. The normal DPW has a sharp systolic up-

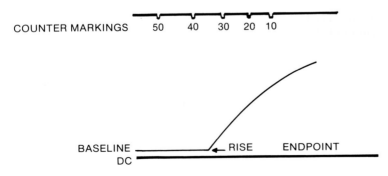

COUNTER MARKINGS   50   40   30   20   10

BASELINE
DC

RISE   ENDPOINT

Figure 17–22. Toe pressure recording using the direct current (DC) mode in extremely low-flow states.

Figure 17–23. Photoplethysmography digit pulse waveforms distal to a moderate obstruction.

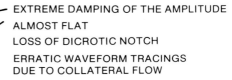

LOSS OF NARROW PEAK
REDUCTION OF AMPLITUDE
ROUNDING OF THE WAVEFORM
LOSS OF DICROTIC NOTCH

sweep, rising rapidly to a peak and dropping towards the baseline. The dicrotic notch is seen on the downslope (Fig. 17–19).

2. Vasoconstriction is shown as a decreased amplitude and rounding of the peak. The normal contour will return with vasodilation or reactive hyperemia to distinguish between the constricted state and occlusive disease.

3. Distal to obstruction, the DPW becomes rounded with a gradual upswing. The downslope bows away from the baseline, and the dicrotic notch disappears (Fig. 17–23).

4. In severely occlusive states, the DPW is extremely low in amplitude, with rounded peaks and absence of the dicrotic notch (Fig. 17–24).

5. Total occlusion presents with no pulsations and a flat waveform (Fig. 17–25).

Assessing Sympathetic Activity

Digit pulse waveform photoplethysmography can be used to demonstrate sympathetic innervation activity. In normal subjects, when a stimulus is applied, there will be a change in volume and waveform amplitude. To verify the sympathetic activity, the DPW technique described previously is used. However, the recorder is set at 5 mm/second, instead of 25 mm/second. The patient performs deep inspiration and expiration maneuvers, and the waveforms are continuously recorded. Markers are placed to signify inspiration and expiration maneuvers.

The normal response to deep inspiration or vasoconstriction is a significant decrease in the pulse amplitude. In expiration, the amplitude returns to normal, representing the vasodilated state. Figure 17–26 demonstrates the normal sympathetic activity.

In cases of Raynaud's disease or advanced arterial disease, there will be attenuation of the response. Sympathetic activity is frequently assessed to determine the value of a sympathectomy. Absence of the sympathetic response is seen in patients who have had a sympathectomy and also is seen in diabetic patients.

Doppler Techniques

Doppler techniques are among the most widely used noninvasive methods for identifying and localizing arterial disease. Doppler examinations provide wave morphology to correlate with the segmental pressures.

The peripheral arterial examination routinely uses a continuous-wave (CW) Doppler unit that transmits a continuous sound wave through the area of interest. These units are simple and inexpensive, but they are somewhat limited because they receive signals from all the vessels in the field of view. This problem can possibly be overcome with proper positioning and manipulation. In some cases, the duplex system with pulsed Doppler and sample volume gating may be necessary to differentiate specific vessels.

For peripheral arterial examinations, the CW Doppler uses a small pencil probe available in frequency ranges from 5 to 10 MHz (Fig. 17–27). The higher-frequency probes are used for superficial vessels; the lower-frequency probes are used for deeper vessels.

The transducer probe houses two piezoelectric crystals, one for sending and another for receiving. Illustration of the CW Doppler probe is seen in Figure 1–9. The use of two properly aligned crystals provides a narrow region of sensitivity while greatly attenuating the signals from other vessels. This beam discrimination aids in identifying the vessel of interest.

The CW Doppler receives boundary reflections from the vessel being insonated. According to

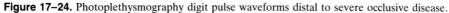

EXTREME DAMPING OF THE AMPLITUDE
ALMOST FLAT
LOSS OF DICROTIC NOTCH
ERRATIC WAVEFORM TRACINGS
DUE TO COLLATERAL FLOW

Figure 17–24. Photoplethysmography digit pulse waveforms distal to severe occlusive disease.

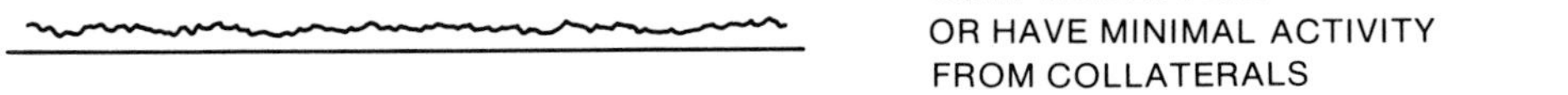

MINIMAL FLUCTUATIONS RESTING
ON THE ZERO BASELINE MAY BE
COMPLETELY FLAT
OR HAVE MINIMAL ACTIVITY
FROM COLLATERALS

Figure 17–25. Photoplethysmography digit pulse waveforms with a total occlusion.

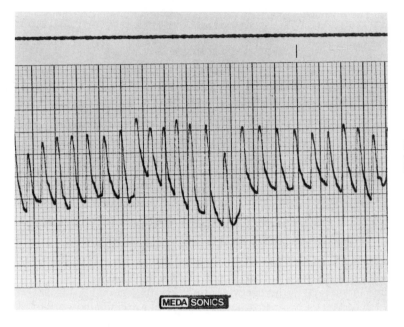

Figure 17–26. Photoplethysmography recording of the normal sympathetic activity.

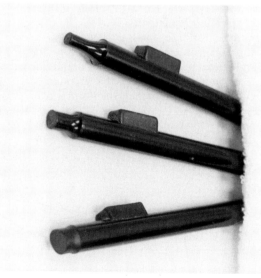

Figure 17–27. Continuous-wave Doppler probes—5, 8, and 10 MHz.

the Doppler principle, boundaries moving towards the transducer reflect a higher frequency than the transmitted frequency. Conversely, boundaries moving away from the transducer reflect a lower frequency. The amount of increase or decrease in frequency (Doppler shift) is proportional to the velocity of the moving boundary.

The received signal can be processed in several forms, including the audio signal, visual meter deflections, and the analog waveform tracing. The audio signal is the simplest form of monitoring and allows the operator to localize the vessel while obtaining the maximum Doppler shift. The meter deflection will indicate the direction of flow as positive or negative and will quantitate the velocity or frequency shift. The strip chart recorder provides the permanent recording of the analog waveform and allows for a more objective analysis. The bi-directional Doppler unit with zero crossing detection allows for identification and separation of blood flowing away from and towards the probe. The blood flow towards the probe is seen as a positive deflection (arterial signal), and the blood flow away from the probe is seen as a negative deflection (venous signal) (Fig. 17–28). Prior to the examination, the Dop-

pler unit is calibrated to ensure the correct size of the waveform and to provide measurement of the Doppler shift. The zero baseline is set at 10 to 20 mm above the bottom line to include the reverse component and forward flow. The running speed of the strip chart recorder is 25 mm/ second.

Doppler examination of the peripheral arteries includes waveform recordings of the common femoral artery, superficial femoral artery, popliteal artery, posterior tibial artery, dorsalis pedis, and anterior tibial artery (Figs. 17–29 and 17–30). Recordings are obtained bilaterally for comparison and evaluation of both extremities.

The transducer face is placed in contact with the skin surface with an acoustical gel as the coupling agent. The probe is held at a 45° angle to the vessel, which is determined by the highest pitch in sound or the maximum deflection of the waveform. The angle of incidence is of primary importance because the Doppler shift is maximal when angle θ is zero and is reduced proportionally when the angle is increased, as demonstrated in Figure 1–8.

Considerable experience is required to become proficient in hearing the multiphasic peripheral

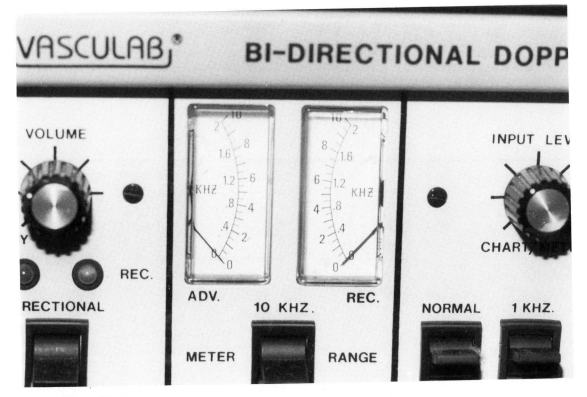

Figure 17–28. Doppler meter display for positive (advancing) and negative (receding) deflections.

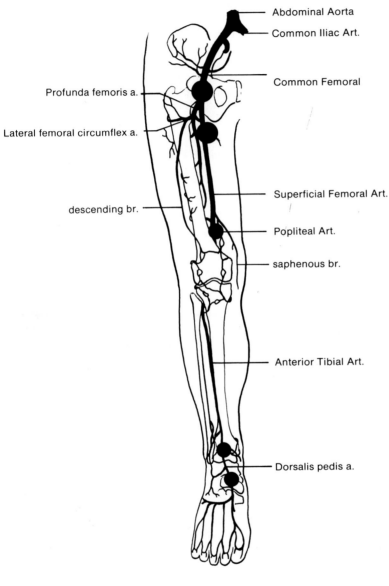

Abdominal Aorta

Common Iliac Art.

Common Femoral

Profunda femoris a.

Lateral femoral circumflex a.

Superficial Femoral Art.

descending br.

Popliteal Art.

saphenous br.

Anterior Tibial Art.

Dorsalis pedis a.

Anterior View

Figure 17–29. Anatomical diagram of the Doppler recording sites, which include the common femoral, superficial femoral, popliteal, dorsalis pedis, and anterior tibial arteries.

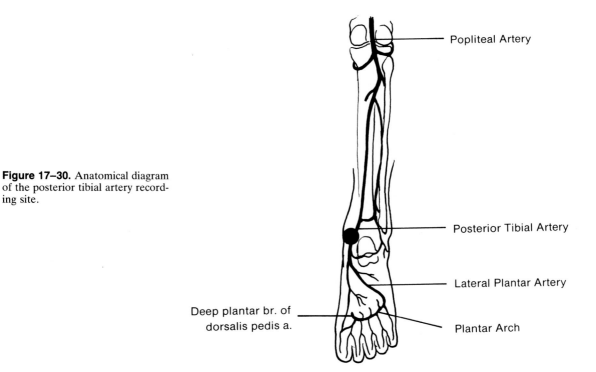

Figure 17–30. Anatomical diagram of the posterior tibial artery recording site.

Popliteal Artery

Posterior Tibial Artery

Lateral Plantar Artery

Deep plantar br. of dorsalis pedis a.

Plantar Arch

sounds and to recognize the changes in sound with arterial disease. Stereophonic headphones provide separation of the arterial and venous signals to assist in the discrimination of the vessels. The arterial sounds (towards the probe) will be heard in the right ear; the venous sounds (away from the probe) will be heard in the left ear. The headphones also eliminate sounds from external sources and increase the hearing sensitivity.

The examiner should be equally skilled in visualizing the analog waveform tracing. The normal peripheral arterial waveform is triphasic or multiphasic with a sharp systolic upsweep, a brief reverse component in early diastole, and a

low forward flow in late diastole. In cases of significant arterial disease, the systolic upsweep will decrease. As the disease advances, the waveform becomes increasingly damped and monophasic, with loss of the diastolic reverse component. The reverse component is dependent on the peripheral resistance; this is why it becomes more prominent during vasoconstrictive states and is reduced or absent during vasodilation and arterial disease. Examples of normal and abnormal Doppler waveforms are shown in Figures 17–31 through 17–33.

The Doppler waveforms are compared bilaterally and correlated with the segmental pressure study. Note the waveform examples in Figures

NORMAL PERIPHERAL ARTERIAL WAVEFORM

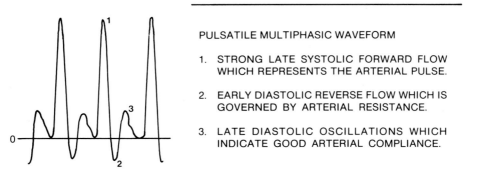

PULSATILE MULTIPHASIC WAVEFORM

1. STRONG LATE SYSTOLIC FORWARD FLOW WHICH REPRESENTS THE ARTERIAL PULSE.

2. EARLY DIASTOLIC REVERSE FLOW WHICH IS GOVERNED BY ARTERIAL RESISTANCE.

3. LATE DIASTOLIC OSCILLATIONS WHICH INDICATE GOOD ARTERIAL COMPLIANCE.

Figure 17–31. Normal peripheral artery analog waveform.

PROXIMAL ARTERIAL STENOSIS

1. REDUCES LATE SYSTOLIC AMPLITUDE

2. INCREASES THE WIDTH OF THE SYSTOLIC FORWARD FLOW

3. ABSENCE OF REVERSE FLOW IN EARLY DIASTOLE

4. REDUCTION OR ABSENCE OF LATE DIASTOLIC OSCILLATIONS

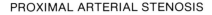
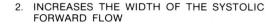

Figure 17–32. Peripheral artery analog waveform proximal to a stenosis.

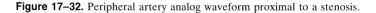
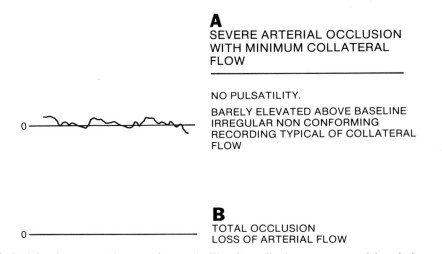

A
SEVERE ARTERIAL OCCLUSION WITH MINIMUM COLLATERAL FLOW

NO PULSATILITY.

BARELY ELEVATED ABOVE BASELINE IRREGULAR NON CONFORMING RECORDING TYPICAL OF COLLATERAL FLOW

B
TOTAL OCCLUSION
LOSS OF ARTERIAL FLOW

Figure 17–33. Peripheral artery analog waveforms. *A*, Waveform distal to severe arterial occlusion and exhibiting minimum collateral flow patterns. *B*, Waveform distal to a total occlusion with a zero-flow pattern.

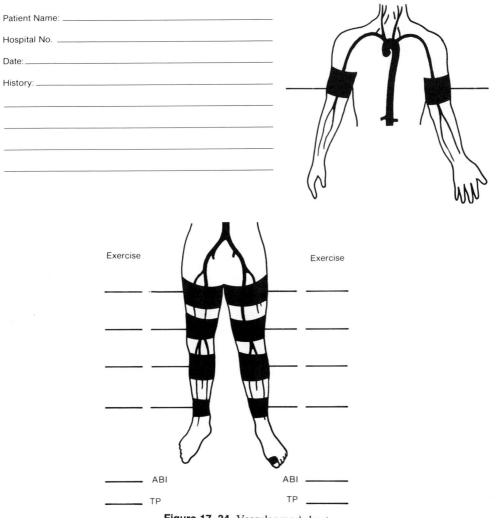

LOUISIANA STATE UNIVERSITY
MEDICAL CENTER - Shreveport
Ultrasound - Radiology

PERIPHERAL ARTERIAL EXAMINATION

Patient Name:

Hospital No.

Date:

History:

Exercise   Exercise

_____ ABI   ABI _____

_____ TP   TP _____

Figure 17–34. Vascular worksheet.

17–10 through 17–12 combined with the systolic pressure studies. Although each test is an independent study, the tests should be correlated to achieve a proper diagnosis. If they do not correlate, the site should be re-evaluated to ensure accuracy. In some cases, the pressure and waveforms will differ, which may be a correct finding. For example, in a patient who has an abdominal aneurysm, the high-thigh pressure will be diminished and common femoral and superficial femoral analog waveforms will be normal. Decreased high-thigh pressures usually indicate inflow disease; however, with normal waveforms, an aneurysm is suspected. An aneurysm can be proved by real-time scanning of the aorta. Calcified vessels will produce abnormally high pressure recordings. The use of analog waveforms will verify the normal or abnormal status of the vessel. The extremity can be further evaluated with the ABI and/or toe pressures to further verify the flow status of the extremity.

Upon completion of the bilateral analog waveform recordings, all information is recorded on a worksheet for interpretation. The worksheet should provide the complete patient data along with a record of all the pressure recordings and analog waveform tracings. Examination computations, such as the ABI and toe pressures, should be calculated. It is advisable to record the date of the examination and to note any vascular surgery or therapeutic procedures before or afterwards in order to have a baseline reference for follow-up examinations. An example of a vascular worksheet is seen in Figure 17–34.

The newest technique for examination of the peripheral arterial system is real-time imaging with duplex scanners. Although these units have been used predominantly in carotid imaging, they are currently being utilized for evaluation and research in the peripheral vessels.

In our laboratory, we perform the baseline peripheral examination that includes the techniques described in the text. Once the area of interest has been isolated, we image that specific area. Real-time imaging is specifically used for examining grafts, arteriovenous fistulas, aneurysms, false aneurysms, hematomas, ruptured vessels, and vessel anatomy.

References

1. Raines J. Noninvasive evaluation of peripheral vascular disease. Med Clin North Am 1980; 64:283–284.
2. Beyers M, Dudas S. The clinical practice of medical surgical nursing. 2nd ed. Boston, Little, Brown & Company, 1964:590–592.
3. Barnes R. Introduction to peripheral vascular disease: a student syllabus. Richmond, Medical College of Virginia, 1979; 15–20.
4. Winsor T. Influence of arterial disease on the systolic blood pressure gradient of the extremity. Am J Med Sci 1950; 220:117.
5. Segmental blood pressure measurements. Sonicaid Publication No. 8220–8504. Chichester, England.
6. Segmental pressure procedure outline. Mountain View, Calif, MedaSonics Publications.
7. Criteria, procedures and instrumentation for the clinical vascular laboratory. Greenwich, Conn, Life Sciences Instruments, 1978.
8. Kempczinski R, Yao J. Practical noninvasive vascular diagnosis. Chicago, Year Book Medical Publishers, 1983: 90.
9. Application of photoplethysmography. Sonicaid Publication No. 8100–8507. Chichester, England.

Introduction

The noninvasive methods used to detect aortoiliac inflow obstructions include (1) the *high-thigh* (HT) systolic pressure,[1-4] (2) the *upper thigh/brachial index* (UTBI),[1-4] and (3) the *Doppler femoral artery velocity waveforms*.[5]

High-Thigh Segment Systolic Pressures

The pressure of the upper thigh is greatly influenced by the size of the limb and the width of the measuring cuffs. Because these dimensions vary according to patient population and type of cuffs used, normal standards will have to be determined by each laboratory. Generally, wide cuffs (15 to 18 cm) and thin thighs produce fewer cuff-limb pressure artifacts than do narrow cuffs (12 cm) and thick thighs. The cuff-limb artifacts caused by narrow cuffs and thick thighs result in overestimation of the HT systolic pressures, whereas those of wide cuffs and thin thighs closely approximate the HT pressures. Actual intra-arterial pressure measurements from the femoral artery at the groin correspond to the brachial artery pressure in the arm. However, HT cuff pressures are higher than brachial artery pressures because of the cuff-limb discrepancy artifact of the thigh. This discrepancy causes the HT pressure to be 20 to 30 mm Hg higher than the brachial artery pressure under normal circumstances.[6]

If the HT pressure is lower than the brachial artery pressure, a significant obstruction is suspected to involve either or both the aortoiliac inflow system and the common femoral, profunda femoral, and superficial femoral artery outflow system. This is because the HT cuff is placed over the proximal segments of the profunda femoral and superficial femoral arteries and not

the common femoral artery in most patients. High-thigh pressures are then recorded during the compression of the profunda femoral and superficial femoral arteries. An obstruction in the aorta, iliac arteries, or common femoral artery will decrease the pressure of these vessels. Likewise, an obstruction of either or both the profunda femoral artery and superficial femoral artery will decrease the HT pressure. When the superficial femoral artery is occluded near its origin and the profunda femoral artery enlarges to provide collateral blood flow to the distal limb, the HT pressure may not be decreased because the measurement gives the high pressure in the enlarged profunda femoral artery.[7]

A normal example (Fig. 18–1) shows a brachial pressure of 107 mm Hg and a HT pressure of 134 mm Hg. A HT pressure 27 mm Hg higher than the brachial pressure is recorded because of the cuff-limb artifact. Obstructions that may cause the HT pressure to be lower than the brachial pressure may be located in any of the following sites:

- abdominal aorta
- common iliac artery
- external iliac artery
- common femoral artery
- profunda femoral artery
- superficial femoral artery

Upper Thigh/Brachial Index

The upper thigh/brachial index is determined by dividing the HT systolic pressure by the brachial systolic pressure. It should be >1.0 in the absence of significant obstructions in the arteries mentioned earlier. Like the ankle/brachial index (ABI) both the HT pressure and the UTBI may be normal in the resting limb and decreased when exercise or reactive hyperemia is used to unmask an underlying obstruction. A UTBI of 1.29 was

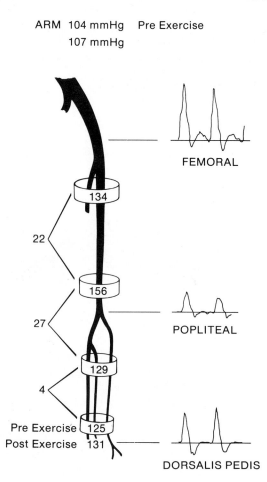

ARM 104 mmHg Pre Exercise
107 mmHg

FEMORAL

POPLITEAL

Pre Exercise
Post Exercise

DORSALIS PEDIS

ABI = 1.16 Pre Exercise
1.22 Post Exercise

Figure 18–1. Normal pattern. CFA = Common femoral artery; HT = high thigh; HT–BK = high thigh to below knee; BK–A = below knee to ankle; UTBI = upper thigh/brachial index.

Extremity	Right	Left
CFA waveforms	Normal	Normal
HT	Normal	Normal
HT–BK	Normal	Normal
BK–A	Normal	Normal
UTBI	Normal	Normal

obtained from the example shown in Figure 18–1. It did not decrease after exercise.

Doppler Femoral Artery Velocity Waveforms

A triphasic velocity waveform indicates a normal arterial inflow proximal to the site of the

Doppler probe. An example of a normal triphasic Doppler velocity waveform is shown in Figure 18–2*A*. Triphasic waveforms are obtained from the common and superficial femoral, popliteal, posterior tibial, and dorsalis pedis arteries in the normal nonvasoconstricted lower extremity at rest. As the Doppler probe site is moved distally towards the feet, the height (H) of the systolic peak (Phase 1) is reduced and the amount of early diastolic reversed flow (Phase 2) is reduced. These changes can be seen on the normal Doppler velocity waveforms shown in Figure 18–1.

Vasoconstriction caused by cool temperatures increases both the systolic peak and the early diastolic reversed flow. It decreases the late diastolic forward flow (Phase 3). These changes can be appreciated by a close examination of the velocity waveforms in Figure 18–1. In the figure, the patient's bare feet were exposed to the air-conditioned environment of the examining room prior to the study. The late diastolic forward flow is absent, and the early diastolic reversed flow is

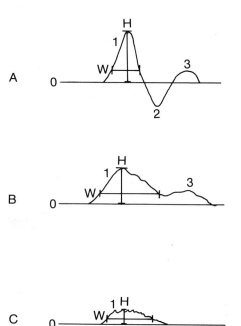

Figure 18–2. Doppler velocity waveforms.

A, Normal triphasic waveform. *1*, Systolic forward flow phase. *2*, Early diastolic reversed flow phase. *3*, Late diastolic forward flow phase. *H*, Height systolic peak. *W*, Width systolic and early diastolic waveform segments.

B, Attenuated biphasic waveform. Height *(H)* decreased, width *(W)* increased, and early diastolic reversed flow phase *(2)* is absent.

C, Attenuated monophasic waveform. Height *(H)* flat, width *(W)* increased, and both early *(2)* and late *(3)* diastolic flow phases are absent.

increased in the foot as compared with the thigh. Vasoconstriction also accounts for the loss of Phase 3 in the popliteal and dorsalis pedis arteries in this patient. The systolic peak in the dorsalis pedis artery is also quite high because of the vasoconstriction.

Vasodilatation caused by exercise produces the opposite effect. It decreases both the systolic peak velocity and the early diastolic reversed flow but increases the late diastolic forward flow.

Variations in the velocity waveforms caused by the effects of either vasoconstriction or vasodilatation can lead to confusing results during the interpretation of the velocity waveforms. To avoid this confusion, the patient should rest for up to 30 minutes before the examination and the bare feet should be covered with a blanket to prevent them from being exposed to cool temperatures.

The effects on the velocity waveform caused by a significant obstruction are shown in Figure 18–2. When a waveform is obtained from an arterial site *distal* to an obstruction, it may be either biphasic or monophasic. An example of a biphasic waveform is shown in Figure 18–2*B*. This waveform is biphasic because the early diastolic reversed flow is absent, whereas both the systolic and late diastolic forward flow phases can still be identified. The waveform becomes monophasic when both the early and late diastolic phases are absent and only the systolic forward flow (Phase 1) can be identified, as shown in Figure 18–2*C*.

An obstruction also attenuates the systolic upslope, the systolic peak, and the early diastolic downslope segments of the Doppler velocity waveform. The systolic upslope is less steep and more gradual than that observed in the waveform of a normal vessel. This distinction is made by comparing the systolic upslopes in Figure 18–2*A* and *B*. The height of the systolic peak becomes flat and round, and it is lower than that observed in the normal vessel. These waveforms can be appreciated by comparing the systolic peak height in Figure 18–2*B* and *C* with the one shown in Figure 18–2*A*. The early diastolic downslope becomes gradual, causing an increase in the width (W) of the waveform segments in Figure 18–2*B* and *C* as compared with Figure 18–2*A*. Figure 18–2*B* and *C* indicates a damping of the arterial pulsatility below the obstruction site.

Pulsatility is the difference between the systolic peak and late diastolic peak flow velocities. High systolic peak and low end-diastolic flow velocities produce good pulsatility; low systolic peak and low end-diastolic flow velocities produce poor

pulsatility. The waveform in Figure 18–2*A* would have good pulsatility, whereas that in Figure 18–2*C* would have poor pulsatility.

The basic Doppler velocity waveform abnormalities distal to a significant obstruction site include (1) disappearance of the early diastolic reversed flow; (2) a flat, round, reduced systolic forward flow peak; and (3) loss of pulsatility.

When the Doppler probe is placed *directly over* a stenosis, it will record an abnormally high systolic peak velocity. This reflects the increased flow velocity passing through the stenosis. The contour of the waveform obtained *proximal* to an obstruction will depend on the capacity of the collateral circulation going around the obstruction site. If the collaterals are well developed, the waveforms may be normal. For example, in a patient with normal iliac and profunda femoral arteries, the common femoral artery waveform may be normal even in the presence of a superficial femoral artery occlusion. The profunda femoral artery acts as the collateral pathway around the superficial femoral artery occlusion site in this example. When the collaterals are poorly developed, the velocity waveform proximal to an obstruction will have a systolic peak but the diastolic phases will be absent. Failure to obtain any of the three velocity waveform phases over a vessel indicates either a complete occlusion or a flow velocity too low to produce a detectable Doppler frequency shift.

Limitations of the Noninvasive Assessment of Aortoiliac Inflow Disease

Unfortunately, the high-thigh segmental systolic pressure measurement, the upper thigh/brachial index, and the common femoral artery Doppler velocity waveform analysis cannot be relied upon to detect significant obstructions in the aortoiliac inflow system. This is because the proximal superficial femoral artery obstructions with poor collateral circulation through the profunda femoral artery cannot be differentiated from isolated aortoiliac inflow disease.[2, 5, 8] An isolated superficial femoral artery obstruction with poor profunda femoral artery collateral circulation will cause the common femoral artery velocity waveforms to be abnormal and will reduce both the HT systolic pressures and the UTBI. Because these are the same parameters used to detect aortoiliac disease, they cannot be used to distinguish aortoiliac obstructions from superficial femoral artery obstructions. This is a significant limitation because femoropopliteal outflow obstructions are often found in combination with aortoiliac inflow obstructions. Therefore, when the common femoral artery waveforms are abnormal and the HT systolic pressures are reduced, the following possibilities must be considered:

1. Abnormal aortoiliac inflow system.
2. Normal aortoiliac inflow system with abnormal femoropopliteal outflow system.
3. Abnormal aortoiliac inflow and femoropopliteal outflow system.

Because of these limitations, direct intra-arterial femoral artery pressure measurements and pressure gradient measurements across aortoiliac obstructions during arteriography with reactive hyperemia or papaverine injection remain the most sensitive methods for determining significant aortoiliac obstructions and differentiating them from superficial femoral artery obstructive disease.

Segmental Pressure and Velocity Waveform Patterns

Examples are provided to illustrate the lower limb segmental pressure and velocity waveform patterns produced by the various combinations of obstructive lesions. The aortoiliac inflow system is considered abnormal when a significant flow-limiting stenosis or a total occlusion exists in either or both the aorta and the iliac arteries. The femoropopliteal outflow system is considered abnormal when these lesions exist in the common femoral, profunda femoral, or superficial femoral arteries in the absence of adequate collateral blood flow to the affected lower extremity. A total occlusion of the superficial femoral artery is certainly abnormal, but it may not be of hemodynamic significance when the profunda femoral artery serves as a well-developed collateral pathway around the obstruction. The noninvasive test may be normal and the patient may remain asymptomatic under these circumstances. This would then be considered a hemodynamically normal lower extremity by the noninvasive vascular procedures.

The example illustrations begin with a relatively normal examination of the left lower extremity. The normal findings may be used as a baseline for comparison with the subsequent abnormal findings. Correlative angiograms are used to show the anatomy and sites of the obstructive lesions.

Normal Patterns

Normal patterns are illustrated in Figure 18–1.

Doppler Velocity Waveforms

The Doppler velocity waveforms of the common femoral artery are used to evaluate the inflow system; those from the superficial femoral and popliteal arteries are used to evaluate the outflow system. The run-off system is evaluated by Doppler velocity waveforms from the anterior and posterior tibial arteries at the ankle and the dorsalis pedis artery over the dorsum of the foot. All of these waveforms are normally triphasic. The late diastolic forward flow is absent in the popliteal, anterior tibial, and dorsalis pedis arteries (Fig. 18–1) because of peripheral vasoconstriction from exposure to cool temperatures.

Pressure Measurements

Four cuffs are used to obtain the segmental Doppler systolic pressure measurements. These are designated as the high-thigh (HT), above-knee (AK), below-knee (BK), and ankle (A) cuffs. The HT pressure is normally 20 to 30 mm Hg higher than the brachial artery (BA) pressure because of the cuff-limb discrepancy artifact of the thigh. A HT pressure <20 mm Hg above the brachial artery pressure is considered abnormal. Pressure gradients between the HT–AK, AK–BK, and BK–A cuff segments should be less than 30 mm Hg.

The ankle/brachial index (ABI) should be 1 or greater than 1. It should not decrease significantly after exercise or reactive hyperemia.

Normally, the ABI does not fall after exercise but it does fall transiently after reactive hyperemia (5 minutes of cuff occlusion). A normal reactive hyperemia test finding is one in which (1) the lowest ABI is >0.80, and (2) the ABI returns to normal within 1 minute following deflation of the thigh cuff.

Upper Thigh/Brachial Index

The HT systolic segmental pressure divided by the highest brachial artery systolic pressure should be 1 or greater in the normal lower extremity. It is 1.29 in Figure 18–1; this value did not decrease after exercise.

Abdominal Aortic Occlusion Pattern

The abdominal aortic occlusion pattern is characterized by grossly abnormal velocity waveforms and segmental pressure in both of the lower extremities. It is illustrated in the following cases.

Case I (Figs. 18–3 and 18–4) is an example of how an aortic occlusion limits the noninvasive vascular examination of the lower extremities. Because the aortic occlusion reduces all the segmental pressures to zero, the arteries in the lower extremities cannot be further evaluated for obstructive lesions. The velocity waveforms are monophasic in all the arteries, indicating an aortoiliac inflow obstruction that affects both of

the lower extremities. This pattern could also be caused by bilateral iliac or common femoral artery obstructions.

Correlative angiograms are shown in Figure 18–4. The abdominal aortogram in Figure 18–4A shows total occlusion of the abdominal aorta. Enlarged lumbar arteries form collateral routes around the inflow obstruction. These vessels are grossly enlarged, indicating that the inflow obstruction is a long-standing process that thrombosed acutely and caused the abnormalities seen on the segmental pressure and velocity waveform examinations. The angiograms of the outflow and run-off systems in Figure 18–4B and C show the arteries in these systems to be patent despite the abnormal waveforms and pressures found on the noninvasive vascular examination.

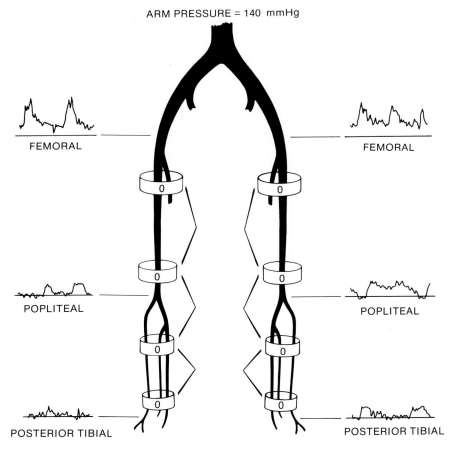

Figure 18–3. *Case I.* Aortic occlusion pattern. CFA = Common femoral artery; HT = high thigh; HT–BK = high thigh to below knee; BK–A = below knee to ankle; UTBI = upper thigh/brachial index.

Extremity	Right	Left
CFA waveforms	Abnormal	Abnormal
HT	Abnormal	Abnormal
HT–BK	Abnormal	Abnormal
BK–A	Abnormal	Abnormal
UTBI	Abnormal	Abnormal

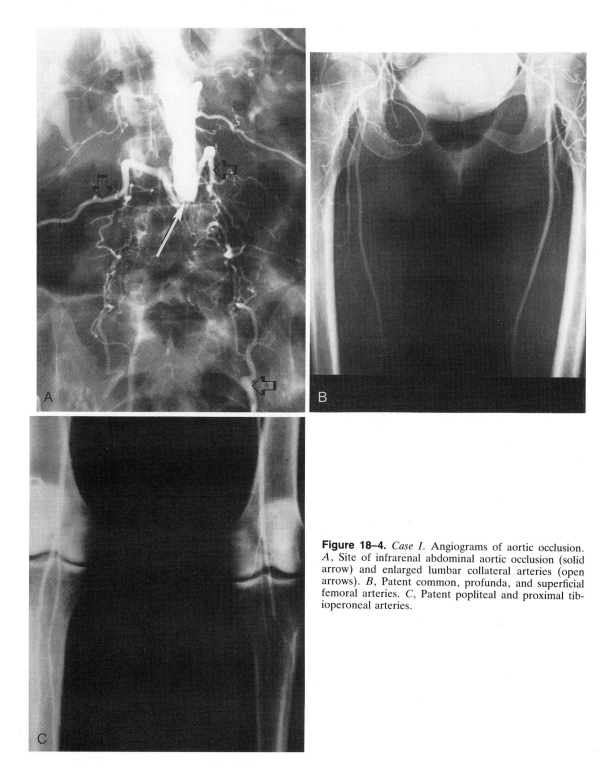

Figure 18–4. *Case I.* Angiograms of aortic occlusion. *A*, Site of infrarenal abdominal aortic occlusion (solid arrow) and enlarged lumbar collateral arteries (open arrows). *B*, Patent common, profunda, and superficial femoral arteries. *C*, Patent popliteal and proximal tibioperoneal arteries.

Case I illustrates how an obstructive process in the inflow system can prevent the high-pressure pulse wave in the aortic root from being transmitted into the peripheral vessels of the lower extremities. This example also shows how the pressures in the vessels of these extremities may be rendered unobtainable, making their evaluation by noninvasive vascular procedures difficult.

Case II (Figs. 18–5 through 18–7) shows how digital photoelectric plethysmography is used to illustrate the severe attenuation of the digital artery pulse waveform caused by an aortic occlusion. A normal digital photoelectric plethysmographic pulse waveform is shown in Figure 18–6. It has a steep upslope, a narrow peak, and a dicrotic notch on a downslope that is concave towards the baseline. The grossly abnormal digital

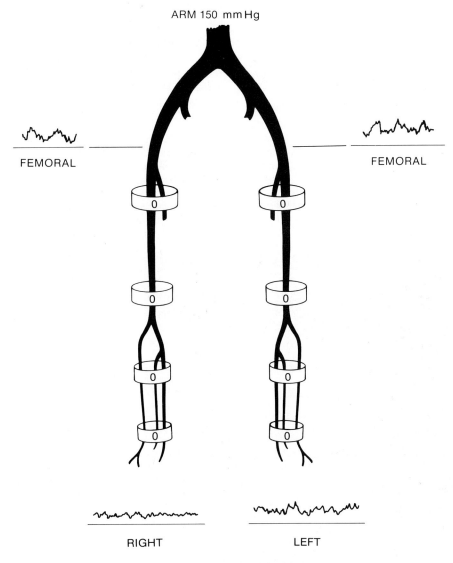

DIGITAL PLETHYSMOGRAPHY

Figure 18–5. *Case II.* Aortic occlusion pattern. CFA = Common femoral artery; HT = high thigh; HT–BK = high thigh to below knee; BK–A = below knee to ankle; UTBI = upper thigh/brachial index.

Extremity	Right	Left
CFA waveforms	Abnormal	Abnormal
HT	Abnormal	Abnormal
HT–BK	Abnormal	Abnormal
BK–A	Abnormal	Abnormal
UTBI	Abnormal	Abnormal

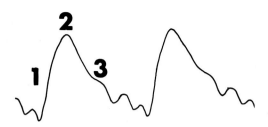

Figure 18–6. Normal digital photoelectric plethysmographic pulse waveform. *1*, Steep upslope. *2*, Narrow peak. *3*, Dicrotic notch.

pulse waveforms in Figure 18–5 exhibit gradual upslopes; rounded, flat peaks; and no dicrotic notch. Aortography of the aortic occlusion in this example is shown in Figure 18–7.

Case III (Figs. 18–8 and 18–9) shows the effect of a total aortic occlusion on toe pressures. Again, the aortic inflow occlusion pattern is demonstrated with abnormal waveforms and depressed segmental pressures throughout both lower extremities. The toe systolic pressures are decreased bilaterally. Normally, these should be approximately 50 mm Hg or either 60% of the ankle systolic pressure or 80 to 90% of the brachial artery systolic pressure.

Abdominal Aortic Aneurysms

An example of an abdominal aortic aneurysm simulating an aortoiliac inflow obstruction is shown in Figures 18–10 and 18–11. The velocity waveforms are normal, but the segmental pressures are abnormal in both of the lower extremities.

Unilateral Iliac Artery Inflow Obstruction Pattern

In the unilateral iliac artery inflow obstruction pattern, the common femoral artery velocity waveforms and HT pressures are abnormal in the affected limb but normal in the unaffected limb. An example of this pattern is shown in *Case I* (Figs. 18–12 and 18–13).

Case I. Figure 18–12 shows that unilateral inflow obstruction causes a monophasic velocity waveform in the left common femoral artery, whereas the waveform in the right common femoral artery remains triphasic. There is also a difference between the right and left HT segmental pressures. The right HT pressure is higher than the arm pressure because of the cuff-limb

Text continued on page 335

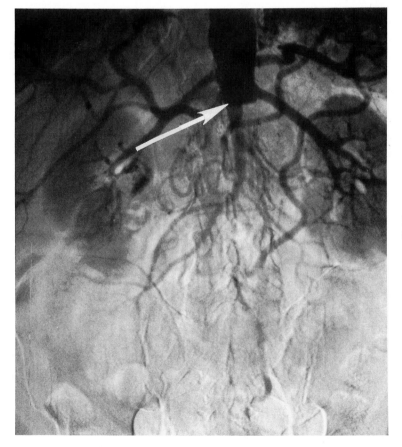

Figure 18–7. *Case II.* Angiogram of aortic occlusion (arrow).

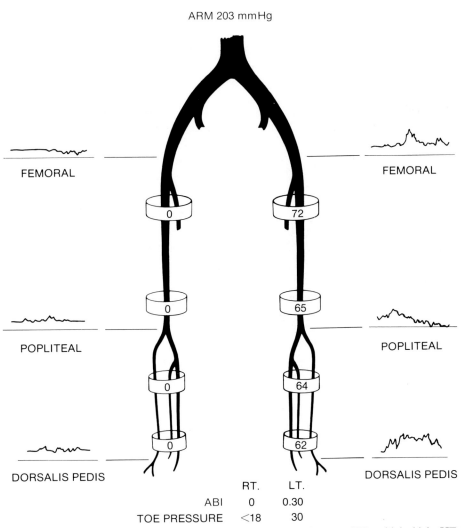

Figure 18–8. *Case III.* Aortic occlusion pattern. CFA = Common femoral artery; HT = high thigh; HT–BK = high thigh to below knee; BK–A = below knee to ankle; UTBI = upper thigh/brachial inflex.

Extremity	Right	Left
CFA waveforms	Abnormal	Abnormal
HT	Abnormal	Abnormal
HT–BK	Abnormal	Abnormal
BK–A	Abnormal	Abnormal
UTBI	Abnormal	Abnormal

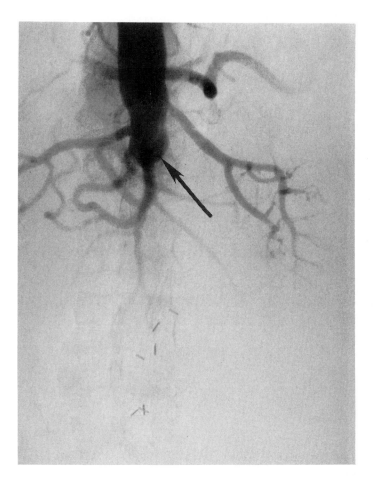

Figure 18–9. *Case III.* Angiogram of aortic occlusion (arrow).

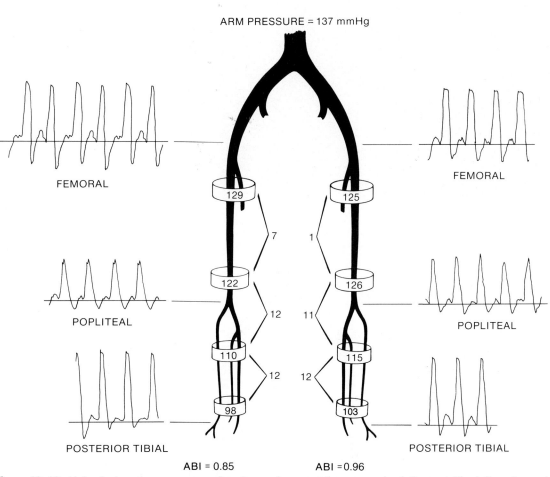

Figure 18–10. Abdominal aortic aneurysm causing abnormal segmental pressures simulating aortoiliac inflow obstructive disease. CFA = Common femoral artery; HT = high thigh; HT–BK = high thigh to below knee; BK–A = below knee to ankle; UTBI = upper thigh/brachial index.

Extremity	Right	Left
CFA waveforms	Normal	Normal
HT	**Abnormal**	**Abnormal**
HT–BK	Normal	Normal
BK–A	Normal	Normal
UTBI	Normal	Normal

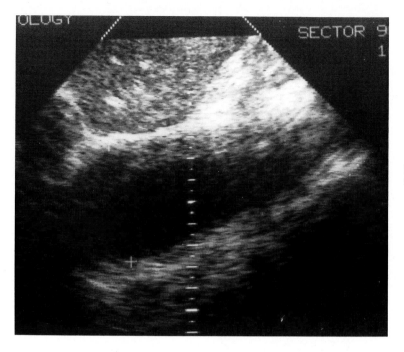

Figure 18–11. Sonogram of abdominal aortic aneurysm.

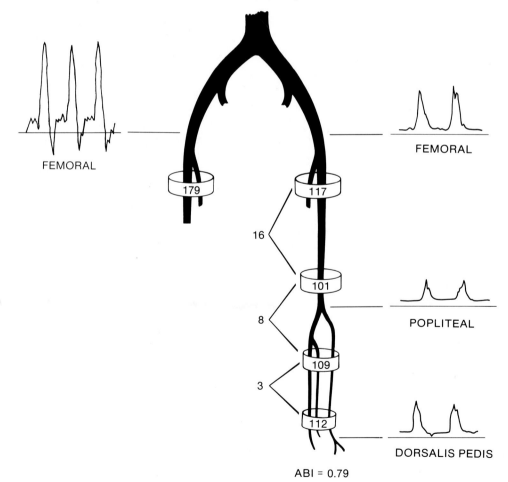

ARM 141 mmHg

FEMORAL

179

117

FEMORAL

16

101

POPLITEAL

8

109

3

112

DORSALIS PEDIS

ABI = 0.79

Figure 18–12 *See legend on opposite page*

334

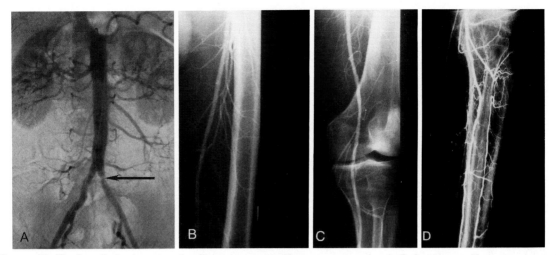

Figure 18–13. *Case I.* Angiograms of unilateral common iliac artery stenosis. *A*, Left common iliac artery stenosis (arrow). *B*, Patent superficial and profunda femoral arteries. *C*, Patent popliteal artery. *D*, Patent tibioperoneal arteries.

discrepancy artifact of the thigh. A decreased HT pressure on the left is caused by the iliac artery stenosis. Monophasic waveforms persist in the popliteal and dorsalis pedis arteries below the level of the iliac artery stenosis. No significant pressure gradients are present between the HT–AK, AK–BK, and BK–A cuffs, indicating the absence of obstructive lesions in the outflow and run-off arterial systems. The resting ABI is reduced to 0.79. Correlative angiograms are shown in Figure 18–13.

Case II (Figs. 18–14 and 18–15) shows another example of the unilateral iliac artery inflow obstruction pattern.

Bilateral Iliac Artery Inflow Obstruction Pattern

When the iliac arteries are occluded bilaterally, the pattern simulates that seen with an abdominal aortic occlusion. An example is shown in Figures 18–16 and 18–17. The velocity waveforms and segmental pressures are grossly abnormal in both of the lower extremities because of the severity of the iliac artery occlusions.

Inflow and Outflow Combination Obstructive Patterns

The most common form of the inflow and outflow combination obstructive pattern is iliac artery disease in association with an obstruction of the superficial femoral artery. This pattern produces a dilemma because both the HT and the common femoral artery waveforms may be abnormal as a result of either the iliac artery obstruction or the superficial femoral artery obstruction. It is then difficult to determine whether the reduced HT pressures and abnormal common femoral artery waveforms are caused by an iliac artery obstruction or a superficial artery obstruction, or both in combination.

Case I in Figures 18–18 and 18–19 illustrates the problem just described. The HT pressure is reduced, and there is no significant pressure gradient between the HT–AK segment cuff pressures. Angiography demonstrated both iliac artery and superficial femoral artery occlusions, as shown in Figure 18–19.

Case II in Figures 18–20 and 18–21 illustrates bilateral iliac artery disease in combination with bilateral

Text continued on page 343

Figure 18–12. *Case I.* Unilateral iliac artery obstruction pattern. CFA = Common femoral artery; HT = high thigh; HT–AK = high thigh to above knee; AK–BK = above knee to below knee; BK–A= below knee to ankle; UTBI = upper thigh/brachial index.

Extremity	Right	Left
CFA waveforms	Normal	**Abnormal**
HT	Normal	**Abnormal**
HT–AK		Normal
AK–BK		Normal
BK–A		Normal
UTBI	Normal	**Abnormal**

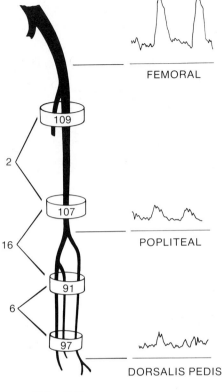

ARM 113 mmHg

FEMORAL

109

2

107

POPLITEAL

16

91

6

97

DORSALIS PEDIS

ABI = 0.85

Figure 18–14. *Case II*. Unilateral iliac artery obstruction pattern. CFA = Common femoral artery; HT = high thigh; HT–AK = high thigh to above knee; AK–BK = above knee to below knee; BK–A = below knee to ankle; UTBI = upper thigh/brachial index.

Extremity	*Left*
CFA waveforms	**Abnormal**
HT	**Abnormal**
HT–AK	Normal
AK–BK	Normal
BK–A	Normal
UTBI	**Abnormal**

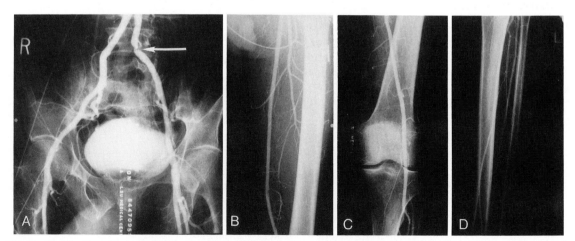

Figure 18–15. *Case II*. Angiograms of unilateral common iliac artery stenosis. *A*, Left common iliac artery stenosis (arrow). *B*, Patent superficial and profunda femoral arteries. *C*, Patent popliteal artery. *D*, Patent tibioperoneal arteries.

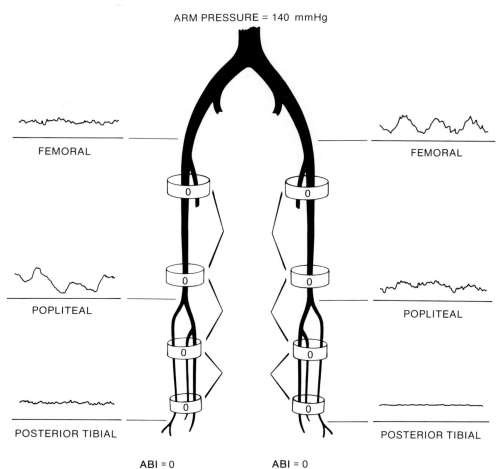

Figure 18–16. Bilateral iliac artery occlusion pattern. CFA = Common femoral artery; HT = high thigh; HT–BK = high thigh to below knee; BK–A = below knee to ankle; UTBI = upper thigh/brachial index.

Extremity	Right	Left
CFA waveforms	Abnormal	Abnormal
HT	Abnormal	Abnormal
HT–BK	Abnormal	Abnormal
BK–A	Abnormal	Abnormal
UTBI	Abnormal	Abnormal

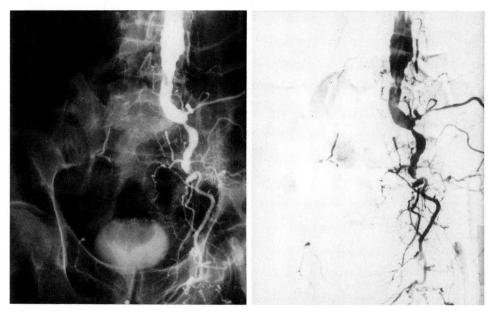

Figure 18–17. Angiogram of bilateral iliac artery occlusions.

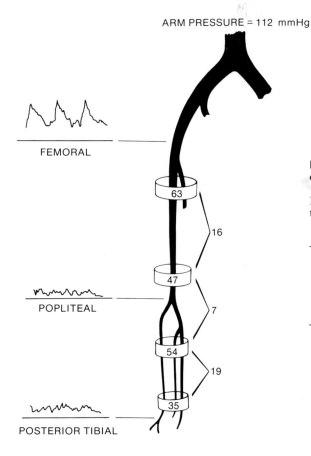

Figure 18–18. *Case I.* Inflow and outflow combination obstruction pattern. CFA = Common femoral artery; HT = high thigh; HT–AK = high thigh to above knee; AK–BK = above knee to below knee; BK–A = below knee to ankle; UTBI = upper thigh/brachial index.

Extremity	Right
CFA waveforms	Abnormal
HT	Abnormal
HT–AK	**Normal**
AK–BK	**Normal**
BK–A	**Normal**
UTBI	Abnormal

ARM PRESSURE = 112 mmHg

FEMORAL

63

16

47

POPLITEAL

7

54

19

35

POSTERIOR TIBIAL

ABI = 0.31

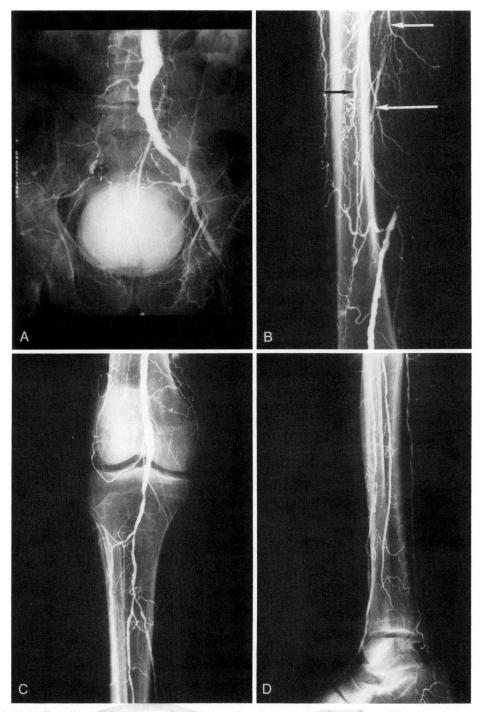

Figure 18–19. *Case I*. Right inflow and outflow combination obstruction angiograms. *A*, Right common and external iliac artery occlusions. Although not shown, the common and profunda femoral arteries were patent on subsequent angiograms. *B*, Occluded superficial femoral artery. Collateral vessels are shown (black arrow) arising from patent profunda femoral artery (white arrows). *C*, Patent popliteal artery. *D*, Patent tibioperoneal arteries.

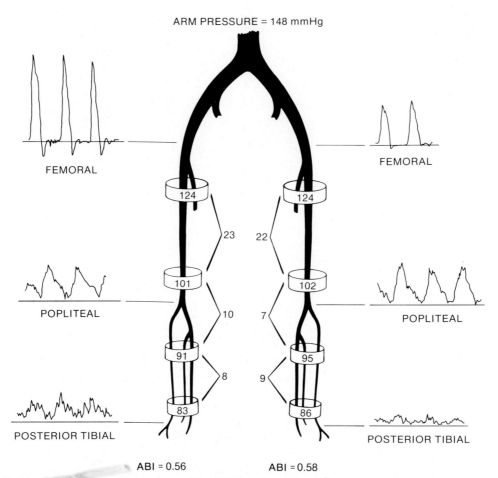

Figure 18–20. *Case II.* Inflow and outflow combination obstructive pattern. CFA = Common femoral artery; Pop = popliteal artery; HT = high thigh; HT–AK = high thigh to above knee; AK–BK = above knee to below knee; UTBI = upper thigh/brachial index.

Extremity	Right		Left	
Waveforms	(CFA)	Normal	(CFA)	Normal
	(Pop)	Abnormal	(Pop)	Abnormal
HT		Abnormal		Abnormal
HT–AK		Normal		Normal
AK–BK		Normal		Normal
UTBI		Abnormal		Abnormal

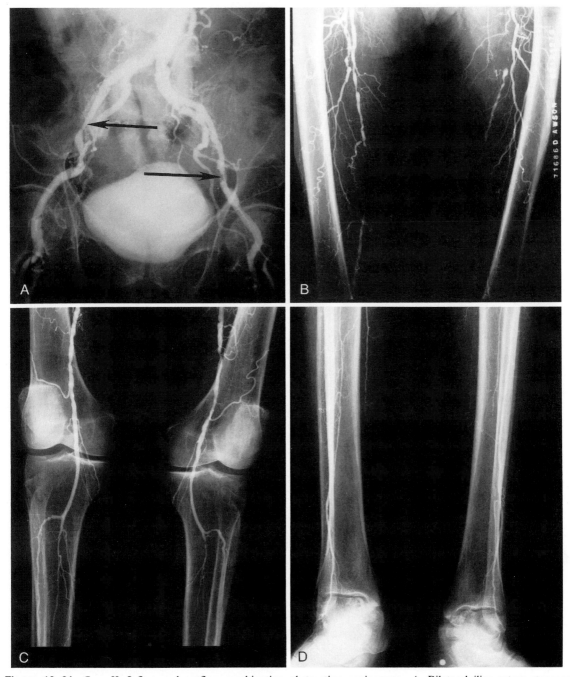

Figure 18–21. *Case II.* Inflow and outflow combination obstruction angiograms. *A*, Bilateral iliac artery stenoses (arrows). *B*, Bilateral superficial femoral artery occlusions. *C*, Patent popliteal arteries. *D*, Patent anterior tibial and peroneal arteries, bilateral view. Both posterior tibial arteries are occluded.

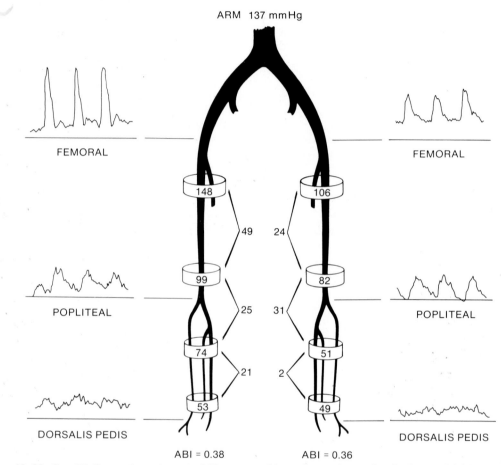

Figure 18–22. *Case III.* Comparison of a normal iliac artery with an abnormal one when both superficial femoral arteries are occluded. CFA = Common femoral artery; HT = high thigh; HT–AK = high thigh to above knee; UTBI = upper thigh/brachial index.

Extremity	Right	Left
CFA waveforms	Abnormal	Abnormal
HT	Abnormal	Abnormal
HT–AK	Abnormal	**Abnormal**
UTBI	**Normal**	Abnormal

superficial femoral artery occlusions. The common femoral artery waveforms are normal, whereas those in the popliteal and tibioperoneal arteries are abnormal. These findings could indicate the absence of significant iliac inflow obstructions and the presence of significant disease in the superficial femoral outflow arteries. However, both the HT pressures and the UTBI are reduced. Such data make it difficult to exclude obstructive lesions in the iliac inflow system. These lesions are present, as shown in the angiograms in Figure 18–21. No significant pressure gradient exists between the HT–AK segment cuffs despite the fact that the superficial femoral artery is occluded in both lower limbs, as shown in Figure 18–21. This case points out the difficulty in assessing the status of the iliac inflow system when the common femoral artery waveforms are in conflict with the HT pressures.

Case III compares normal iliac artery inflow with abnormal inflow when both superficial femoral arteries are occluded (Figs. 18–22 and 18–23). The common femoral artery waveforms and the HT pressures are abnormal bilaterally, as shown in Figure 18–22, making it difficult to exclude bilateral iliac inflow system disease. A significant pressure gradient exists between the right HT–AK segment cuffs, indicating right superficial femoral artery disease. However, no such pressure gradient exists between the left HT–AK segment cuffs even though the left superficial femoral artery is occluded. The abnormal right common femoral artery waveforms and the reduced HT pressure are caused

by the superficial artery occlusion. The abnormal left common femoral artery waveforms and the reduced HT pressure are caused by the iliac artery stenosis and the superficial femoral artery occlusion. Despite the fact that the right UTBI could be considered normal at 1.08, it would be difficult to exclude right iliac artery inflow disease because of the abnormal common femoral artery waveforms and the reduced HT pressure.

Normal Inflow, Abnormal Outflow Pattern

The normal inflow, abnormal outflow pattern shows the effect on the common femoral artery waveform, the HT pressure, and the UTBI from an isolated superficial femoral artery occlusion when the superficial femoral artery is occluded at its origin. The left common femoral artery waveform is normal because of outflow into the collateral profunda femoral artery, as shown in *Case I* (Figs. 18–24 and 18–25).

Case I. The HT pressure is reduced, and the UTBI is abnormal. No pressure gradient exists across the HT–AK segment cuffs because the superficial femoral artery is occluded at its origin, which is above the level of the HT cuff. The profunda femoral artery collateral blood flow is not adequate because the ankle/brachial index is 0.63.

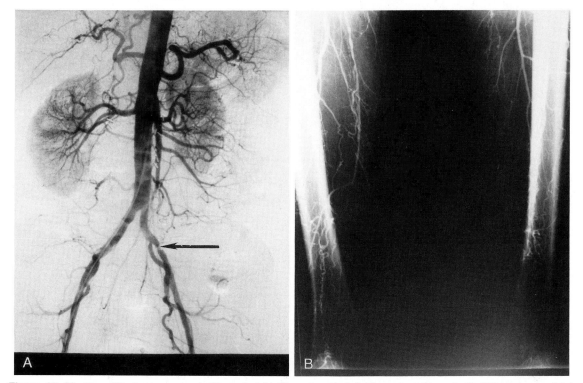

Figure 18–23. *Case III*. Angiograms. *A*, Normal right iliac, stenotic left iliac artery (arrow). *B*, Bilateral superficial femoral artery occlusion.

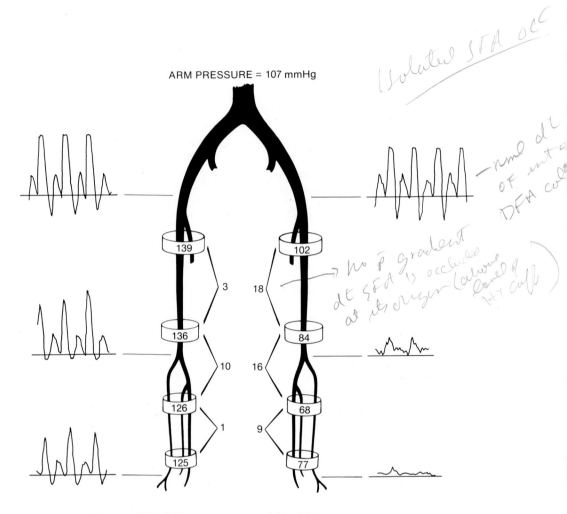

Figure 18–24. *Case I.* Normal inflow, abnormal outflow pattern. CFA = Common femoral artery; HT = high thigh; HT–AK = high thigh to above knee; AK–BK = above knee to below knee; UTBI = upper thigh/brachial index.

Extremity	Right	Left
CFA waveforms	Normal	Normal
HT	Normal	**Abnormal**
HT–AK	Normal	Normal
AK–BK	Normal	Normal
UTBI	**Abnormal**	**Abnormal**

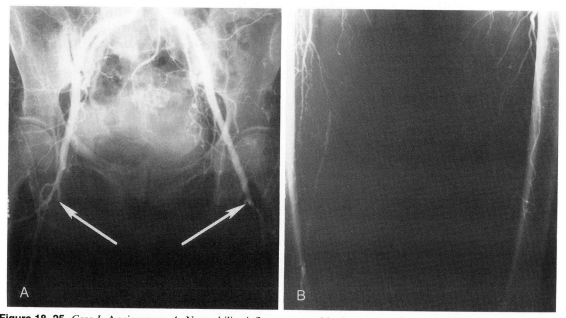

Figure 18–25. *Case I.* Angiograms. *A*, Normal iliac inflow system with abnormal outflow secondary to occlusion of both superficial femoral arteries at origin (arrows). *B*, Occlusion of both superficial femoral arteries. Patent profunda femoral arteries provide collaterals.

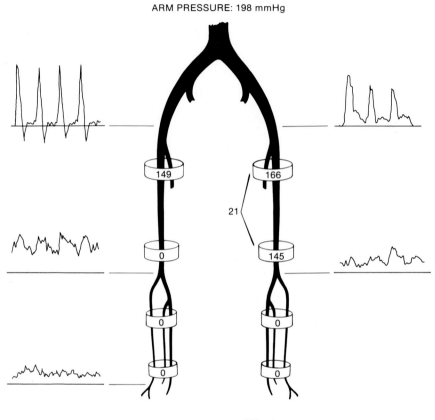

Figure 18–26. *Case II*. Normal inflow, abnormal outflow pattern. CFA = Common femoral artery; HT = high thigh; HT–AK = high thigh to above knee; UTBI = upper thigh/brachial index.

Extremity	Right	Left
CFA waveforms	**Normal**	Abnormal
HT	Abnormal	Abnormal
HT–AK	Abnormal	**Normal**
UTBI	Abnormal	Abnormal

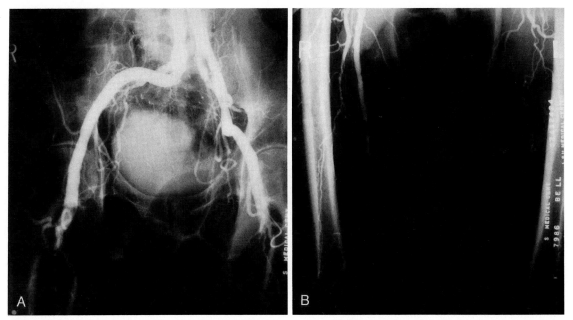

Figure 18–27. *Case II*. Angiograms. *A*, Normal iliac inflow system. *B*, Bilateral superficial femoral artery occlusions.

Case II shows a normal iliac inflow system with embolic occlusions of the superficial femoral arteries (Figs. 18–26 and 18–27). The profunda femoral arteries remain patent. Both the HT pressures and the UTBI are abnormal in both lower extremities. Because these are abnormal, iliac inflow disease would be suspected despite the normal right common femoral artery waveform. Left iliac inflow obstruction would be suspected because of the associated abnormal left common femoral artery waveform.

References

1. Heintz SE, Bone GE, Slaymaker EE, Hayes AC, Barnes RW. Value of arterial pressure measurements in the proximal and distal part of the thigh in arterial occlusive disease. Surg Gynecol Obstet 1978; 146:337–343.

2. Flanigan DP, Gray B, Schuler JJ, Schwartz JA, Post KW. Correlation of Doppler-derived high thigh pressure and intra-arterial pressure in the assessment of aortoiliac occlusive disease. Br J Surg 1981; 68:423–425.

3. Flanigan DP, Gray B, Schuler JJ, Schwartz JA, O'Connor RJA, Williams LR. Utility of wide and narrow blood pressure cuffs in the hemodynamic assessment of aortoiliac occlusive disease. Surgery 1982; 92:16–20.

4. Bauer GM, Zupan TL, Gates KH, Porter JM. Blood flow in the common femoral artery. Evaluation in a vascular laboratory. Am J Surg 1983; 145:585–588.

5. Baird RN, Bird DR, Clifford PC, Linsby RJ, Skidmore R, Woodcock JP. Upstream stenosis. Its diagnosis by Doppler signals from the femoral artery. Arch Surg 1980; 115:1316–1322.

6. Fronek A, Johansen KH, Dilley RB, Bernstein EF. Noninvasive physiologic tests in the diagnosis and characterization of peripheral arterial occlusive disease. Am J Surg 1973; 126:205–214.

7. Carter SA. Indirect systolic pressures and pulse waves in arterial occlusive disease of the lower extremities. Circulation 1968; 37:624.

8. Brener BJ, Frief DK, Alpert J, Goldenkranz RJ, Parsonnet V. Clinical usefulness of noninvasive arterial studies. Contemp Surg 1980; 16:41–55.

19 • Obstructive Disease of the Femoropopliteal Outflow and Tibioperoneal Run-Off Systems

Introduction

The femoral and popliteal arteries comprise the outflow system because they receive the outflow from the aortoiliac inflow system (Fig. 19–1A and B). The run-off system, which receives run-off blood from the aortoiliac inflow and femoropopliteal outflow systems, consists of the anterior tibial, posterior tibial, and peroneal arteris (Fig. 19–1C). Atherosclerosis is the most common cause of obstruction. Embolism is another common cause of obstruction. The most frequent obstructive sites secondary to atherosclerosis have been shown in Figures 16–4 and 16–9. The noninvasive methods of detecting obstructive lesions within these vessels are listed below:

- Doppler arterial waveforms
- segmental systolic pressures
- ankle/brachial index

These methods have been discussed in detail in Chapter 18.

Case presentations will be discussed to illustrate how these methods are used to diagnose obstructive arterial disease in the femoropopliteal and tibioperoneal run-off systems. The normal pattern is demonstrated in Case I and Figure 19–2A and B.

Doppler Arterial Waveforms

Doppler arterial waveforms from the common femoral and popliteal arteries are utilized to assess the outflow system; those from the anterior tibial, posterior tibial, and dorsalis pedis arteries are used to appraise the run-off system. Normally, arterial waveforms from these arteries are triphasic. Often the third component of the late diastolic forward flow is absent in the distal vessels if the examination is performed in a cold room or if the extremity itself is cold. This should not be mistaken for occlusive disease. This error

can be resolved by repeating the examination after covering the extremity with a warm blanket.

Segmental Systolic Pressure Measurements

Three or four cuffs are employed to obtain segmental systolic pressures. The advantage of the four-cuff method over the three-cuff technique is that it has the capability of differentiating obstructive disease in the aortoiliac segment from that in the superficial femoral artery. The technique has been described in detail in Chapter 17. Normally, the pressure gradients between the various contiguous segments should be <20 mm Hg. The pressure gradients of 20 to 30 mm Hg are borderline, and those greater than 30 mm Hg are definitely abnormal. Figure 19–2 demonstrates normal pressure gradients between various segments and indicate an absence of a hemodynamically significant obstructive lesion in the lower limbs.

Ankle/Brachial Index

The ankle systolic pressure divided by the highest brachial artery pressure is known as the ankle/brachial index (ABI). Normally, it should be equal to or greater than 1.0. The ABI of 1.1 in Figure 19–2 is within the normal range and indicates an absence of hemodynamically significant obstructive disease in the arteries of the lower extremity.

Obstruction of the Femoral Arteries

Common Obstructive Patterns

The femoropopliteal segment is the most common site of obstruction in the arteries of the

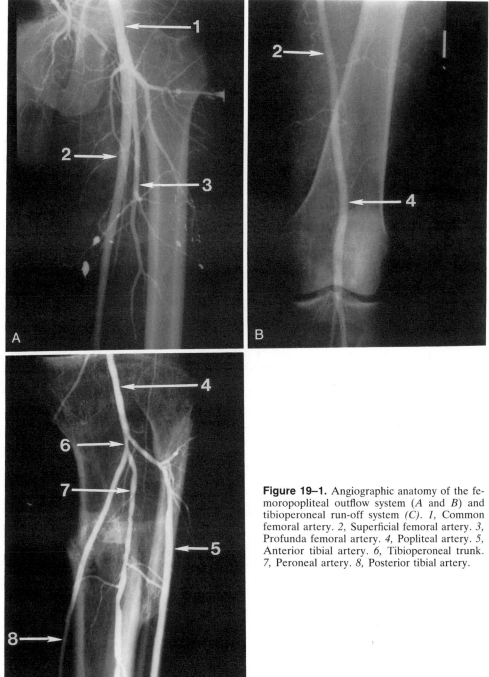

Figure 19–1. Angiographic anatomy of the femoropopliteal outflow system (*A* and *B*) and tibioperoneal run-off system *(C)*. *1,* Common femoral artery. *2,* Superficial femoral artery. *3,* Profunda femoral artery. *4,* Popliteal artery. *5,* Anterior tibial artery. *6,* Tibioperoneal trunk. *7,* Peroneal artery. *8,* Posterior tibial artery.

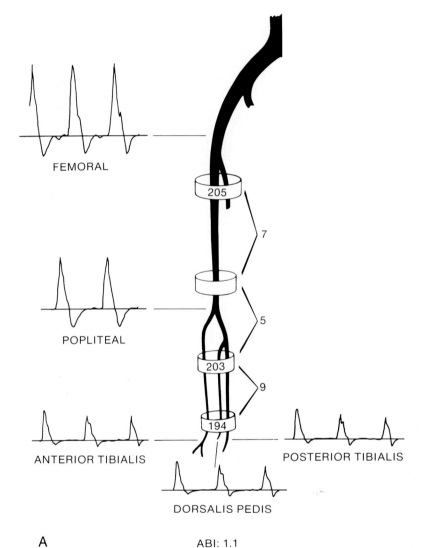

ARM PRESSURE: 170 mmHg

Figure 19–2. *Case I.* Doppler arterial waveforms and segmental pressures of normal femoropopliteal outflow and tibioperoneal run-off system. Right *(A)*, left *(B)*.

	Right	*Left*
Arterial Waveforms		
Common femoral artery	Normal	Normal
Popliteal	Normal	Normal
Anterior tibial artery	Normal	Normal
Posterior tibial artery	Normal	Normal
Dorsalis pedis artery	Normal	Normal
Segmental Pressures and Gradients		
ankle/brachial index (ABI)	Normal	Normal

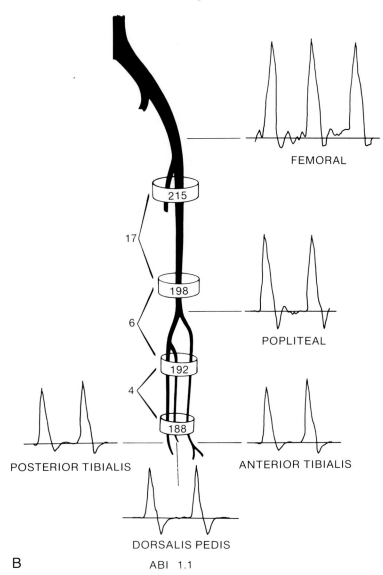

ARM PRESSURE: 170 mmHg

FEMORAL

215

17

198

POPLITEAL

6

192

4

188

POSTERIOR TIBIALIS

ANTERIOR TIBIALIS

DORSALIS PEDIS

B

ABI 1.1

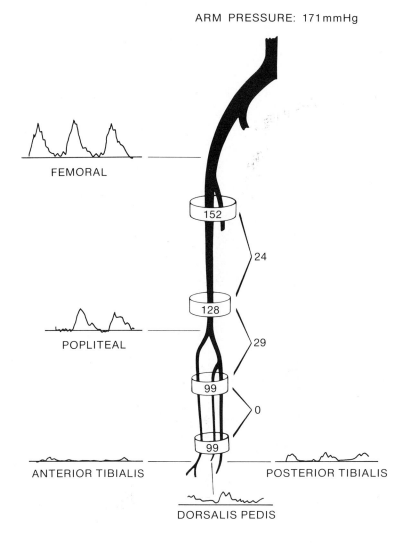

ARM PRESSURE: 171mmHg

FEMORAL

152

24

128

POPLITEAL

29

99

0

99

ANTERIOR TIBIALIS

POSTERIOR TIBIALIS

DORSALIS PEDIS

ABI: 0.57

Figure 19–3. *Case II.* Common femoral artery obstructive pattern. CFA = Common femoral artery; HT = high thigh; HT–BI = high-thigh/brachial index; HT–AK = high thigh to above knee; AK–BK = above knee to below knee; BK–A = below knee to ankle; ABI = ankle/brachial index.

	Right Extremity
Arterial Waveforms	
CFA waveforms	Abnormal
Distal arterial waveforms	Abnormal
Pressures and Gradients	
HT pressure	Abnormal
HT–BI	Abnormal
HT–AK pressure gradient	Borderline
AK–BK pressure gradient	Borderline
BK–A pressure gradient	Normal
ABI	Abnormal

lower limb.[1, 2] The extent and location of lesions in this area are variable. An obstructive lesion can vary from a focal area of mild stenosis to the commonly encountered total occlusion of the entire superficial femoral artery.[2] The superficial femoral artery in the adductor canal (or at the adductor magnus hiatus) is the most common site of obstruction. The origin of the artery is another common location for an obstructive lesion in the superficial femoral artery. The common femoral artery, the deep femoral artery at its origin, and the superficial femoral artery in the midthigh region are other sites of obstruction.[3, 4] Diffuse stenotic changes may occur in the superficial femoral artery in about 20% of cases. Isolated lesions are often seen in nondiabetic patients.

Common Femoral Artery Obstructive Pattern

A common femoral artery (CFA) obstruction simulates an aortoiliac inflow obstruction on non-invasive tests, as illustrated in *Case II* and Figure 19–3. The Doppler arterial waveform from the common femoral artery is affected in a manner similar to a waveform from a diseased inflow system and varies from a monophasic to a collateral flow pattern, depending upon the severity of the obstruction (Fig. 19–3). High-thigh (HT) pressure is reduced, with a high-thigh/brachial pressure difference of less than 30 mm Hg. The ABI is also reduced to 0.57, indicating proximal obstruction.

Monophasic arterial waveforms from distal arteries and normal distal pressure gradients suggest the absence of a hemodynamically significant lesion in the distal vessels. The correlative arteriogram is displayed in Figure 19–4. The aortoiliac inflow system showed no obstructive lesion (Fig. 19–4A), whereas the common femoral artery showed a stenosis. Multiple areas of stenosis in the superficial femoral artery (Fig. 19–4B) were perhaps of no hemodynamic significance because the waveform from the popliteal artery did not differ significantly from the common femoral artery waveform and the distal pressure gradients were within the normal range. A two-vessel run-off is shown in Figure 19–4C and D.

Profunda Femoral Artery Obstructive Pattern

A profunda femoral artery obstruction is seen more frequently in diabetics than in nondiabetics. Obstruction usually occurs in the form of a stenosis (Fig. 19–6A), although complete occlusion rarely does occur.[5]

An isolated lesion of the profunda femoral artery usually does not affect segmental systolic pressures. The high-thigh–above-knee (HT–AK) pressure gradient also remains normal. When the cuff is applied over a region containing two or more vessels of equal size, the acquired pressure measurement will reflect the pressure in the artery with the highest pressure.[1] Therefore, in the presence of a patent superficial femoral artery, a stenosis or an occlusive lesion of the profunda femoral artery may be obscured. If both the superficial and deep femoral arteries have obstructive lesions, the findings may mimic aorto-iliac inflow disease.

Superficial Femoral Artery Obstructive Pattern

Obstructive lesions of the superficial femoral artery most commonly are marked by a normal Doppler arterial waveform from the common femoral artery and an abnormal waveform from the popliteal and distal arteries on the affected side. The HT pressure is often normal, but distal pressures are frequently reduced. These findings are associated with an abnormal pressure gradient between the HT–AK segment and a normal gradient between the above-knee–below-knee (AK–BK) and the below-knee–ankle (BK–A) segments. This situation is illustrated in *Case III*.

Case III (Figs. 19–5 and 19–6)
A middled-aged woman presented with intermittent claudication of the right leg. The Doppler arterial waveform from the right common femoral artery was triphasic and normal. This indicated an absence of a hemodynamically significant obstructive lesion in the aortoiliac inflow system on the symptomatic side. The Doppler arterial waveforms from the popliteal and distal vessels were monophasic, indicating a hemodynamically significant obstructive lesion between the aortoiliac segment and the popliteal artery (Fig. 19–5).

The proximal thigh pressure of 145 mm Hg was greater than the brachial artery pressure by 30 mm Hg. The HT brachial index was 1.26. Both of these parameters were within normal limits and suggested a normal aortoiliac system. The pressure gradient of 56 mm Hg between the HT–AK segment was abnormal, whereas that between the AK–BK and BK–A was normal. All of these findings indicate an obstructive lesion of hemodynamic significance in the outflow system in the region of the superficial femoral artery. This patient showed a mild decrease in the ABI, which is often seen with outflow obstructive disease.

The correlative arteriogram shown in Figure 19–6 shows complete occlusion of the right superficial femoral artery with normal right inflow and distal vessels. The arteriogram confirmed the findings of the Doppler arterial waveform and segmental systolic pressures. If the pressure gradient is mildly abnormal, a stenotic

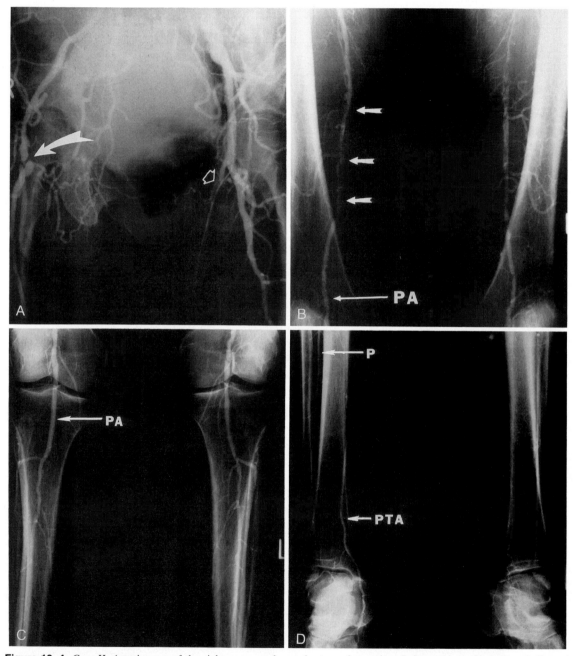

Figure 19–4. *Case II.* Arteriogram of the right common femoral artery obstruction. Inflow *(A)*, outflow *(B and C)*, and run-off *(C and D)*. *A*, A high-grade stenosis in the terminal portion of the right common femoral artery (arrow). The left superficial femoral artery is totally obstructed (open arrow). *B and C*, Multiple areas of stenosis in the right superficial femoral artery (arrows). PA = Patent popliteal artery. *C and D*, Two-vessel run-off: posterior tibial artery (PTA) and peroneal artery (P).

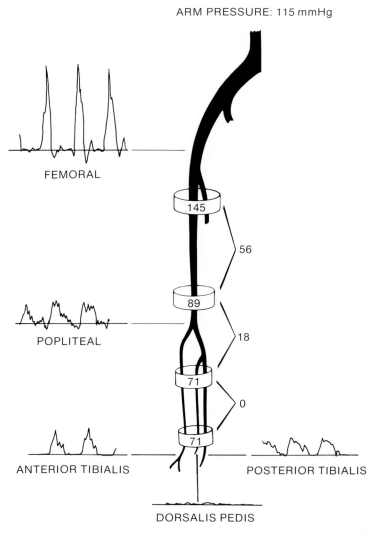

ARM PRESSURE: 115 mmHg

FEMORAL

POPLITEAL

ANTERIOR TIBIALIS

POSTERIOR TIBIALIS

DORSALIS PEDIS

ABI: 0.61

145

56

89

18

71

0

71

Figure 19–5. *Case III.* Doppler arterial waveforms and segmental pressures of the right superficial femoral artery obstruction. CFA = Common femoral artery; HT = high thigh; HT–BI = high-thigh/brachial index; HT–AK = high thigh to above knee; AK–BK = above knee to below knee; BK–A = below knee to ankle; ABI = ankle/brachial index.

	Right Extremity
Arterial Waveforms	
CFA waveforms	Normal
Popliteal and distal	
arterial waveforms	Abnormal
Pressures and Gradients	
HT pressure	Normal
HT–BI	Normal
HT–AK pressure gradient	Abnormal
AK–BK pressure gradient	Normal
BK–A pressure gradient	Normal
ABI	Abnormal

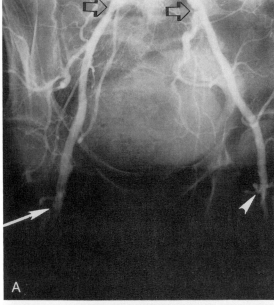

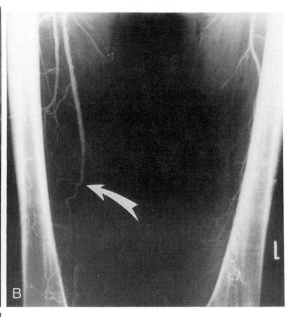

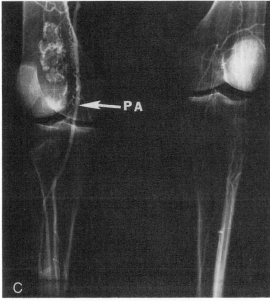

Figure 19–6. *Case III.* Arteriogram of the right superficial femoral artery obstruction: inflow *(A)*, outflow *(B and C)*, and outflow run-off *(C)*. *A*, Stenosis of the common iliac arteries bilaterally (open arrows) with stenosis of the right deep femoral artery at its origin (arrow) and total occlusion of the left superficial femoral artery (arrowhead). *B*, Total occlusion of the right superficial femoral artery in the midthigh (arrow). *C*, Patent right popliteal artery (PA) with three-vessel run-off.

lesion is more likely; highly abnormal pressure gradients indicate a total occlusion. In this patient, the pressure gradient was highly abnormal between the HT–AK segment, indicating total occlusion.

Other examples of superficial femoral artery obstruction are shown in *Cases IV* and *V*.

Case IV (Figs. 19–7 and 19–8)

The Doppler arterial waveform from the left common femoral artery was triphasic, suggesting that a normal inflow system was present on the left side (Fig. 19–7). The popliteal arterial waveform was monophasic with slow acceleration and deceleration of the systolic component and absence of the diastolic phase. This

finding suggested the presence of an obstructive lesion between the popliteal artery and the inflow system. The arterial waveforms from the tibial vessels were monophasic, indicating good run-off with no additional obstruction.

The proximal thigh pressure was greater than the arm pressure by only 18 mm Hg. This raised the suspicion of inflow disease. However, the pressure gradient between the HT–AK segment was abnormal, which is a usual finding with an obstructive lesion of the superficial femoral artery. The distal pressure gradients were within normal limits, indicating the absence of obstructive lesions in the distal vessels. The ABI was mild-to-moderately reduced in this case.

The correlative arteriogram (Fig. 19–8) revealed an

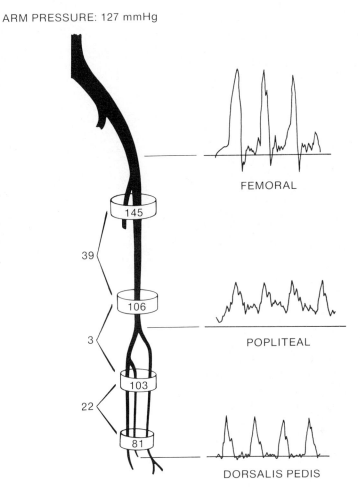

ARM PRESSURE: 127 mmHg

FEMORAL

145

39

106

POPLITEAL

3

103

22

81

DORSALIS PEDIS

ABI: 0.63

Figure 19–7. *Case IV*. Doppler arterial waveforms and segmental pressures of left superficial femoral artery obstruction. CFA = Common femoral artery; HT = high thigh; HT–BI = high-thigh/brachial index; HT–AK = high thigh to above knee; AK–BK = above knee to below knee; BK–A = below knee to ankle; ABI = ankle/brachial index.

	Left Extremity
Arterial Waveforms	
CFA waveforms	Normal
Distal arterial waveforms	Abnormal
Pressures and Gradients	
HT pressure	Abnormal
HT–BI	Normal
HT–AK pressure gradient	Abnormal
AK–BK pressure gradient	Normal
BK–A pressure gradient	Borderline
ABI	Abnormal

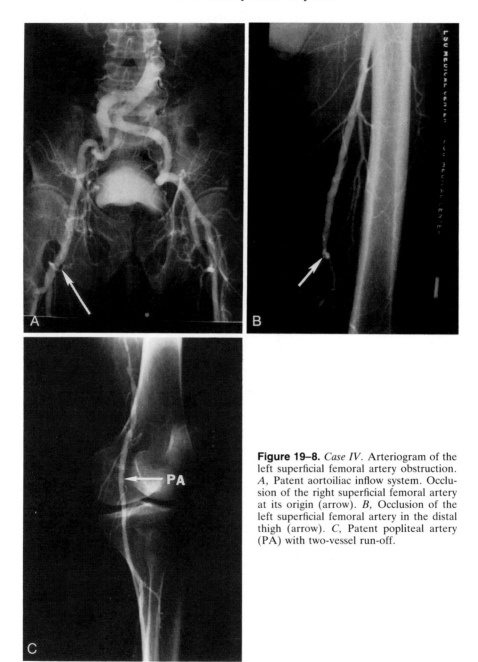

Figure 19–8. *Case IV.* Arteriogram of the left superficial femoral artery obstruction. *A,* Patent aortoiliac inflow system. Occlusion of the right superficial femoral artery at its origin (arrow). *B,* Occlusion of the left superficial femoral artery in the distal thigh (arrow). *C,* Patent popliteal artery (PA) with two-vessel run-off.

obstructive lesion in the distal portion of the superficial femoral artery and thus confirmed the findings of the noninvasive tests.

Case V (Figs. 19–9 and 19–10)

A middle-aged man presented with intermittent claudication of the left lower extremity. The Doppler arterial waveform of the left common femoral artery was triphasic, indicating normal inflow (Fig. 19–9). The arterial waveforms from the popliteal and distal arteries were monophasic, indicating obstruction of the outflow system on the left side. The ABI was also mildly

reduced, which is often seen with outflow system obstruction.

A normal proximal thigh pressure and high-thigh/brachial index suggests the absence of aortoiliac inflow disease. The abnormal pressure gradient of 63 mm Hg between the HT–AK segment indicates a superficial femoral artery obstruction. This abnormal finding was associated with a normal pressure gradient between the AK–BK and the BK–A segments, indicating a patent popliteal artery with good run-off.

The correlative arteriogram illustrated in Figure 19–10 confirmed the findings of the noninvasive tests and

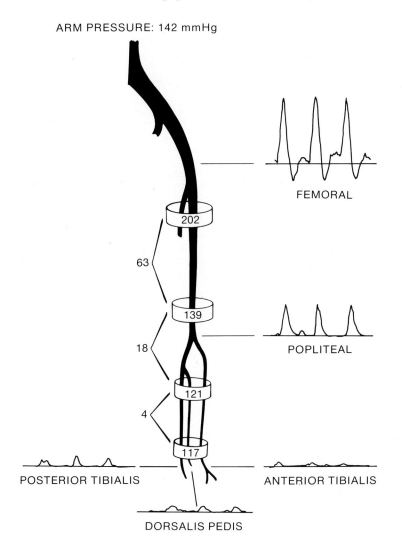

ARM PRESSURE: 142 mmHg

FEMORAL

202

63

139

POPLITEAL

18

121

4

117

POSTERIOR TIBIALIS

ANTERIOR TIBIALIS

DORSALIS PEDIS

ABI: 0.83

Figure 19–9. *Case V.* Doppler arterial waveforms and segmental pressures of left superficial femoral artery obstruction. CFA = Common femoral artery; HT = high thigh; HT–BI = high-thigh/brachial index; HT–AK = high thigh to above knee; AK–BK = above knee to below knee; BK–A = below knee to ankle; ABI = ankle/brachial index.

	Left Extremity
Arterial Waveforms	
CFA waveforms	Normal
Popliteal and distal arterial waveforms	Abnormal
Pressures and Gradients	
HT pressure	Normal
HT–BI	Normal
HT–AK pressure gradient	Abnormal
AK–BK pressure gradient	Normal
BK–A pressure gradient	Normal
ABI	Abnormal

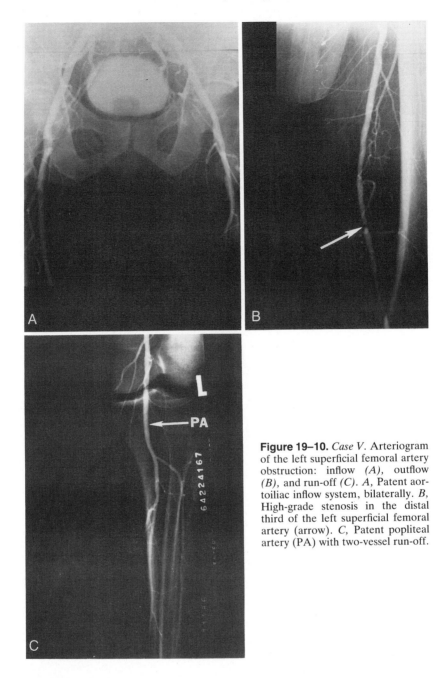

Figure 19–10. *Case V.* Arteriogram of the left superficial femoral artery obstruction: inflow *(A)*, outflow *(B)*, and run-off *(C)*. *A,* Patent aortoiliac inflow system, bilaterally. *B,* High-grade stenosis in the distal third of the left superficial femoral artery (arrow). *C,* Patent popliteal artery (PA) with two-vessel run-off.

demonstrated a superficial femoral artery obstructive lesion with patent inflow system and two-vessel run-off.

Superficial Femoral Artery Obstruction Mimicking Aortoiliac Inflow Disease

Some cases of superficial femoral artery obstruction may be associated with an abnormal Doppler arterial waveform of the common femoral artery and an abnormal proximal thigh pressure. The high-thigh/brachial index is also abnormal in these patients. This situation frequently occurs when the superficial femoral artery is obstructed in its proximal portion or at its origin. A similar pattern is also seen when both superficial and deep femoral arteries are involved in an obstructive process. The pressure gradient between the HT–AK segment may be normal or abnormal, depending upon the size of the deep femoral artery and the presence of collateral vessels. This pattern is discussed in *Case VI.*

Case VI (Figs. 19–11 and 19–12)

The patient is the same as in *Case IV.* However, in this instance, the right superficial femoral artery was

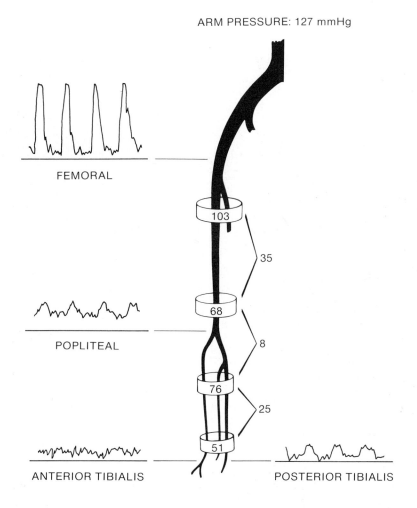

ARM PRESSURE: 127 mmHg

FEMORAL

103

35

POPLITEAL

68

8

76

25

51

ANTERIOR TIBIALIS

POSTERIOR TIBIALIS

ABI: 0.40

Figure 19–11. *Case VI.* Doppler arterial waveforms and segmental pressures of the right superficial femoral artery obstruction mimicking inflow disease. CFA = Common femoral artery; HT = high thigh; HT–BI = high-thigh/brachial index; HT–AK = high thigh to above knee; AK–BK = above knee to below knee; BK–A = below knee to ankle; ABI = ankle/brachial index.

	Right Extremity
Arterial Waveforms	
CFA waveform	Abnormal
Distal arterial waveforms	Abnormal
Pressures and Gradients	
HT pressure	Abnormal
HT–BI	Abnormal
HT–AK pressure gradient	Abnormal
AK–BK pressure gradient	Normal
BK–A pressure gradient	Borderline
ABI	Abnormal

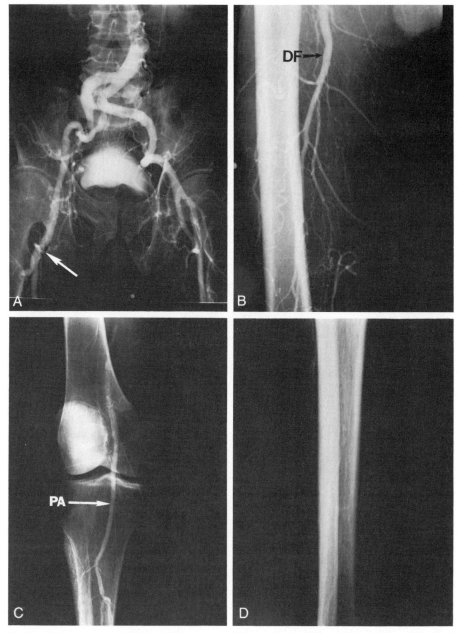

Figure 19–12. *Case VI.* Arteriogram of the right superficial femoral artery obstruction: inflow *(A)*, outflow *(B)*, and outflow run-off *(C and D)*. *A,* Patent inflow system with total occlusion of the right superficial femoral artery at its origin (arrow). *B,* Occlusion of the entire right superficial femoral artery with patent deep femoral artery (DF). *C and D,* Patent popliteal artery (PA) with one-vessel run-off.

occluded, simulating inflow disease. The Doppler arterial waveform of the right common femoral artery was monophasic with loss of the diastolic component (Fig. 19–11). Distal arterial waveforms were also monophasic and more damped. These waveforms suggested the presence of obstruction in the right inflow system.

The proximal thigh pressure was lower than the arm pressure yielding a high-thigh/brachial index of less than 1.0. This finding substantiates the diagnosis of inflow disease suggested by the arterial waveforms. However, an abnormal pressure gradient of 35 mm Hg between the HT–AK segment supports the diagnosis of a superficial femoral artery obstruction because the distal waveforms did not change significantly from the common femoral artery to suggest additional obstruction. The ABI was markedly reduced to 0.4.

The correlative arteriogram shown in Figure 19–12 confirmed the diagnosis of a superficial femoral artery obstruction.

Superficial Femoral Artery Obstruction Mimicking Popliteal Artery Disease

This pattern is associated with a normal pressure gradient between the HT–AK segment and an abnormal gradient across the knee similar to a popliteal artery obstruction. This situation usually occurs when an obstruction is present in the distal superficial femoral artery. An example is provided in *Case VII.*

Case VII (Figs. 19–13 and 19–14)
A 65-year-old woman presented for evaluation of peripheral vascular disease. The HT pressure and the pressure gradients between the HT–AK and BK–A segments were normal on the right side (Fig. 19–13). The pressure gradient across the knee (AK–BK) was abnormal. This finding suggested a popliteal artery obstruction of hemodynamic significance.

The Doppler arterial waveform from the right common femoral artery was triphasic, excluding a diagnosis of aortoiliac inflow disease. The popliteal artery waveform showed a monophasic pattern, indicating outflow disease. The damped and collateral flow pattern of the Doppler arterial waveforms from the tibioperoneal run-off vessels suggested run-off disease. The ABI was minimally reduced, suggesting a single lesion.

The correlative arteriogram (Fig. 19–14) revealed a stenosis in the distal one third of the superficial femoral artery. This finding was associated with a single-vessel run-off to the leg. The popliteal and iliac arteries had no significant obstructive lesions. The abnormal pressure gradient across the knee was believed to be secondary to the diminished tibioperoneal run-off.

Superficial Femoral Artery Occlusion with a Nonobstructive Pattern

Some cases of isolated superficial femoral artery obstruction are associated with normal pressures and normal pressure gradients in the affected lower limb. These patients remain asymptomatic. This situation usually occurs when the superficial femoral artery is obstructed and the deep femoral artery takes over the blood supply to the leg. In these patients, the deep femoral artery is usually enlarged to the size of the superficial femoral artery. Also, there are extensive collateral vessels to the distal leg.

Popliteal Artery Obstructive Pattern

Obstructive lesions of the popliteal artery are usually associated with disease in the femoral artery or tibioperoneal trunk. Isolated popliteal artery obstructive lesions are uncommon, but they occur most frequently in nondiabetic patients. Initially, obstructive disease is usually segmental and is seen as a focal area of stenosis or total occlusion. The most common site of the obstruction is the midportion of the popliteal artery behind the femoral condyles at the level of the knee joint. Other frequent sites are at the origin of the popliteal artery from the superficial femoral artery and the termination of the popliteal artery into the tibioperoneal trunk. The proximal half of the vessel is affected more often than is its distal half. Diabetics frequently have more advanced disease, which often extends to the femoral and tibial vessels.

Popliteal artery obstruction is characterized by abnormal Doppler arterial waveforms from the popliteal and distal arteries, abnormal segmental systolic pressures at the below-knee and ankle levels with an abnormal pressure gradient between the AK–BK segment, and an ABI of <1.0. Popliteal artery obstruction is illustrated in *Case VIII.*

Case VIII (Figs. 19–15 and 19–16)
A middle-aged man presented with intermittent claudication of the left leg. The Doppler arterial waveform of the left common femoral artery was triphasic, whereas the waveforms from the popliteal and distal vessels were monophasic (Fig. 19–15). These findings implied a normal aortoiliac inflow system and an abnormal femoropopliteal outflow system.

The high-thigh pressure was slightly low, but this may have been related to cuff artifact. The pressures at the BK and A levels, along with the abnormal pressure gradient of 44 mm Hg across the knee, were reduced. The pressure gradients between the HT–AK and BK–A segments were within the normal range. These tests confirmed the findings of the Doppler arterial waveforms and localized the obstructive process in the popliteal artery. As in patients with superficial femoral artery obstructive disease, the ABI was minimally reduced.

Text continued on page 368

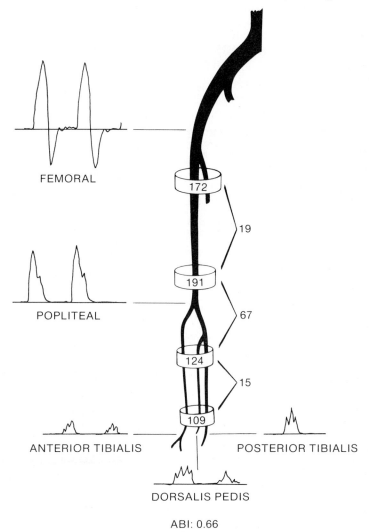

ARM PRESSURE: 165 mmHg

FEMORAL

172

19

POPLITEAL

191

67

124

15

109

ANTERIOR TIBIALIS

POSTERIOR TIBIALIS

DORSALIS PEDIS

ABI: 0.66
TBI: 0.47
TOE PRESSURE: 78 mmHg

Figure 19–13. *Case VII.* Doppler arterial waveform and segmental pressures of the right superficial femoral artery obstruction mimicking popliteal artery disease. CFA = Common femoral artery; HT = high thigh; HT–BI = high-thigh/brachial index; HT–AK = high thigh to above knee; AK–BK = above knee to below knee; BK–A = below knee to ankle; ABI = ankle/brachial index.

	Right Extremity
Arterial Waveforms	
CFA waveforms	Normal
Popliteal and distal arterial waveforms	Abnormal
Pressures and Gradients	
HT pressure	Abnormal
HT–BI	Normal
HT–AK pressure gradient	Normal
AK–BK pressure gradient	Abnormal
BK–A pressure gradient	Normal
ABI	Abnormal

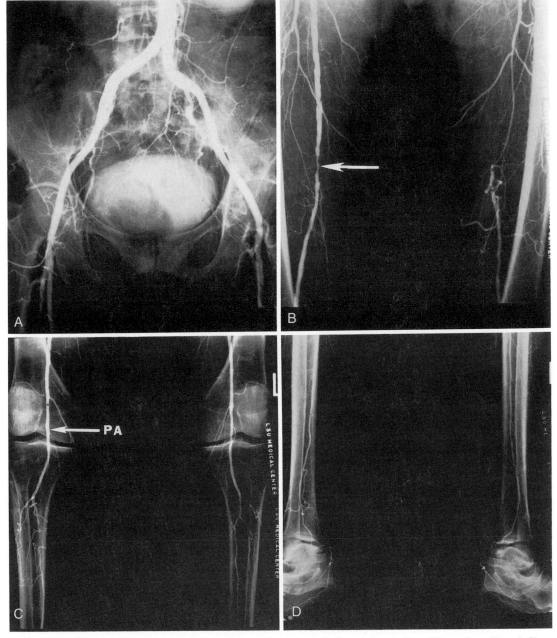

Figure 19–14. *Case VII.* Arteriogram of the right superficial femoral obstruction: inflow *(A)*, outflow *(B* and *C)*, and run-off *(C* and *D)*. *A*, Patent aortoiliac inflow system. *B* and *C*, Stenosis in the middle third of the right superficial femoral artery (arrow) with patent popliteal artery (PA). *C* and *D*, Patent popliteal artery with one-vessel run-off.

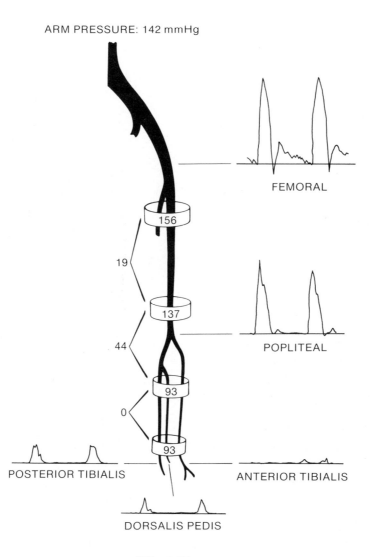

ARM PRESSURE: 142 mmHg

FEMORAL

156

19

137

POPLITEAL

44

93

0

93

POSTERIOR TIBIALIS

ANTERIOR TIBIALIS

DORSALIS PEDIS

ABI = 0.65

Figure 19–15. *Case VIII.* Doppler arterial waveforms and segmental pressures of the left popliteal artery obstruction. CFA = Common femoral artery; HT = high thigh; HT–BI = high-thigh/brachial index; HT–AK = high thigh to above knee; AK–BK = above knee to below knee; BK–A = below knee to ankle; ABI = ankle/brachial index.

	Left Extremity
Arterial Waveforms	
CFA waveforms	Normal
Popliteal and distal arterial	
waveforms	Abnormal
Pressures and Gradients	
HT pressure	Abnormal
HT–BI	Abnormal
HT–AK pressure gradient	Normal
AK–BK pressure gradient	Abnormal
BK–A pressure gradient	Normal
ABI	Abnormal

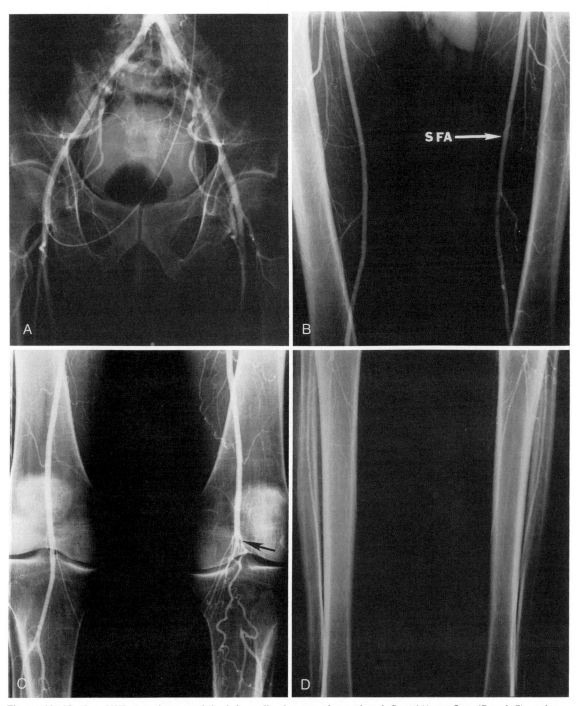

Figure 19–16. *Case VIII.* Arteriogram of the left popliteal artery obstruction: inflow *(A)*, outflow *(B* and *C)*, and run-off *(C* and *D)*. *A,* Patent inflow system. *B* and *C,* Left popliteal artery obstruction at the knee joint level (black arrow) with patent superficial femoral artery (SFA). *C* and *D,* Total occlusion of the left distal popliteal artery with two-vessel run-off.

The correlative arteriogram is shown in Figure 19–16. The abdominal arteriogram showed a normal inflow system (Fig. 19–16A). The common, superficial, and deep femoral arteries were patent and showed no obstructive lesions (Fig. 19–16B). The left popliteal artery was totally obstructed at the level of the knee joint and behind the femoral condyles (Fig. 19–16C). This obstruction was associated with good run-off into the tibioperoneal vessels (Fig. 19–16D). This example showed excellent correlation between the noninvasive tests and the arteriogram.

Another example of a popliteal artery obstruction is demonstrated in *Case IX*.

Case IX (Figs. 19–17 and 19–18)

A 60-year-old woman presented with right leg pain. The systolic pressures at the HT and AK levels, the high-thigh/brachial index, and the HT–AK pressure gradients were within normal limits (Fig. 19–17). These pressure measurements suggested the absence of a hemodynamically significant obstructive lesion in the inflow system or in the common and superficial femoral arteries. The reduced systolic pressure at the BK and A levels indicated an obstructive lesion in the popliteal and tibioperoneal vessels. The pressure gradients of 81 mm Hg between the AK–BK segment and 47 mm Hg between the BK–A segment reflected the presence of a hemodynamically significant obstruction in the popliteal and tibioperoneal vessels.

The monophasic arterial waveforms from the popliteal artery and the markedly damped abnormal waveforms from the tibioperoneal vessels also confirmed the findings of popliteal artery obstructive disease with poor run-off.

The correlative arteriogram is shown in Figure 19–18. The abdominal arteriogram showed no aortoiliac inflow disease (Fig. 19–18A). The common, superficial, and deep femoral arteries revealed no obstruction bilaterally (Fig. 19–18B). A short segment of the right popliteal artery at its origin within the adductor canal was totally obstructed (Fig. 19–18C). The distal popliteal artery was patent. The tibioperoneal vessels were occluded proximally (Fig. 19–18D). As in this case, popliteal artery obstruction with extension into the tibioperoneal vessels is often seen in diabetic patients.

Uncommon Obstructive Patterns

Popliteal Artery Obstructive Disease Simulating Tibioperoneal Run-off Disease

Sometimes popliteal artery obstruction may mimic tibioperoneal run-off disease on noninvasive tests. This situation usually occurs when the popliteal artery is obstructed either in its distal portion or at its termination. Similar situations arise when extensive disease involves the entire vessel. In this case, the systolic pressure at the BK level, along with an abnormal pressure gradient

between the BK–A segment, may be reduced. The pressure gradient across the knee may be normal. However, the Doppler arterial waveform from the popliteal artery may be abnormal and thus may assist in localizing the exact obstructive site. These findings are shown in *Case X*.

Case X (Figs. 19–19 and 19–20)

A 60-year-old woman with diabetes presented with a foot ulcer. The ABI was reduced to 0.73, suggesting proximal obstruction. A normal HT pressure and HT–AK pressure gradient helped to exclude the diagnosis of an obstructive lesion of hemodynamic significance in the aortoiliac inflow system and in the common and superficial femoral arteries (Fig. 19–19). The pressure gradient across the knee was borderline; the BK–A segment was abnormal. These findings suggested obstruction in the tibioperoneal run-off system.

However, monophasic Doppler arterial waveforms from the popliteal artery suggested the presence of obstruction in the popliteal artery. Normal common femoral arterial waveforms indicated the absence of obstruction in the inflow system.

The correlative arteriogram is displayed in Figure 19–20. The aortogram showed a patent inflow system (Fig. 19–20A). The superficial femoral artery was without significant obstructive lesions (Fig. 19–20B), whereas the popliteal artery was obstructed at the level of the knee joint (Fig. 19–20C). Only the proximal portion of the anterior tibial artery was obstructed (Fig. 19–20C).

Tibioperoneal Run-Off Obstructive Pattern

Obstructive disease of the tibioperoneal vessels is frequently associated with femoropopliteal disease. All three vessels are often involved in various combinations. Extensive or combined outflow run-off disease is more common in diabetic patients; mild, isolated, or focal disease is more prevalent in nondiabetic patients. The peroneal artery is affected less frequently by obstructive processes than are the other two vessels of the leg.

Common Obstructive Pattern

Obstructive disease of the tibioperoneal run-off system is characterized most commonly by normal Doppler arterial waveforms from the common femoral and popliteal arteries and abnormal waveforms from the tibioperoneal vessels. The systolic pressures at the HT, AK, and BK segments are frequently normal, whereas those at the ankle are often reduced. These test results are associated with an abnormal pressure

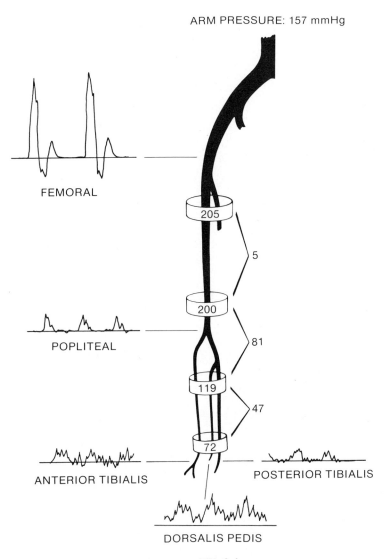

ARM PRESSURE: 157 mmHg

FEMORAL

POPLITEAL

ANTERIOR TIBIALIS

POSTERIOR TIBIALIS

DORSALIS PEDIS

ABI: 0.4

Figure 19–17. *Case IX.* Doppler arterial waveforms and segmental pressures of the right popliteal artery obstruction. CFA = Common femoral artery; HT = high thigh; HT–BI = high-thigh/brachial index; HT–AK = high thigh to above knee; AK–BK = above knee to below knee; BK–A = below knee to ankle; ABI = ankle/brachial index.

	Right Extremity
Arterial Waveforms	
CFA waveforms	Normal
Popliteal arterial waveforms	Abnormal
Tibioperoneal arterial waveforms	Abnormal
Pressures and Gradients	
HT pressure	Normal
HT–BI	Normal
HT–AK pressure gradient	Normal
AK–BK pressure gradient	Abnormal
BK–A pressure gradient	Abnormal
ABI	Abnormal

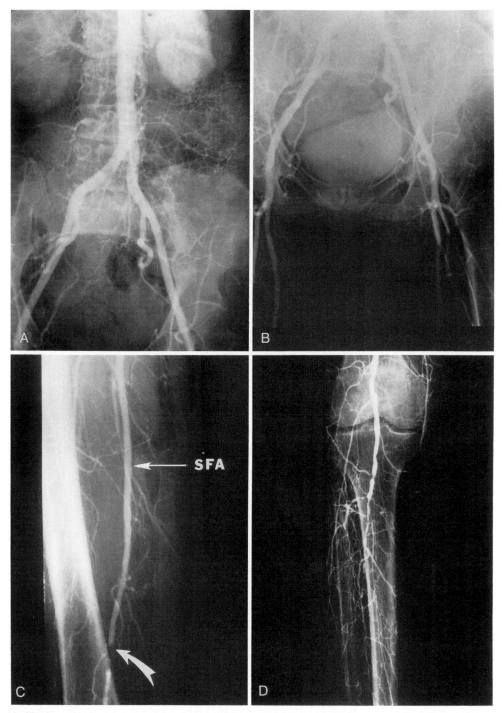

Figure 19–18. *Case IX.* Arteriogram of the right popliteal artery obstruction: inflow *(A and B)*, outflow *(B and C)*, and outflow run-off *(D)*. *A,* and *B,* Patent aortoiliac inflow system. *C,* Patent right superficial femoral artery (SFA) with total occlusion of the short segment of the right popliteal artery at its origin (arrow). *D,* Patent distal popliteal artery with poor run-off.

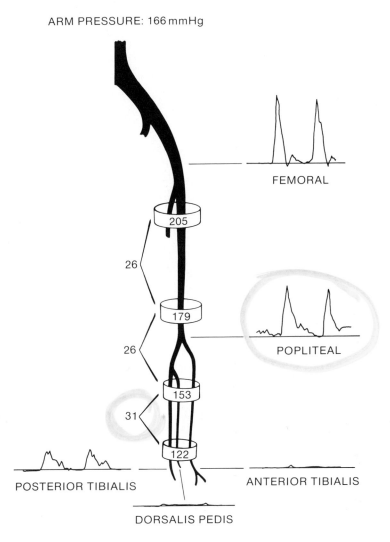

ARM PRESSURE: 166 mmHg

FEMORAL

POPLITEAL

205

26

179

26

153

31

122

POSTERIOR TIBIALIS

ANTERIOR TIBIALIS

DORSALIS PEDIS

ABI: 0.73

Figure 19–19. *Case X.* Doppler arterial waveforms and segmental pressures of the left popliteal artery obstruction. CFA = Common femoral artery; HT = high thigh; HT–BI = high-thigh/brachial index; HT–AK = high thigh to above knee; AK–BK = above knee to below knee; BK–A = below knee to ankle; ABI = ankle/brachial index.

	Left Extremity
Arterial Waveforms	
CFA waveforms	Normal
Popliteal artery waveforms	Abnormal
Tibioperoneal waveforms	Abnormal
Pressures and Gradients	
HT pressure	Normal
HT–BI	Normal
HT–AK pressure gradient	Borderline
AK–BK pressure gradient	Borderline
BK–A pressure gradient	Abnormal
ABI	Abnormal

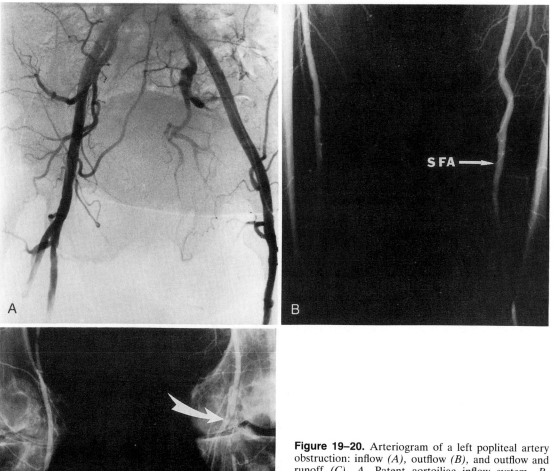

Figure 19–20. Arteriogram of a left popliteal artery obstruction: inflow *(A)*, outflow *(B)*, and outflow and runoff *(C)*. *A*, Patent aortoiliac inflow system. *B*, Patent superficial femoral artery (SFA). *C*, Obstruction of the popliteal artery at the level of the knee joint (arrow). Patent peroneal (P) and posterior tibial arteries (PTA). Occlusion of the anterior tibial artery (arrowhead).

gradient between the below-knee–ankle (BK–A) segment. The ABI is usually mildly reduced. These findings are illustrated in *Case XI*.

Case XI (Figs. 19–21 and 19–22)

A middle-aged man presented with pain in the right lower extremity. The patient had aortoiliac disease and bypass surgery 6 months prior to the present complaint. Doppler ultrasonography demonstrated monophasic waveforms from the right common femoral and popliteal arteries, suggesting an obstructive process in the

inflow system (Fig. 19–21). The arterial waveform was damped from the anterior tibial artery; the Doppler signal was absent from the right dorsalis pedis and posterior tibial arteries. These findings indicated poor run-off.

The high-thigh pressure of 113 mm Hg was greater than the brachial artery pressure by 25 mm Hg. This finding was borderline normal. The high-thigh/brachial index (HT/BI) was within the normal range. The monophasic waveform from the common femoral artery could have been related to the transmission of the

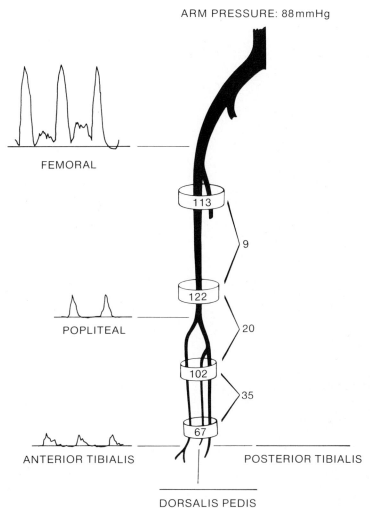

ARM PRESSURE: 88mmHg

FEMORAL

113

9

122

POPLITEAL

20

102

35

67

ANTERIOR TIBIALIS

POSTERIOR TIBIALIS

DORSALIS PEDIS

ABI: 0.76

Figure 19–21. *Case XI.* Obstructive pattern of the right tibioperoneal vessels. CFA = Common femoral artery; HT = high thigh; HT–AK = high thigh to above knee; AK–BK = above knee to below knee; BK–A = below knee to ankle; ABI = ankle/brachial index.

	Right Extremity
Arterial Waveforms	
CFA waveforms	Abnormal
Popliteal artery waveforms	Abnormal
Tibioperoneal arterial waveforms	Abnormal
Pressures and Gradients	
HT pressure	Normal
HT–AK pressure gradient	Normal
AK–BK pressure gradient	Normal
BK–A pressure gradient	Abnormal
ABI	Abnormal

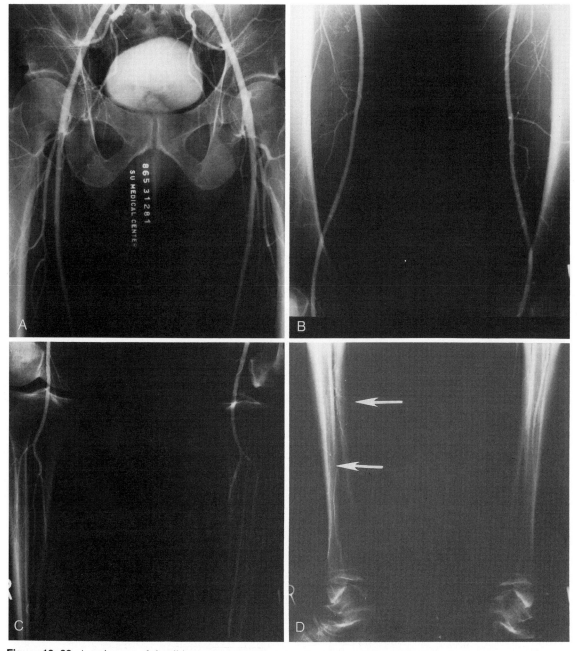

Figure 19–22. Arteriogram of the tibioperoneal run-off obstruction: inflow *(A)*, outflow *(B and C)*, and run-off *(D)*. *A,* Patent inflow system. *B and C,* Patent femoropopliteal outflow system. *D,* Obstruction of the tibioperoneal vessels (arrows).

pressure waveform through the graft or related to a mild degree of stenosis at the anastomotic site. The pressure gradients between the HT–AK and the AK–BK segments were within normal limits, suggesting an absence of a hemodynamically significant lesion in the femoropopliteal outflow system. The pressure gradient between the BK–A segment was abnormal, indicating tibioperoneal disease on the affected side.

The correlative arteriogram is shown in Figure 19–22. The aortoiliac inflow and femoropopliteal outflow system were patent and were without any significant obstructive lesions. All three arteries in the leg were obstructed in their midportion and showed poor collateral vessels. The pressure gradient was abnormal because of the poor collateral vessels in the affected leg.

Another example of tibioperoneal obstructive disease is illustrated in *Case IX* (Figs. 19–17 and 19–18), and a third example is demonstrated in *Case XII*.

Case XII (Figs. 19–23 and 19–24)

A middle-aged man presented with symptoms of peripheral vascular disease in both lower extremities. The ABI was normal on the left side and abnormal on the right side (Fig. 19–23), indicating the presence of an obstructive lesion on the right side and no lesions on the left. The proximal thigh pressure and HT/BI were normal on the left side, but they were abnormal on the right. These findings suggested aortoiliac inflow disease on the right side and a normal system on the left side.

A normal pressure gradient between the HT–AK segment on the left side excluded the diagnosis of outflow disease. A borderline pressure gradient between the HT–AK segment suggested a lesion in the right outflow system. A diagnosis of obstructive disease in the popliteal artery was excluded by a normal pressure gradient between the AK–BK segment. The pressure gradient between the BK–A segment was at the upper limits of normal, indicating possible disease in the tibioperoneal run-off system.

The Doppler arterial waveforms from the common femoral artery were normal (triphasic) on the left side but were abnormal (monophasic) on the right side. These findings suggested obstruction in the right aortoiliac system and confirmed the findings of the segmental pressures.

Severely damped arterial waveforms from the right popliteal artery suggested an additional lesion in the right outflow system. A normal left outflow system was indicated by normal arterial waveforms from the left popliteal artery.

Severely damped waveforms from the right lower leg vessels indicated run-off disease. Doppler arterial waveforms were normal from the left posterior tibial and dorsalis pedis arteries but were damped from the anterior tibial artery. These findings suggested an obstructive lesion in the left anterior tibial artery.

The correlative arteriogram (Fig. 19–24) showed severe stenosis in the right external iliac artery. The

left inflow system was without an obstructive lesion. The superficial femoral artery was totally obstructed in the midthigh on the right side and was patent on the left side. The obstructive lesion on the right extended to the popliteal and tibioperoneal vessels. The left popliteal artery was patent but had poor run-off, thus confirming the findings of the segmental pressures and Doppler arterial waveforms.

This case illustrates the difficulty encountered in precisely locating an obstruction when multi-level occlusive disease is present. The pressure gradient between the HT–AK was borderline, whereas that between the AK–BK segments was normal on the right side even in the presence of extensive disease. This case also shows how a proximal lesion can obscure distal obstructive disease.

Uncommon Obstructive Pattern

The pressure gradient and distal pressure may be within the normal range if only one vessel remains patent in the distal leg. This situation can be attributed to the formation of excellent collateral vessels between the lower leg vessels. However, when two or more vessels run parallel under the pressure cuff, the vessel with the higher pressure is usually the one recorded. Therefore, if one vessel is patent, the pressure from the patent vessel may result in normal segmental pressure measurements. This error can be avoided by recording the ankle pressure with the Doppler probe over each of the three vessels in the foot. If there is a pressure difference of greater than 15 mm Hg between the three vessels, the vessel with the lower pressure is known to be obstructed.

Another alternative is acquiring and comparing Doppler arterial waveforms from the individual vessels. When an obstructive lesion of hemodynamic significance is present, the Doppler arterial waveform from the affected vessel may show an abnormal waveform, which can vary from a monophasic to a collateral flow pattern. This is shown in *Case XIII*.

Case XIII (Figs. 19–25 and 19–26)

A middle-aged man with intermittent claudication of the right lower limb was evaluated by noninvasive tests. The Doppler arterial waveforms from the right common femoral, popliteal, and posterior tibial arteries were normal (Fig. 19–25). The anterior tibial artery waveform was monophasic and damped, whereas the waveform from the dorsalis pedis artery was monophasic.

The HT pressure and pressure gradients between the HT–AK, AK–BK, and BK–A segments were

Text continued on page 380

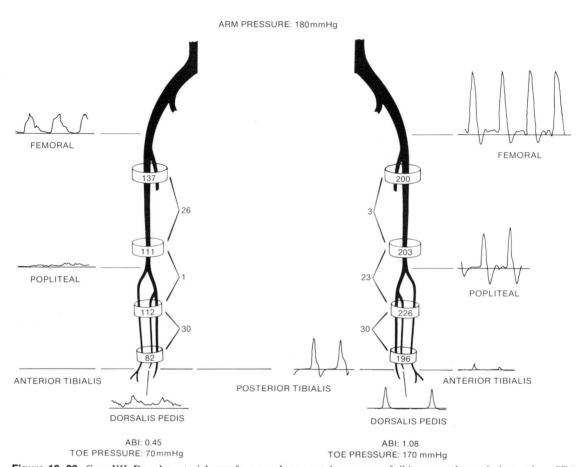

ARM PRESSURE: 180mmHg

FEMORAL

137

26

111

POPLITEAL

1

112

30

82

ANTERIOR TIBIALIS

DORSALIS PEDIS

ABI: 0.45
TOE PRESSURE: 70mmHg

FEMORAL

200

3

203

23

POPLITEAL

226

30

196

POSTERIOR TIBIALIS

ANTERIOR TIBIALIS

DORSALIS PEDIS

ABI: 1.08
TOE PRESSURE: 170 mmHg

Figure 19–23. *Case XII.* Doppler arterial waveforms and segmental pressures of tibioperoneal vessel obstruction. CFA = Common femoral artery; HT = high thigh; HT–BI = high-thigh/brachial index; HT–AK = high thigh to above knee; AK–BK = above knee to below knee; BK–A = below knee to ankle; ABI = ankle/brachial index.

	Right	*Left*
Arterial Waveforms		
CFA waveforms	Abnormal	Normal
Popliteal arterial waveforms	Abnormal	Normal
Posterior tibial arterial waveforms	Abnormal	Normal
Anterior tibial arterial waveforms	Abnormal	Abnormal
Dorsalis pedis arterial waveforms	Abnormal	Normal
Pressures and Gradients		
HT pressure	Abnormal	Normal
HT–BI	Abnormal	Normal
HT–AK pressure gradients	Borderline	Normal
AK–BK pressure gradients	Normal	Borderline
BK–A pressure gradients	Abnormal	Abnormal
ABI	Abnormal	Normal

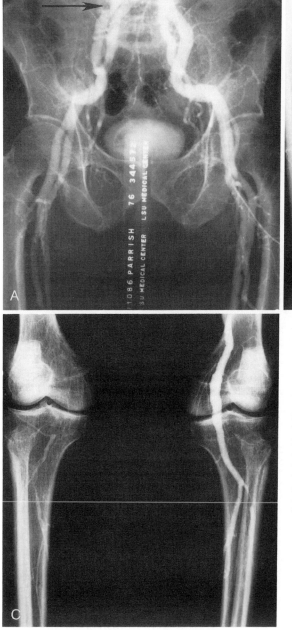
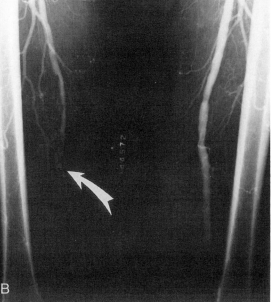

Figure 19–24. Arteriogram of the right tibioperoneal vessel obstruction: Inflow *(A)*, outflow *(B* and *C)*, and run-off *(C)*. *A*, Severe stenosis of the right external iliac artery (arrow). *B* and *C*, Total occlusion of the middle one third of the right superficial femoral artery (arrow) with extension into the popliteal artery. *C*, Total occlusion of the proximal portion of the right popliteal artery with one-vessel run-off. Patent left popliteal artery with one-vessel run-off.

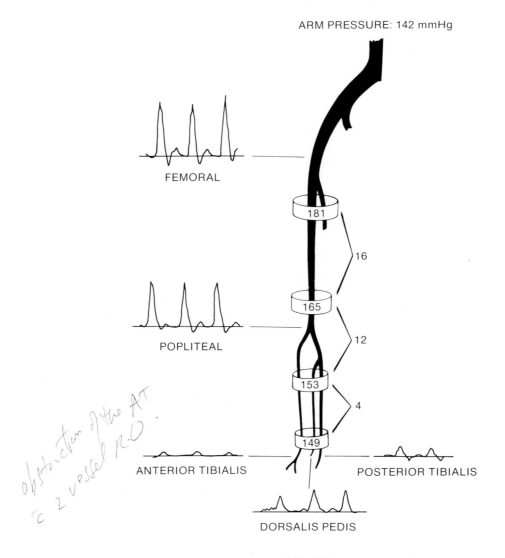

ARM PRESSURE: 142 mmHg

FEMORAL

181

16

POPLITEAL

165

12

153

4

ANTERIOR TIBIALIS   149   POSTERIOR TIBIALIS

DORSALIS PEDIS

Obstruction of the AT c 2 vessel R.O.

ABI: 1.04

Figure 19–25. *Case XIII.* Doppler arterial waveforms and segmental pressures of tibioperoneal obstructive disease. CFA = Common femoral artery; HT = high thigh; HT–BI = high-thigh/brachial index; HT–AK = high thigh to above knee; AK–BK = above knee to below knee; BK–A = below knee to ankle; ABI = ankle/brachial index.

	Right Extremity
Arterial Waveforms	
CFA waveforms	Normal
Popliteal arterial waveforms	Normal
Posterior tibial arterial waveforms	Abnormal
Dorsalis Pedis arterial waveforms	Abnormal
Anterior tibial arterial waveforms	Abnormal
Pressures and Gradients	
HT pressure	Normal
HT–BI	Normal
HT–AK pressure gradients	Normal
AK–BK pressure gradients	Normal
BK–A pressure gradients	Normal
ABI	Normal

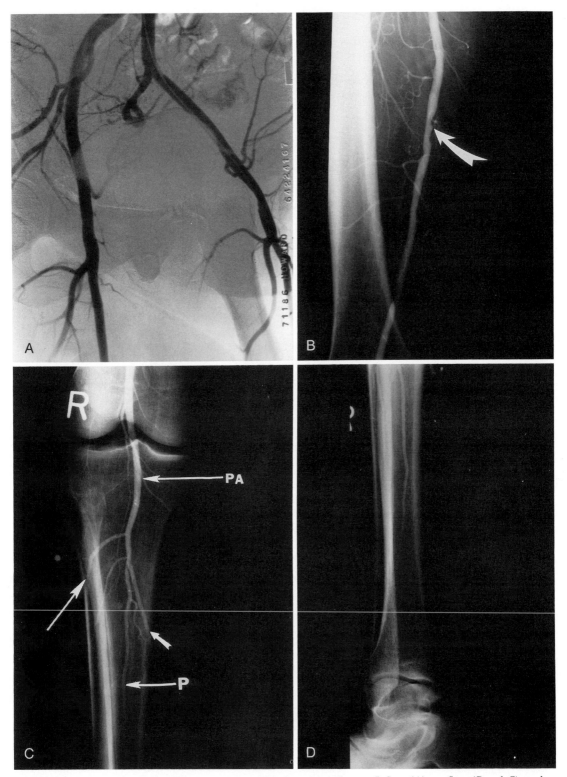

Figure 19–26. Arteriogram of right tibioperoneal arterial obstructive disease: Inflow *(A)*, outflow *(B* and *C)*, and run-off *(C* and *D)*. *A*, Patent aortoiliac inflow system. *B* and *C*, Mild stenosis in the middle third of the right superficial femoral artery (arrow) with patent popliteal artery (PA). *C* and *D*, Occlusion of the anterior tibial (large arrow) and posterior tibial (small arrow) arteries with patent peroneal (P) artery.

within normal limits. The patient was asymptomatic with an ABI of 1.04, which is normal.

The correlative arteriogram obtained for the symptomatic right lower limb is shown in Figure 19–26. It shows two-vessel run-off with obstruction of the proximal anterior tibial artery. The other vessels were without any hemodynamically significant lesions.

References

1. Carter SA. Indirect systolic pressures and pulse waves in arterial occlusive disease of the lower extremities. Circulation 1968; 37:624.

2. Haimovici H. Patterns of atherosclerotic lesions of the lower extremity. Arch Surg 1967; 95:118.

3. Strandness DE. The role of noninvasive procedures in the management of the lower extremity arterial disease. *In* Zwiebel WJ (ed). Introduction to vascular ultrasonography. 2nd ed. Orlando, Fla, Grune & Stratton, 1986; 281–286.

4. Stieghorst MF, Crummy AB. Lower extremity arterial anatomy and collateral routes. *In* Zwiebel WJ (ed). Introduction to vascular ultrasonography. 2nd ed. Orlando, Fla, Grune & Stratton, 1986; 287–303.

5. Haimovici H. Femoropopliteal arteriosclerotic occlusive disease. *In* Vascular surgery: Principles and techniques. New York, McGraw-Hill, 1976; 422–456.

20 • Noninvasive Testing of Transluminal Angioplasty for Lower Extremity Ischemia

Introduction

Uses for Noninvasive Tests

Noninvasive vascular testing can provide valuable information in the evaluation of lower extremity obstructive arterial lesions. This is particularly true when noninvasive tests are used in conjunction with angioplasty procedures.

To be successful, the angioplasty procedure must ameliorate the patient's symptoms. To do this, the obstructive lesion or lesions causing the patient's symptoms must be treated. Successful treatment cannot be achieved by correcting asymptomatic obstructive lesions, no matter how beautiful the arteriographic result turns out to be. One problem then is identifying the lesion that is causing the patient's symptoms.

It is now recognized that arteriography cannot always result in successful assessment of the hemodynamic significance of a lesion. This difficulty presents a real problem when multiple lesions are scattered throughout various levels of the lower extremity circulation. It must be decided which lesion, or lesions, is causing the patient's symptoms. Single-plane arteriography may add confusion to this decision-making process because it often results in an underestimation of the degree of arterial obstruction present. This is because atherosclerotic plaques often begin in the posterior wall of the vessel and can be very extensive before they are appreciated in the anteroposterior (AP) view. Use of the arteriogram as a guide may lead to a significant lesion going unnoticed even though other, more apparent lesions are successfully dilated. This problem may be addressed by using biplane and oblique views of the aorta and pelvic vessels. However, these views are more cumbersome to obtain in the other vessels of the lower extremities.

Another solution is to dilate all of the stenoses in an attempt to locate the one causing the patient's symptoms. Unfortunately, this type of an approach may only prolong the procedure and produce unnecessary trauma to the vessels. Optimally, the offending lesion or lesions should be diagnosed with as little contrast medium as possible so that all efforts can be directed towards the most expedient, least traumatic treatment method possible. The combination of arteriographic anatomy and noninvasive hemodynamics may be used to achieve this goal.

Noninvasive techniques may be used to assess the intraprocedural or immediate post-procedural results of an angioplasty. For instance, if a residual stenosis remains present after multiple dilatation attempts, it may be important to assess the hemodynamic significance of such a stenosis before further attempts to re-dilate it are made. Further attempts to dilate the residual stenosis may be avoided when the noninvasive studies show that it is not hemodynamically significant. On the other hand, further attempts to re-dilate the residual stenosis may be indicated when the noninvasive studies show that it is hemodynamically significant. Knowing when to stop can be a problem when one is performing angioplasty procedures. This difficulty arises from the fact that continuing to re-dilate a stenosis site could lead to extensive damage of the vessel wall. Continuing to re-enter and re-dilate a stenosis could be avoided if it were known that the stenosis had been rendered hemodynamically insignificant by the previous dilatations. Again, the combination of arteriographic anatomy and noninvasive hemodynamics may be used to achieve this goal.

Noninvasive techniques may also be used to provide a quantitative follow-up assessment of patients after angioplasty. Repeat studies are obtained 24 to 48 hours after the procedure. An immediate improvement of these studies is indicative of a positive response to the procedure. A poor result should be detected immediately so that the proper therapy may be planned. Long-term follow-up consists of repeating the noninvasive studies every 3 months for the first 6 months and every 6 months thereafter. If the studies show a decrease in the hemodynamics, a repeat arteriogram is indicated to look for recurrence of the lesion or progression of the disease. The goal of the immediate testing is to make sure that the hemodynamics of the lower extremity are improved by the angioplasty and to provide a quantitative baseline for comparison with subsequent follow-up examinations. Long-term follow-up testing allows recurrent stenoses or disease progressions to be detected early so that they can be treated with the minimal amount of risk and discomfort to the patient. The goal here is to diagnose the lesions before they are complicated by total vessel occlusions and impending tissue loss. Once again, the combination of arteriographic anatomy and noninvasive hemodynamics may be used to achieve these goals.

Types of Noninvasive Tests

There are a wide variety of noninvasive vascular tests and indices available to evaluate the lower extremity hemodynamics before, during, and after the angioplasty procedure. Some of these include:

- segmental limb pressures
- exercise testing
- reactive hyperemia testing
- segmental volume plethysmography
- doppler blood flow velocity waveform analysis
- duplex scanning
- toe pressure measurements
- digital photoplethysmography (PPG) waveform analysis
- ankle/brachial index
- thigh/brachial index
- toe/brachial index
- ankle–toe difference pressure measurements.

Although this ever-growing list is incomplete, it is presented in this introduction to show how impractical it would be to use all of these tests and indices in each and every patient undergoing an angioplasty procedure. To do so would overburden a busy noninvasive vascular laboratory, add additional expense, provide redundant data, prolong hospitalization, and perhaps interfere with the angioplasty procedure itself. This by no means detracts from the importance of any of these tests and indices. They are all important in assessing the hemodynamics of the lower extremity circulation and may be used in the initial diagnosis of an obstructive disease process. Once the diagnosis is made, we use only a limited number of these tests in conjunction with the angioplasty procedure.

Exactly which test and indices to use will depend upon the noninvasive test equipment available and the skill and preference of the operators. Because the content of this chapter has been derived from the experience gained in our own particular laboratory, it reflects our personal preferences. The purpose of this chapter, then, is not to dictate which test to use. Instead, its function is to illustrate how noninvasive vascular testing can provide additional and useful information concerning the management of patients undergoing angioplasty procedures. To obtain the best results from these tests, it is necessary to understand the basic principles controlling blood flow in a vessel. These will be reviewed briefly here because they have already been described in detail in other chapters of this text.

Basic Principles

Pressure Dynamics

Blood flows from an area of high pressure to areas of low pressure. This phenomenon is governed by Poiseuille's law:

$$Q = \frac{\pi P \cdot r^4}{8nL} \qquad (20\text{–}1)$$

where Q = flow; r = vessel radius; P = pressure drop across the segment; n = blood viscosity; and L = vessel length.

Blood viscosity can be considered constant, making the vessel length and radius the two major determinants of flow. Of these, the radius is the most important.

Because this chapter concerns angioplasty procedures, Equation (20–1) is rewritten to express the blood flow hemodynamics when a stenosis is present in the lower extremity circulation:

$$Q = \frac{P_1 - P_2}{R_s + R_p} \qquad (20\text{–}2)$$

In this equation, $P_1 - P_2$ represents the pressure drop in millimeters of mercury (mm Hg) across the stenosis, R_s is the resistance to blood flow caused by the stenosis, and R_p is the resistance to blood flow produced by the peripheral vascular resistance. The presence of a stenosis in the system increases R_s and decreases the blood flow (Q). Two occurrences can keep Q at a constant level: the peripheral resistance (R_p) can decrease or the pressure drop across the stenosis ($P_1 - P_2$) can increase. Measuring the $P_1 - P_2$

increase is the basis for using segmental limb pressure testing to diagnose the resistance (R_s) decrease caused by dilating the stenosis with an angioplasty procedure.

The resistance (R_s) caused by a stenosis can be expressed by the following equation:

$$R_s = \frac{L}{r^4} \qquad (20\text{--}3)$$

From this equation, it can be seen that the resistance (R_s) of a stenosis goes up when its length (L) increases and its radius (r^4) decreases. A short stenosis with a small reduction of its radius may have only a minimal pressure drop ($P_1 - P_2$) across it in order to keep the flow (Q) constant in the extremity at rest. Generally, the pressure drop across the stenosis must be more than 20 mm Hg before it is considered significant by segmental limb pressure measurements.

Looking at Equation (20–2), we can see that lowering the peripheral resistance (R_p) would increase the pressure drop ($P_1 - P_2$) across a stenosis when Q remains constant. If the flow (Q) increases in response to the lowering of the peripheral resistance (R_p), there may be no increase in the pressure drop ($P_1 - P_2$) across the stenosis. The increase in Q compensates for the decrease in peripheral resistance (R_p) under these circumstances. This is what happens when an extremity containing a mild stenosis like the one just described is subjected to exercise testing. A stenosis of this type would be considered insignificant by segmental limb pressure measurements done at rest and after exercise.

Next, consider a somewhat longer stenosis with a moderate reduction of its radius. Equation (20–3) shows that the resistance (R_s) created by the stenosis goes up when its length increases and its radius decreases. An increase in R_s in Equation (20–2) would lower the flow (Q) unless the increase in R_s is compensated for by the other factors in this equation. A decrease in the peripheral resistance (R_p) could allow the flow to remain constant without increasing the pressure drop ($P_1 - P_2$) across the stenosis. Segmental limb pressures on this extremity at rest would reveal the stenosis to be insignificant. However, segmental limb pressure of this same extremity after exercise could reveal the stenosis to be significant. Here is why.

Exercise lowers the peripheral resistance (R_p) even further and causes the flow (Q) to increase. In order for Q to increase, the factors in Equation (20–2) must change. The resistance of the stenosis (R_s) cannot change because it is fixed in length and radius. Exercise has already opened up the peripheral resistance (R_p) as much as possible so that it cannot be lowered any further. The only factor left to change is the pressure drop ($P_1 - P_2$) across the stenosis. It then increases as the blood flow (Q) through the stenosis increases. Segmental limb pressures on this extremity after exercise will detect the increase in the pressure drop ($P_1 - P_2$) and will reveal the stenosis to be significant.

Finally, consider a long stenosis with a severely reduced radius. Actually, it does not have to be long. Equation (20–3) shows that the radius reduction has a more profound effect on the resistance created by the stenosis than does its length because the radius is raised to the fourth power. Therefore, consider the stenosis to have a severely reduced radius. The resistance (R_s) in Equation (20–2) now increases dramatically. This causes the peripheral resistance to become wide open in order to keep the flow (Q) constant. However, the resistance (R_s) created by this stenosis is so high that R_s cannot be compensated for by decreasing the peripheral resistance (R_p) to its lowest value. Something else in Equation (20–2) must change to keep Q constant. The only factor left is the pressure drop ($P_1 - P_2$) across the stenosis. It increases in an attempt to keep the flow (Q) constant. Segmental limb pressure measurements will detect the increase in the pressure drop across the stenosis and will reveal it to be significant even when the extremity is at rest. Because the peripheral vascular resistance is already wide open, there may be no need to use exercise testing under these circumstances.

Admittedly, these equations grossly simplify the real hemodynamics of a stenosis placed in a complex pulsatile circulation. They do, however, serve as a model that can be used to understand some of the interplay between blood flow, pressure drops across stenoses, peripheral vascular resistance, and the resistance created by the stenosis.

The noninvasive vascular tests used to detect the increase in the pressure drop ($P_1 - P_2$) created by obstructive lesions located in the lower extremity arterial circulation include:
- segmental limb pressures
- ankle–toe difference pressure measurements
- thigh/brachial index
- toe pressures
- ankle/brachial index
- toe/brachial index

All of these may be used in conjunction with either exercise or reactive hyperemia testing to unmask an obstructive lesion that does not have an increased pressure drop ($P_1 - P_2$) in the extremity at rest. The above list of tests may be further subdivided into those that localize the obstruction to a specific location in the lower extremity vasculature and those that do not.

The tests used to localize the obstruction site to a specific location in the lower extremity vasculature include:

- segmental limb pressures
- ankle–toe difference pressure measurements
- thigh/brachial index

Segmental limb pressures are used to localize lesions located in the aortoiliac inflow system, the femoropopliteal outflow system, or the tibioperoneal run-off system. The thigh/brachial index is used to localize lesions in the aortoiliac inflow system and the proximal portion of the femoropopliteal outflow system. Obstructive lesions located below the ankle level are localized by the ankle–toe difference pressure measurements.

The tests that are used to determine whether an arterial obstructive lesion exists but that do not localize the lesion to any specific site within the lower extremity vasculature include:

- ankle/brachial index
- toe pressures
- toe/brachial index

Because all of these tests have been described in other chapters, they will not be discussed in further detail here.

So far, this discussion has focused mainly on the pressure drop ($P_1 - P_2$) across a stenosis. Yet, there is another important factor that must be considered—the pressure inside of the stenotic segment itself. This pressure is important because it helps to keep the wall of the stenotic or occluded segment open after it has been dilated by the balloon catheter. It may also explain why there may be continued improvement of the stenosis following dilatation. Therefore, it is the pressure inside of the dilated stenotic segment opposing the vessel wall that keeps the vessel open. This can be further explained by the law of Laplace. This law states that the circumferential force expanding the vessel wall and keeping the vessel open is proportional to the diameter of the vessel multiplied by the pressure inside the vessel, or $F = D \times P$. Reducing the diameter of the dilated segment increases its resistance, as shown in Equation (20–3). As the resistance (R_s) increases, the pressure in the previously dilated stenotic segment decreases, causing an increase in the pressure drop ($P_1 - P_2$) across the segment, as shown in Equation (20–4) and Figure 20–1A.

$$R_s = P_1 - P_2 \qquad (20\text{–}4)$$

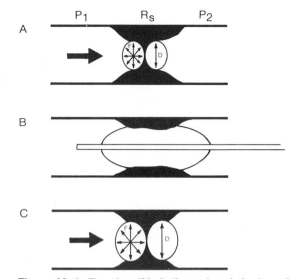

Figure 20–1. Equation (20–4) (in text) and the law of Laplace applied to a dilated stenosis site. *A,* As the stenosis resistance R_s goes up, the pressure in its lumen goes down, causing an increase in the pressure drop P_1–P_2 across it. Arrow denotes blood flow direction in vessel. *B,* Stenosis dilated by balloon catheter. *C,* As the stenosis resistance R_s goes down, the pressure in its lumen goes up, causing a decrease in the pressure drop P_1–P_2 across it. Force (F) expanding the stenosis wall goes up because both (D) and (P) are increased.

This situation can set into motion a vicious circle that may result in the occlusion of the dilated segment. This circle may occur because as the pressure in the lumen of a previously dilated stenosis is lowered, the walls begin to oppose each other, reducing its diameter. This diameter reduction lowers the expansion force still more, causing a further decrease in the diameter of the dilated segment. If this continues, the site of the previously dilated stenosis may close off totally. A decrease in the pressure drop ($P_1 - P_2$) across an angioplasty site then means (1) its resistance (R_s) is reduced, (2) its radius is increased, (3) its internal pressure is elevated, and (4) the circumferential force expanding its wall is increased (Fig. 20–1C).

Pulse Pressure Wave Dynamics

Pulse pressure waves generated in the proximal aortic root segment during cardiac systole propel the blood flow throughout the arterial circulation. These waves travel through the vessels, forming a series of alternating high-to-low pressure zones. As the blood flows from these high-to-low pressure zones, it is propelled through the circulation at varying velocities. Because of its weight, blood flow velocity is quite sluggish as compared with the velocity of the pulse pressure wave, which travels rapidly throughout the arterial circulation. Because the blood is heavy and does not want to move, the pulse pressure waves are fighting constantly against the inertia of blood in order to propel it through the vessels. As a result, multiple pulse pressure waves are required to move blood each centimeter down the lumen of a vessel.

These pulse pressure waves are generated by the pumping action of the heart. At the end of diastole, blood is moving at a low velocity in the low-pressure zone of the proximal aortic root segment adjacent to the aortic valve. When the heart begins to eject blood into the aorta at a high velocity during early systole (Fig. 20–2A) the blood is blocked by the high-inertia/low-velocity blood flow in the proximal aortic root segment. This results in the high-velocity blood flow combining with the low-velocity blood flow to increase the total blood volume in the proximal aortic root segment. This expands the proximal aortic root segment, causing it to become a high-pressure zone, whereas the relaxed aortic segment immediately above it is a low-pressure zone (Fig. 20–2B).

The left ventricle also becomes a low-pressure zone as its walls begin to relax at the end of systole (Fig. 20–2C). The blood under high pressure in the distended proximal aortic root segment must have a place to go. Immediately, the blood flows into the low-pressure zone in the left ventricle and moves back towards the aortic valve. The pressure in the left ventricle is lower than that of the aorta below the aortic root segment because it is momentarily empty of blood. Blood is always present in the aorta above the level of the proximal aortic root segment, so it has a higher end-systolic pressure than the empty left ventricle. Blood then flows in a reversed direction towards the aortic valve, and it snaps shut (Fig. 20–2C). Again, the blood, still under high pressure in the proximal aortic root segment, must have a place to go. Now the blood moves at a high velocity towards the low-pressure zone in the relaxed aortic segment above it. However, the high-velocity blood flow from the proximal aortic root segment is blocked by the low-velocity blood flow in the relaxed, low-pressure segment above it (Fig. 20–2D). These two blood volumes combine to distend the walls of the proximal aortic root segment, creating a new high-pressure zone (Fig. 20–2E).

By now, the proximal aortic root segment has become a high-pressure zone again because of the pumping action of the heart and the ejection

of blood into it during systole (Fig. 20–2F). Only the amount of blood necessary to snap the aortic valve shut can reverse the direction of the blood and cause it to flow back from the newly created high-pressure zone to the proximal aortic root segment. As a result, the blood in the newly created high-pressure segment must now flow in a forward direction towards the relaxed, low-pressure aortic segment beyond it. In doing so, the blood is blocked again by the inertia of the low-velocity blood flow in the low-pressure segment beyond it (Fig. 20–2G). It again combines with this blood flow to create a new high-pressure zone farther out in the aorta (Fig. 20–2G).

Pulse pressure waves are important because they propel blood flow away from the heart in a forward direction throughout the arterial system. Furthermore, they are important in noninvasive testing because arterial obstructions can damp these waves as they propagate along the arterial tree (Fig. 20–3A). Damping of the pulse pressure waves, in turn, interferes with their ability to propel blood flow through the arterial circulation. For example, an obstructive lesion in the superficial femoral artery will cause damping of the pulse pressure waves at that site. This, in turn, will interfere with the blood flow at the site of the lesion and impede its progress into the popliteal artery. Noninvasive vascular tests, such as Doppler blood flow velocity waveform analysis, do not directly measure the damping of the pulse pressure wave caused by arterial obstructive lesions. Instead, they measure the changes in the velocities of the blood flow that result from damping of the pulse pressure waves caused by an obstructive arterial lesion.

As shown in Figure 20–2, the pulse pressure waves cause blood to flow at varying velocities throughout each phase of the cardiac cycle. Doppler velocity waveform analysis presents a graphic representation of how blood is flowing through the artery. In the peripheral artery of a normal limb, there is a rapid forward flow of blood during systole (Fig. 20–2B), followed by slowing and then a small amount of reverse flow at the end of systole (Fig. 20–2C). The graphic representation created by the Doppler tracing presents a waveform that shows this. There is a rapid upstroke, a sharp peak, a rapid downstroke, and a short peak below the baseline representing reverse flow. A stenosis in the arterial circulation damps the pulse pressure waveform, as shown in Figure 20–3A. This alters the blood flow velocities distal to the site of the stenosis. The Doppler velocity waveforms reveal these alterations. At this point, the upstroke is slower and the systolic

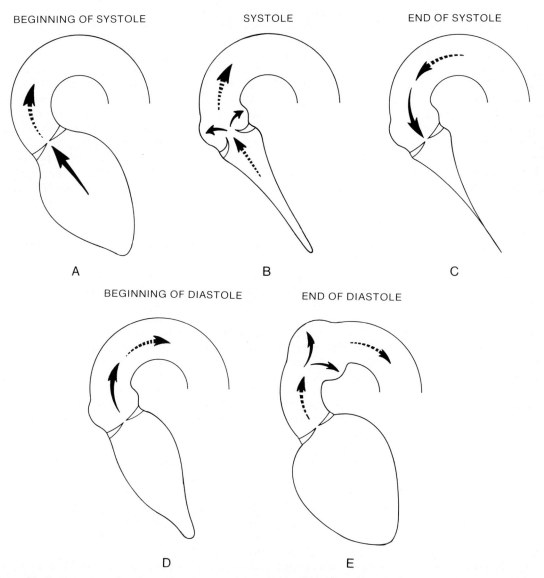

Figure 20–2. Formation of pulse pressure waves used to propel blood flow through the arteries. Solid arrows denote high-pressure, high-velocity flow; dashed arrows denote low-pressure, low-velocity flow.

A, As the left ventricle begins to eject high-pressure, high-velocity flow in the aorta, it is blocked by the inertia of the low-pressure, low-velocity flow in the proximal aortic root segment.

B, High-pressure, high-velocity left ventricular flow combines with the low-pressure, low-velocity flow of proximal aortic root segment to form a high-pressure zone distending its walls.

C, High-pressure, high-velocity flow of proximal aortic root segment goes towards the low, left ventricle; pressure snaps aortic valve shut.

D, High-pressure, high-velocity flow of proximal aortic root segment blocked by low-pressure, low-velocity flow in aortic segment above it.

E, Blood volumes combine, creating new high-pressure, high-velocity flow in the aortic segment.

SYSTOLE   END OF SYSTOLE

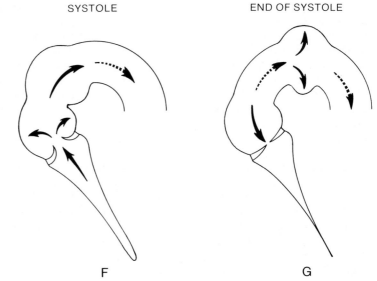

Figure 20–2 *Continued. F,* Both the proximal aortic root segment and the aortic segment above it become high-pressure, high-velocity flow zones, propelling blood flow further out in the aorta.

G, Pulse pressure wave propagates along aorta, propelling blood flow in front of it down the aorta and into the peripheral vessels of the lower extremities.

F   G

peak is rounded. There is no peak below the baseline level. The more severe the obstructive disease is proximal to the vessel being examined, the more dramatic the waveform changes. A flat Doppler tracing indicates a lack of blood flow in the vessel. Opening up the stenosis with a balloon catheter will prevent the pulse pressure wave from being damped and will restore the Doppler velocity waveform to its normal configuration (Fig. 20–3*B*).

The noninvasive vascular tests used to detect blood flow velocity changes caused by pulse pressure wave damping resulting from obstructive lesions located in the lower extremity arterial circulation include:

1. Doppler blood flow velocity waveform analysis.

2. Digital photoplethysmography waveform analysis.

3. Segmental volume plethysmography.

4. Duplex scanning.

Digital PPG waveform analysis does not show the localization of the obstructive lesion to any specific site in the lower extremity arterial circulation. It merely denotes that an obstructive lesion (or lesions) exists somewhere in this circulation. The other tests may be used to localize the lesion to a specific site in the lower extremity circulation.

Applications of Testing

Exactly how the hemodynamics of these noninvasive tests may be applied to angioplasty procedures will now be described. These noninvasive tests can be used for pre-procedural, intraprocedural, and post-procedural testing.

Pre-procedural Testing

Pre-procedural tests are used for baseline measurements. These measurements are then compared with findings obtained in the immedi-

A

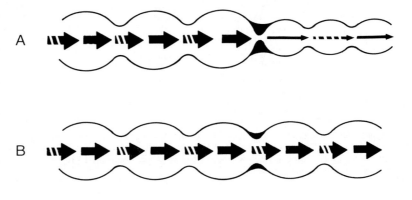

Figure 20–3. Pulse pressure wave damped by stenosis. *A,* Stenosis damps pulse pressure waves and alters blood flow velocity waveforms below it. *B,* Dilating stenosis restores propagation of pulse pressure wave through it and blood flow velocity waveforms below it.

B

ate post-angioplasty period to evaluate the results of the angioplasty procedure. The immediate post-angioplasty period occurs within 24 to 48 hours following the procedure. Because the use of multiple duplicate tests on the same patient are required, we prefer to use as few tests as possible. Our pre-procedural assessment includes the (1) *ankle/brachial index*, (2) *segmental limb pressure measurements*, and (3) *Doppler velocity waveform analysis*. These tests are not repeated after exercise or after reactive hyperemia when the results of the resting test are grossly abnormal. They are used, when the test results are either normal or borderline, to unmask the hemodynamic significance of any lesion that can manifest itself during exercise.

The pre-procedural segmental limb pressures from the left lower extremity of the patient in Figure 20–4 localized an obstruction between the above-knee (AK) and below-knee (BK) segmental limb cuffs. Figure 20–4A shows a pressure drop ($P_1 - P_2$) of 81 mm Hg between these two cuff levels. The Doppler velocity waveforms ob-

tained from the popliteal artery are damped, as shown by the low amplitude of the systolic waveforms and by the absence of the reversed flow peak in Figure 20–4A. The arteriographic anatomy of the arterial obstructions is shown in Figure 20–5A. There are two stenotic segments and one totally occluded segment. One of the stenoses is located in the superficial femoral artery; the other is located in the popliteal artery. The totally occluded segment is located at the junction between the superficial femoral and popliteal arteries in the adductor hiatus. An attempt was made to dilate all three of these lesions. Figure 20–5B shows incomplete dilatation of the stenosis in the superficial femoral artery segment and complete dilatation of the other two lesions.

The question now arises as to what hemodynamic effect the residual superficial femoral artery stenosis has on the lower-extremity circulation. This is an important question, because if the residual stenosis is hemodynamically significant, either it will have to be re-dilated or it will have to be treated surgically to improve the lower

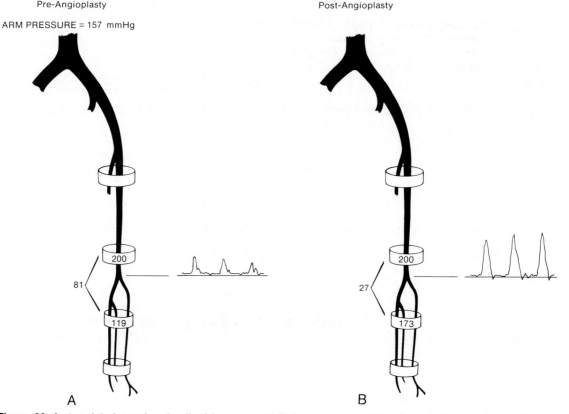

Pre-Angioplasty

ARM PRESSURE = 157 mmHg

Post-Angioplasty

A

B

Figure 20–4. Arterial obstructions localized by segmental limb pressures and Doppler velocity waveform testing. *A*, Pressure drop of 81 mm Hg localized obstructions between above-knee and below-knee segment cuff levels. Popliteal artery waveforms damped below obstruction sites. *B*, Decreased pressure drop and restored waveforms indicate good response to angioplasty procedure.

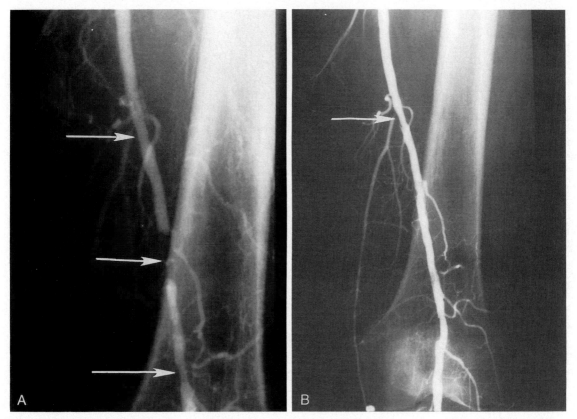

Figure 20–5. Pre-angioplasty and post-angioplasty arteriograms. *A*, Sites of obstructive lesions (arrows). *B*, Post-angioplasty residual stenosis (arrow).

extremity circulation. To answer this question, the pre-procedural baseline test results can be compared with the post-procedural test results in Figure 20–4. The comparison shows the pressure drop ($P_1 - P_2$) between the AK and BK cuffs decreased from 81 mm Hg to 27 mm Hg with restoration of the Doppler velocity waveforms below the level of the treated arterial segments. These findings indicate a good response to the angioplasty procedure, and no further treatment of the residual stenosis was done. Should subsequent follow-up testing reveal an increase in the pressure drop between the AK and BK cuffs compared with the findings of the post-procedural assessment, the residual stenosis could be re-evaluated arteriographically and re-dilated at that time.

Isolated, short iliac artery stenoses like the one in Figure 20–6 may necessitate only minimal pre-procedural assessment. The arteriograms of this patient were normal except for the tight right common iliac artery stenosis shown in Figure 20–6A. The stenosis was considered hemodynamically significant because the right resting ankle/brachial index was 0.7. The stenosis was dilated,

as shown in Figure 20–6B. This resulted in a resting ankle/brachial index of 0.97 twenty-four hours after the angioplasty procedure. Segmental limb pressures and Doppler waveform analysis are not really necessary in this type of lesion. Instead, noninvasive vascular procedures should be directed towards exercise or reactive hyperemia testing. The purpose of this type of testing is to determine whether the flow-limiting, hemodynamically significant iliac artery stenosis has been successfully eliminated by the angioplasty. If it has, the ankle/brachial index should not decrease following exercise or reactive hyperemia testing. It should either stay the same or increase slightly after exercise. Such a finding means that the flow and pressure-limiting hemodynamics of the right iliac artery stenosis have been successfully treated by the angioplasty procedure.

Both resting and post-exercise ankle/brachial indices are used to follow up the treatment results in patients such as those just discussed. If an abnormally low ankle/brachial index is found on subsequent follow-up evaluations, the patient is referred for segmental limb pressures and Doppler waveform analysis. These follow-up tests are

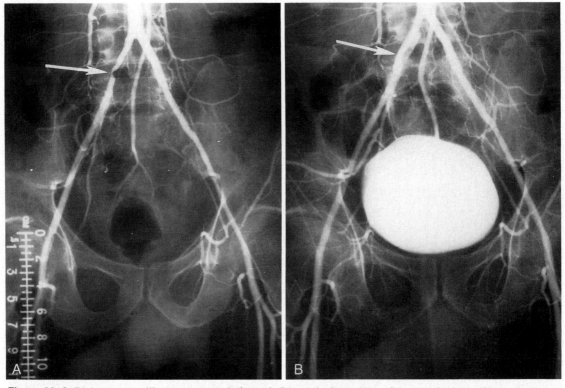

Figure 20–6. Right common iliac artery stenosis (arrow). Pre-angioplasty *(A)* and post-angioplasty *(B)* arteriograms.

used to determine whether the obstruction is due to a recurrence of the iliac artery stenosis or to the development of new obstructions in the lower extremity arteries. No other noninvasive tests are used when both the resting and post-exercise ankle/brachial indices are found to be normal and the patient remains asymptomatic on subsequent follow-up evaluations.

The pre-procedural assessment of a patient with an isolated, long, proximal popliteal artery segment that is occluded is shown in Figure 20–7A. The figure shows an ankle/brachial index of 0.7 with damping of the Doppler velocity waveforms obtained from the popliteal and dorsalis pedis arteries below the level of the occlusion site. The waveforms from these vessels are abnormal because they remain high above the zero baseline level throughout the cardiac cycle. These abnormal waveforms result because flow below the level of the obstruction is more continuous than normal. Angioplasty was used to treat the occlusion, as shown in Figure 20–8. After angioplasty, the ankle/brachial index increased from 0.7 to 1.07 and the Doppler velocity waveforms dropped down to the zero baseline level. The restored reversed flow peaks from both the popliteal and dorsalis pedis arteries are also present.

These changes indicate a good response to the angioplasty procedure.

The pre-procedural assessment of a patient with an isolated stenosis located at the junction between the right external iliac artery and the common femoral artery is shown in Figure 20–9. Both of the lower extremities are included in this illustration so that the abnormal waveforms from the right can be compared with the normal ones from the left lower extremity. Also, note the lower segmental limb pressures in the right lower extremity compared with the left. The proximally located stenosis has lowered the systolic pressure measurements in all the right lower extremity arteries below it. There are no significant pressure drops between the segmental limb cuffs because there are no other obstructive lesions in the arteries of this lower extremity. All of the Doppler velocity waveforms are damped below the level of the stenosis. The arteriographic anatomy of the stenosis is shown in Figure 20–10A. The stenosis was dilated with the balloon catheter, as shown in Figure 20–10B. After angioplasty, the Doppler velocity waveforms were restored to their normal configurations (Fig. 20–11A) and the segmental limb systolic pressure measurements increased. The ankle/brachial in-

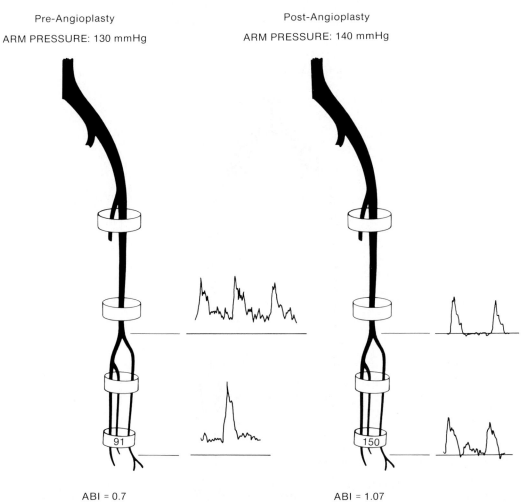

Pre-Angioplasty
ARM PRESSURE: 130 mmHg

Post-Angioplasty
ARM PRESSURE: 140 mmHg

91

150

ABI = 0.7
A

ABI = 1.07
B

Figure 20–7. Pre-angioplasty *(A)* and post-angioplasty *(B)* Doppler velocity waveforms. *A*, Waveforms damped in popliteal and dorsalis pedis arteries below level of proximal popliteal artery occlusion. Waveforms are high above baseline level. *B*, Waveforms at baseline level with return of reversed-flow peak below baseline.

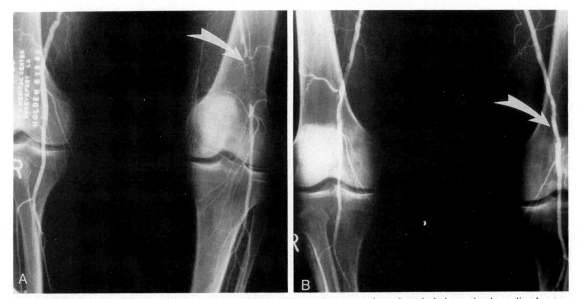

Figure 20–8. Pre-angioplasty *(A)* and post-angioplasty *(B)* arteriograms of total occluded proximal popliteal artery segment (arrow).

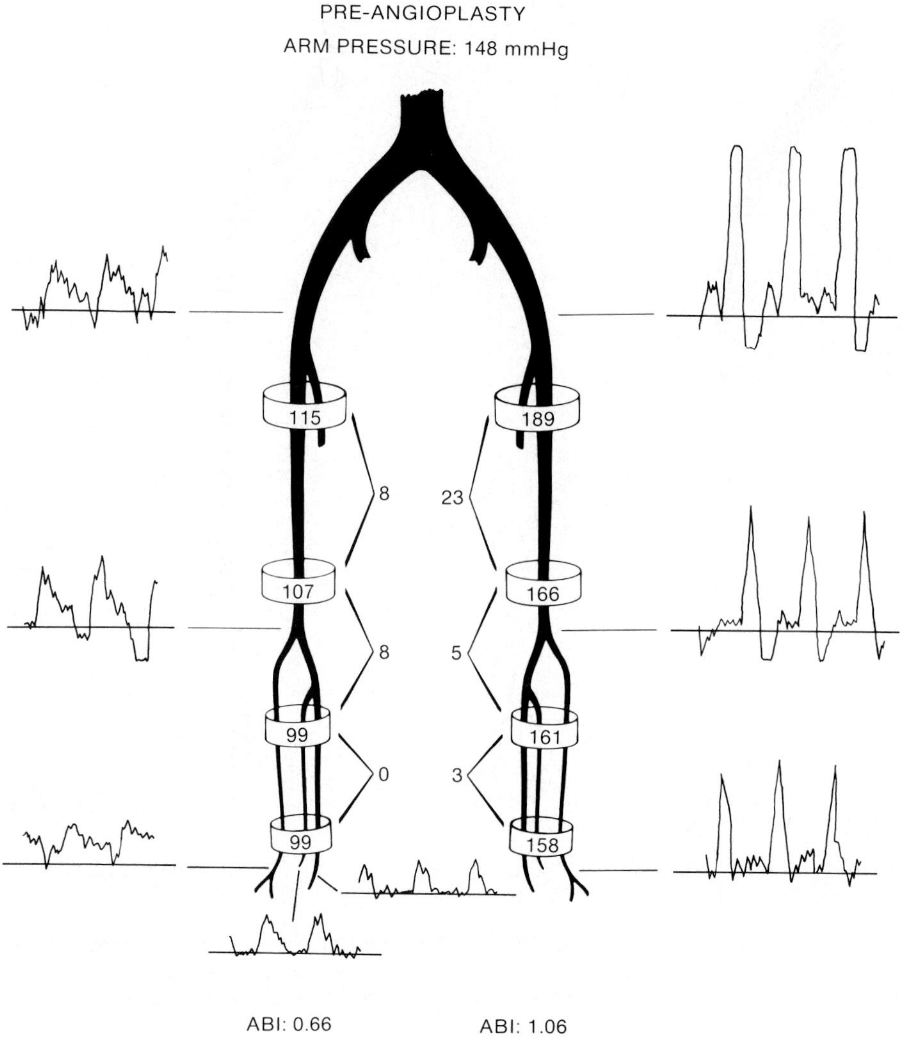

PRE-ANGIOPLASTY
ARM PRESSURE: 148 mmHg

115   189

8   23

107   166

8   5

99   161

0   3

99   158

ABI: 0.66   ABI: 1.06

Figure 20–9. Doppler velocity waveforms and segmental limb pressures below level of stenosis are located at the junction between the right external iliac and common femoral arteries.

dex also increased from 0.66 to 0.84. The patient was then subjected to exercise testing. Immediately after exercise, the ankle/brachial index rose to 1.07, indicating an excellent response to the angioplasty procedure. The post-angioplasty arteriogram is shown in Figure 20–11*B*.

Intraprocedural Testing

Intraprocedural testing is used to determine whether the dilatation procedure has reduced the pressure drop across the lesion before the catheter is removed from the patient. Because a catheter is already in the vessel, it is used to obtain the pressure measurements. Pressures on both sides of the lesion should be obtained before

and after the dilatation procedure. Ideally, two catheters should be used. One is positioned proximal to the lesion, and the other is placed distal to the lesion. The use of this two-catheter method allows the pressure both proximal and distal to the lesion to be recorded simultaneously. This approach is practical in the iliac vessels because the aortic catheter can be inserted on the contralateral side to measure the pressure proximal to the lesion and the other catheter can be placed in the ipsilateral femoral artery to measure the pressure below the lesion. This technique is illustrated in Figure 20–12*A*.

A single catheter may be used to obtain a pullback pressure across the lesion as shown in Figure 20–12*B*. This single-catheter method uses a No.

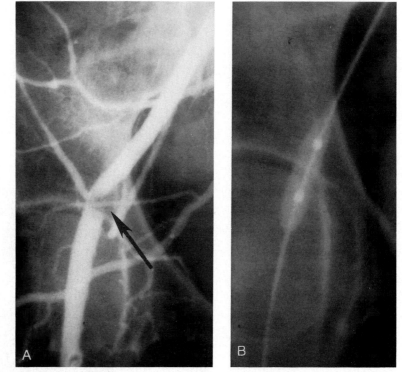

Figure 20–10. Pre-angioplasty arteriogram of stenosis located at junction between the right external iliac and common femoral arteries *(A)* (arrow) and shown dilated with balloon catheter *(B)*.

5 French catheter that takes a 0.038 inch guide wire. Once the catheter is advanced through the stenosis, the larger 0.038 inch guide wire is exchanged for a smaller 0.025 inch guide wire. Using a Y adaptor, the pressures are obtained as the catheter tip is pulled back across the stenosis. The guide wire remains across the stenosis site during this maneuver. The wire is small enough to prevent damping of the pressure measurements and large enough to pass the catheter over it should there be a need to traverse the stenosis site again. The guide wire is then used to guide the catheter tip back and forth across the stenosis or post-dilatation site when recording multiple pull-back pressure measurements.

The single-catheter method was used to obtain the pull-back pressure measurements in Figure 20–13. The arteriogram in this figure shows a stenosis in the left external iliac artery. Pull-back pressures across the stenosis were first obtained without the use of any blood flow augmentation techniques. These systolic pressure measurements were 166 mm Hg above the stenosis and 158 mm Hg below the stenosis. This represents a pressure drop $(P_1 - P_2)$ of 8 mm Hg across the stenosis in this patient at rest. A systolic pressure drop $(P_1 - P_2)$ of 10 to 15 mm Hg or greater at rest is considered significant in the iliac system.

Because this patient complained of left leg pain when walking, the stenosis was challenged with a blood flow augmentation technique to simulate exercise. In this case, papaverine (30 mg) was injected intra-arterially below the stenosis site. This maneuver simulates exercise, which lowers the peripheral resistance (R_p) and increases the demand for flow (Q), as shown in Equation (20–2). As this equation demonstrates, the pressure drop $(P_1 - P_2)$ across the stenosis increases as the blood flow (Q) through the stenosis increases. The pull-back pressures in Figure 20–13 indicate this change. After the peripheral resistance (R_p) was lowered by papaverine, the systolic pressure above the stenosis was 171 mm Hg and 125 mm Hg below the stenosis. This resulted in a pressure drop $(P_1 - P_2)$ of 46 mm Hg across the stenosis, which is significant. Dilating the stenosis eliminated the pressure drop, as shown in Figure 20–14.

Intra-arterial pressure measurements of this type tell a great deal about the pressure drop across the stenosis site, but they reveal little about how eliminating this pressure drop affects the pressures and blood flow in the remaining lower extremity arteries. This information is important because the patient with the iliac artery stenosis in Figures 20–13 and 20–14 also had

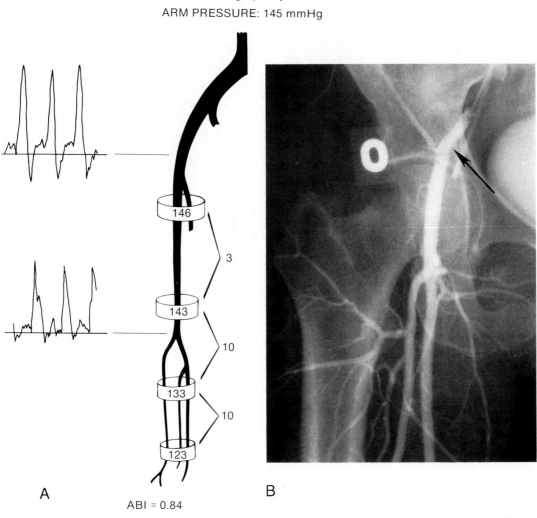

Post-Angioplasty
ARM PRESSURE: 145 mmHg

A

ABI = 0.84

B

Figure 20–11. Post-angioplasty Doppler velocity waveforms, segmental limb pressures *(A)*, and arteriograms *(B)*. *A*, Restored waveforms with sharp, pointed systolic peaks and good flow reversal below baseline level. High-thigh systolic pressure improved from 115 mm Hg pre-angioplasty to 146 mm Hg post-angioplasty. *B*, Post-angioplasty arteriogram of dilatation site (arrow).

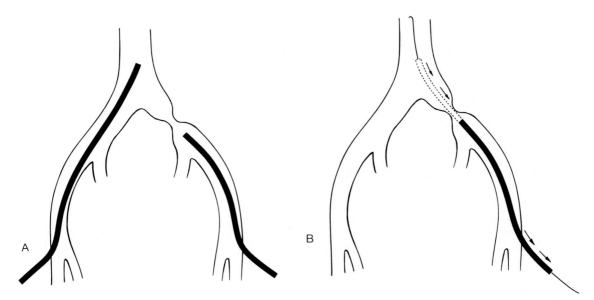

Figure 20–12. Intra-arterial catheter methods used to measure pressure drops across iliac artery stenoses. *A*, Two-catheter method allows the pressure above and below the stenosis to be measured simultaneously. *B*, Single-catheter method used to measure a pull-back pressure drop across the stenosis. Dotted line catheter denotes position above stenosis; solid line catheter denotes position below stenosis.

Figure 20–13. Pull-back systolic pressure drops across left external iliac artery stenosis before and after blood flow augmentation with vaso-dilator drug.

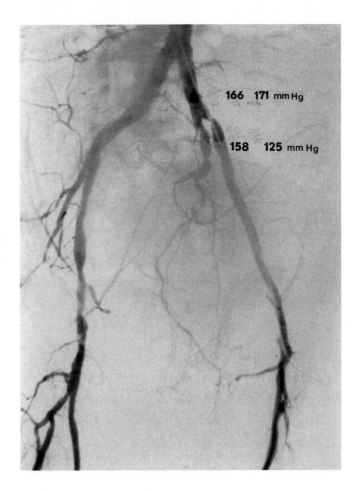

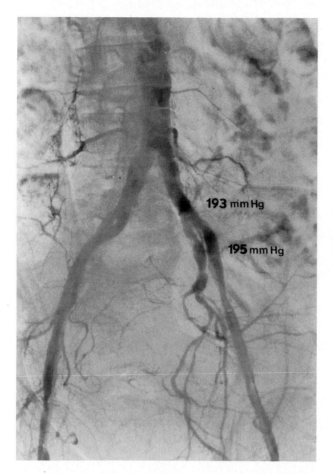

193 mmHg

195 mmHg

Figure 20–14. Post-angioplasty pull-back pressures show no pressure drop across dilatation site after blood flow augmentation with vasodilator drug.

PRE-ANGIOPLASTY

A

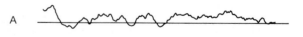

Figure 20–15. Intraprocedural digital photoplethysmographic waveforms from left great toe. *A,* Pre-angioplasty waveforms damped by iliac artery stenosis. *B,* Waveforms improve after first balloon inflation and deflation. *C,* Waveforms continue to improve after two more balloon inflations and deflations.

CATHETERIZATION DURING ANGIOPLASTY

B

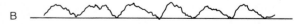

POST-ANGIOPLASTY

C

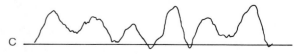

multiple vascular occlusions of the tibial and peroneal arteries. If eliminating the iliac artery stenosis does not improve the blood flow to the leg, a more aggressive approach may be required. Such an approach could include dilating the tibial and peroneal stenoses in addition to eliminating the iliac artery lesion.

Intraprocedural noninvasive monitoring may be used in this type of a decision-making process. Digital photoplethysmography waveform analysis (see Chapter 21, "Toe Pressures and Digital Plethysmography") can be used for this purpose. This type of monitoring was used during the iliac artery angioplasty of the patient in Figures 20–13 and 20–14. The results of the digital PPG waveforms in this patient are presented in Figure 20–15. Figure 20–15A shows damping of the digital PPG waveform obtained from the left great toe prior to dilating the iliac artery stenosis. This waveform improved after the first balloon inflation and deflation, as shown in Figure 20–15B. Two more balloon inflations caused further improvement in the waveforms, as shown in Figure 20–15C. This figure shows the amplitude of the PPG waveform increasing as the balloon is deflated. No further dilatations were attempted once the digital PPG waveforms in Figure 20–15C were obtained. The angiogram in Figure 20–14 indicated a good anatomical result, and both the intra-arterial pressures and the digital PPG waveforms indicated a good hemodynamic response to the procedure.

The digital PPG waveforms in Figure 20–16 were obtained during an attempt to dilate the left iliac artery stenosis shown in Figure 20–17. During the catheterization procedure, there was complete loss of the digital PPG waveform (Fig. 20–16B). This was caused by spasm of the proximal superficial femoral artery, deep femoral artery, and common femoral artery at the catheter insertion site (Fig. 20–18). The spasm is obvious on the arteriogram in Figure 20–18 when the contrast media opacification and the size of the involved vessels on the left are compared with those on the right. Note that the spasm persisted after the catheter was removed, as indicated by the digital PPG waveform in Figure 20–16C. This type of a complication must be recognized early to prevent occlusion of the vessel and angioplasty site. A digital PPG waveform pattern like the one in Figure 20–16 may also be seen when thrombosis occludes the vessel at the puncture site or when atherosclerotic debris is dislodged during the course of an angioplasty procedure and causes distal embolization of the peripheral vessels. Distal embolization of athero-

sclerotic debris was suspected in the patient whose digital PPG waveforms are shown in Figure 20–16. However, the follow-up arteriogram in Figure 20–19, obtained after the intra-arterial administration of vasodilators, revealed diseased vessels but no evidence of embolization.

Another characteristic digital PPG waveform pattern that may be seen during an angioplasty procedure is illustrated in Figure 20–20. The pre-angioplasty waveform in Figure 20–20A is further damped during the procedure in Figure 20–20B. A waveform tracing of this type occurs when the balloon is not completely deflated during the recording of the waveform tracing. Fully deflating the balloon and removing it from the dilatation site result in the PPG waveforms in Figure 20–20C. The balloon damping is now absent. However, comparison between the pre-angioplasty and post-angioplasty waveforms shows that minimal hemodynamic improvement was achieved by the procedure.

Digital PPG waveform analysis offers a means of following the blood flow pulse waveforms during the course of an angioplasty procedure. Because arterial obstructions block the pulse pressure waves and interfere with blood flow, the digital PPG waveforms can be used to determine when blood flow is restored after these obstructions are opened up by angioplasty. Digital PPG is simple to use. Monitoring devices are placed on the great toe and out of the field of operation, as shown in Figure 20–21.

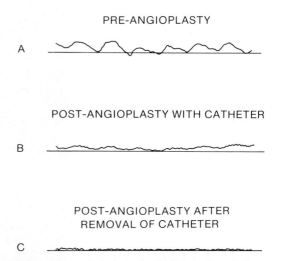

Figure 20–16. Intraprocedural digital photoplethysmographic waveforms from left great toe. A, Pre-angioplasty waveforms damped by iliac artery stenosis. B, Loss of waveform pulsations caused by arterial spasm at catheter site. C, Waveform pulsations remain absent after catheter is removed.

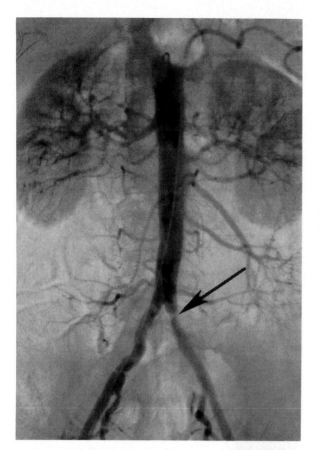

Figure 20–17. Pre-angioplasty arteriogram of left common iliac artery stenosis (arrow).

Figure 20–18. Spasm of proximal superficial femoral, profunda femoral, and common femoral arteries at catheter insertion site (arrows).

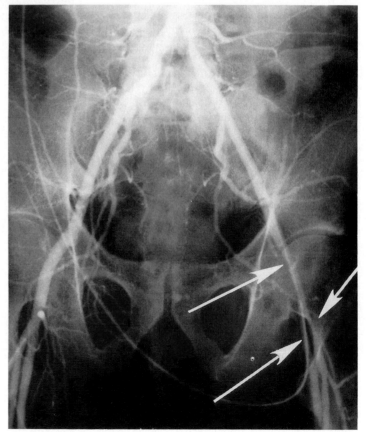

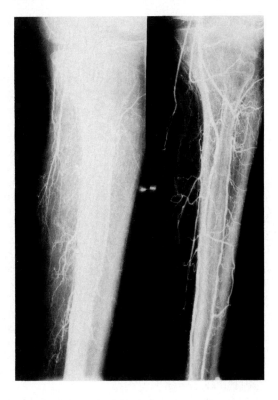

Figure 20–19. Leg arteriogram shows no evidence of distal embolization.

PRE-ANGIOPLASTY

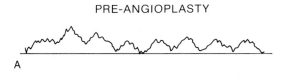

A

CATHETERIZATION DURING ANGIOPLASTY

B

POST-ANGIOPLASTY

C

Figure 20–20. Digital photoplethysmographic waveforms damped by balloon catheter at stenosis site. *A*, Pre-angioplasty waveforms. *B*, Waveforms damped because of incomplete balloon deflation at stenosis site. *C*, Waveforms return after balloon is fully deflated and removed from dilation site.

Figure 20–21. Instrumentation for toe pressure measurement and digital photoplethysmographic waveform monitoring during angioplasty.

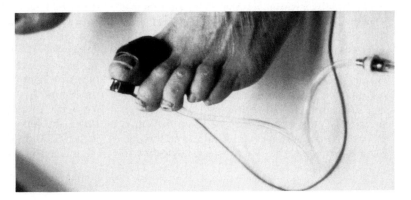

Follow-up Testing

Follow-up testing is used to detect the recurrence of a lesion that has been dilated or the progression of new disease in the lower extremity arteries. As stated previously, a baseline study is done prior to angioplasty. Recordings can be obtained during the procedure to monitor progress. Repeat studies done 24 to 48 hours after the procedure are compared with the pre-procedural baseline test to evaluate the immediate results of the angioplasty. The immediate post-procedural test results are also used in the subsequent follow-up evaluations of the patients. Follow-up studies may be obtained every 3 months for the first 6 months and every 6 months thereafter. When results of these studies show a decrease in the hemodynamic flow, a repeat angiogram is indicated to look for recurrence of the lesion or progression of the disease.

The purpose of follow-up testing is to detect obstructive lesions early before they are later complicated by extensive thrombotic occlusions. By detecting these lesions early, they may be amenable to angioplasty, thus circumventing surgical intervention.

An example of serial long-term, follow-up noninvasive vascular testing is presented in Figure 20–22. The patient presented with bilateral lower extremity intermittent claudication, which adversely affected her work as a waitress. The symptoms were worse in the left lower extremity than the right. Arteriography showed total occlusion of the left iliac system and stenoses in the right common iliac artery (Fig. 20–23). Fibrinolytic therapy was used to lyse the clot in the occluded left iliac system. This was followed by angioplasty of stenoses located in both the right and left common iliac arteries (Fig. 20–24). The arteriographic anatomical results of this therapy are shown in Figure 20–25. Both iliac arterial systems are now widely patent.

Follow-up testing was helpful for this patient because of the extensive amount of disease present in the iliac arterial system. Follow-up testing began with the pre-angioplasty evaluation (Figure 20–22). This follow-up evaluation showed a depressed ankle/brachial index of 0.50 with monophasic damped Doppler velocity waveforms below the level of the occluded left iliac arterial system. All of the segmental limb systolic pressure measurements were low and were without any significant pressure drop between the cuffs. The obstructive lesions were localized to the iliac vessels in this patient. There was no evidence of significant obstructive lesions in the remainder of the lower extremity arterial circulation.

The immediate post-procedural testing done at 1 day after angioplasty showed that the ankle/brachial index increased from 0.50 to 0.87 (Fig. 20–22). Although this indicated improvement, it was still abnormally low. The ankle/brachial index, however, did remain stable after exercise testing. The segmental limb pressures also improved, as shown in Figure 20–22. Doppler velocity waveforms from the femoral and posterior tibial arteries also improved. However, the femoral waveform was still abnormally damped, as noted by its high position above the zero baseline level (Fig. 20–22). Its reversed flow component is absent. The posterior tibial artery waveform is also located above the zero baseline level.

Based on the improved hemodynamic results present on the comparison between the pre-procedural and post-procedural noninvasive assessments, the patient was discharged from the hospital to be followed up in the noninvasive laboratory after 1 month. The 5-week follow-up revealed continued improvement in the hemodynamic status of the lower extremity (Fig. 20–22). Triphasic Doppler velocity waveforms began to appear in the femoral, popliteal, and posterior tibial arteries. These continued to improve, as shown on the 11-month follow-up evaluation. The ankle/brachial index was normal at 1. This currently asymptomatic waitress is to be followed up at 6-month intervals and is to be examined for recurrence of the iliac artery stenosis or for progression of disease in the remainder of the lower extremity vessels.

The patient whose noninvasive studies are shown in Figure 20–26 had obstructive lesions in both the aortoiliac inflow and femoropopliteal outflow systems. By means of arteriography, the obstruction of the aortoiliac inflow system was found to be located in the left external iliac artery (Fig. 20–27). The obstructive lesion in the left femoropopliteal outflow system consisted of totally occluded superficial femoral and proximal popliteal arterial segments (Fig. 20–28A). There were no obstructive lesions in the tibioperoneal run-off system below the knee (Fig. 20–28B). Angioplasty was used to dilate the iliac artery stenosis prior to a femoropopliteal surgical bypass graft procedure. The pre-angioplasty assessment in Figure 20–26 showed (1) ankle/brachial index of 0.36; (2) damped Doppler velocity waveforms from the femoral, popliteal, and posterior tibial arteries; and (3) low-segment limb pressures with significant pressure drops between the high-thigh,

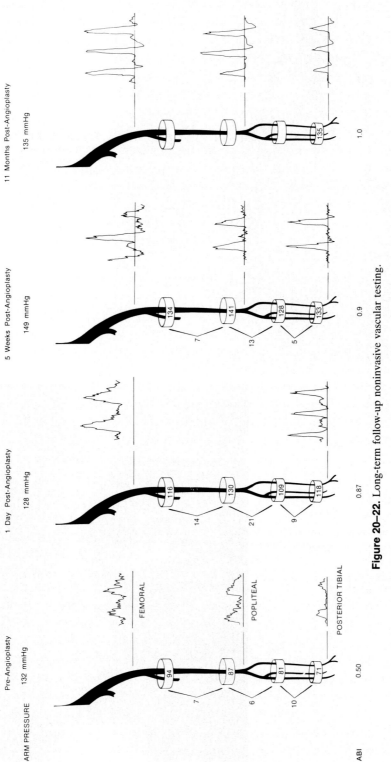

Figure 20–22. Long-term follow-up noninvasive vascular testing.

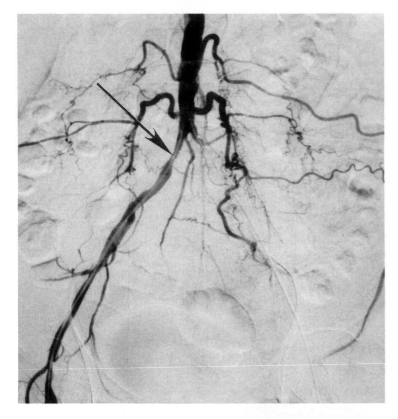

Figure 20–23. Pre-treatment arteriogram showing total left iliac system occlusion and right common iliac artery stenosis (arrow).

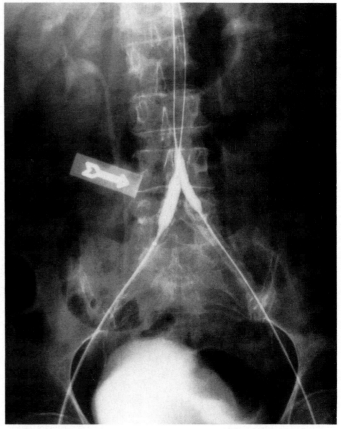

Figure 20–24. Balloon catheters (arrow) used to dilate common iliac arteries.

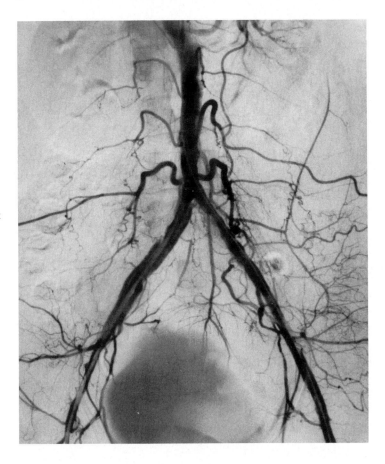

Figure 20–25. Iliac arterial systems patent post-therapy.

above-knee, and below-knee cuffs. Follow-up studies performed 21 and 27 days after the angioplasty procedure showed no improvement when compared with the pre-angioplasty evaluation.

Due to the presence of the occluded superficial femoral artery and proximal popliteal arterial segment, it is difficult to evaluate the hemodynamic results of the iliac angioplasty procedure for the following reasons:

1. An obstruction of either or both the superficial femoral and deep femoral arteries will damp the Doppler velocity waveforms from the common femoral artery above and the popliteal and posterior tibial arteries below the level of the obstruction.

2. Obstructions of the superficial femoral artery and proximal popliteal arterial segment will lower the ankle/brachial index and segmental limb pressures and will cause a pressure drop between the high-thigh, above-knee, and below-knee cuffs.

Thus, eliminating the iliac artery stenosis may not be reflected in improved noninvasive test results as long as the other obstructions exist in the arterial system. For this reason, the actual intra-arterial measurement of the pressure drop across a lesion before and after it has been dilated remains the most accurate method of assessing its hemodynamic significance when other obstructions exist in the arterial system. The methods for this type of pressure drop assessment are given in Figures 20–12 and 20–13. Without these pressure measurements, it is difficult to know whether or not the angioplasty eliminated the pressure drop across the iliac artery stenosis prior to the femoropopliteal artery bypass surgical procedure. This is important, because if the pressure drop across the iliac artery stenosis is not eliminated, the blood flow through the iliac artery stenosis may not be adequate enough to keep the femoropopliteal bypass graft open, thus resulting in its occlusion.

Noninvasive testing after femoropopliteal bypass surgery of the patient in Figure 20–26 showed marked improvement of the common femoral artery Doppler velocity waveform as compared with the pre-surgical evaluations. The high-thigh segmental limb pressures increased from 106 to 140 mm Hg, and the ankle/brachial index increased from 0.36 to 0.75. A normal

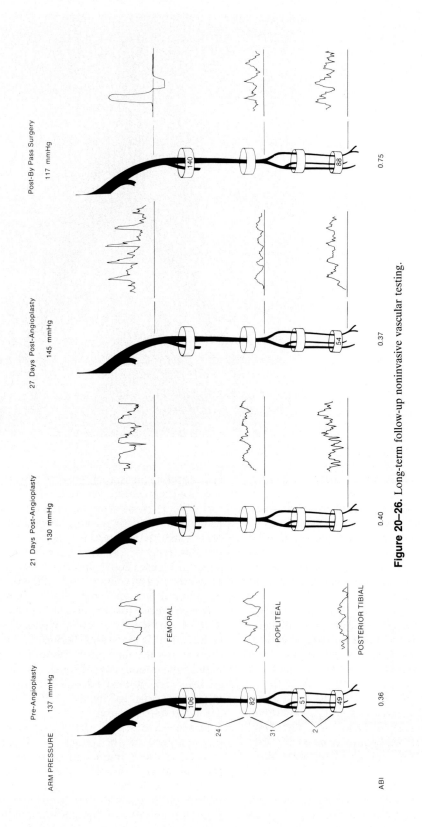

Figure 20–26. Long-term follow-up noninvasive vascular testing.

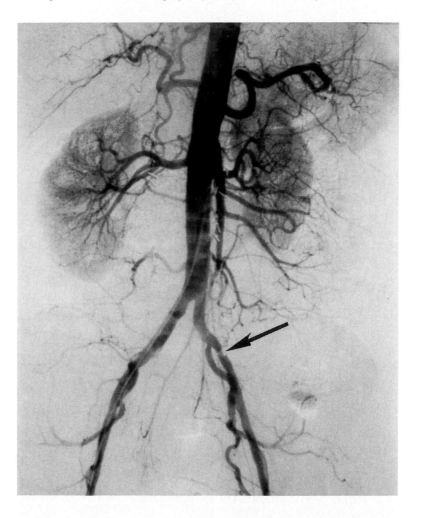

Figure 20–27. Pre-angioplasty arteriogram of left external iliac artery stenosis (arrow).

high-thigh systolic pressure in this patient at the time of the post-bypass evaluation (Figure 20–26) should be 147 mm Hg (i.e., brachial arm pressure + 30 = 147). The normal-appearing triphasic femoral artery Doppler velocity waveform and the high-thigh pressure of 140 mm Hg are good indicators that blood flow through the dilated iliac artery stenosis is adequate to keep the bypass graft open. However, the Doppler velocity waveforms below the level of the femoropopliteal bypass graft remain damped (Fig. 20–26). This, together with the ankle systolic pressure of 88 mm Hg and an ankle/brachial index of 0.75, indicates obstruction at the site of the femoropopliteal bypass graft. The graft eventually became occluded, as shown in Figure 20–29. Arteriograms performed to show the graft occlusion also revealed the site of the previously dilated iliac artery stenosis to be widely patent (Fig. 20–30).

In summary, this case is presented to illustrate several points. First, it is difficult to evaluate the hemodynamic improvement resulting from an iliac artery angioplasty by noninvasive vascular testing when other obstructive lesions exist in the lower extremity arterial circulation. Second, the hemodynamic improvement of an iliac artery angioplasty can be determined by noninvasive vascular testing when the lower extremity arterial obstruction is relieved by surgical bypass graft procedures. Third, early developing obstructions of the surgical bypass graft site can be distinguished from obstructions developing at the site of a previously dilated iliac artery stenosis. However, when the graft becomes totally occluded, the hemodynamics of the lower extremity change drastically, as shown in Figure 20–31. The Doppler velocity waveforms in Figure 20–31 resemble those seen in the pre-angioplasty assessment in Figure 20–22. The femoral artery waveforms and

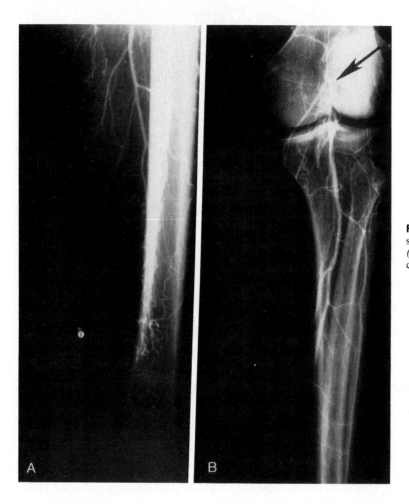

Figure 20–28. Arteriograms showing superficial femoral artery occlusion *(A)* and proximal popliteal artery occlusion (arrow) *(B)*.

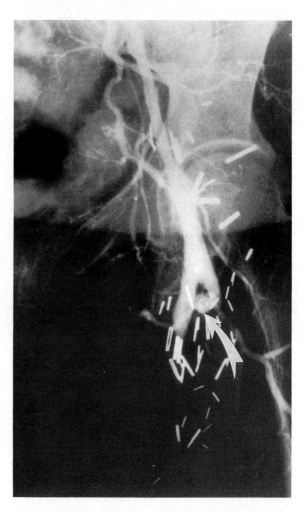

Figure 20–29. Arteriogram showing occluded femoro-popliteal artery bypass graft (arrow).

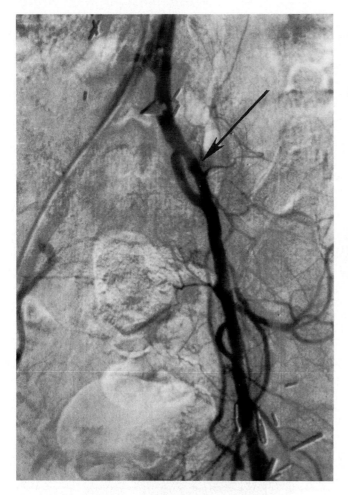

Figure 20–30. Follow-up arteriogram showing patency of iliac artery at site of previous stenosis angioplasty (arrow).

high-thigh pressures become abnormal again, making it impossible to distinguish an occluded graft from an occlusion at the site of the iliac artery angioplasty under these circumstances.

The patient whose arteriograms are shown in Figure 20–32 was treated with fibrinolytic therapy for thromboembolic occlusions of the origins of the anterior and posterior tibial arteries (Fig. 20–32A). Figure 20–32A shows the catheter tip positioned at this site. Continuous digital PPG waveforms were used to monitor the pulsatile blood flow in the left great toe during the infusion of the fibrinolytic agent. The pre-infusion damped waveforms are shown in Figure 20–33A. These can be compared with those obtained after 3 hours of infusion treatment (Fig. 20–33B). This comparison shows that the fibrinolytic agent has opened up the occlusion site, as indicated by the increase in the pulsatile blood flow waveforms obtained from the left great toe. Based upon this

finding, the fibrinolytic agent infusion was discontinued and angiograms were re-taken to evaluate the occlusion site. As shown in Figure 20–32B, the thrombus is lysed and the origins of both the anterior and posterior tibial arteries are open.

Follow-up noninvasive vascular testing was used in this patient to evaluate the continued patency of the previously occluded tibial artery segments. The results of the baseline pre-infusion studies are given in Figure 20–34A. These studies showed the following results:

1. Damped posterior tibial artery Doppler velocity waveforms below the occlusion site.

2. Segmental limb pressure drop of 47 mm Hg between the above-knee and ankle cuffs.

3. Ankle/brachial index of 0.70.

Comparison of the waveforms from the popliteal artery with those from the posterior tibial artery shows the damping effect on the Doppler

GRAFT OCCLUSION

6 MONTHS POST BYPASS

ARM PRESSURE: 126 mmHg

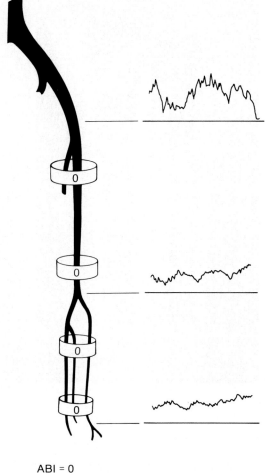

Figure 20–31. Doppler velocity waveforms and segmental limb pressure measurements of left lower extremity with occluded femoropopliteal artery bypass graft. Note that the damped femoral artery waveforms resemble those seen on the pre-angioplasty examination in Figure 20–22.

ABI = 0
TBI = 0.26

velocity waveforms created by the occlusion in the proximal tibial vessels. The waveforms from the popliteal artery are triphasic, whereas those from the posterior tibial artery are damped and monophasic. A systolic pressure of 115 mm Hg was recorded from the popliteal artery when the above-knee (AK) cuff was deflated, and a pressure of only 68 mm Hg was recorded from the tibial vessels when the ankle cuff was deflated. This pressure drop of 47 mm Hg indicated an occlusion site located in the proximal tibial vessels.

The immediate follow-up noninvasive test performed 1 day after infusion (Fig. 20–34B) shows that the Doppler velocity waveforms from the posterior tibial artery are now triphasic. Compare these waveforms with the monophasic ones ob-

tained from the posterior tibial artery on the pre-infusion evaluation in Figure 20–34A. This comparison shows that the previously noted damping effect caused by the proximal tibial artery occlusions is now absent. The segmental limb pressures also reflect a resolution of the obstructing process. A systolic pressure of 120 mm Hg is recorded from the popliteal artery when the AK cuff is deflated, and a pressure of 96 mm Hg was recorded from the tibial vessel when the ankle cuff was deflated. The pressure drop between these two cuff levels is only 24 mm Hg. This represents considerable improvement from the previously recorded pre-infusion pressure drop of 47 mm Hg across these cuff levels. The ankle/brachial index also increased from 0.70 to 0.96.

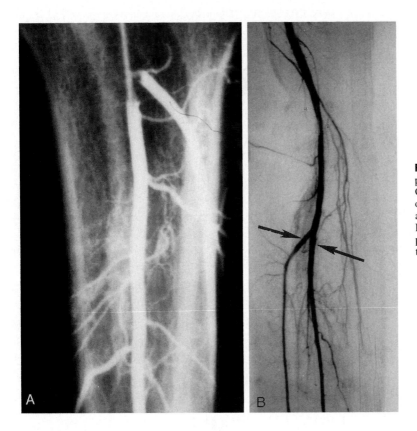

Figure 20–32. Pre-infusion and post-infusion arteriograms. *A,* Catheter tip positioned in thrombus occlusion at origins of the anterior and posterior tibial arteries. *B,* Post-infusion arteriogram showing patency of anterior and posterior tibial artery origins (arrows).

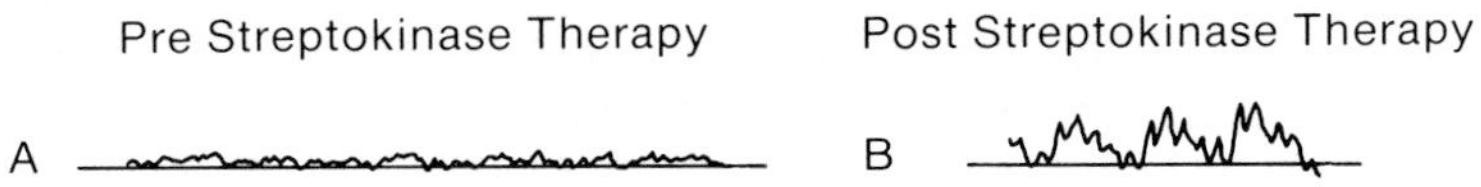

Figure 20–33. Pre-infusion digital photoplethysmographic waveforms are damped *(A)*; post-infusion waveforms show increased pulsatile blood flow *(B)*.

Pre Streptokinase Therapy

Post Streptokinase Therapy

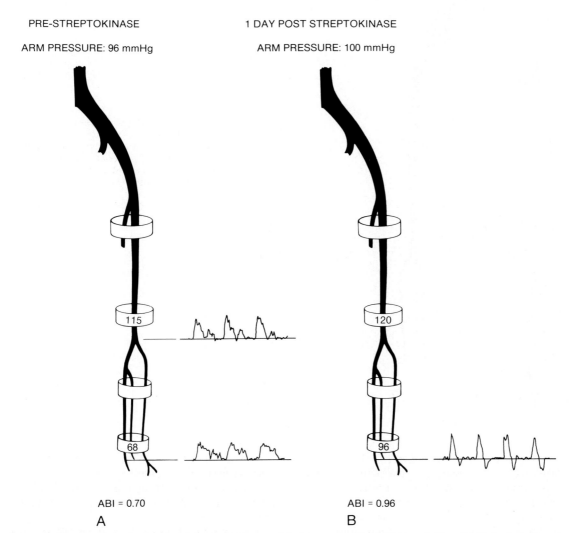

PRE-STREPTOKINASE

ARM PRESSURE: 96 mmHg

1 DAY POST STREPTOKINASE

ARM PRESSURE: 100 mmHg

115

68

ABI = 0.70

A

120

96

ABI = 0.96

B

Figure 20–34. Doppler velocity waveforms and segmental limb pressures before *(A)* and after *(B)* fibrinolytic therapy. *A,* Pre-infusion: Damped, monophasic waveforms in posterior tibial artery and pressure drop of 47 mm Hg between above-knee and ankle cuff levels. *B,* Post-infusion: Triphasic waveforms in posterior tibial artery and pressure drop decreased to 24 mm Hg between above-knee and ankle cuff levels.

4 MONTHS POST-STREPTOKINASE

ARM PRESSURE: 135 mmHg

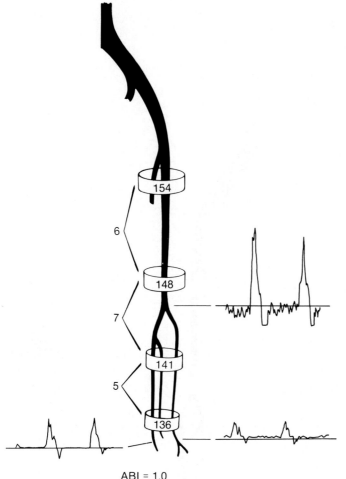

ABI = 1.0

Figure 20–35. Doppler velocity waveforms and segmental limb pressures 4 months after infusion show triphasic waveforms in popliteal, anterior, and posterior tibial arteries. No significant pressure drop exists between any of the segmental cuff levels.

Because the findings from these studies showed considerable improvement in the hemodynamics of the lower extremity, this currently asymptomatic patient was discharged from the hospital to be followed up in the noninvasive vascular laboratory. These follow-up examinations were used to observe the status of the previously occluded tibial artery segments as well as to check for evidence of recurrent embolic arterial occlusions. The test results from a 4-month follow-up evaluation are shown in Figure 20–35. These were interpreted as follows:

1. Triphasic Doppler velocity waveforms from the popliteal, anterior, and posterior tibial arteries.

2. No significant pressure drops between the segmental limb pressure measurements.

3. Normal ankle/brachial index of 1.0 before exercise and after exercise.

The results of these noninvasive tests indicate absence of obstructive disease in the lower extremity vessels.

In summary, this case was presented to illustrate several points. First, continuous digital PPG waveform analysis may be used to monitor the results of fibrinolytic agents during their infusion. Second, continuous digital PPG waveform analysis may also be used during the course of the infusion to determine when repeat arteriography should be used to thoroughly examine the patency of the vessels. Third, as with angioplasty procedures, noninvasive testing can be used to follow up patients after treatment with fibrinolytic agents.

21 • Toe Pressures and Digital Photoplethysmography

Introduction

Toe pressure measurements and photoplethysmographic (PPG) waveform analysis provide important information about blood flow distal to the ankle.[1, 2] How these procedures are used in the initial evaluation and follow-up of patients with peripheral vascular disease will be illustrated throughout this chapter by case presentations. Angiograms are included so that the anatomy of the obstructive arterial lesions can be correlated with the results of the noninvasive procedures.

Toe Pressure Measurement Techniques

Several methods are available for measuring toe pressures. A Doppler probe,[3] a strain gauge plethysmograph,[2, 4, 5] or a photoplethysmograph[6-10] is used to detect the pulse changes altered by an occlusion cuff placed around the toe. Of these, the photoplethysmograph is the most adaptable for routine use because it is simple to use, it is associated with fewer variables, and it provides the most consistently reproducible results.

Doppler Probe. The Doppler probe technique is hampered by the inability of the operator to hold the probe steadily at the proper angle on the digital artery while the cuff on the toe is being inflated and deflated.[10]

Strain Gauge Plethysmography. Strain gauge plethysmography may also be unacceptable because once the cuff is placed on the toe, there may be no room left to apply the strain gauge. As a result, the cuff often lies over the strain gauge, producing artifactual measurements. This does not occur with PPG because the photoelectric cell is placed on the tip of the toe, beyond the distal margin of the cuff. Since PPG is the most commonly used method for obtaining toe

pressures, the technique for its use will be described in further detail.

Photoplethysmography.[1] A small (2 to 3 cm wide) occlusion cuff is placed around the proximal phalanx of the great toe, as shown in Figure 21–1. The second and third toes may be used when the great toe is absent or severely ulcerated (Fig. 21–2). Toe pressure measurements from the fourth and fifth toes are avoided because these toes are too small to accommodate both the photoelectric cell and the cuff. Optimally, the proximal edge of the cuff should not be farther than 1 cm from the base of the toe. There is no significant difference in the toe pressure measurement when the proximal edge of the cuff is placed either at the base of the toe or 1 cm from the base of the toe. Air is pumped in and out of the cuff, and its pressure measured during total occlusion and re-opening of the digital arteries. The alterations in the digital artery pulses during the inflation and deflation of the cuff are detected by the photoelectric cell placed on the toe (Figs. 21–1 and 21–2). This photoelectric cell is attached to the skin surface over the plantar aspect of both the great toes with transparent, double-coated adhesive cellophane tape. A permanent record of the toe pressure measurements is made with a strip chart recorder. An example of this type of recording is given in Figure 21–3. The cuff pressures are recorded simultaneously with the pulse waveforms. Figure 21–3 shows that the pulses in the digital arteries of both toes disappear when the cuffs are inflated to a pressure of 100 mm Hg. Deflation of the cuffs results in re-appearance of the PPG pulse waveforms, as shown in Figure 21–3. The cuff pressures at the re-appearance point of the PPG waveforms represent the systolic pressure measurements of the toe. In this case, the values are 87 mm Hg for the right great toe and 99 mm Hg for the left great toe (Fig. 21–3).

Photoplethysmographic pulse waveforms may

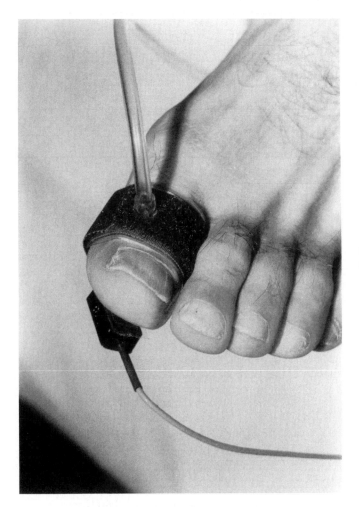

Figure 21–1. Pressure cuff and photocell on the great toe for pressure measurement.

Figure 21–2. Amputated great toe with pressure cuff and photocell placed on the second toe for toe pressure measurement.

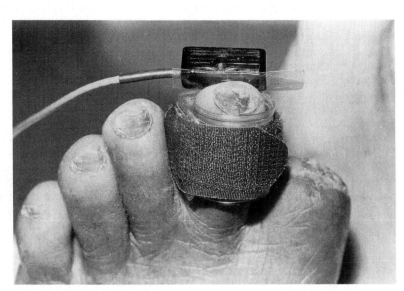

NORMAL BILATERAL TOE PRESSURES

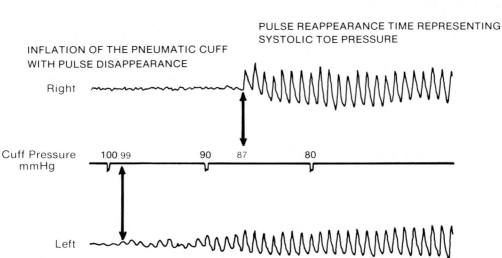

Figure 21–3. Photoplethysmography in alternating current (AC) mode. The re-appearance of pulse corresponds to toe systolic pressure (arrows). Right toe pressure is 87 mm Hg. Left toe pressure is 99 mm Hg.

be recorded from the toes by means of either the alternating current (AC) or direct current (DC) modes. The AC mode is used to detect the rapid movement of the red blood cells (RBCs) through the microvascular skin circulation during arterial pulsations. When the PPG measurements are unobtainable with the AC mode, the DC mode is used to detect the slow movement of the RBCs through the microvascular skin circulation, which occurs when the arterial pulsations are damped by severe obstructive vascular disease. Under these circumstances, the end point of the toe systolic pressure measurement is approximated by a sudden rise of the waveform on the tracing as blood enters the toe during deflation of the cuff. An example of this type of tracing is given in Figure 21–4.

Figure 21–4 shows that a sharp rise in the DC mode PPG waveform tracing occurred when the cuff pressure was deflated to 35 mm Hg. This indicates that the systolic pressure measurement in this toe is 35 mm Hg. The DC mode is then used to measure toe systolic pressures when they are extremely low. It is important to carry out these measurements with the patient comfortable in a warm room. Exposing the feet to the cool air from an air-conditioning duct, for example, may induce vasospasm, resulting in low toe pressure measurements that could be misinterpreted as an indication of organic occlusive disease.

TOE PRESSURE IN DC MODE DUE TO LOW FLOW STATUS

Figure 21–4. Photoplethysmography in direct current (DC) mode. A sharp rise in tracing corresponds to toe systolic pressure (arrow) of 35 mm Hg.

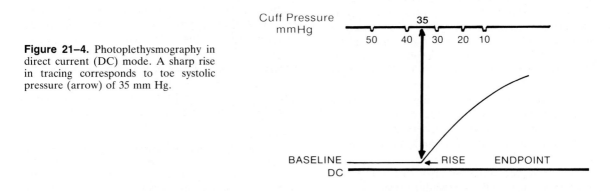

Normal and Abnormal Systolic Toe Pressure Measurements

Toe pressures are normally lower than those found in either the brachial arteries of the arms or the tibial arteries of the ankles. One explanation for this is that the high resistance created by the small digital arteries damps the pressure wave as it travels down the aorta towards the toes. This damping causes a progressive drop in the pressure energy used to propel the blood flow through the legs, ankles, feet, and into the toes.[10, 11]

Two toe pressure measurements use the ankle pressure as a reference point. These are the toe/ankle index (TAI) and the ankle–toe difference (ATD). Barnes reports that a normal toe pressure should be 60% of the ankle pressure or greater.[12] Therefore, the toe/ankle index should equal 0.60 or greater. Mathematically, the normal toe pressure and the TAI may be expressed as follows:

$$\text{toe pressure} = 0.60 \times \text{ankle pressure}$$

or

$$\text{TAI} = \frac{\text{toe pressure}}{\text{ankle pressure}} = 0.60$$

It is interesting to note the effect of ankle pressure in these equations. Increasing the ankle pressure raises the limit of the normal value for the toe pressure measurement while it decreases the toe/ankle index.

The ATD is the difference between the ipsilateral systolic ankle and toe pressures. This difference should not exceed 70 mm Hg.[11] An abnormally high ATD (greater than 70 mm Hg) suggests an obstruction located in either or in both the plantar arch and digital arteries. We have encountered some problems when ankle pressure was used as a reference point in diabetic patients with peripheral vascular disease. These patients may have medial arterial wall calcific disease, rendering the tibial arteries totally incompressible or extremely difficult to compress with the occlusion cuff. Total noncompressibility of the tibial arteries makes it impossible to obtain the ankle pressure measurement in these patients. Tibial arteries that are difficult to compress often lead to distortedly high ankle pressure measurements when they are obtained by the occlusion cuff technique. This could cause discrepancies in both the TAI and ATD measurements.

For example, a patient with distortedly high ankle pressures and normal toe pressures could show an ATD >70 mm Hg, giving the false impression that obstructive disease exists in the foot or toe vessels. Furthermore, in patients with systemic hypertension but without peripheral vascular disease, the ATD may be >70 mm Hg.[11] Therefore, an ATD >70 mm Hg may not indicate arterial obstruction in the presence of either or both diabetes and systemic hypertension. This becomes a problem because both these conditions may coexist in the same patient and these patients are often referred to the noninvasive vascular laboratory for the evaluation of peripheral vascular disease.

To avoid this problem, the toe pressure may be expressed as a percentage of the highest brachial artery pressure. The rationale for using the brachial artery as a reference point is that it is less frequently involved with medial arterial wall calcifications than are the arteries of the lower extremities. Normal systolic toe pressures are approximately 80 to 90% of the highest brachial artery systolic pressure (e.g., toe/brachial index [TBI] = 0.80 to 0.90).[1] The toe/brachial index, then, offers a method for obtaining consistency in the toe pressure measurement when it is used to follow patients for either the progression or the regression of peripheral vascular disease.

Toe pressures, not expressed as either the toe/ankle index or the toe/brachial index, have also been used in the evaluation of peripheral vascular disease. Sumner, using the PPG technique to measure the toe pressures in 200 patients with arterial disease, found that in those patients with no symptoms the toe pressure measurements were 90 to 100 mm Hg.[13] Pressure measurements averaged about 20 mm Hg when the feet were ischemic. There was little difference between the toe pressures of diabetics and nondiabetics. This point is significant because the ankle pressures are often quite different in these two groups of patients. Nielsen and colleagues observed that the normal toe pressures in supine young individuals averaged 4.8 mm Hg (plus or minus 6.6) below the brachial arm pressure.[5] In older individuals, the toe pressures were 9.8 mm Hg (plus or minus 10.7) below the brachial arm pressures.

This review of the normal and abnormal toe pressure measurements offers some guidelines to be used in the evaluation and follow-up of patients with peripheral vascular disease, as illustrated in the following cases.

Case I

A middle-aged diabetic woman with systemic hypertension presented with symptoms of intermittent right lower extremity claudication. The results of noninvasive vascular testing are shown in Figure 21–5. These can be correlated with the angiograms in Figures 21–6 and 21–7.

The strip chart recording in Figure 21–5 was interpreted as showing a right great toe pressure of 82 mm Hg and a left great toe pressure of 114 mm Hg. Both the toe/ankle indices and the ATDs are normal, which suggests absence of obstructive disease in the foot and toe vessels. The toe/brachial indices are abnormal bilaterally with more obstructive disease in the right lower extremity than the left. This is also demonstrated by comparing the right and left toe pressure measurements with the ankle/brachial indices. According to the values established by Nielsen and colleagues, both toe pressure measurements are abnormally low. Applying their values to this particular case shows that the toe pressures should not be lower than 148 mm Hg (brachial arm pressure = 169 − [9.8 ± 10.7] = 148 mm Hg). It is also interesting to note that the toe pressure of 82 mm Hg in the symptomatic right lower extremity falls below the 90 to 100 mm Hg toe pressure levels observed by Sumner in asymptomatic patients with peripheral vascular disease.[13]

In summary, the noninvasive test results in Figure 21–5 indicate bilateral lower extremity arterial obstructive disease, which is located proximal to the foot and toe vessels. The disease is more severe on the right. The correlative angiograms in Figures 21–6 and 21–7 show two obstructive lesions in the right femoropopliteal outflow system, whereas the condition of the left is essentially normal. Evaluation of the right tibioperoneal run-off system shows extension of the popliteal artery obstructive disease process into both the anterior tibial and peroneal arteries and total occlusion of the right posterior tibial artery. The left tibioperoneal run-off system shows total posterior tibial artery occlusion, segmental anterior tibial artery occlusion, and patency of the peroneal artery.

Case II

Percutaneous transluminal angioplasty was used to manage the extensive peripheral vascular disease present. A hypertensive middle-aged diabetic woman presented with a nonhealing ulcer on the dorsum of her right foot and with symptoms of right lower-extremity intermittent claudication. The pertinent results from the initial pre-angioplasty noninvasive vascular test are given in Figure 21–8. These consist of Doppler velocity waveforms, systolic toe pressure measurements, and toe/brachial indices. No segmental Doppler pressures are presented because the arteries are so rigid that they could not be occluded by the cuffs placed at the high-thigh, above-knee, below-knee, and ankle levels.

Noncompressibility of the lower extremity arteries is seen in patients with arterial wall calcifications caused by diabetes, chronic corticosteroid therapy, renal dialysis, and renal transplantation.[13] Because these rigid arteries cannot be adequately compressed by the segmental occlusion cuffs, both the segmental Doppler pressure measurements and the ankle/brachial indices may be artifactually abnormal or impossible to obtain in these patients. This problem was encountered during the noninvasive vascular examination of this patient.

Toe pressure measurements offer a solution to this problem because the small digital arteries of the toes are not generally as extensively affected by the disease

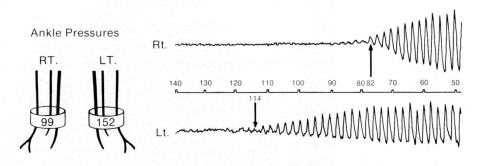

Pressures & Indexes	Right	Left	Normal Values	
Toe Pressures	82	114	< 9.8 ± 10.7 below brachial pressure	(10)
Toe/Ankle Index	0.83	0.75	0.60 or greater	(12)
Toe/Brachial Index	0.48	0.67	0.80 - 0.90	(1)
Ankle-Toe Difference	17	55	< 70	(11)
Ankle/Brachial Index	0.58	0.90	1 or greater	

Figure 21–5. *Case I.* Arterial obstructive disease. Noninvasive vascular test results.

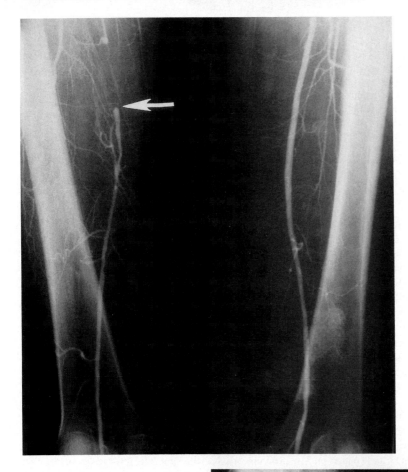

Figure 21–6. *Case 1.* Arterial obstructive disease. Arteriogram of right superficial femoral artery occlusion site (arrow).

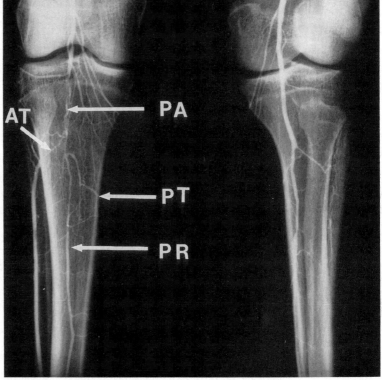

Figure 21–7. *Case 1.* Arteriogram of right popliteal artery (PA) obstructive disease extending into the anterior tibial (AT) and peroneal arteries (PR). Both posterior tibial (PT) arteries are occluded. Segmental left anterior tibial artery occlusions with patency of the left peroneal artery are shown.

process as are the larger arteries of the thighs and legs. As shown in Figure 21–8, the initial pre-angioplasty right great toe pressure was 62 mm Hg (38% of brachial arm pressure) with a toe/brachial index of 0.38. This is considerably less than the 80 to 90% of the brachial pressure levels proposed by Carter and Lezack.[1] It is also lower than the normal values established by Sumner[13] and Nielsen and colleagues.[5] Carter and Lezack reported that the systolic toe pressures averaged 62 mm Hg and 43% of the brachial systolic pressure in their patients with intermittent claudication secondary to arteriosclerosis obliterans.[1] The right great toe pressure in this case is abnormally low and coincides with the pressure measurements previously reported in patients with intermittent claudication.

Because the segmental Doppler pressures could not be obtained in this case, Doppler velocity waveforms were used to determine the locations of the arterial obstructions. A distinct difference between the common femoral and popliteal artery waveforms can be seen (Figure 21–8). Those from the common femoral artery are multiphasic with a high amplitude; those from the popliteal artery are monophasic with a low amplitude. The differences between these two waveforms indicate obstructive disease in the femoropopliteal outflow system. The correlative arteriograms in Figures 21–9 and 21–10 show the anatomy and sites of the arterial obstructions. These consist of stenoses located in the profunda femoral (Fig. 21–9A) and superficial femoral arteries (Fig. 21–10A).

Doppler velocity waveforms from the posterior tibial arteries are also abnormal. The waveforms are wide with damped, rounded systolic peaks at low amplitude. A comparison between the posterior tibial and popliteal artery waveforms indicates that additional obstructive disease is present in the tibioperoneal run-off system. The site and anatomy of the obstructive lesions in this system are shown in Figure 21–11. There is no proximal opacification of either the posterior tibial or peroneal arteries (Fig. 21–11A) because the posterior tibioperoneal trunk is totally occluded at its origin from the popliteal artery. The anterior tibial artery is now the main vessel supplying the leg, ankle, foot, and toes with blood. The artery also supplies the anastomotic collateral network at the ankle. The distal portions of the posterior tibial and peroneal arteries are opacified by the retrograde flow of blood from these anastomotic ankle collaterals (Fig. 21–11B).

Increasing blood flow through the anterior tibial artery should permit more blood to flow through the collateral network into the peroneal and posterior tibial arteries. It should also increase the blood flow through the vessels in the foot and toes. As seen on the arteriograms, the inflow of blood into the anterior tibial artery is limited by the stenoses in the profunda femoral and superficial femoral arteries. Opening these stenoses should then increase the inflow of blood into the leg, ankle, foot, and toes through the anterior tibial artery.

Percutaneous transluminal angioplasty was used to

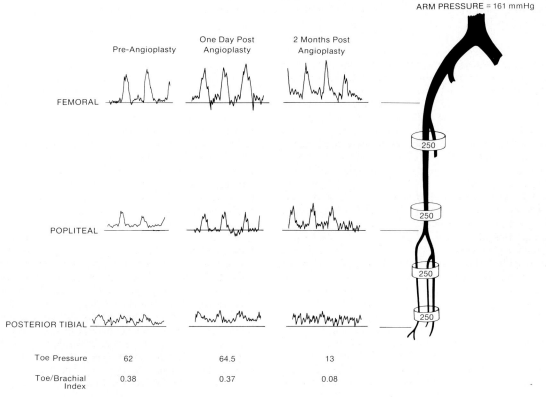

Figure 21–8. *Case II.* Noninvasive vascular test results.

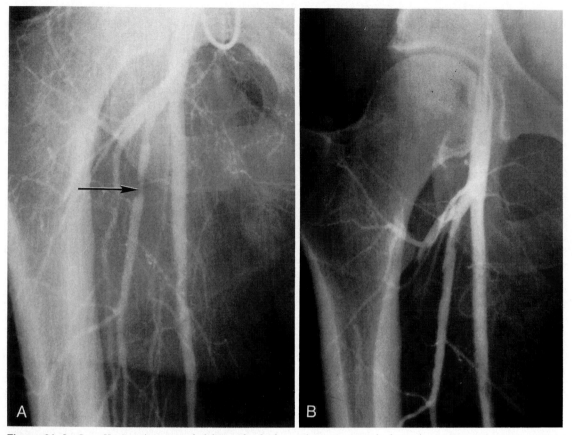

Figure 21–9. *Case II.* Arteriograms of right profunda femoral artery stenosis (arrow). *A*, Pre-angioplasty. *B*, Post-angioplasty.

open the stenoses, and noninvasive vascular testing was used to monitor the results of the procedure. Anatomically, the angioplasty procedure was successful because it dilated the stenoses, as shown on the arteriograms in Figures 21–9*B* and 21–10*B*. Although it is important to observe the anatomical result of the procedure, it is more important to observe its hemodynamic results. This was accomplished with Doppler velocity waveforms, toe pressure measurements, and the toe/brachial index.

For the angioplasty procedure to be hemodynamically successful, it must increase the blood flow from the femoropopliteal outflow system into the tibioperoneal run-off system. An increase in this blood flow would then be indicated by an increase in the amplitude of Doppler velocity waveforms of the popliteal artery, which closely approximate those seen in the common femoral artery. Increased blood flow should also improve the posterior tibial artery Doppler velocity waveform, toe systolic pressure measurement, and the toe/brachial index. Unfortunately, the angioplasty procedure was unsuccessful in correcting any of these parameters, as shown by the results of the noninvasive test done 1 day after angioplasty (Fig. 21–8). The Doppler velocity waveforms from both the popliteal artery and

the posterior tibial artery remain abnormal, and the toe pressure and toe/brachial index remain depressed.

This case example illustrates how noninvasive vascular testing may be used to monitor the hemodynamic success or failure of an angioplasty procedure in a patient with severe peripheral vascular disease. It also illustrates how these tests may be used to follow the progression of the obstructive arterial disease process. This is shown by the noninvasive test results obtained 2 months after the angioplasty procedure. The 2-month follow-up examination reveals a further deterioration in the posterior tibial artery Doppler velocity waveforms, toe pressure measurement, and toe/brachial index. In fact, the toe pressure of 13 mm Hg means that the foot is ischemic and offers a poor prognosis for healing of the foot ulcer and limb salvage in this patient. Paaske and Tonnesen reported that the prognosis for limb salvage was poor when the toe pressure was less than 8% of the brachial pressure.[14] The toe pressure in this case is only slightly above this reported figure. Eight percent of the highest brachial arm pressure at the time of the examination equalled 12 mm Hg (8% of 152 mm Hg). The actual toe pressure measurement in this case was 13 mm Hg. It is also known that only 34% of the foot lesions heal spontaneously when the toe pressure is less than 30 mm Hg, whereas 91% of lesions heal spontaneously when the toe pressures are greater than 30 mm Hg.[15]

Why the toe pressure measurements declined from 64.5 mm Hg to 13 mm Hg 2 months after the angioplasty procedure was of considerable concern. Of particular concern was whether or not the angioplasty procedure had resulted in a thrombosis of either or both the profunda femoral and superficial femoral arteries. An occlusion of either one of these vessels, in this already compromised lower extremity, would certainly cause a drop in the toe pressure measurements. A review of the noninvasive test results (Fig. 21–8) shows that this did not occur. There is no change between the common femoral and popliteal artery Doppler velocity waveforms made 1 day after the angioplasty procedure and those made 2 months after the procedure. The correlative arteriograms made 2 months after the angioplasty procedure support these findings because both the profunda femoral and superficial femoral arteries are patent (Fig. 21–12). There was also no change in the arteriographic appearance of the anterior tibial artery over the 2-month interval. It must be speculated, then, that the drop in the toe pressure measurement was caused by a progression of the obstructive disease process at the ankle, foot, and toe level vessels. The ankle toe difference pressure measurements would have been helpful in confirming this suspicion. Unfortunately, because of noncompressibility of these rigid, diseased vessels, no ankle pressure measurements could be made in this patient.

In summary, toe pressure measurements offer a means of detecting lower extremity vascular insufficiency, as illustrated in *Cases I and II*. Carter and Hamel found a good correlation between the toe pressures and angiographic findings.[11] Toe pressures were abnormal in 97% of the extremities with complete arterial obstructions and in 74% of the extremities with arterial stenoses.

The success of toe or transmetatarsal amputation and healing of the foot lesion can also be predicted by toe pressures. The clinical findings of the skin condition and temperature, pulse level, and operative wound bleeding have been found to be associated with an error rate of 18 to 46%.[16–19] Raines and colleagues utilized ankle

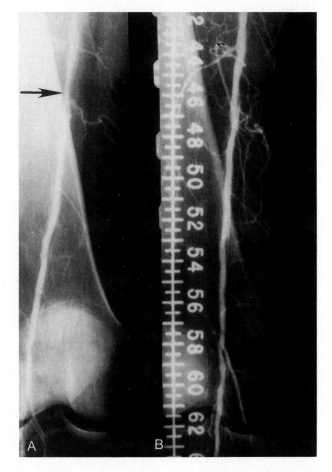

Figure 21–10. *Case II*. Arteriograms of right superficial femoral artery stenosis (arrow). *A*, Pre-angioplasty. *B*, Post-angioplasty.

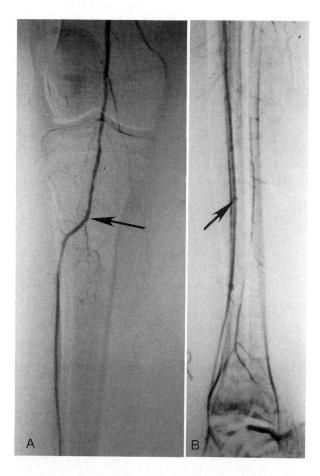

Figure 21–11. *Case II.* Arteriograms. *A*, Posterior tibioperoneal trunk occluded at its origin (arrow) from the popliteal artery. The anterior tibial artery is patent. *B*, Retrograde blood flow fills the peroneal and posterior tibial arteries through collateral anastomoses at the ankle. These collaterals are supplied with blood from the patent anterior tibial artery (arrow).

pressures to predict the healing of foot lesions.[20] According to Raines, the healing of foot lesions was unlikely when an ankle pressure was less than 80 mm Hg in diabetic subjects and less than 55 mm Hg in nondiabetics. In a series by Ramsey and colleagues, only 55% of the lesions healed when the ankle pressure was greater than 80 mm Hg.[7] Thus, a high ankle pressure is not reliable for predicting healing of these lesions; however, low ankle pressure is associated with a grave prognosis. The reason why high ankle pressure is not reliable is because it can be falsely elevated in the presence of rigid or calcified arterial walls, which are often present in these patients.

Both Holpstein[15] and Sumner[13] found the toe pressure to be more reliable than the ankle pressure for determining the success of an amputation and the healing of foot lesions. Foot lesions failed to heal in 66 to 95% of cases when the toe pressure was less than 30 mm Hg. Ulcers healed better (86 to 91%) when the toe pressure was higher than 30 mm Hg. Toe pressure measurements are more reliable than ankle pressures because the measurement location is adjacent to the amputation site.

Digital Photoplethysmographic Waveform Analysis

Instrumentation for digital photoplethysmography consists of a photocell, an amplifier, and a strip chart recorder. This is the same instrumentation used for obtaining the toe systolic pressure measurements. As described previously, the appearance of a waveform following the deflation of an occlusion cuff placed around the toe indicates the systolic pressure in that toe. Once the toe pressure measurement is made, the waveform itself may also be analyzed for the presence or absence of obstructive peripheral vascular disease. Figure 21–1 shows how the PPG photocell is attached to the toe in order to obtain these waveforms. Most PPG photocells consist of two components. These are an infrared light-emitting diode and an infrared light-receiving photosensor. An example of a typical PPG photocell is shown in Figure 21–13. Infrared light is emitted into the skin, where a portion of it is reflected back towards the infrared light-receiving photosensor. Blood reflects more light back to the photosensor than does the surrounding tissue.

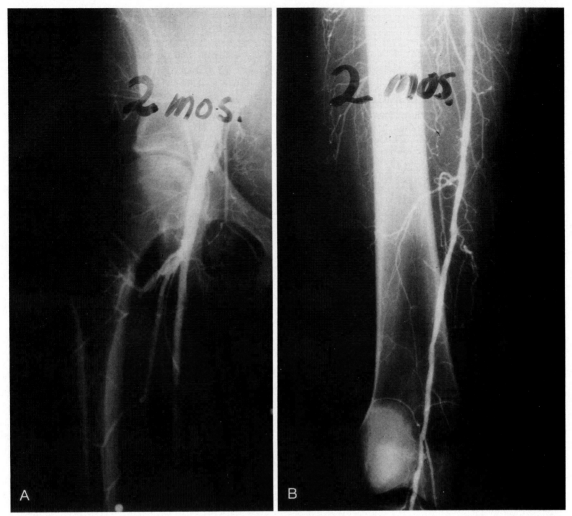

Figure 21–12. *Case II*. Profunda femoral *(A)* and superficial femoral *(B)* arteries are patent on 2-month post-angioplasty follow-up arteriogram.

Figure 21–13. Photoplethysmographic transducer. *1*, Infrared light-emitting diode. *2*, Infrared light-receiving photosensor.

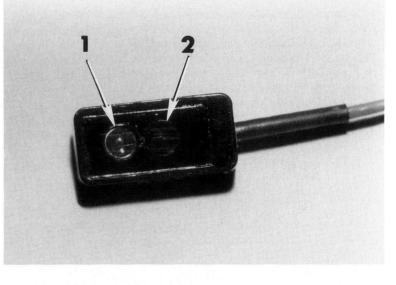

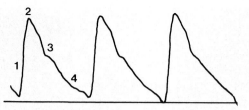

Figure 21–14. Normal photoplethysmography digital pulse waveform. *1*, Steep systolic upslope. *2*, Narrow systolic peak. *3*, Dicrotic notch on diastolic downslope. *4*, Diastolic downslope is concave towards baseline.

This occurs because blood is more opaque to red and near-infrared light than are the surrounding tissues. The amount of light reflected back towards the photosensor is proportional to the amount of blood in the microvascular skin circulation. Because the amount of blood in the skin microvasculature changes rapidly with each phase of the cardiac cycle, the light is reflected back towards the photosensor in a pulsatile manner.

Light pulses received by the photosensor may be amplified in either the AC or DC mode. The AC mode is used to detect rapidly changing blood content in the skin microvasculature, whereas the DC mode is used to detect slowly changing blood content in the skin microvasculature. This explains why the arterial toe pulsations are amplified in the AC mode and venous filling or emptying of the skin microvasculature is amplified in the DC mode. Extremely poor arterial perfusion of the toe may also be evaluated by DC mode amplification. This is used when systolic toe pressures cannot be obtained in the AC mode by the methods described previously. DC mode amplification is used, in these circumstances, in an attempt to obtain a systolic toe pressure measurement. It is not used to obtain the PPG waveform.

Once the light pulses are processed by AC mode amplification, they are sent to the strip chart recorder, where a graphic output of the PPG waveforms is produced, like the ones shown in Figures 21–14 and 21–15. A comparison between these two figures shows the waveforms to be quite different. The one in Figure 21–14 is characteristic of a normal, nonobstructive digital PPG waveform pattern; the one in Figure 21–15

is characteristic of an abnormal, obstructive waveform pattern. How these waveforms are generated is of considerable importance in analyzing their configurations. This is described in detail in Chapter 16, "Hemodynamic Arterial Anatomy of the Lower Extremity." However, because it is important, the method by which pulse waves are generated will be briefly reviewed in this chapter. In this review, a distinction must be made between the generation and the detection of the pulse waveform. Pulsatile waveforms are generated by the pumping action of the heart. They are detected by Doppler probes and photoelectric cells placed over the arteries under investigation. Doppler probes measure the velocities of RBC movement, whereas photoelectric cells measure the density of RBCs in a given circulation. Because the Doppler shift principle has been explained in Chapter 1, it will not be described here. Instead, how the photoelectric cell detects the pulsatile waves generated by the pumping action of the heart will be explored.

The digital PPG waveform in Figure 21–14 represents a graphic display of the pulsatile blood flow through the microvascular circulation in the skin over the toe. To understand each of the components of this waveform, the arterial tree should be considered as a vast network of liquid-filled elastic tubes that are set into motion by each heart beat. When the left ventricle contracts during systole, it ejects even more blood volume into the proximal aortic root segment, which is already filled with blood. Blood entering the proximal aortic root segment pushes the blood already present in this segment ahead of it in a forward direction down into the descending aorta and out into the peripheral arteries of the lower extremities. This, in turn, pushes more blood into the digital arteries and out into the skin microvasculature of the toes. The elastic arterial walls of the skin microvasculature become distended as the increased blood volume enters them during systole. This occurs because the increased blood volume entering the digital arteries during systole cannot immediately flow out into the venous circulation because of the resistance created by the arterioles. The arteries of the skin microvasculature then become high-pressure storage reservoirs filled with the in-

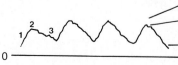

LOSS OF NARROW PEAK
REDUCTION OF AMPLITUDE
ROUNDING OF THE WAVEFORM
LOSS OF DICROTIC NOTCH

Figure 21–15. Abnormal photoplethysmography digital pulse waveform (DPW) with moderate occlusive disease. *1*, Gradual ascent of systolic upslope. *2*, Broad systolic peak. *3*, Gradual descent of diastolic downslope; the dicrotic notch is absent.

creased blood volume pumped into them during systole.

This increase in blood volume and RBCs causes more light to be reflected back towards the photosensor cell, which is recorded as a steep systolic upslope on the PPG waveform (Fig. 21–14). The systolic upslope ends at the systolic peak, which marks the end of left ventricular contraction. Because the left ventricle is momentarily empty of blood at the end of systole, the pressure in the left ventricle drops sharply. This sudden drop in pressure allows the blood under high pressure in the proximal aortic root segment to flow backward through the open aortic valve cusps into the left ventricle. The reversal in blood flow snaps the aortic valve cusp shut, producing the dicrotic notch. As long as the arterial tree between the aortic root segment and the digital arteries of the toes remains unobstructed, the dicrotic notch will travel throughout this system, and it is recorded on the PPG digital waveform. However, the dicrotic notch is either damped or lost completely when an obstruction exists between the aortic root segment and the digital arteries of the toes. An obstruction will also alter the steep systolic upslope component of the PPG digital waveform. The obstruction damps the

forward pulsatile blood flow, producing a gradual ascent of the systolic upslope, as shown in Figures 21–15 and 21–16.

Figure 21–16 shows a damped PPG digital waveform caused by obstructive lesions located at the origins of the tibial vessels from the popliteal artery. The PPG waveforms in this figure exhibit absence of the dicrotic notch and a gradual ascent of the systolic upslope. Also, note that the height of the systolic peak is depressed and that the systolic peak is broad and rounded. A total arterial occlusion may prevent the pulsatile pressure wave from traveling from the aortic root segment down into the digital arteries of the toes. No digital PPG waveform will be obtained under these circumstances.

There must be an open pathway between the proximal aortic root segment and the digital arteries for the pulse wave to travel through before it can be detected by the photoelectric cell placed on the toe. Any obstruction, occlusion, or tangle of collateral vessels anywhere along this route will alter the configuration of the PPG waveform recorded at the toe. The pressure pulse wave is damped as it travels from the proximal aortic root segment out into the peripheral vessels. The systolic components of the PPG

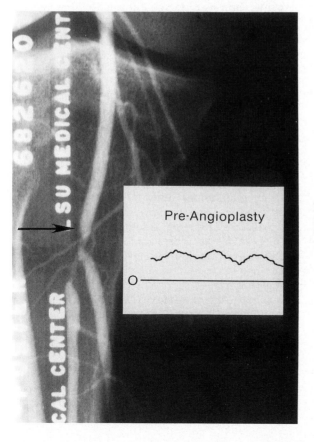

Figure 21–16. Abnormal photoplethysmography waveform caused by arterial obstructive disease. Arteriogram shows stenosis (arrow) located at the origins of the tibial vessels from the popliteal artery.

waveform, then, offer a sensitive method for detecting damping of the pulse wave caused by the various types of arterial obstructive lesions.

The diastolic component of the PPG waveform seems to be less important in this regard. It is formed as the elastic recoil of the distended elastic arterial reservoirs begins to push the flow of blood forward through the arterioles and out into the venous circulation. The blood volume and the number of RBCs present in the skin microvasculature of the toes decrease during diastole. This causes less light to be reflected back towards the photosensor cell, resulting in the diastolic downslope component of the PPG waveform towards the zero baseline level. Optimally, the diastolic downslope component should be concave towards the baseline, as illustrated in Figure 21–14. It should also drop down to the zero baseline level (Fig. 21–14). Rounding of the diastolic downslope in a convex manner away from the baseline and failure of this component to drop down to the zero baseline level are indicators of diastolic waveform damping caused by proximal arterial obstructive disease. These findings are illustrated by the PPG waveforms in Figures 21–15 and 21–16.

There is obviously a broad range of applications for the use of digital PPG waveform analysis. However, we have found it most useful for patients in whom pulses could not be evaluated by any other practical methods. This is demonstrated in the following cases.

Case III

A 60-year-old man presented with the symptoms of bilateral lower extremity rest pain. No pulses were palpable in either of the lower extremities. Noninvasive vascular studies are shown in Figure 21–17. The correlative arteriograms in Figures 21–18 and 21–19 show an adequate aortoiliac inflow system, but the femoropopliteal outflow and tibioperoneal run-off systems are obstructed bilaterally. There is almost total absence of blood flow to the left lower extremity. A small profunda femoral artery supplies the right lower extremity. This vessel terminates in a network of collateral arteries about the knee. These collateral vessels carry blood around the totally occluded popliteal artery into the proximal tibial vessels. Unfortunately, the distal segments of the tibial vessels are also occluded. A surgical limb salvage procedure would be difficult under these circumstances. Instead, this patient is a candidate for bilateral lower extremity amputations.

It is generally agreed that a below-knee (BK) amputation is preferable from the standpoint of rehabilitation. However, it is also recognized that significant morbidity and mortality rates are associated with such a procedure. This is particularly true when the BK amputation fails to heal and results in a second operative procedure. Predicting whether or not a BK amputation site will heal on the basis of the information obtained from the clinical and arteriographic examination is a difficult task. It thus appears that noninvasive vascular testing could be used to minimize the morbidity from amputations performed through ischemic tissue.

Both the calf systolic pressure obtained below the knee and the ankle systolic pressure measurements have been used to predict healing following lower extremity amputations. However, neither of these is completely reliable. In patients with a calf systolic pressure of 50 to 70 mm Hg, several studies have confirmed that primary healing of BK amputations can be expected in 88 to 100%.[20-22] Conversely, healing has occurred in 10% of patients with calf systolic pressures below 50 mm Hg.[22] Healing of BK amputation sites has also been reported in patients with unobtainable pressures at the BK and ankle levels.[23]

It is also recognized that rigid noncompressible arteries may yield falsely elevated pressure measurements that may be misleading in predicting amputation wound healing. Therefore, the decision of whether or not to do an above-knee or below-knee amputation should not be based on the pressure measurements alone. The measurements, however, do add information that may be used in conjunction with the clinical and arteriographic examinations to determine the amputation level.

Likewise, cutaneous microvascular circulation photoplethysmography may add information. It has been used to predict healing of skin ulcers.[24] If cutaneous blood flow is vigorous, as demonstrated by good pulsatile PPG waveforms in the skin immediately surrounding the ulcer, the ulcers usually heal spontaneously.

This type of information may also eventually prove to be helpful in minimizing the morbidity from amputations performed through ischemic skin tissues. For example, the Doppler velocity waveforms of the major lower extremity arteries in *Case III* are correlated with the cutaneous PPG waveforms in Figure 21–17. They show good cutaneous circulation about the right inguinal region but poor cutaneous circulation in the left inguinal region. There is also poor cutaneous circulation about the knees and toes in this case. This is to be expected because both the popliteal and tibial artery Doppler velocity waveforms are grossly abnormal. Putting all of the clinical, arteriographic, and noninvasive vascular test information together, this patient had bilateral above-knee amputations, despite the right calf systolic pressure measurement of 59 mm Hg.

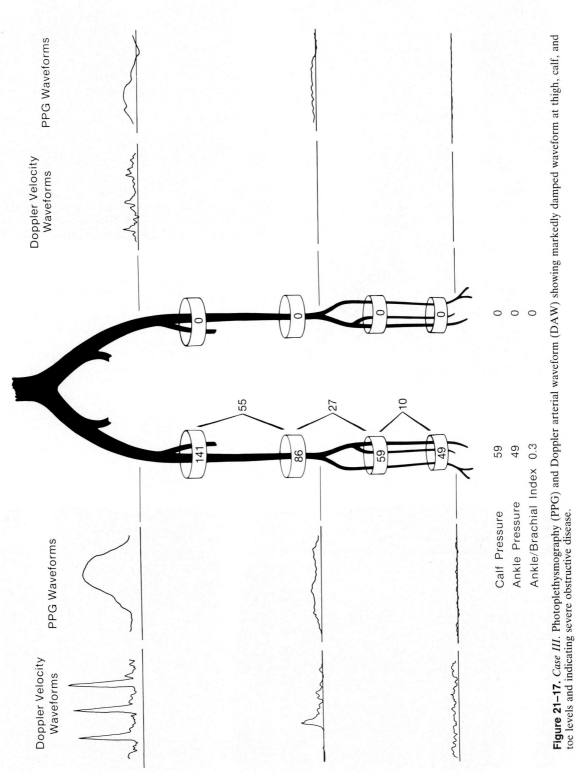

Figure 21–17. *Case III.* Photoplethysmography (PPG) and Doppler arterial waveform (DAW) showing markedly damped waveform at thigh, calf, and toe levels and indicating severe obstructive disease.

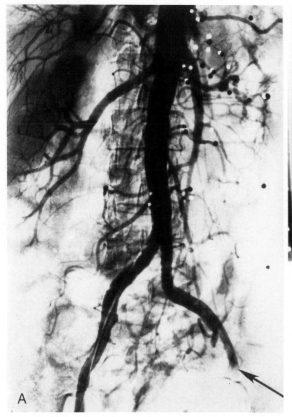

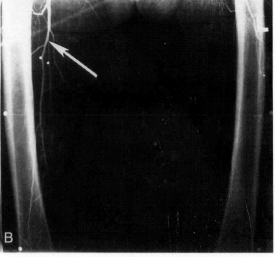

Figure 21–18. *Case III.* Arteriogram showing severe bilateral obstructive disease at multiple levels. *A*, Arteriogram of the abdominal aorta and iliac vessels showing total occlusion of the left external iliac artery (arrow). *B*, Arteriogram at the thigh level showing occlusion of both superficial femoral and left deep femoral arteries. Right profunda femoral artery is patent (arrow).

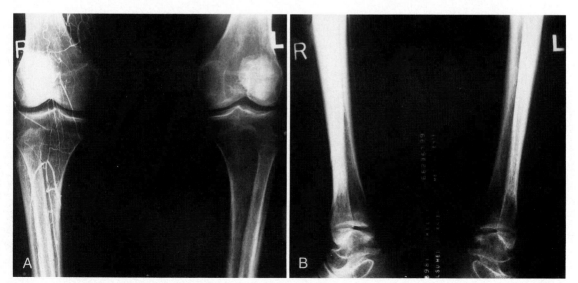

Figure 21–19. *Case III.* Arteriogram at knee levels *(A)* showing occlusion of both popliteal arteries with poor run-off *(B)*.

The decision to perform bilateral AK amputations in this case was not decided based upon the PPG waveform data alone. This case example is presented only to illustrate how the cutaneous PPG waveforms may be used to supply information about the skin circulation at the site of a proposed amputation. Further investigations must be undertaken before this type of information can be considered of any clinical value.

Case IV
Case IV illustrates how the PPG waveforms are used to gain information about the lower extremity circulation when it cannot be obtained by any other practical means. A premature infant was found to have absent peripheral pulses in the right lower extremity after the exchange of an umbilical artery catheter. Neither the segmental Doppler pressures nor the Doppler velocity waveforms were recordable from the right lower extremity. Although they were damped considerably, PPG waveforms were found to be present in the microvascular circulation of the skin over the thigh, calf, and foot levels, as shown in Figure 21–20. Figure 21–20 shows good PPG waveforms from the left lower extremity cutaneous microvasculature; the waveforms are damped in the right lower extremity cutaneous

microvasculature. Based on the fact that there was some blood flow in the cutaneous circulation of the right lower extremity, this infant was treated conservatively and subsequently improved.

Case V
There will be instances in which it is impractical to use the Doppler velocity flow probe for evaluating peripheral pulses. Such a situation is illustrated in *Case V*. Here it was desired to monitor the peripheral pulses during an angioplasty procedure for multiple superficial femoral artery obstructions (Fig. 21–21). Because it was impractical to hold a Doppler probe over the dorsalis pedis artery during the procedure, a photocell was used for this purpose. The photocell was taped to the great toe so that the continuous PPG waveforms could be observed on a strip chart recorder before, during, and after the balloon inflations. This provides immediate hemodynamic information about the results of the procedure. A strip chart recorder is used to make a permanent record of this information.

The patient is a middle-aged hypertensive diabetic man who had already undergone a left BK amputation. He now presents with right lower-extremity rest pain. His pre-angioplasty arteriogram in Figure 21–21A shows multiple superficial artery obstructive lesions. The numbers in these illustrations are used to precisely

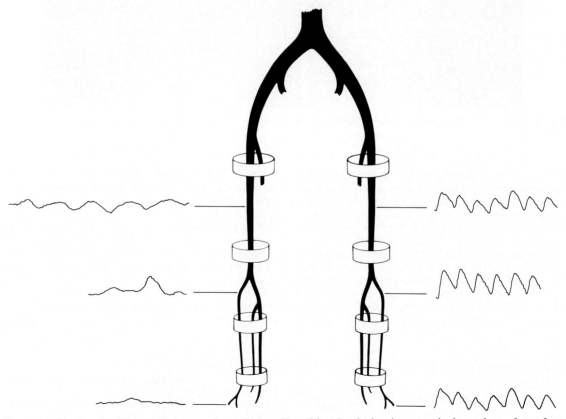

Figure 21–20. *Case IV*. Photoplethysmography at thigh, calf, and foot levels showing severely damped waveforms from the right leg and normal waveforms from the left leg.

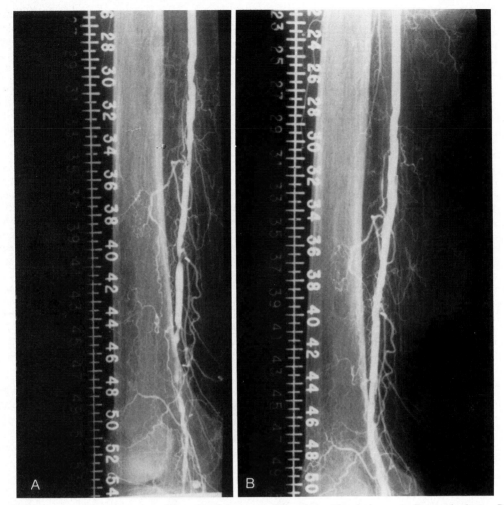

Figure 21–21. *Case V.* Arteriograms of superficial femoral artery obstructive lesions. *A*, Pre-angioplasty. *B*, Post-angioplasty.

locate the sites of the lesions under fluoroscopy during the angioplasty procedure. Stenoses are located at numbers 30, 33, 35, 41, 45, 46, and 50. A total occlusion is located between the numbers 47 and 49.

The angioplasty procedure is begun by dilating the stenosis at number 50. Then the balloon catheter is sequentially pulled back and the balloon inflated and deflated until all of the obstructive lesions are dilated. During these maneuvers, there should be continued improvement of the PPG waveforms. A complete loss of the PPG waveform when the balloon is deflated may be used to alert the operator of possible compli-

cations. These include arterial dissection, arterial spasm, and distal embolization of atherosclerotic debris. Arteriography may then be used to define the anatomy and the site of the complication immediately before continuing the procedure. An example is given in Figure 21–22. Figure 21–22*A* shows a markedly damped PPG waveform resulting from arterial spasm. This spasm was treated by the intra-arterial administration of a vasodilator medication, which prompted a return of the PPG waveform (Fig. 21–22*B*).

Besides being used to monitor for complications, the PPG waveforms can be used to assess the hemody-

PRE-VASODILATOR DRUG   POST-VASODILATOR DRUG

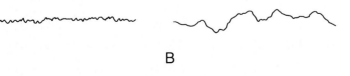

A   B

Figure 21–22. *Case V.* Arterial spasm treated by vasodilator medications. *A*, Pre-vasodilator drug. *B*, Post-vasodilator drug.

PRE-ANGIOPLASTY   POST-ANGIOPLASTY

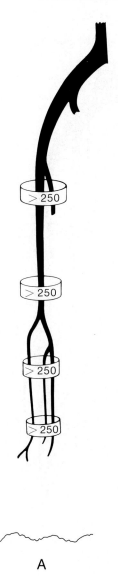

Figure 21–23. *Case V.* Photo-plethysmography digital waveforms. *A*, Pre-angioplasty. *B*, Post-angioplasty.

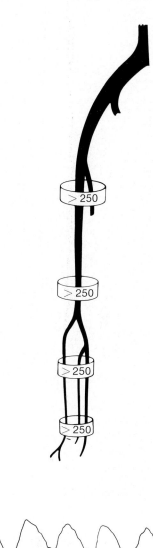

A   B

namic response of the angioplasty procedure. A comparison between the PPG waveforms in Figure 21–23*A* and *B* shows a marked improvement in the PPG waveform following the completion of the angioplasty procedure. This indicates a good hemodynamic response. The post-angioplasty arteriogram in Figure 21–21*B* shows a good anatomical result.

Case VI

A 42-year-old man was evaluated for patency of a right femoroperoneal bypass graft. Low systolic pressures and a low ankle/brachial index indicated an obstruction of the graft (Fig. 21–24). Obstruction was also suggested by a low toe pressure of 24 mm Hg and by damped Doppler arterial waveforms from the right

popliteal and distal vessels. The Doppler arterial waveform displayed the loss of pulsatility; the PPG waveform was damped, along with a rounded peak and loss of the dicrotic notch. Arteriography confirmed the obstruction of the bypass graft at the proximal end (Fig. 21–25). The graft was cleaned out surgically.

The patient subsequently returned after 8 months for re-evaluation of bypass patency. At this time, the segmental pressures were not recordable. The toe pressure of 31 mm Hg was low, and the Doppler arterial waveforms were damped in the distal arteries (Fig. 21–26). The PPG was more damped than on the previous examination. The graft occlusion was confirmed at surgery.

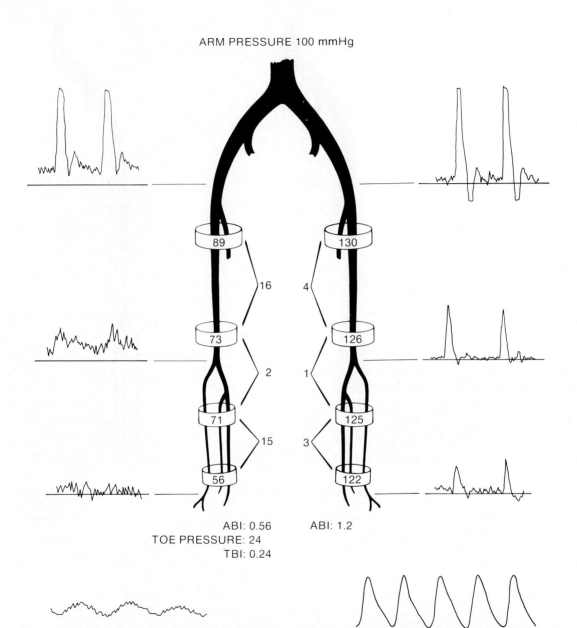

Figure 21–24. *Case VI.* Right femoroperoneal graft occlusion. SP = Systolic pressure; ABI = ankle/brachial index; TP = toe pressure; TBI = toe/brachial index; DAW = Doppler arterial waveform; PPG = photoplethysmography.

	Right	*Left*
SP	Abnormal	Normal
ABI	Abnormal	Normal
TP	Abnormal	—
TBI	Abnormal	—
PPG	Abnormal	Normal
DAW	Abnormal	Normal

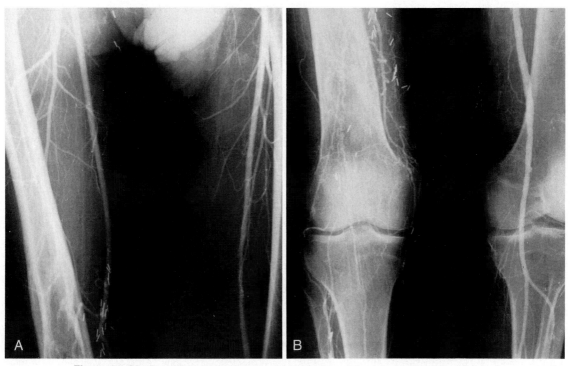

Figure 21–25. *Case VI.* Arteriogram showing occlusion of the femoroperoneal graft.

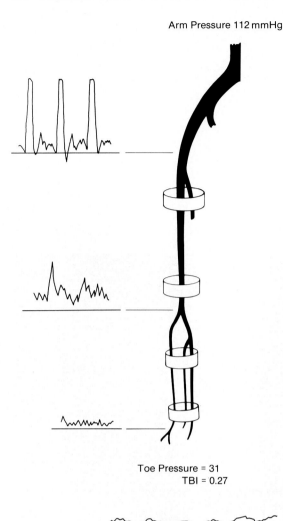

Arm Pressure 112 mmHg

Toe Pressure = 31
TBI = 0.27

Figure 21–26. *Case VI.* Femoroperoneal graft re-occlusion. Ankle/brachial index, toe pressure, toe/brachial index, Doppler arterial waveform, and photoplethysmography are all abnormal.

In summary, photoplethysmography and toe pressures can provide valuable information about the vascular system and can complement arteriography and other noninvasive vascular examinations to achieve the diagnosis and to assess the results of surgical and medical management.

References

1. Carter SA, Lezack JD. Digital systolic pressures in the lower limb in arterial disease. Circulation 1971; 43:904–914.
2. Gunderson J. Diagnosis of arterial insufficiency with measurement of blood pressure in in fingers and toes. Angiology 1971; 22:191.
3. Strandness DE, Sumner DS. Hemodynamics for surgeons. New York, Grune & Stratton, 1975:545.
4. Lezack JD, Carter SA. Systolic pressures in the extremities of man with special reference to the toes. Can J Physiol Pharmacol 1970; 48:469.
5. Nielsen PE, Bell G, Lassen NA. The measurement of digital systolic blood pressure by strain gauge technique. Scan J Clin Lab Invest 1972; 29:371.
6. Bone GE, Pomajzl MJ. Toe blood pressure by photoplethysmography: An index of healing in forefoot amputation. Surgery 1981; 89:569–574.
7. Ramsey DE, Manke DA, Sumner DS. Toe blood pressure: A valuable adjunct to ankle pressure measurement for assessing peripheral arterial disease. J Cardiovasc Surg 1983; 24:43.
8. Vollrath KD, Salles-Cunha SX, Vincent D, et al. Noninvasive measurement of toe systolic pressures. Bruit 1980; 4:27.
9. Vincent DG, Salles-Cunha SX, Bernhard VM, et al. Noninvasive assessment of toe systolic pressures with special reference to diabetes mellitus. J Cardiovasc Surg 1983; 24:22.
10. Lamb SL, Anderson J, Geifert KB, Blackshear WN Jr. The optimum method of toe pressure measurement. Bruit 1983; 7:26–32.
11. Carter SA, Hamel ER. Role of pressure measurements in vascular disease. *In* Bernstein EF (ed). Noninvasive diagnostic techniques in vascular disease. St Louis, CV Mosby 1985:513–544.

12. Barnes RW. Segmental blood pressures and digital plethysmography. *In* Barnes RW (ed). Noninvasive diagnostic techniques in peripheral vascular disease. Little Rock, Ark, Barnes RW, 1980:29–40.

13. Sumner DS. Digital plethysmography and pressure measurements. *In* Hershey RB, Barnes RW, Sumner DS (eds). Noninvasive diagnosis of vascular disease. Pasadena, Calif, Appleton-Davies, 1984:35–42.

14. Paaske WP, Tonnesen KH. Prognostic significance of distal blood pressure measurements in patients with severe ischaemia. Scand J Thorac Cardiovasc Surg 1980; 14:105.

15. Holstein P, Noer I, Tonnesen KH, et al. Distal blood pressure in severe arterial insufficiency. *In* Bergan JJ, Yao JST (eds). Gangrene and severe ischemia of the lower extremities. New York, Grune and Stratton, 1978:95–114.

16. Baker WH, Barnes RW. Minor forefoot amputation in patients with low ankle pressure. Am J Surg 1977; 133:331–332.

17. Gibbons GW, Wheelock FC, Siembieda C, Hoar CS, et al. Noninvasive prediction of amputation level in diabetic patients. Arch Surg 1979; 114:1253–1257.

18. Verta MJ, Gross WS, Bellen B, et al. Forefoot perfusion pressure and minor amputation for gangrene. Surgery 1976; 80:729–734.

19. Johnson WC, Patten DH. Predictability of healing of ischemic leg ulcers by radioisotopic and Doppler ultrasonic examination. Am J Surg 1977; 133:485–489.

20. Raines JK, Darling RC, Buth J, et al. Vascular laboratory criteria for the management of peripheral vascular disease of the lower extremities. Surgery 1976; 79:212.

21. Dean RH, Yao JST, Thompson RG, et al. Predictive value of ultrasonically derived arterial pressure in determination of amputation level. Am J Surg 1975; 41:731–734.

22. Barnes RW, Shanik GD, Slaymaker EE. An index of healing in below-knee amputations: leg blood pressure by Doppler ultrasound. Surgery 1976; 79:13–16.

23. Barnes RW, Thornhill B, Nix L, et al. Prediction of amputation wound healing. Roles of Doppler ultrasound and digital photoplethysmography. Arch Surg 1981; 116:80.

24. Lee BY, Trainer FS, Kavner D, et al. Assessment of the healing potentials of ulcers of the skin by photoplethysmography. Surg Gynecol Obstet 1979; 148:233–235.

Part V • Noninvasive Assessment of Upper Extremity Vascular Lesions

22 • Upper Extremity Arterial and Venous Abnormalities

Introduction

A wide variety of vascular abnormalities can affect the upper extremities. Most of these may be diagnosed by the noninvasive vascular procedures described in this chapter. What procedures to use, how to use them, and what findings may be obtained will all be described. Pathological anatomy will be illustrated by comparing arteriograms and venograms with the findings on the noninvasive vascular procedures. The noninvasive vascular procedures to be demonstrated include:

- segmental systolic pressure measurements
- Doppler arterial waveform analysis
- photoplethysmography (PPG)
- duplex ultrasonography

Examination of the Upper Extremity Arteries

Anatomy

The upper extremity arteries to be evaluated by noninvasive testing are shown in Figure 22–1. They include the subclavian and axillary arteries of the shoulder girdle; the brachial artery of the arm; and the radial, ulnar, and interosseous arteries of the forearm.[1] Other arteries that may be examined include those that form the palmar arches of the hands and the digital arteries of the fingers. The anatomy of these arteries must be understood before they can be properly examined by noninvasive testing. Understanding the anatomy allows the examiner to know which artery is being examined and precisely where to locate the abnormality in the artery under investigation. Because collateral pathways are commonly encountered around either stenotic or total arterial occlusive lesions, it is necessary to be familiar with these as well. The anatomy of

the major arteries will now be described, along with the potential collateral pathways that may form around stenotic or occlusive lesions in the vessels. Arterial anatomy is used to define which vessel is being studied and where the lesion is located; the anatomy of the collateral pathway is used to diagnose an underlying obstructive lesion.

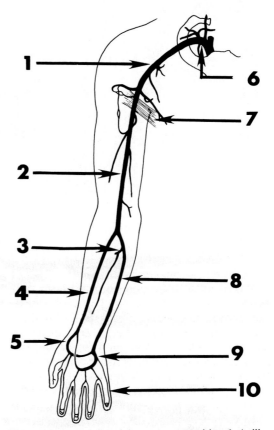

Figure 22–1. Arteries of the upper extremities. *1*, Axillary artery. *2*, Brachial artery. *3*, Common interosseous artery. *4*, Radial artery. *5*, Deep palmar arch. *6*, Subclavian artery. *7*, Teres major muscle. *8*, Ulnar artery. *9*, Superficial palmar arch. *10*, Digital arteries.

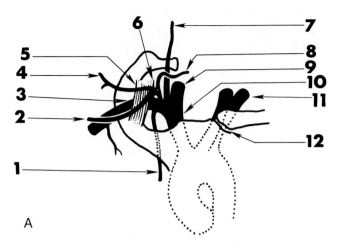

A

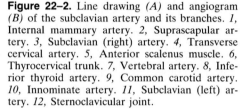

B

Figure 22–2. Line drawing *(A)* and angiogram *(B)* of the subclavian artery and its branches. *1,* Internal mammary artery. *2,* Suprascapular artery. *3,* Subclavian (right) artery. *4,* Transverse cervical artery. *5,* Anterior scalenus muscle. *6,* Thyrocervical trunk. *7,* Vertebral artery. *8,* Inferior thyroid artery. *9,* Common carotid artery. *10,* Innominate artery. *11,* Subclavian (left) artery. *12,* Sternoclavicular joint.

Subclavian Artery

The right subclavian artery originates from the innominate or brachiocephalic trunk; the left subclavian artery arises directly from the aortic arch, as shown in Figure 22–2. These arteries lie posterior to the subclavian veins. The proximal origins of the subclavian arteries are difficult to examine by either Doppler or B-mode ultrasonography because of their deep intrathoracic positions behind the sternoclavicular joints. However, as they exit the thorax, they pass between the anterior and middle scalene muscles to lie in a superficial location above and anterior to the first rib. Here arterial pulses may be palpated and the arteries are accessible for evaluation by noninvasive vascular techniques. The subclavian artery ends and the axillary artery begins at the lateral border of the first rib.

Because the subclavian arteries lie in close proximity to the clavicles, first ribs, and scalene muscles, they may be extrinsically compressed by these structures, producing the vascular component of the *thoracic outlet syndrome.*

Subclavian artery stenoses and occlusions may be bypassed through collateral pathways formed from its major branches. The major branches of the subclavian artery forming these collaterals are shown in Figure 22–2 and consist of the vertebral, thyrocervical trunk branches, and internal mammary arteries.

Collateral Pathways around Subclavian Artery Obstruction

Subclavian artery obstructions can be divided into two types, according to whether the obstructions are proximal or distal to the origin of the

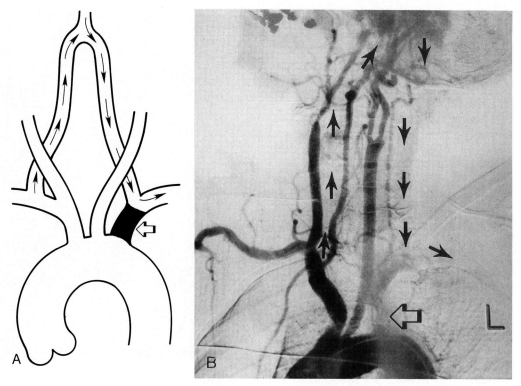

Figure 22–3. Subclavian artery obstruction proximal to origin of the vertebral artery. Line drawing *(A)* and angiogram *(B)* demonstrate obstruction of the left subclavian artery (open arrow) with collateral flow from the vertebral arteries (arrows).

vertebral arteries. Those that occur proximal to the vertebral artery origins form collaterals through the vertebral arteries, as shown in Figure 22–3. This type of collateral flow constitutes the *subclavian steal syndrome* because blood is "stolen" from the vertebrobasilar circulation to supply the affected upper extremity. Subclavian artery obstructions distal to the vertebral artery origins are bypassed by collateral pathways formed from the branches of the thyrocervical trunk and internal mammary arteries. These collateral pathways transport blood flow around the subclavian artery occlusion site into the subscapular branches of the axillary artery (Figure 22–4).

Axillary Artery

The axillary artery begins on the superolateral margin of the first rib and courses through the axilla to become the brachial artery at the lower margin of the teres major muscle. These landmarks, along with the major branches of the axillary artery, are presented in Figure 22–5. Because the axillary artery is located superficially, it can be readily palpated and examined

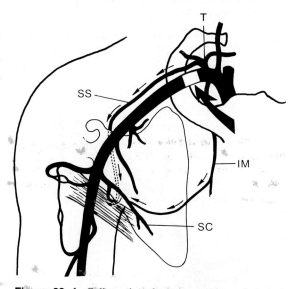

Figure 22–4. Collateral pathways around a subclavian artery obstruction distal to the vertebral artery origin (large arrow). Collateral flow is from the thyrocervical trunk (T) through the suprascapular artery (SS) into the subscapular branch of the axillary artery (SC) and from the internal mammary artery (IM) into the subscapular branch of the axillary artery. Arrows denote collateral blood flow direction.

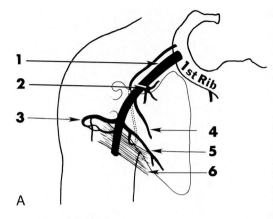

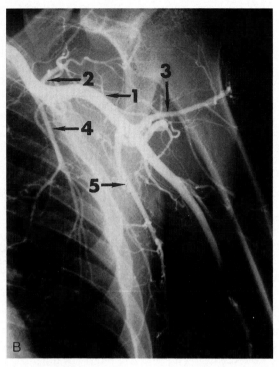

Figure 22–5. Line drawing *(A)* and angiogram *(B)* of the axillary artery and its branches. *1,* Axillary artery. *2,* Thoracoacromian artery. *3,* Humeral circumflex artery. *4,* Lateral thoracic artery. *5,* Subscapular artery. *6,* Teres major muscle.

by Doppler and B-mode ultrasound imaging techniques throughout its entire course.

Collateral Pathways around Axillary Artery Obstruction

The collateral pathway patterns around proximal axillary artery obstructions are shown in Figures 22–6 and 22–7. These are the same patterns as those found in the subclavian artery when the obstruction occurs distal to the origin of the vertebral artery (Fig. 22–4). Under these circumstances, a vast network of rich collaterals can be formed between the branches of the thyrocervical trunk, internal mammary, and subscapular arteries. However, this rich collateral network is completely lost when a distal axillary artery obstruction occurs below the level of the

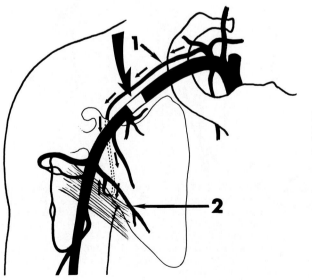

Figure 22–6. Axillary artery obstruction (large arrow) proximal to the origin of the thoracoacromian branch with collaterals between the suprascapular *(1)* branch of the thyrocervical trunk and the subscapular branch *(2)* of the axillary artery.

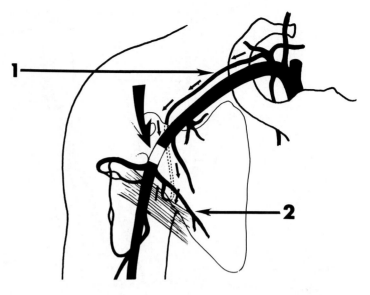

Figure 22–7. Axillary artery obstruction (large arrow) between thoracoacromian and subscapular arteries with collaterals between the suprascapular *(1)* branch of the thyrocervical trunk and the subscapular *(2)* branch of the axillary artery.

subscapular and humeral circumflex arteries, as shown in Figure 22–8. This figure shows that the only collateral pathway that is readily available is between the humeral circumflex branch of the axillary artery and the profunda branch of the brachial artery. Distal axillary artery obstructions, then, are extremely important to recognize. They can seriously jeopardize the blood flow to the affected upper extremity because of the lack of adequate collateral pathways. Of clinical significance is the fact that the axillary artery is often punctured at this site when catheters are introduced through the axilla for angiographic procedures and the administration of chemotherapeutic agents. Patients who develop upper limb ischemia following these procedures should be investigated thoroughly for a distal axillary artery obstruction below the level of the humeral circumflex and subscapular axillary artery branches, as shown in Figure 22–8.

Brachial Artery

The brachial artery extends from the lower margin of the teres major muscles in the axilla to the level of its bifurcation in the cubital fossa

Figure 22–8. Distal axillary artery obstruction (large arrow) with few collateral pathways between the humeral circumflex branch of the axillary artery and the profunda branch of the brachial artery. *1,* Humeral circumflex artery. *2,* Collateral pathway. *3,* Profunda brachial artery.

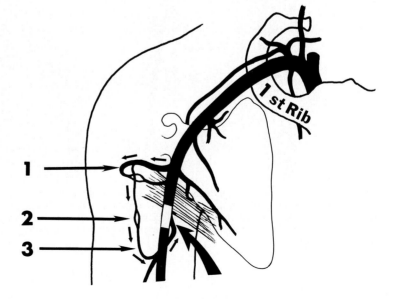

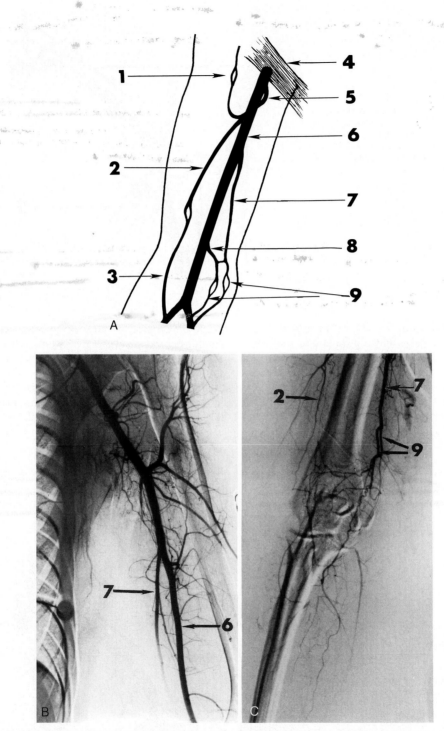

Figure 22–9. Line drawing *(A)* and angiograms *(B* and *C)* of the brachial artery, its branches, and its collateral routes. *1,* Ascending profunda brachial artery (collateral route). *2,* Descending profunda brachial artery (collateral route). *3,* Radial recurrent artery (collateral route). *4,* Teres major muscle. *5,* Profunda branchial artery. *6,* Brachial artery. *7,* Superior ulnar artery (collateral route). *8,* Inferior ulnar artery (collateral route). *9,* Anterior and posterior ulnar recurrent arteries.

at the elbow. It is palpable throughout its course, which runs along the medial aspect of the humerus down to the elbow. Like the axillary artery, the brachial artery is a frequent site for the introduction of catheters during angiography and may become occluded as a result of these procedures. Collateral pathways around these occlusions are shown in Figure 22–9. These collateral pathways may not be adequate to prevent forearm ischemia when the brachial artery is occluded. Therefore, it is important to detect brachial artery occlusions so that they can be surgically corrected.

Ulnar and Radial Arteries

The ulnar artery is the larger of the two distal branches of the brachial artery. It begins in the cubital fossa at the elbow and runs along the medial aspect of the forearm to the wrist, where it passes into the palm of the hand to form the superficial palmar arch, as shown in Figure 22–10. A major branch of the ulnar artery is the common interosseous artery. Its branches lie deep within the muscles and do not normally supply blood to the hand; they are not generally examined by noninvasive vascular techniques. The ulnar artery is palpable in the cubital fossa and over the anterior medial surface of the wrist.

The radial artery begins in the cubital fossa at the elbow and runs along the lateral aspect of the forearm to the wrist, where it is palpable and divides into the dorsal carpal arch and the deep palmar arch.

Arteries of the Hand

Three arterial arches are found in the hand. They are (1) the dorsal carpal arch, (2) the deep palmar arch, and (3) the superficial palmar arch.

The *dorsal carpal arch* is found on the back or dorsum of the hand and is one of the first terminal

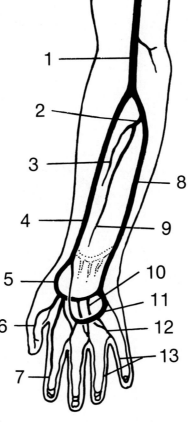
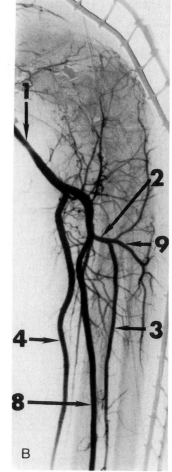

Figure 22–10. Line drawing *(A)* and angiogram *(B)* of the radial and ulnar arteries and their branches. Dashed lines outline the location of the dorsal carpal arch and its three dorsal metacarpal branches. *1,* Brachial artery. *2,* Common interosseous artery. *3,* Anterior interosseous artery. *4,* Radial artery. *5,* Deep palmar arch. *6,* Princeps pollicis artery. *7,* Radialis indicis artery. *8,* Ulnar artery. *9,* Posterior interosseous artery. *10,* Palmar metacarpal artery. *11,* Superficial palmar arch. *12,* Common palmar digital artery. *13,* Proper palmar digital artery.

A

B

branches of the radial artery. It gives rise to the three dorsal metacarpal branches that supply the intrinsic hand muscles. The location of this arch and its branches is denoted by the dashed lines in Figure 22–10.

The *deep palmar arch* is found in the proximal palm of the hand and is the second major terminal branch of the radial artery. Its branches are (1) the princeps pollicis artery of the thumb, (2) the radialis indicis artery of the index finger, and (3) the three palmar metacarpal arteries.

The *superficial palmar arch* is formed by the distal curved portion of the ulnar artery. It anastomoses with the three palmar metacarpal arteries of the deep palmar arch to form the three common palmar digital arteries. These then give rise to the proper palmar digital arteries that supply the third, fourth, and fifth fingers and the medial aspect of the index or second finger, as shown in Figure 22–10. The fact that the digital arteries receive blood flow from both the superficial and deep palmar arches is important because these branches continue to be perfused with blood when either the ulnar artery or the radial artery is totally occluded.

Arterial Examination Techniques

Segmental Systolic Pressure Measurements

Upper extremity segmental blood pressures are obtained by means of the Doppler technique. It is a simple, reliable method of detecting arterial disease. This method has previously been de-scribed in Chapter 17, "Noninvasive Vascular Examination of the Lower Extremity Arteries." Basic equipment requirements are four 14 × 40 cm pneumatic cuffs coupled to an automated inflation system and a bi-directional Doppler unit with 5, 8, and 10 MHz probes.

The patient is placed in a supine or sitting position with the arms extended in a resting state. Pneumatic cuffs are placed around both upper arms and forearms. The Doppler probe is positioned over the radial or ulnar artery, whichever exhibits the strongest arterial signal. It should be noted that the site of the pressure measurement recording is at the level of the cuff and not the Doppler probe site. The pneumatic cuff is inflated above the systolic blood pressure until systolic sounds are absent and the arterial flow is occluded. The cuff is then allowed to slowly deflate until the first systolic Doppler sound is heard. The return of the systolic Doppler sound represents the systolic arterial pressure, which is documented. Bilateral pressures are obtained for comparison and for evaluating both extremities for arterial disease.

Normally, there is no more than 10 mm Hg difference in the pressures between both arms (Fig. 22–11).[2, 3] If the difference is greater than 10 mm Hg, stenosis or occlusion of the innominate, subclavian, axillary, or proximal arteries is indicated on the side with lower pressure. There should be no more than 10 mm Hg difference in any gradient between cuffs, and the forearm pressure should be equal to or slightly higher than the arm pressure (Fig. 22–11). If exercise

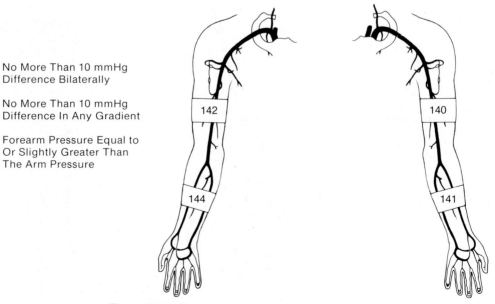

No More Than 10 mmHg
Difference Bilaterally

No More Than 10 mmHg
Difference In Any Gradient

Forearm Pressure Equal to
Or Slightly Greater Than
The Arm Pressure

142

140

144

141

Figure 22–11. Normal segmental systolic pressure values.

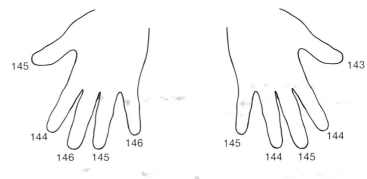

Figure 22–12. Normal digital segmental pressure values.

No more than 15 mmHg difference between digits.
Equal to or slightly higher than the Brachial Pressure. Brachial Systolic Pressure is 140 mmHg in this illustration.

or reactive hyperemia testing is performed in a patient with significant stenosis or occlusion, there will be an increase in the pressure drop distal to the lesion.

Digit pressures can be obtained with Doppler or photoplethysmographic techniques. However, digital pressures with PPG techniques are easier to obtain and to reproduce. Using the PPG technique, the examiner places a digit pneumatic cuff (3 cm) around the proximal forefinger and secures the photocell to the distal portion. The strip chart recorder is set at 5 mm/second with the waveform centered and the height adjusted to 20 or 30 mm. The digit cuff is inflated above the systolic pressure until the pulse disappears, then is slowly deflated until the pulse re-appears. As the cuff is deflated, counter markings are placed on the strip recording for obtaining numerical values. The pulse re-appearance time represents the systolic digit pressure. The normal finger pressure is 13 mm Hg higher than the toe pressure and is equal to or slightly higher than that found in the forearm.[4] There should be no more than 15 mm Hg pressure difference between digits (Fig. 22–12).[5]

Doppler Arterial Examination with Velocity Waveform Analysis

The bi-directional continuous-wave Doppler examination is combined with the segmental blood pressure study for correlation and for providing flow characteristics at specific arterial levels.

The physical principles of Doppler ultrasonography were presented in Chapter 1, "Sound spectral Analysis Instrumentation." The same exam-

ination techniques and principles are used in the arterial examination of the upper extremities as are described for lower extremities in Chapter 17. However, there are some differences in the characteristics of the velocity waveforms between the upper and lower extremities, in addition to the specialized examination techniques required for evaluating subclavian steal syndrome, Raynaud's symptoms, thoracic outlet syndrome, and palmar arch testing.

A bi-directional continuous-wave Doppler unit with 5, 8, and 10 MHz probes is utilized. The higher frequencies are used for the smaller, superficial vessels, such as the radial and ulnar arteries; the lower frequencies are used for penetration of deeper vessels. The Doppler probe is positioned with a 30 to 45° angle into the forward flow to demonstrate a positive velocity waveform. The sound is audibly heard, which enables the examiner to hear the maximum pitch and to achieve the correct angle for demonstrating the highest Doppler shift. The strip chart recorder is engaged to provide an analog velocity waveform tracing for final analysis and interpretation. The recorder is set at 25 mm/second with the zero baseline approximately 20 mm above the paper edge to allow for recording of the reverse component as well as the forward systolic portion. The recorder can be calibrated and set at 1 kHz to enable the operator to calibrate the frequency levels from the printed waveform. The recorder has multiple size levels for decreasing or increasing the velocity waveform size while the recorder remains calibrated at 1 kHz. This allows the operator to quickly change size levels to display all of the waveform without changing the calibration of the recorder.

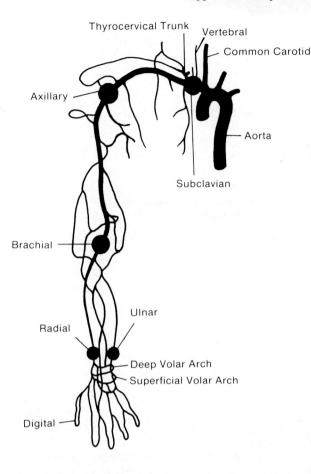

Figure 22–13. An anatomical diagram of the upper extremity demonstrating arterial Doppler positions used to acquire waveforms.

The patient is examined in either a supine or a sitting position, depending upon the patient's physical condition and access to the vessels. However, the extremities must be in a resting state prior to evaluation. An anatomical diagram of the Doppler examination sites is shown in Figure 22–13. The probe positions of these various sites are demonstrated in Figure 22–14. Examination sites for the upper extremity are determined as follows:

1. The subclavian artery is located by directing the probe medial and inferior to the proximal end of the clavicle (Fig. 22–14A).

2. The axillary artery is located by directing the probe below the distal clavicle in the notch between the head of the humerus and the clavicle (Fig. 22–14B). The axillary artery is also examined in the axilla (Fig. 22–14C).

3. The brachial artery is located above the antecubital fold and anterior to the medial condyle (Fig. 22–14D).

4. The radial artery is located at its distal point slightly above the wrist (Fig. 22–14E).

5. The ulnar artery is located at its distal point slightly above the wrist (Fig. 22–14F).

Waveform analysis of the blood flow velocity in the subclavian artery normally exhibits strong pulsatility with a sharp, rapid upsweep, a prominent reverse flow component below the zero baseline level, and a very small diastolic forward flow (Fig. 22–15). The remaining upper-extremity vessels exhibit a similar pattern, with slightly decreasing amplitude in the distal vessels. Both extremities are evaluated and their blood flow velocity waveforms compared.

A significant hemodynamic stenosis proximal to the probe site will produce a velocity waveform with low pulsatility and a reduction or absence of the reverse component. At the site of the stenosis, there will be an increase in the waveform amplitude with turbulent sounds and loss of the reverse component. Distal to the site of the stenosis, the waveform becomes monophasic with no reverse component. Also, there will be a decrease in waveform amplitude (damping) that is proportional to the severity of the disease.

Total occlusion presents with complete absence of the velocity waveform at the site of obstruction and decreased amplitude proximal to the lesion. The site should be carefully observed to identify any collateral flow profiles distal to the obstruction (Fig. 22–16).

Palmar Arch Testing

There are several methods of verifying the patency of the radial and ulnar arteries. The simplest method, which requires no equipment, is the Allen test. The patient is placed in a sitting position with the hands in the lap and is instructed to clench the fist. The examiner compresses the radial artery firmly as the patient opens and relaxes the hand. Upon release of the compression, the palms should turn pink quickly; if not, occlusion of the ulnar artery is suspected. The test is then repeated with compression of the ulnar arteries to verify radial artery patency.[6, 7]

Doppler ultrasonography can also be used to verify palmar arch patency. A 10 MHz probe is positioned over the radial artery while the ulnar artery is compressed. The position is then reversed; the probe is positioned over the ulnar artery, and the radial artery is compressed (Fig. 22–17). Normally, there is stable flow with no augmentation. In cases of stenosis or occlusion, the flow is augmented or absent, depending upon the severity of the disease.

Photoplethysmography is the third method of evaluating the palmar arch continuity and is one of the easiest techniques to reproduce. The patient is placed in a sitting position with the hands resting in the lap. The PPG photocell is attached to the distal portion of each forefinger using double-stick tape (Fig. 22–18A). A strip chart recorder is set in the PPG format and is activated with a running speed of 5 mm/second. The baseline is placed in the center of the tracing with the amplitude adjusted to 20 or 30 mm. Compression maneuvers are performed on the radial artery and then the ulnar artery while the strip chart recorder is running.

Normally, there is no change in the amplitude during the compression maneuvers (Fig. 22–18B). However, in cases of stenosis or occlusion of either the radial artery or the ulnar artery, the pulse volume recording will be augmented or absent.

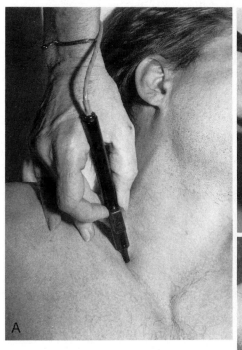

Figure 22–14. Doppler probe positions on the patient to obtain the following arterial waveforms: *A,* Subclavian artery. *B,* Axillary artery. *C,* Axillary artery.

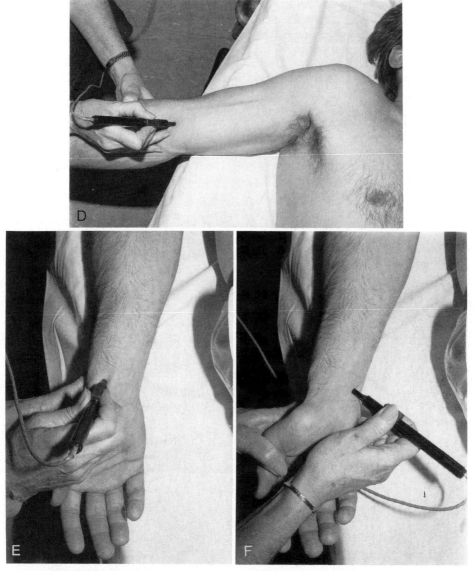

Figure 22–14 *Continued D*, Brachial artery. *E*, Radial artery. *F*, Ulnar artery.

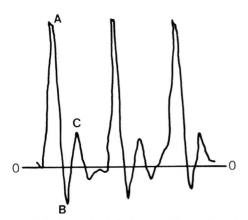

Figure 22–15. Normal subclavian arterial waveform showing a sharp systolic upsweep *(A)*, a prominent reverse component *(B)* below the zero baseline, and a small diastolic forward component *(C)*.

Real-time Imaging and Duplex Examination

Real-time imaging of the upper extremity provides an additional method of identifying pathology and of determining the tissue characteristics of specific lesions. If duplex imaging is employed, anatomical evaluation combined with Doppler analysis is provided. Currently, excellent images are produced with high-resolution systems and high-performance transducers. The duplex systems use a 7.5 or 10 MHz transducer combined with a Doppler frequency of 4.5 or 5 MHz for the best resolution in the axial and lateral fields. The axial resolution is approximately 0.2 mm to 0.5 mm, and the lateral resolution is 0.8 mm. It is preferable to have a combined continuous-wave and pulsed Doppler system integrated into one transducer. This allows the operator to survey the area with the continuous Doppler mode and to specifically delineate the individual vessels with the pulsed Doppler mode.

Real-time imaging is an art in itself and must be completely mastered. Equal time and effort should be spent on mastering imaging techniques and Doppler applications. Imaging principles include the placement of the transducer at a 90° angle to the structure for maximum reflection and for the best delineation. This is in direct contrast to the Doppler applications in which minimum signals are obtained at a 90° angle. It should also be emphasized that the structure of interest is examined in multiple planes so that all areas are imaged. The frequency employed should be the highest (for maximum resolution) that can penetrate the structure of interest. Superficial structures usually require 7.5 or 10 MHz frequencies. The focal depth, which is defined by the manufacturer, should be known, and the structure of interest placed within the near field range. Also, the operator should be aware that exceeding the focal ranges will cause a degradation of the image and possible loss of information. The time-gain compensation and power controls should be properly utilized to achieve the best sensitivity and to define the true tissue characteristics. Needless to say, improper machine settings can greatly distort the images and, in some instances, cause misdiagnosis.

Pathology of the Upper Extremity

Aneurysms

Aneurysms are found less frequently in the upper extremity arterial system than in the lower extremity arterial system. In the upper extremity, the subclavian and axillary arteries are the two most common sites for aneurysm. Aneurysms of

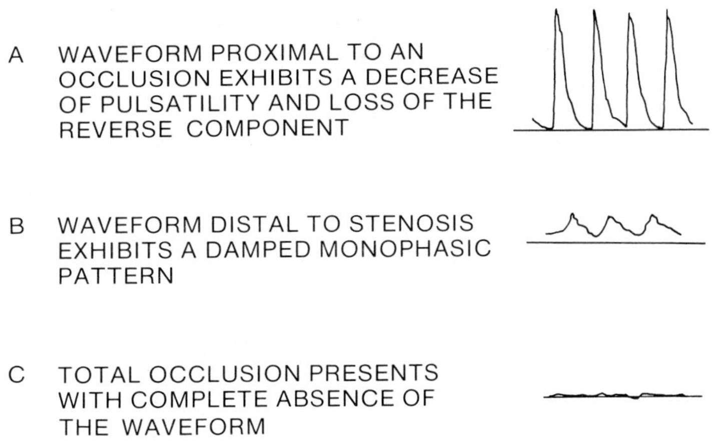

Figure 22–16. Doppler analog arterial velocity waveforms of obstructive arterial lesions. *A,* Waveform proximal to an occlusion. *B,* Waveform distal to a stenosis. *C,* Waveform distal to an occlusion.

A   WAVEFORM PROXIMAL TO AN OCCLUSION EXHIBITS A DECREASE OF PULSATILITY AND LOSS OF THE REVERSE COMPONENT

B   WAVEFORM DISTAL TO STENOSIS EXHIBITS A DAMPED MONOPHASIC PATTERN

C   TOTAL OCCLUSION PRESENTS WITH COMPLETE ABSENCE OF THE WAVEFORM

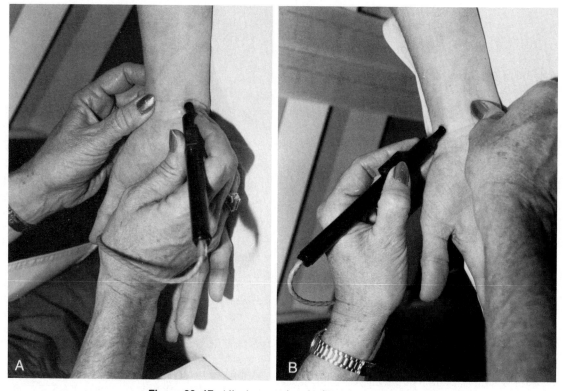

Figure 22–17. Allen's test using the Doppler technique.

the brachial and distal vessels are relatively uncommon.[8]

Upper extremity aneurysms are frequently traumatic in origin.[8] The trauma may occur in the form of direct penetration or blunt-type injury. Lacerations of the vessel caused by these types of injuries consequently may result in pseudoaneurysm formation. More recently, aneurysms have occurred because of the increased utilization of angiographic catheterization procedures.[9, 10] However, Braunwald found only 10 local arterial complications and no traumatic aneurysms in 12,367 cardiac catheterizations.[11] Traumatic aneurysm may also occur in drug addicts. Other, less common, causes are atherosclerosis, arteritis (mycotic, necrotic, and giant cell), congenital, periarteritis nodosa, and Takayasu's disease.[12]

Most patients with aneurysms present with symptoms secondary to vascular or neurological complications; others may either remain asymptomatic or present with a palpable pulsatile mass. Vascular complications usually occur because of thrombo-embolic phenomena from mural thrombosis in the aneurysm. These complications may

be associated with ischemia or gangrene and may lead to amputation of the upper extremity if adequate treatment is not provided in time. Aneurysms may rupture or produce compression of the nerve or adjacent veins.[8]

A tortuous subclavian artery can also present as a palpable pulsatile mass and mimic an aneurysm. It is important clinically to differentiate the two entities because aneurysms are associated with the complication of distal ischemia of the hand and digits. A post-stenotic dilatation beyond the extrinsic compression defect caused by either a cervical rib or a tight scalenus muscle is the most frequent type of subclavian artery aneurysm.[13] These aneurysms are often small and frequently contain thrombus, which may be the source of emboli to the distal arteries. The following clinical maneuver may be helpful in distinguishing a tortuous artery from an aneurysm. The patient is asked to take a deep breath and hold it; if there is significant decrease or absence of pulsation in the mass, the diagnosis is most likely a tortuous artery. The pulsation will persist or remain unchanged when an aneurysm is present.[8]

Figure 22–18. Allen's test. *A,* Photoplethysmograph technique. *B,* Arterial waveform tracing exhibiting no change in blood flow.

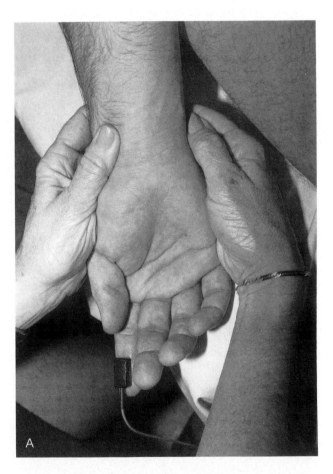

Arteriography still prevails as the diagnostic examination of choice for the assessment of aneurysms. It serves the following functions:

1. Determines the exact location of the aneurysm.

2. Delineates the presence or absence of adequate collateral vessels.

3. Distinguishes atherosclerotic thrombotic obstruction from embolic obstruction.

However, because arteriography is an invasive procedure, it cannot be repeated frequently. In this respect, noninvasive tests can play a complementary role. They may not only be used to confirm the diagnosis, but they may also be used to evaluate the remainder of the circulation for sites of distal obstruction.[3]

Duplex sonography is a simple, rapid noninvasive examination that can directly visualize the normal artery as well as aneurysms. Thrombus, which is not directly visualized by arteriography, is well demonstrated within an aneurysm by means of real-time ultrasonography. These noninvasive tests can differentiate tortuous arteries from aneurysms and can follow the course, as illustrated in *Case I.*

Case I

A 45-year-old man presented to the hospital with a pulsatile neck mass. Real-time sonography of the neck revealed a tortuous right subclavian artery without aneurysm (Fig. 22–19). Segmental systolic pressures and Doppler arterial velocity waveforms also determined the absence of distal obstruction (Fig. 22–20).

The topic of tortuous subclavian arteries simulating supraclavicular and cervical masses is fully described in Chapter 24 "Duplex Sonography of Superficial Masses."

The sonographic appearance of subclavian, brachial, or distal arterial aneurysms depends upon their type (saccular or dissecting). Examples of saccular and dissecting aneurysms are shown in *Cases II* and *III*, respectively.

Case II

A 69-year-old man presented with soft tissue swelling in the right cubital fossa after a brachial artery puncture for an angiographic procedure. A sonogram demonstrated a 21 mm long pulsatile, sonolucent mass (Fig. 22–21A) representing a saccular aneurysm in the right cubital fossa that was free of any internal echoes, indicating the absence of thrombus.

The 1 month follow-up ultrasonogram revealed an increase in the size of the aneurysm (Fig. 22–21B). The blood flow was detected within the mass by Doppler ultrasonography (Fig. 22–21C). Normal segmental pressures and arterial waveforms indicated the patency of the distal vessels (Fig. 22–21D).

Case III

A middle-aged man presented with pain in the right distal upper arm following cardiac catheterization through the brachial artery. Ultrasonography of the right distal arm revealed a dissecting aneurysm of the distal brachial artery. The aneurysm was suggested by two lumens that were separated by an echogenic intimal flap (Fig. 22–22A). One lumen was sonolucent; the other lumen had moving internal echoes representing slow-flowing blood. These findings were confirmed by arteriography (Fig. 22–22B). In some patients, internal echoes may be due to the presence of thrombosis. Other patients may show two sonolucent lumens, normal segmental systolic pressure, and nor-

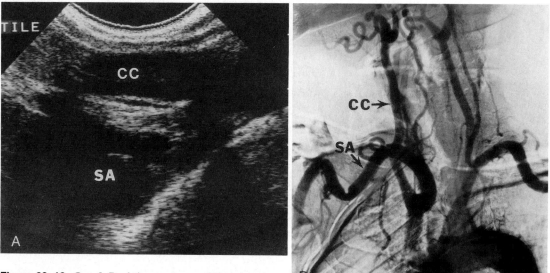

Figure 22–19. *Case I.* Real-time sonogram *(A)* and angiogram *(B)* of the palpable pulsatile mass in the right supraclavicular fossa showing tortuous subclavian artery (SA) and common carotid artery (CC).

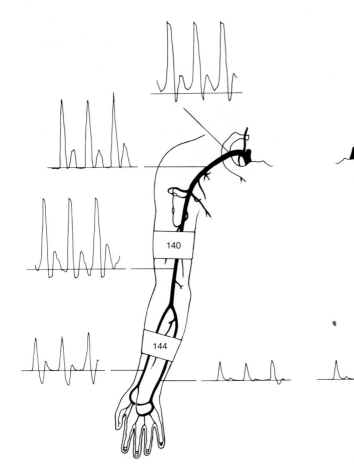

Figure 22–20. *Case I.* Segmental pressures and Doppler arterial waveforms.

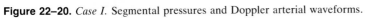

	Right	*Left*
Segmental Pressures		
Brachial Pressures	Normal	Normal
Forearm Pressures	Normal	Normal
Arm/Forearm Gradient	Normal	Normal
Arterial Waveforms		
Subclavian	Normal	Normal
Brachial	Normal	Normal
Radial/Ulnar	Normal	Normal

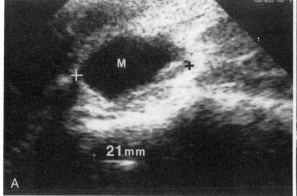

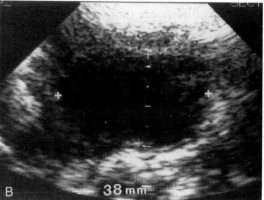

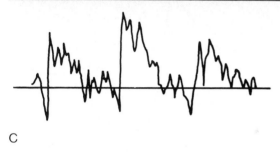

C

Figure 22–21. *Case II.* Real-time ultrasound image *(A and B)*, Doppler ultrasound waveform *(C)*, and segmental pressures and arterial waveform *(D)* of a brachial artery aneurysm. *A*, Real-time ultrasonogram demonstrating a sonolucent mass (M) measuring 21 mm along the long axis. *B*, Follow-up real-time ultrasonogram showing increase in the size (38 mm) of the aneurysm. *C*, Doppler ultrasound waveform showing the presence of arterial-blood flow within aneurysm. *D*, Normal segmental pressures and arterial waveform.

	Right
Segmental Pressures	
Brachial Pressure	Normal
Forearm Pressure	Normal
Arm/Forearm Gradient	Normal
Arterial Waveforms	
Subclavian	Normal
Brachial	Normal
Radial/Ulnar	Normal

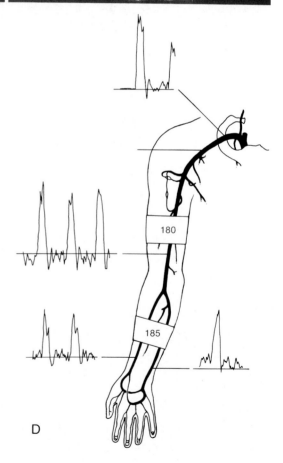

D

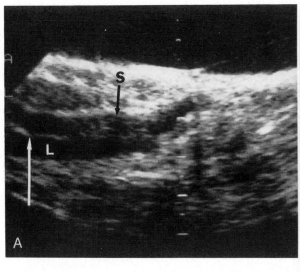

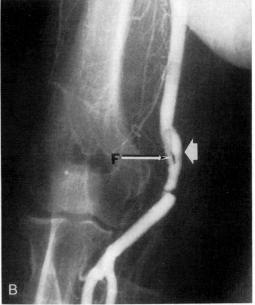

Figure 22–22. *Case III.* Real-time ultrasonogram *(A)* and angiogram *(B)* of the dissecting aneurysm of the brachial artery. *A,* Aneurysm with two lumens separated by an echogenic intimal flap (white arrow). One lumen is sonolucent (L), and the second contains low-level echoes from the slow blood flow (S). *B,* Dissecting aneurysm (large arrow) with intimal flap (F).

mal arterial velocities, findings that exclude distal obstruction.

Case IV illustrates the use of duplex ultrasonography in differentiating hematoma from aneurysm.

Case IV

A 50-year-old man presented with soft tissue swelling in the right cubital fossa after having undergone a brachial artery puncture for an angiographic procedure. Duplex ultrasonography demonstrated a sonolucent mass in the right cubital fossa with absence of pulsations, indicating the mass was a hematoma (Fig.

22–23*A*). This finding was confirmed by Doppler examination in which no flow could be detected within the mass (Fig. 22–23*B*).

The cases just presented indicate how the noninvasive tests were useful in achieving the proper diagnosis of either aneurysm or hematoma and following its course.

Duplex examination of aneurysms can be complemented by segmental pressures and Doppler arterial waveform analysis to determine any distal obstruction. These noninvasive tests can also be used to follow the results of reconstructive sur-

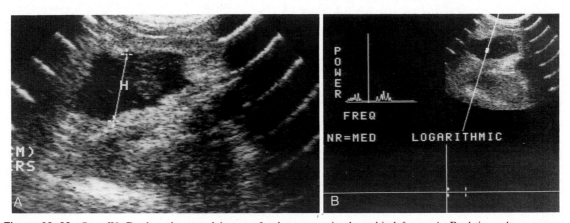

Figure 22–23. *Case IV.* Duplex ultrasound image of a hematoma in the cubital fossa. *A,* Real-time ultrasonogram illustrates a sonolucent mass (H) representing a hematoma. *B,* Doppler ultrasonogram shows an absence of blood flow in the hematoma.

gery consisting of excision of the aneurysm, with continuity maintained by either direct end-to-end anastomosis or vein graft placement.

Arterial Obstruction

The two most common causes of arterial obstruction in the upper extremity are embolism[14-16] and traumatic injury.[16, 17] Because it is situated in a vulnerable location, the brachial artery is easily injured. The incidence of trauma to various arteries is shown in Figure 22–24. Penetrating trauma is more frequent than blunt injuries. More recently, brachial, axillary, and subclavian arterial thrombosis with subsequent occlusion is caused by angiographic and cardiac catheteriza-

tion. Other causes of arterial trauma are drug abuse and fractures.

The incidence of emboli to the upper extremity arteries has been reported to occur in 17% of cases, and the distribution of emboli at various sites is illustrated in Figure 22–25 and Table 22–1.[14] The brachial artery bifurcation and its middle one-third portion are the two most frequent sites of arterial embolism in the upper extremity.

Atrial fibrillation, myocardial infarction, and bacterial endocarditis are the most common sources of embolism from the heart. Other sources include paradoxical embolism from systemic venous thrombosis, pulmonary venous thrombosis, and post-stenotic aneurysm.

Atherosclerosis is observed more frequently in

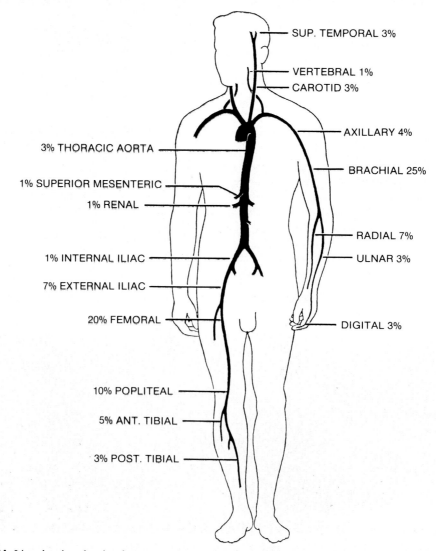

Figure 22–24. Line drawing showing frequency of arterial injuries. (From Jackson BB. Surgery of Acquired Vascular Disorders. Springfield, Ill, Charles C Thomas, 1969; 186, by permission.)

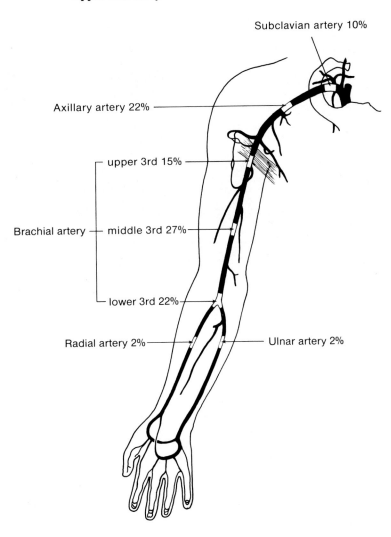

Subclavian artery 10%

Axillary artery 22%

upper 3rd 15%

Brachial artery — middle 3rd 27%

lower 3rd 22%

Radial artery 2%

Ulnar artery 2%

Figure 22–25. Line drawing showing the distribution (in percent) of embolisms in the upper extremity arterial system. (From Baird RJ, Lajos TZ. Emboli to the arm. Ann Surg 1964; 160:905, by permission.)

the lower extremities than in the upper extremities. When it does occur in the upper extremities, the subclavian and axillary arteries are affected more than any other distal vessels. An example of atherosclerotic plaque in the subclavian artery is shown in Figure 22–26. Brachial artery occlusion by atherosclerosis is uncommon.

The least common causes of upper extremity arterial obstruction are arteritis, Takayasu's disease, scalenus anticus syndrome, cervical rib syndrome, costoclavicular syndrome, pressure from a tumor, and congenital atresia of the intrathoracic segment of the left subclavian artery.[18, 19]

The clinical features vary with the location and degree of obstruction. The patient may present with cerebrovascular symptoms if the subclavian artery is obstructed before the origin of the vertebral artery. This is known as subclavian steal syndrome and is discussed in detail in Chapter 23. Other patients may remain asymptomatic, and the occlusion may be later discovered incidentally during a routine examination. Some subjects may present with weakness, pain at rest, cold hands, and paresthesia in the hand or forearm. Distal pulsations may be reduced or absent, depending upon the degree of obstruction and the presence or absence of collateral vessels. A bruit may be present in the supraclavicular region if the subclavian artery is partially occluded.

The use of noninvasive vascular techniques in

Table 22–1. Distribution of Emboli in Upper Extremity Arteries

Artery	Haimovici	Baird & Lajos
Subclavian	0%	10%
Axillary	28.3%	22%
Brachial	56.6%	64%
Radial	6.7%	2%
Ulnar	7.6%	2%

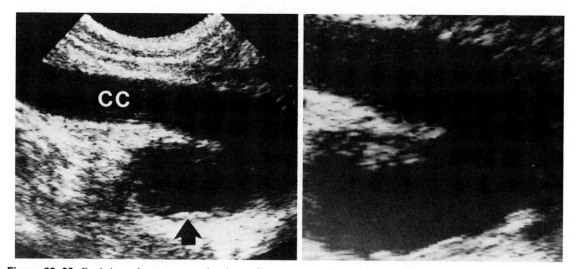

Figure 22–26. Real-time ultrasonogram showing a fibrous plaque (arrow) in the subclavian artery. CC = Common carotid artery.

the diagnosis of upper extremity obstructive arterial lesions is demonstrated in *Cases V* and *VI*.

Segmental Pressures

Normally, the brachial artery pressure is either equal to or within 10 mm Hg to that on the contralateral side.[2] The pressure gradient between the brachial artery and the radial or ulnar artery on the same side is also less than 10 mm Hg.[2] When the subclavian, axillary, or brachial artery is partially or completely obstructed, the systolic pressure distal to the obstruction is reduced. This results in an increased pressure difference greater than 10 mm Hg between the brachial arteries, with the pressure lower on the side of the obstruction. However, a low brachial pressure measurement cannot be used to determine the precise site of the obstructive lesion, and it cannot used to determine whether the

lesion is present in the subclavian, axillary, or brachial artery. This distinction can be made by determining the forearm pressure at the wrist. If the pressure gradient between the brachial and forearm on the same side is greater than 10 mm Hg, an obstructive lesion is present in the brachial artery. If this gradient is normal, the obstruction is present in the axillary or subclavian artery. These findings are shown in *Cases V* and *VI*.

Case V
A 51-year-old woman presented with vertebrobasilar symptoms. The brachial systolic pressures were obtained during the duplex carotid examination. The left brachial pressure (71 mm Hg) was significantly lower than the right brachial pressure (108 mm Hg) (Fig. 22–27A). The brachial pressure difference (37 mm Hg), along with the absolute pressure (71 mm Hg) on the left, was abnormal. This suggested the presence of an obstructive lesion in the left subclavian, axillary, or brachial artery. The arm/forearm pressure gradient was

Figure 22–27. *Case V.* Stenosis originating from left subclavian artery with abnormal segmental pressures. *A*, Velocity waveforms.

	Right	Left
Segmental Pressures		
Brachial Pressures	Normal	Abnormal
Forearm Pressures	Normal	Normal
Arm/Forearm Gradient	Normal	Normal
Arterial Waveforms		
Subclavian	Normal	Abnormal
Brachial	Normal	Abnormal
Radial/Ulnar	Normal	Abnormal

B, Angiogram showing stenosis (arrow) of the left subclavian artery.

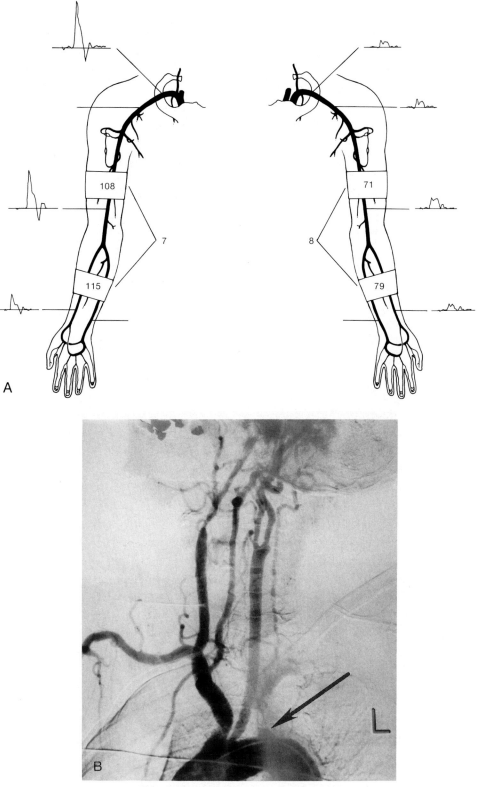

Figure 22–27 *See legend on opposite page*

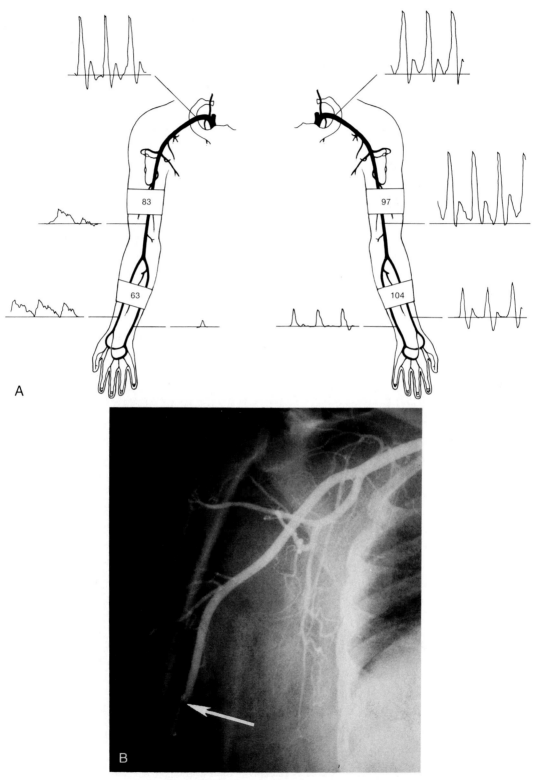

Figure 22–28 *See legend on opposite page*

normal bilaterally, which eliminated the brachial artery as a location for the lesion (Fig. 22–27A). The lesion was localized further by means of arterial velocity waveforms, which showed a monophasic pattern from the left subclavian artery and indicated that the site of obstruction was located in this artery (Fig. 22–27A). This was confirmed by arteriography (Fig. 22–27B).

Case VI

A middle-aged man presented with reduced pulsations of the radial and ulnar arteries of the right wrist following trauma to the brachial artery. The right brachial systolic pressure of 83 mm Hg was lower than the left brachial systolic pressure (97 mmHg) (Fig. 22–28A). These findings indicate an obstructive lesion present in the innominate, right subclavian, axillary, or brachial artery. The right forearm pressure of 63 mm Hg was lower than the brachial artery pressure; normally it is either equal to or higher than the brachial artery pressure. An abnormal pressure gradient of 20 mm Hg between the right brachial artery and the forearm suggests an obstructive lesion located in the right brachial artery (Fig. 22–28A). This diagnosis was further confirmed by Doppler arterial velocity waveforms, which were normal from the right subclavian and axillary arteries, monophasic from the right brachial artery, and markedly damped at the distal radial and ulnar arteries. An arteriogram showed right brachial artery occlusion (Fig. 22–28B).

Doppler Arterial Velocity Waveform

Doppler arterial velocity waveforms complement the systolic segmental pressure measurement as a means of achieving an accurate diagnosis.

The arterial velocity waveform obtained from a normal peripheral artery is usually multiphasic. It consists of a systolic component, a reversed early diastolic component, and a forward late diastolic component. The waveform distal to an obstruction may be monophasic, continuous, or absent, depending upon the severity of obstruction and the presence or absence of the collateral vessels. When an obstructive lesion is present in the subclavian artery, the arterial waveform from the ipsilateral subclavian and distal vessels will be abnormal, as shown in *Case V* and Figure 22–27A. If an obstruction is located in the axillary artery, the waveform from the subclavian artery will be normal on the same side, whereas waveforms from the axillary, brachial, and distal vessels will be abnormal. A brachial artery obstruction will be associated with a normal waveform from the subclavian artery and the axillary artery; an abnormal waveform will be obtained from the obstructed artery and distal vessels, as shown in *Case VI* and Figure 22–28A.

Duplex Ultrasonography

Real-time ultrasonography, by means of a high-frequency transducer for imaging, directly visualizes the vessel lumen and, thereby, is able to demonstrate the patency or occlusion of blood vessels. Real-time sonography can also show changes in the surrounding tissue. A thrombus in the lumen of a vessel may vary in appearance, depending upon its age. The Doppler component of a duplex system may be helpful in the early stage when the thrombus is usually sonolucent and cannot be identified by real-time imaging. Later, when the thrombus is older, it is often seen as an echogenic area occupying the lumen of a vessel (Fig. 22–29A). The use of duplex sonography, in conjunction with segmental pressures and arterial waveforms is demonstrated in *Case VII*.

Case VII

A 49-year-old man complained of arm pain following an angiographic procedure performed through the brachial artery. The real-time ultrasonogram of the puncture site showed an echogenic area representing thrombus in the lumen of the distal brachial artery (Fig. 22–29A). Hypoechoic areas were also seen surrounding

Figure 22–28. *Case VI.* Right brachial artery occlusion with abnormal segmental pressures. *A,* Velocity waveforms and segmental pressures.

	Right	*Left*
Segmental Pressures		
Brachial Pressures	Abnormal	Normal
Forearm Pressures	Abnormal	Normal
Arm/Forearm Gradient	Abnormal	Normal
Arterial Waveforms		
Axillary	Normal	Normal
Brachial	Abnormal	Normal
Radial/Ulnar	Abnormal	Normal

B, Angiogram demonstrating brachial artery occlusion (arrow).

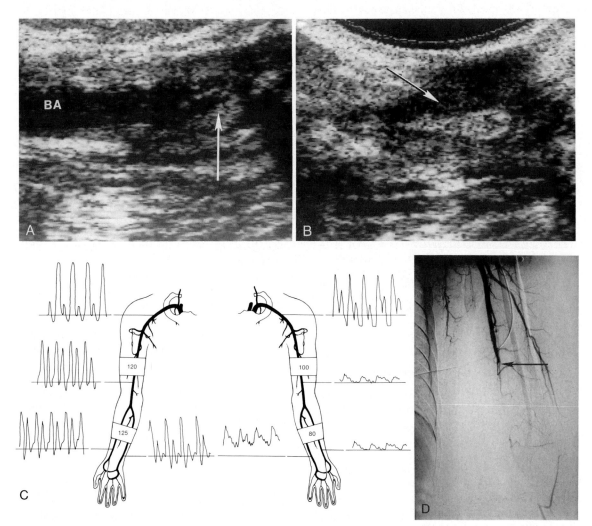

Figure 22–29. *Case VII.* Real-time ultrasonogram (*A* and *B*), Doppler arterial waveform *(C)* and angiogram *(D)* demonstrating hematoma.

A, Echogenic thrombus (arrow) in the brachial artery (BA).

B, Inhomogeneous hypoechoic area (arrow) representing hematoma.

C, Velocity waveforms and segmental pressures.

	Right	*Left*
Arterial Waveforms		
Axillary	Normal	Normal
Brachial	Normal	Abnormal
Radial/Ulnar	Normal	Abnormal
Segmental Pressures		
Brachial Pressures	Normal	Abnormal
Forearm Pressures	Normal	Abnormal
Arm/Forearm Gradient	Normal	Abnormal

D, Brachial artery occlusion (arrow).

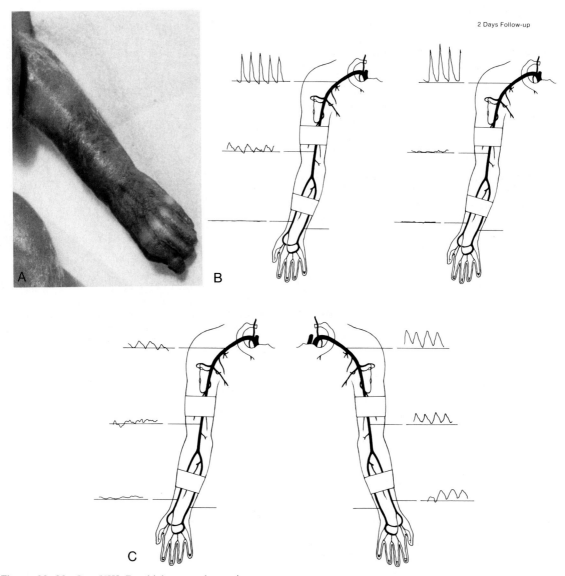

Figure 22–30. *Case VIII.* Brachial artery obstruction.
  A, Photograph showing skin color changes in the forearm caused by ischemia.
  B, Doppler arterial waveforms.

Arterial Waveforms	*Right*	
Axillary	Normal	
Brachial	Abnormal	
Radial	Abnormal	

C, Photoplethysmographic (PPG) waveforms.

PPG Waveforms	*Right*	*Left*
Axillary	Normal	Normal
Brachial	Abnormal	Normal
Radial	Abnormal	Normal

the blood vessel at the site of the thrombosis (Fig. 22–29B). These tissues changes were due to resolving hematoma from the brachial artery catheterization. Normal Doppler arterial waveforms from the subclavian and axillary arteries on the ipsilateral side were normal, whereas those from the brachial artery were monophasic, indicating the site of the obstruction (Fig. 22–29C). The radial and ulnar arterial waveforms were markedly damped; the arterial waveforms from the contralateral vessels were normal. The site of brachial artery obstruction is shown on the angiogram in Figure 22–29D.

Photoplethysmography

Photoplethysmography can be utilized to complement Doppler ultrasonography. PPG can also be utilized as the primary examination when the Doppler examination proves cumbersome or when a patient's condition limits its use. A PPG examination is shown in *Case VIII*.

Case VIII
A premature newborn weighing 600 gm was found to have color changes in the right forearm (Fig. 22–30A) along with an absent radial artery pulsation following brachial artery catheterization. Doppler ultrasonography showed a normal arterial waveform

from the right axillary artery. The right brachial artery waveform was monophasic; waveforms from the radial and ulnar arteries were absent (Fig. 22–30B). These findings suggested the presence of obstruction in the right brachial artery. A Doppler ultrasonographic follow-up taken 2 days later revealed no significant change in the appearance of the arterial waveforms (Fig. 22–30B). Photoplethysmography of the right upper extremity also confirmed the Doppler findings (Fig. 22–30C). Amputation of the right forearm was subsequently performed.

Case IX
A 72-year-old man complained of pain in his right arm. The brachial, radial, and ulnar pulsations were normal. Photoplethysmographic waveforms from the middle and ring fingers were normal; those from the thumb, index finger, and little fingers were damped. The digital pressures were low in the thumb, index fingers, and little fingers (Fig. 22–31), which signified obstruction. An arteriogram confirmed the PPG findings (Fig. 22–32).

Case X
A 24-year-old man presented with a canine bite of the left arm. The left brachial and radial pulsations were absent on physical examination. The preoperative arteriogram revealed a left brachial artery occlusion for which the patient underwent bypass surgery. The

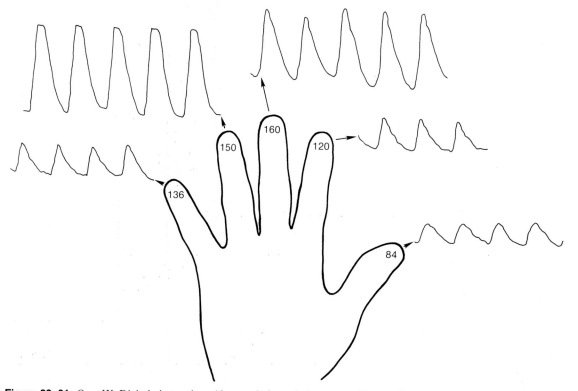

Figure 22–31. *Case IX.* Digital obstruction. Abnormal photoplethysmographic waveforms and digital pressures from the thumb, index finger, and little finger. Normal pressures and waveform from the middle and ring fingers.

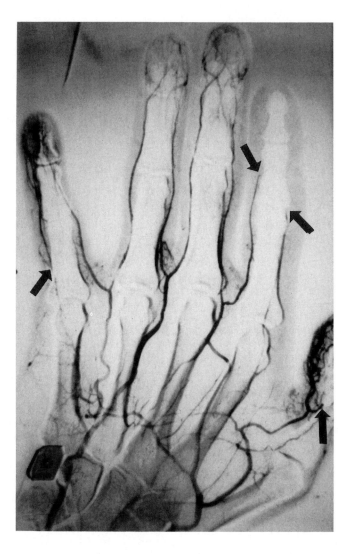

Figure 22–32. *Case IX.* Angiogram shows obstructed digital vessels (arrows).

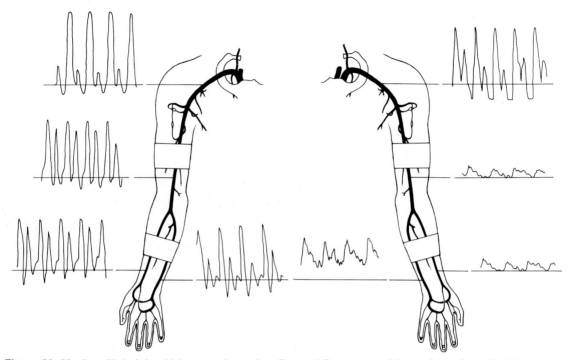

Figure 22–33. *Case X.* Left brachial artery obstruction. Damped Doppler arterial waveforms from the left brachial, radial, and ulnar arteries.

post-bypass Doppler examination showed normal arterial waveforms from the arteries of the right extremity and the left axillary artery. The Doppler waveforms from the left brachial, left radial, and left ulnar arteries were damped (Fig. 22–33). The PPG waveforms of the digits of the left hand showed damped waveforms in the thumb and little finger (Fig. 22–34).

The PPG waveform from the index finger was definitely normal, and the waveforms from the middle and ring finger were mildly abnormal. Waveforms from the middle and ring fingers lacked the normal concavity towards the baseline along the descending limb. The postoperative arteriogram revealed brachial artery obstruction (Fig. 22–35A) with patent radial and ulnar arteries (Fig. 22–35B). The arteriogram of the hand demonstrated obstruction of digital vessels to the first, third, fourth, and fifth digits (Fig. 22–35C). Subsequently, surgery was again performed to relieve the obstruction of the brachial artery.

Thoracic Outlet Syndrome

Thoracic outlet syndrome (TOS) occurs from compression of the neurovascular structures that course through the neck to supply the upper extremities. Thoracic outlet syndrome is further subdivided into various syndromes, based on the underlying defects and on the signs and symptoms. Other syndromes include *cervical rib syndrome, scalenus anticus* and *scalenus medius syn-*

dromes, costoclavicular syndrome, pectoralis minor syndrome, and *Wright's syndrome.*

Patients usually present with a dull, aching pain radiating from the point of compression to the neck, shoulder girdle region, arm, forearm, and hand. Thoracic outlet syndrome is often associated with paresthesia and numbness in the distribution of C8 to T1 dermatomes (volar aspect of the fourth and fifth digits) when the patient abducts the arm to 90° and externally rotates it. These symptoms are frequently relieved when the subject places the arm in the neutral position. They become exaggerated with prolonged use of the affected extremity. A bruit is often present in the supraclavicular fossa when the arm is abducted to 90°. Occasionally, patients with TOS may have subclavian artery aneurysms and may present with further complications.

Patients who are suspected of having TOS are usually evaluated during physical examination with special maneuver techniques that include:

1. *Adson's maneuver.* The patient takes a deep breath and holds it while extending the neck upward and turning the chin to the right and left. This maneuver assesses the compression of the scalenus muscle or the cervical rib (Fig. 22–36A and B).

2. *Costoclavicular maneuver.* The patient draws the shoulders downward and backward in

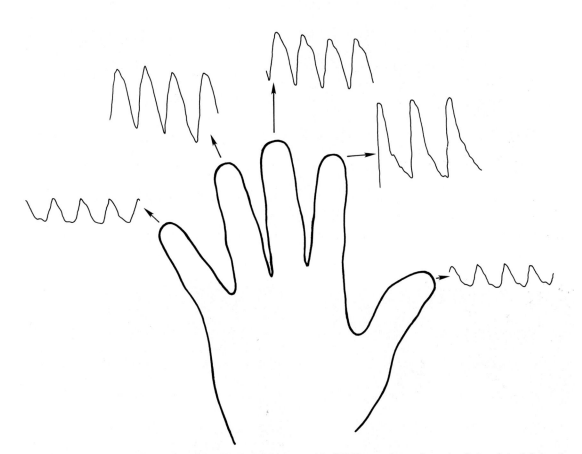

Figure 22–34. *Case X.* Digital obstruction. Photoplethysmographic (PPG) waveforms from the digits of the left hand.

Digits	PPG Waveform
Thumb	Abnormal
Index	Normal
Middle	Abnormal
Ring	Abnormal
Little	Abnormal

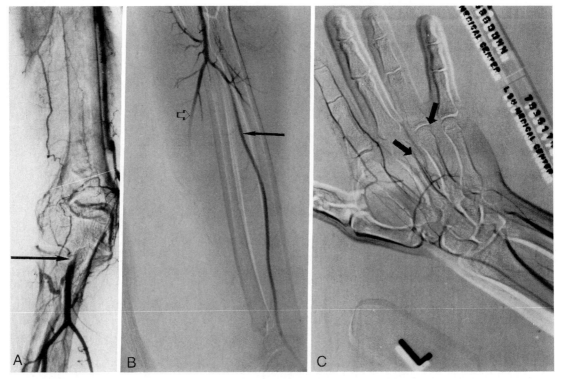

Figure 22–35. Case X. Angiograms of the arm *(A)*, forearm *(B)*, and hand *(C)*. *A*, Brachial artery obstruction (arrow). *B*, Patent radial (arrow) and ulnar (open arrow) arteries. *C*, Obstruction of the digital arteries (arrows).

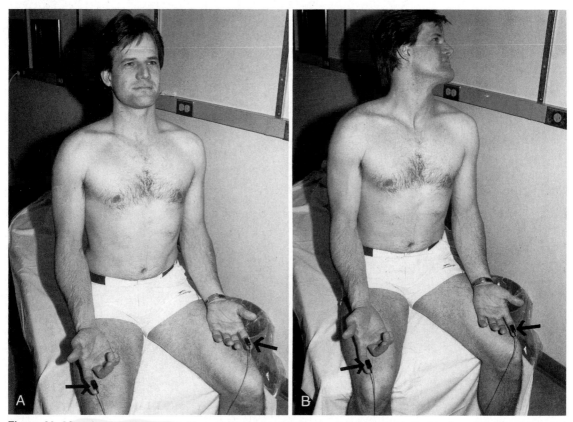

Figure 22–36. Adson's maneuver. *A*, Photoplethysmographic photocells (arrows) attached to fingers for the Adson test. *B*, Adson's maneuver. The neck is extended upward, and the chin is turned to the right or left.

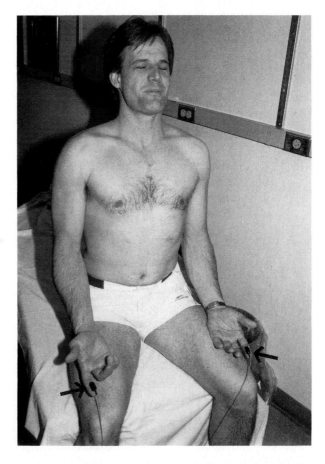

Figure 22–37. Costoclavicular position with photoplethysmographic photocells (arrows) attached to fingers. Shoulders are forced downward and backward in a military posture.

a military fashion. This maneuver assesses neurovascular compression between the clavicles and the first rib (Fig. 22–37).

3. *Hyperabduction.* The patient externally rotates the arm with the palm upward and then extends the arm upward to 90° and 180°, respectively. This maneuver assesses neurovascular compression by the coracoid process or the pectoralis minor muscle (Fig. 22–38A and B).

These same maneuvers are used in the noninvasive examinations to evaluate the vascular component of the TOS. Blood flow characteristics are monitored by means of Doppler or PPG techniques.

A 10 MHz Doppler probe is positioned over the brachial or radial artery at a 30 to 45° angle into the forward flow. The strip chart recorder is set at 5 mm/second and is run continuously throughout the maneuver. Normally, there is only a slight increase or no change in the signal. However, in the presence of TOS, there is attenuation or absence of arterial flow.[21, 22]

The PPG technique is the simplest method for reproducing and maintaining contact with the artery during maneuvers. The photocells are attached bilaterally to the forefingers using double-stick tape or Velcro straps. The chart strip recorder is set at 5 mm/second for the tracing. PPG monitoring is continuous throughout all of the maneuvers. Normally, there is only a slight increase or change in the amplitude of the waveform (Fig. 22–39A). However, in the presence of TOS, there is a marked decrease or an absence of flow (Fig. 22–39B).

The noninvasive study may be equivocal in some cases, requiring further testing. However, it has been found that using the criteria of complete obliteration of flow and reproduction of the patient's symptoms during maneuvers makes the noninvasive testing a valuable procedure. One must remember that the normal Doppler examination cannot rule out TOS because some patients may only have neurological involvement without the vascular component. If these patients have subclavian artery aneurysms, real-time ultrasonography may be helpful in achieving the diagnosis. Segmental systolic pressures and arterial waveforms from the distal arteries should also be used to determine distal obstruction that is present as a complication of the syndrome.

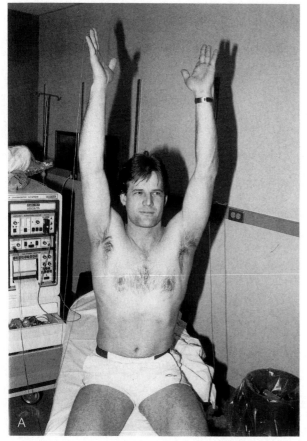

Figure 22–38. Hyperabduction maneuver *(A)* and corresponding photoplethysmographic (PPG) waveforms *(B)*. *A,* Hyperabduction position with PPG photocells attached to fingers. *B,* Analog waveform tracing during hyperabduction maneuver. The various position changes are reflected in the change in amplitude of the waveform.

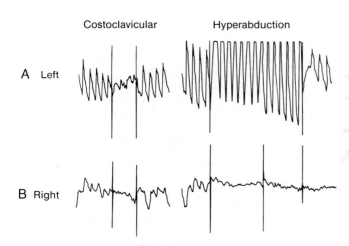

Figure 22–39. Normal photoplethysmographic (PPG) waveforms *(A)* compared with those found in thoracic outlet syndrome (TOS) *(B)*. *A,* Normal PPG waveform during various maneuvers indicates an absence of the vascular component of TOS. *B,* Thoracic outlet syndrome (TOS) suggested by marked diminished amplitude of waveform during costoclavicular and hyperabduction maneuvers. (From Barnes RW. Noninvasive diagnostic techniques in peripheral vascular disease. Records of the Medical College of Virginia, 1980, with permission.)

Arteriography may also assist in localizing and determining the cause of obstruction. The nerve conduction velocity of the peripheral nerve of the upper extremity provides the definite diagnosis.

Ischemia of the Hand and Digits

Ischemia of the hands and digits is an infrequent occurrence that is most commonly caused by vasospastic abnormalities.[24] Patients suffering from these abnormalities may be evaluated in the noninvasive vascular laboratory for the presence of either *Raynaud's disease* or *Raynaud's phenomenon*. Unfortunately, the terms themselves are confusing and lead to considerable misunderstanding about these conditions. To avoid this confusion, several terms must be defined before discussing the noninvasive vascular examinations.

Raynaud's Symptoms. Raynaud's symptoms are characterized by sensitivity to cold resulting in pain and color changes in the skin. They occur most commonly in the fingers and hands and are related to cold and emotional stimuli.

Raynaud's Syndrome. Raynaud's syndrome is defined as episodic vasoconstriction of the arteries and arterioles of the extremities in response to cold or emotional stimuli, which produces the Raynaud's symptoms. The term Raynaud's symptoms is used to describe the patient's complaints. The term Raynaud's syndrome is used in an attempt to define the pathophysiology of these complaints. For example, the skin changes observed by the patient with Raynaud's symptoms would include the skin color turning white, then blue, and finally red. These changes must be caused by episodic vasoconstriction in response to cold or emotional stimuli in order to constitute Raynaud's syndrome. The skin turning white or pallor in the early stages of an attack is caused by a severe vascular spasm, which results in an absence of blood flow in the skin capillary bed. Anaerobic metabolites then begin to build up in the ischemic tissues, causing a slight relaxation of the arteriolar spasm. This results in a small trickle of blood entering into the dilated capillary bed of the skin. The capillary bed soon becomes depleted of its oxygen content, which causes the blue skin color of cyanosis. Further relaxation of the arterioles causes more and more blood to enter the capillary bed until the skin turns red (rubor). The attack terminates with the passage of a normal volume of blood through the relaxed arterioles, and the skin color regains its normal appearance. These attacks may occur with either Raynaud's disease or Raynaud's phenomenon.

Raynaud's Disease. Raynaud's disease is defined as Raynaud's syndrome occurring in conjunction with an anatomically normal, *nonobstructive* arterial system. The disease usually follows a benign course, but in long-standing cases, trophic changes develop, causing atrophy of the skin, subcutaneous tissue, and muscles. Ulceration and ischemic gangrene are rare. Raynaud's disease occurs almost exclusively in young females with onset in the second or third decade. Bilateral involvement is almost always present. The true etiology of Raynaud's disease remains unknown. It is postulated to be related to some form of hyperlability of the sympathetic neuromuscular synaptic end-plate in the arterial muscle. However, numerous studies have failed to demonstrate any consistent abnormality of sympathetic nerve function in the arteries of patients suffering from Raynaud's syndrome.

It is to be emphasized, then, that Raynaud's disease is an idiopathic vasospastic disorder affecting the small arteries and arterioles of the extremities and occurs mainly in young, apparently healthy, women. The symptoms are due to vasoconstriction, and there are no true obstructive lesions within the arterial walls.

Criteria for the diagnosis of Raynaud's disease include:

1. Skin over digits turning white, blue, and red in response to cold.
2. Bilateral or symmetrical involvement.
3. History of intermittent attack episodes over 2 years.
4. No primary cause is found.
5. Nutritional changes in skin only.

Raynaud's Phenomenon. Raynaud's phenomenon is defined as Raynaud's syndrome occurring in conjunction with an anatomically abnormal, *obstructive* arterial system. The arterial obstructions decrease the blood pressure in the affected tissues of the hands and fingers. This decrease in arterial pressure allows the normal vasoconstrictive response to cold temperatures or emotional stimuli to produce an absence of blood flow in the skin capillary beds of the affected tissues. As a result, the same symptoms that are found in Raynaud's disease are also present in Raynaud's phenomenon. The obstructive lesions that may lead to the Raynaud's phenomenon include arteriosclerosis, arterial trauma, and autoimmune diseases affecting the digital arteries. Of these, the diagnosis of Raynaud's phenomenon is particularly important in the diagnosis of scleroderma because this phenomenon may precede the skin changes by months or even years. A detailed list of the underlying disorders that can

Table 22–2. Causes of Raynaud's Phenomenon

Collagen vascular disorders
  Scleroderma
  Systemic lupus erythematosus
  Dermatomyositis
Trauma
  Hypothenar hammer syndrome
  Arteriovenous fistula
  Thrombosis
  Ulnar artery aneurysm
  Drug abuse
Occupational and industrial exposure
  Vibrating instruments
Poisoning
  Arsenic
  Lead
Drug ingestion
  Ergotamine preparation
  Methysergide
  Propranolol
Chronic arterial disease
  Thromboangiitis obliterans
Hematologic disorders
  Cryoglobins
  Cold agglutinins
  Dysproteinemia
Iatrogenic
  Catheterization procedures
  Arteriography
  Arterial puncture
  Dialysis access
Bilateral thoracic outlet syndrome
Bilateral frostbite
Primary pulmonary hypertension
Occult malignancy

cause Raynaud's phenomenon is given in Table 22–2.[24, 26] Because these disorders may not affect all of the arteries in the hands and fingers, Raynaud's phenomenon can be unilateral and may involve only one or two digits. This is an important point in distinguishing it from Raynaud's disease, which affects all of the digits of both hands.

Raynaud's Disease versus Raynaud's Phenomenon

Patients are usually known to have Raynaud's syndrome before they are referred to the noninvasive vascular laboratory. This is because they have already gone to a physician with the chief complaint of an uncomfortable sensation of numbness in their hands or fingers, which is aggravated by exposure to cool temperatures or emotional stress. The examining physician may then refer the patient to the noninvasive vascular laboratory to determine whether the suspected Raynaud's syndrome is caused by Raynaud's

disease or Raynaud's phenomenon. It is important to make this distinction because Raynaud's disease is a benign condition with a good prognosis and Raynaud's phenomenon is often associated with a serious underlying disorder (Table 22–2) with a poor prognosis.

The noninvasive vascular procedures used to distinguish Raynaud's disease from Raynaud's phenomenon include:

1. Segmental systolic pressure measurements.
2. Doppler arterial velocity waveform analysis.
3. Digital systolic pressure measurements.
4. Digital PPG waveform analysis.

The examination is begun by obtaining segmental systolic pressure measurements of the brachial, radial, and ulnar arteries in both upper extremities, as previously described. When these pressure measurements are normal (Fig. 22–11), Raynaud's phenomenon caused by an obstructive lesion in the subclavian, axillary, brachial, radial, or ulnar artery is excluded. Pressure measurements do not exclude Raynaud's phenomenon caused by digital artery obstructive lesions or Raynaud's disease caused by a diffuse vasoconstriction of digital arteries containing no obstructive lesions. To exclude these possibilities, the use of digital systolic pressure measurements and digital PPG is required.

Digital systolic pressure measurements are normal in patients with Raynaud's disease but are decreased in patients with Raynaud's phenomenon. The normal digital systolic pressure measurements are given in Figure 22–12. In patients with Raynaud's phenomenon, the decrease in the systolic pressure measurements is either unilateral or localized to a few digits of the affected hand. This, of course, depends upon the cause of the digital artery obstructive lesions that are, in turn, producing the Raynaud's phenomenon. For example, Raynaud's phenomenon caused by arteriosclerotic, traumatic, or embolic digital artery occlusions is characterized by decreased systolic pressure measurements that are generally localized to two or three digits of the involved hand. Digital artery occlusions caused by collagen diseases, Buerger's disease (thromboangiitis obliterans), or frostbite are associated with decreased systolic pressure measurements in all of the digits. The digital systolic pressure measurements are considered decreased when they are 20 mm Hg below the brachial artery systolic pressure.

Digital photoplethysmographic waveforms are normal in Raynaud's disease and abnormal in Raynaud's phenomenon. The techniques for using digital PPG in obtaining both the digital systolic pressure measurements and the digital blood flow waveforms have been previously described in discussions on palmar arch testing and the TOS. These methods are used to localize arterial obstructions in the subclavian arteries during the various test maneuvers for TOS or in the palmar arches during Allen's test maneuvers. These same methods are also applied in the detection of digital artery obstructive lesions and represent a powerful tool to be used in distinguishing Raynaud's phenomenon from Raynaud's disease in patients with Raynaud's syndrome.

Although it is used profusely in the literature, the term photoplethysmography is a misnomer because the technique does not measure volume changes. Instead, it measures the rapid changes in the blood content of the skin, which produce a pulsatile waveform that follows the cardiac cycle. Photoplethysmography is accomplished by attaching the probe or photoelectric cell to the finger tip, as shown in Figure 22–18A. Infrared light is emitted from the probe into the skin, where it is reflected back towards the probe face. The amount of infrared light that is reflected back toward the probe face is proportional to the number of red blood cells (RBCs) in the microvasculature of the skin. The actual quantity being measured by photoelectric plethysmography is the number of RBCs in the skin microvasculature. Because the number of RBCs increases during systole and decreases during diastole, the probe records a pulsatile waveform that follows the cardiac cycle. A greatly diminished or absent waveform is recorded by the probe when blood ceases to flow through the microvasculature of the skin. In the absence of blood flow, few, if any, RBCs are present in the skin microvasculature to reflect the emitted infrared light back towards the probe face. This principle then makes photoelectric plethysmography an excellent method to be used in the detection of blood flow in skin surfaces, such as the finger tips.

An example of a normal, pulsatile blood flow waveform recorded from the finger tip is shown in Figure 22–40A. It has a rapid systolic upswing, a sharp systolic peak, and a dicrotic notch on the diastolic downslope. These waveforms are seen in patients with Raynaud's disease.

Patients with obstructive arterial lesions producing the Raynaud's phenomenon will exhibit digital PPG waveforms like the one shown in Figure 22–40B. This figure demonstrates an abnormal obstructive waveform characterized by a slow systolic upswing; a rounded, flat systolic peak; and loss of the dicrotic notch on the gradual diastolic downslope. The peaked PPG waveform in Figure 22–40C represents another abnormal waveform that may be seen in Raynaud's phenomenon with underlying digital artery obstructive disease.[27-31] This waveform is characterized by a slightly delayed systolic upswing, an irregular rounded systolic peak, and a diastolic downslope that is bowed away from the baseline. The peaked portion of the waveform is caused by an anacrotic notch that occurs before the systolic peak and a dicrotic notch that occurs after the systolic peak. Together the anacrotic and dicrotic notches cause the peaked portion of this waveform. Another small dicrotic notch may be observed on the downslope of the waveform in late diastole.

It is possible to have an abnormal PPG waveform in a digit that exhibits a normal digital pressure measurement. This occurs when the digital artery obstruction is located near the finger tip and beyond the site of the occlusion cuff.[1] A lesion of this type is readily detected by PPG waveform analysis because the photoelectric cell is placed on the finger tip beyond the site of the digital artery occlusion. Photoplethysmographic waveform analysis, then, offers an effective

Figure 22–40. Normal and abnormal photoplethysmographic waveforms.

A, Normal waveform with rapid systolic upswing (S), sharp systolic peak (P), and a dicrotic notch (N) on the diastolic downslope (D).

B, Abnormal obstructive waveform with slow systolic upswing (S), rounded flat systolic peak (P), and loss of the dicrotic notch on the gradual diastolic downslope (D).

C, "Peaked" waveform with slightly delayed systolic upswing (S), anacrotic notch (A), irregular systolic peak (P), and dicrotic notches (N) on the diastolic downslope (D).

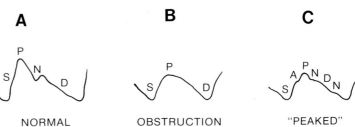

method for detecting digital artery occlusions that occur in the extreme distal portions of the finger tips.

Both digital pressure measurements and PPG waveform analysis offer a method for detecting the underlying arterial obstructive lesions associated with Raynaud's phenomenon, but, used alone, they are nonspecific for the diagnosis of Raynaud's disease. This problem arises because there are no underlying arterial obstructive lesions associated with Raynaud's disease. Unless vasoconstriction is stimulated in these patients, their digital pressures and PPG waveforms will be normal. A simple way to stimulate vasoconstriction is to immerse the hand in ice water. We simply call this the "ice water" test.

Ice Water Test

Normally, the microvasculature in the skin over the finger tips is very sensitive to changes in temperature and emotional stimuli. This fact causes many of the pitfalls seen with PPG waveform analysis of the blood flow in the skin of the finger tips. Patients who arrive in the noninvasive vascular laboratory on a cold winter day to find themselves surrounded by strange equipment will often exhibit an abnormal PPG waveform. To avoid this pitfall, allow the patient to sit in the examining room for a while and to become familiar with the surroundings. Optimally, the room should be warmed to at least 25° C. The use of an electric blanket to provide supplementary warming of the hands and fingers prior to the examination is extremely helpful.

After the patient has become familiar with the surroundings and the hands and fingers are warm, perform baseline testing to exclude Raynaud's phenomenon caused by arterial obstructive disease. These baseline tests should include digital and thumb systolic pressure measurements and PPG waveforms. If these are normal, immerse the patient's hand in ice water for 3 minutes if this can be tolerated by the patient. Remove the patient's hand from the ice water, wipe it dry with a towel, and immediately obtain PPG waveforms and pressure measurements on the four digits of the hand. Measurements after ice water immersion are not made on the thumb because it is usually not involved in Raynaud's disease.[32] The index finger is most frequently involved, followed by the middle, ring, and little fingers.

When the ice water test provokes an attack of complete digital artery closure in a patient with Raynaud's disease, the digital pressure will be zero and the PPG waveform will be absent. If this does not occur, it must be assumed that the ice water test has failed to provoke an acute attack of complete digital artery closure in a patient with the symptoms of Raynaud's disease. An ice water test with positive results and loss of the digital pressure and PPG waveforms supports the diagnosis of Raynaud's disease, whereas a test with negative results cannot be used to exclude the diagnosis of this disease. This is because it is difficult to provoke the episodic nature of the vascular spasm associated with Raynaud's disease in a laboratory setting.

When the ice water test causes an abnormal decrease in the digital artery pressures below the pre-cooling baseline levels, some degree of pathological vasospasm must be suspected. Whether or not this degree of vasospasm is actually responsible for the patient's symptoms is difficult, if not impossible, to assess from the results of the ice water test alone. Normally, the digital systolic pressures do not drop more than 5% of the pre-cooling levels.[33, 39]

Patients with Raynaud's phenomenon exhibit a substantial decrease in digital artery systolic pressures after body and digital cooling.[35, 36] A drop in the digital pressures greater than 20% of the pre-cooling levels indicates significant digital artery vasospasm. When this is observed immediately after ice water immersion, the hand is allowed to rewarm at room temperature for 5 minutes. The digital pressure measurements and PPG waveforms are then obtained from each of the four digits of the hand to see whether they are beginning to return to the pre-cooling baseline levels. If these measurements remain abnormal, further evidence that a pathological vasospastic condition exists is provided. Further testing may then be considered to determine whether or not the vasospastic abnormality would respond to therapy that blocks the sympathetic stimuli to the digital artery vascular bed. These tests are easy to perform and center around the PPG waveform changes that occur in response to deep breathing, breath holding, and reactive hyperemia.

Sympathetic Response Testing

Sympathetic response tests are easy to perform in the noninvasive vascular laboratory once the mechanism for control of blood flow through the fingers is understood. Blood flow through the fingers increases when the digital arteries and arterioles are open (dilated) and decreases when these vessels are closed (constricted). The opening and closing of these vessels are regulated through the autonomic nervous system by a mechanism known as *sympathetic tone.* Sympathetic tone normally keeps almost all of the blood vessels in the body constricted to approximately half their maximum diameter. An increase in sympathetic tone causes further constriction of these vessels; a decrease in sympathetic tone results in dilatation. The concept of the sympathetic tone mechanism is important because it explains how a single nervous system can cause both constriction and dilatation of an arterial vascular bed. In this case, the sympathetic nervous system regulates the sympathetic tone in the digital arteries and arterioles of the fingers. This is accomplished through alpha-adrenergic receptor sites that constrict these vessels and decrease the blood flow through the fingers. These receptor sites are not excited when sympathetic nerve stimulation is either absent or blocked. The absence or blockage of sympathetic nerve stimulation allows the muscular walls of the vessels to relax so that they can open up and increase the blood flow through the fingers. Blocking sympathetic nerve stimulation of the alpha-adrenergic receptor sites, then, constitutes one of the major forms of treatment in patients with Raynaud's syndrome.

To review, sympathetic nerve stimulation excites alpha-adrenergic receptors, which increases the sympathetic tone mechanism. This decreases blood flow through the fingers by constricting the digital arteries and arterioles. When the sympathetic nerve stimulation is either absent or blocked, the alpha-adrenergic receptors are not excited and the sympathetic tone mechanism is decreased. This increases blood flow through the fingers by dilating the digital arteries and arterioles.

It is the purpose of the noninvasive vascular laboratory to determine whether the sympathetic nerve stimuli are present or absent. If they are present in a patient with Raynaud's syndrome, the patient may benefit from the blockage of these stimuli either by cutting the sympathetic nerve fibers in the sympathetic chain at T2 and T3 (sympathectomy) or through the use of medications. If sympathetic nerve stimuli are absent in a patient with Raynaud's syndrome, the patient may receive little benefit from either of these forms of treatment. An example is the patient with Raynaud's phenomenon in whom the underlying obstructive arterial disease process has already resulted in maximum dilatation of the digital arteries and arterioles. The sympathetic tone mechanism is already reduced to achieve the maximum dilatation of these vessels.

There may be no need to attempt blocking of the sympathetic nerve stimulation under these circumstances. Sympathetic response testing in the noninvasive vascular laboratory may then be used in an attempt to determine which group of patients is most likely to benefit from some type of sympathetic nerve-blocking therapy.

Sympathetic response testing is also used to determine whether the therapy is effective in blocking sympathetic stimuli. If the therapy is effective, sympathetic stimuli should be absent. The persistence of sympathetic stimuli, of course, means that the therapy is ineffective and some other form of treatment might be of more benefit to the patient.

Respiratory Testing

Respiratory testing makes use of the principle that changes in the cardiac output can alter the sympathetic tone mechanism of the peripheral vascular system. An increase in the cardiac output raises the blood pressure, whereas a decrease in cardiac output lowers the blood pressure. One of the purposes of the sympathetic tone mechanism is to keep the blood pressure constant in the circulatory system during periods when the cardiac output increases or decreases. As the cardiac output increases, sympathetic stimulation decreases and the arterioles dilate to normalize pressure by allowing more blood to run off into the venous system. Conversely, as the cardiac output decreases, the sympathetic stimulation increases and the arterioles constrict to normalize pressure by stopping the run-off of blood flow into the venous system.

Because respiratory maneuvers offer a method of increasing and decreasing cardiac output, they are used to test for sympathetic stimulation. Begin the test by placing a photoelectric plethysmographic probe on the tip of the index finger, as shown in Figure 22–18A. Place the amplifier in the alternating current (AC) mode, and record a baseline strip (Fig. 22–41) with the patient quiet and breathing normally. Then ask the patient to take a deep breath and hold it. Immediately, the PPG waveform will change in amplitude in comparison with the quiet breathing level (Fig. 22–41A). This change occurs because inspiration momentarily lowers the intrathoracic pressure, causing more blood to rush into the heart and increasing the cardiac output. The increase in cardiac output raises the blood pressure, causing a decrease in the sympathetic stimuli, which lowers the sympathetic tone mechanism and dilates the small arteries and arterioles of the

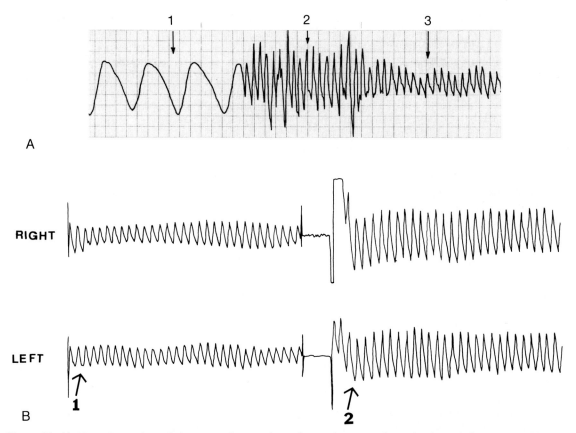

Figure 22–41. Normal test photoplethysmography waveforms for respiratory and reactive hyperemia.

A, Respiratory test for sympathetic stimuli. *1,* Quiet breathing PPG waveform. *2,* Inspiration PPG waveform goes up as sympathetic stimuli are decreased. *3,* Valsalva maneuver PPG waveform goes down as sympathetic stimuli are increased.

B, Reactive hyperemia response. *1,* Baseline PPG waveform. *2,* Reactive hyperemic response to ischemia causes PPG waveforms to increase.

fingers. This allows more RBCs to flow through the finger tips, creating an elevation in the PPG waveform.

Soon the waveform begins to fall as the patient begins to strain against the closed vocal cords in an attempt to hold the deep breath in the lungs (Valsalva maneuver) (Fig. 22–41*A*). This fall in the waveform occurs because the Valsalva maneuver momentarily elevates the intrathoracic pressure, causing less blood to flow to the heart and decreasing cardiac output. The decrease in cardiac output lowers the blood pressure, causing an increase in sympathetic stimuli, which increases the sympathetic tone mechanism and constricts the small arteries and arterioles of the fingers. Few RBCs begin to flow through the microvascular circulation of the finger tips, and the PPG waveform drops down towards or below the baseline level, as shown in Figure 22–41*A*.

In summary, deep inspiration decreases sympathetic stimulation, whereas the Valsalva ma-

neuver increases sympathetic stimulation. Both of these sympathetic responses can readily be evaluated in the noninvasive vascular laboratory. They should be markedly depressed or absent in patients undergoing therapy to block sympathetic stimuli.

Reactive Hyperemia Response

The reactive hyperemia test makes use of the principle that sympathetic stimuli are decreased and sympathetic tone is lowered in response to the metabolic changes in ischemic tissues. Begin the test by placing a photoelectric plethysmographic probe on the tip of the index finger, as shown in Figure 22–18*A*, and then obtain a baseline PPG waveform in the AC amplifier mode (Fig. 22–41*B*). Place an occlusion cuff around the wrist and inflate until the PPG waveform disappears. This indicates that the hand and finger are rendered ischemic by the cuff, which is kept inflated for 3 to 5 minutes. Release the cuff with the strip chart recorder running to observe reactive hyperemic changes in the PPG waveform in response to the 3 to 5 minutes of ischemia. A normal reactive hyperemic response results in a PPG waveform that is higher than the pre-ischemic baseline levels, as shown in Figure 22–41*B*. No reactive hyperemic response to ischemia will be observed in vascular beds that are already maximally dilated as a result of obstructive disease. In such cases, a patient may not benefit from sympathetic blocking medications or surgical sympathectomy.

Examination of the Upper Extremity Veins

Anatomy

Like the veins of the lower extremity, those of the upper extremity are also divided into the superficial and deep venous systems.[37]

Superficial Venous System

The superficial venous system (SVS) arises from a vast network of veins located on the dorsum of the hand. This network is formed from the digital veins that drain the blood from the fingers into the dorsal venous arch on the dorsum of the hand. Arising from this venous arch are the two main superficial veins of the upper extremity. They are the *cephalic* and *basilic veins* (Fig. 22–42). Compressing the fingers and dorsum of the hand will increase the blood flow through the cephalic and basilic veins, augmenting their velocity waveforms on the Doppler examination. Unlike the veins in the deep system, the cephalic and basilic superficial veins do not accompany the major arteries in the forearm and arm.

Cephalic Vein. The cephalic vein originates from the radial (outer) side of the dorsal venous arch and ascends along the lateral aspect of the wrist, forearm, and arm (Fig. 22–42). It runs between the deltoid and the pectoralis major muscles, perforates the costocoracoid membranes, and enters the axillary vein just below the clavicle. The cephalic vein communicates with the basilic vein through the median cubital vein in the cubital fossa at the elbow.

Basilic Vein. The basilic vein, the second major superficial vein in the upper extremity, arises from the medial side (inner) of the dorsal venous arch. The vein runs along the ulnar aspect of the forearm and arm (Fig. 22–42). It penetrates the

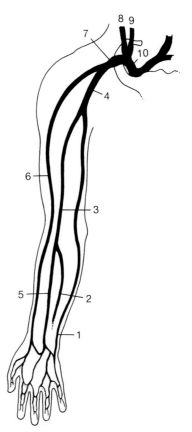

Figure 22–42. Line drawing showing venous anatomy of the upper extremity. *1,* Basilic vein. *2,* Ulnar vein. *3,* Brachial vein. *4,* Axillary vein. *5,* Radial vein. *6,* Cephalic vein. *7,* Subclavian vein. *8,* External jugular vein. *9,* Internal jugular vein. *10,* Innominate (brachiocephalic) vein.

deep fascia of the arm and unites with the brachial vein to form the axillary vein. There are numerous valves scattered throughout the cephalic and basilic superficial veins.

Deep Venous System

The veins of the deep venous system (DVS) usually accompany the arteries from which they receive their corresponding names. These veins are often paired structures and run along each side of the corresponding artery.

The small digital veins drain into the superficial and deep palmar venous arches, which correspond with the superficial and deep palmar arterial arches. The deep radial and ulnar veins of the forearm join at the elbow to form the brachial vein.

Brachial Vein. The brachial veins (Fig. 22–42) may be paired and course along the brachial artery to join with the basilic vein, forming the axillary vein at the lower border of the teres major muscle. The brachial vein receives tributaries corresponding with the branches given off from the brachial artery. The brachial veins contain numerous valves.

Axillary Vein. The axillary vein begins at the lower border of the teres major muscle and becomes larger as it courses upward in the arm (Fig. 22–42). This vein is located medial to the axillary artery and is separated from the latter by the medial cord of the brachial plexus. It receives tributaries corresponding with the branches of the artery. The cephalic vein enters the axillary vein before its termination into the subclavian vein at the outer border of the first rib. Usually, only one valve is found in the axillary vein.

Subclavian Vein. The subclavian vein is a continuation of the axillary vein at the outer border of the first rib (Fig. 22–42). It joins the internal jugular vein near the medial end of the clavicle to form the innominate vein. The subclavian artery lies behind and superior to the subclavian vein, which is usually located anterior to the anterior scalenus muscle and the phrenic nerve. Valves are present in the subclavian veins. The valves are generally located in the venous angle at the junction of the subclavian vein with the internal jugular vein.

Innominate Vein. The innominate or brachiocephalic vein is formed by the subclavian and internal jugular veins (Fig. 22–42). The left innominate vein is longer than the right innominate vein, and the two join to form the superior vena cava. The vein lies anterior and lateral to the innominate artery and receives the vertebral vein, the internal mammary vein, the inferior thyroid vein, and sometimes the superior intercostal vein. There are no valves in the innominate veins. Valves are present in both the external and internal jugular veins, as shown in Figure 22–59.

Venous Examination Techniques

Begin the examination by placing the patient in the supine position with the arm raised to permit access to the axilla, as shown in Figure 22–43A. With the probe placed high in the axilla, locate the axillary vein, which is anterior or superficial to the axillary artery. Then move the probe to the brachial position (Fig. 22–43B) and locate the basilic and brachial veins. As the probe is moved from the axilla down towards the elbow, the axillary vein is seen to bifurcate into the brachial and basilic veins. An example of this bifurcation is shown on the real-time images in Figure 22–43B. This bifurcation is important be-

cause it allows the axillary, brachial, and basilic veins to be identified.

Another important bifurcation is that of the brachial vein into the radial and ulnar veins. This bifurcation is located by placing the probe in the cubital fossa position, as shown in Figure 22–43C. Once the bifurcation is identified, the radial and ulnar veins can be examined by slowly moving the probe down the forearm towards the wrist. The radial and ulnar veins are paired, are very small, and lie adjacent to the radial and ulnar arteries.

An important vein to be evaluated by noninvasive vascular techniques is the subclavian vein. This vein receives both the superficial and deep venous systems of the upper extremity. Because an occlusion of the subclavian vein blocks these two major systems, acute pain, swelling, and edema of the entire upper extremity often result. Under these circumstances, the noninvasive vascular laboratory is used to evaluate the subclavian vein for thrombosis and, if present, to follow its course during anticoagulation therapy.

The subclavian vein is located by placing the probe in the deltopectoral triangle, as shown in Figure 22–43D. This triangle is found at the shoulder and is formed from a depression between the inferior boundary of the clavicle, the medial boundary of the deltoid muscle, and the superior boundary of the pectoralis muscles.

Veins may be examined with either a continuous-wave, bi-directional Doppler probe or a duplex scanner that contains both Doppler and real-time imaging capabilities.

Continuous-Wave Doppler Technique

The continuous-wave Doppler technique makes use of a bi-directional continuous-wave Doppler unit with a 5 to 10 MHz probe. A strip chart recorder provides the permanent waveform recording for interpretation. The recorder is calibrated at 1 kHz with the baseline set approximately 20 mm below the top of the paper. This enables the examiner to record negative profiles with spacing for positive reflux demonstration. The probe is held at a 30 to 45° cephalad position into the forward flow, producing a negative waveform.

The veins exhibit five characteristic qualities, which are routinely evaluated by Doppler, as illustrated in Figure 22–44:

1. Spontaneity. (Venous sounds are automatically elicited at the proper location.)
2. Phasicity. (The vein cycles with respiration.)
3. Augmentation. (Compression or Valsalva

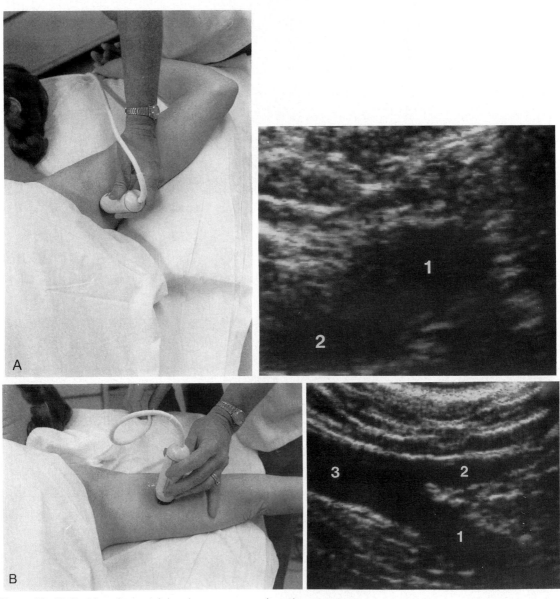

Figure 22–43. Positions for examining the upper extremity veins.

A. Left. Axillary position. *Right.* Vessels on B-mode images include *1,* axillary vein, and *2,* axillary artery.

B. Left. Brachial position. *Right.* Vessels on B-mode include *1,* brachial vein, *2,* basilic vein, and *3,* axillary vein.

C. Left. Cubital fossa position. *Right.* Vessels on B-mode images include *1,* radial vein, *2,* ulnar vein, and *3,* brachial vein.

D. Left. Deltopectoral position. *Right,* Vessels on B-mode image. Probe denotes locations of supraclavicular fossa and deltopectoral triangle. *1,* Subclavian vein. *2,* Subclavian artery.

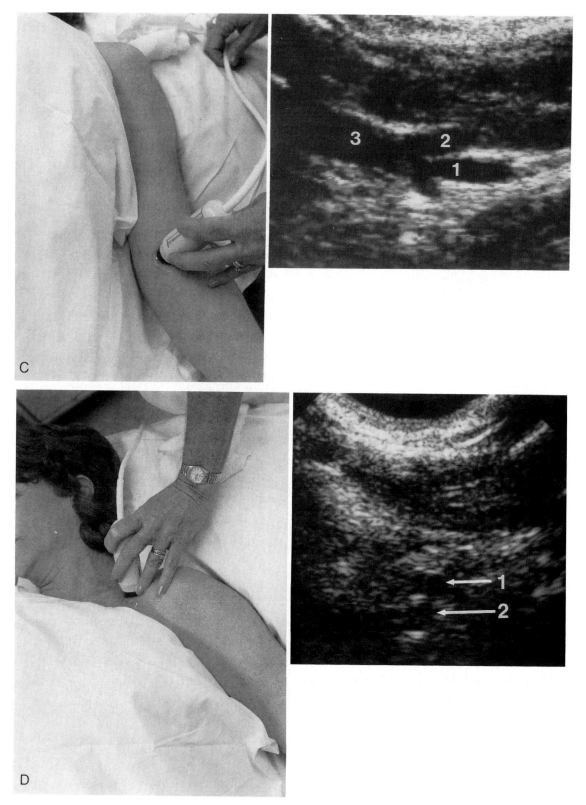

Figure 22–43 *Continued*

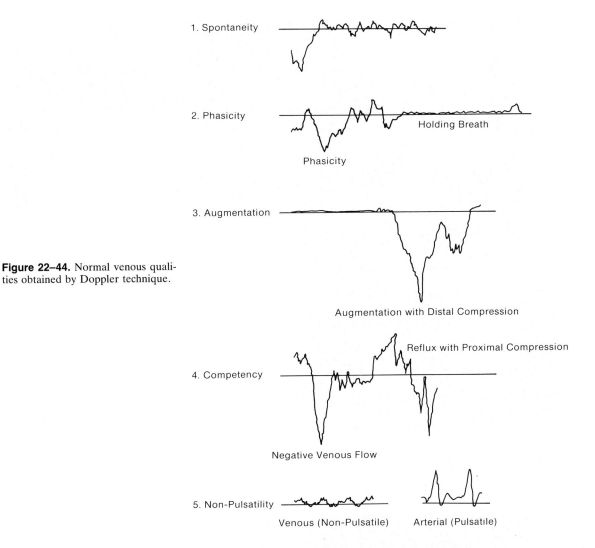

Figure 22–44. Normal venous qualities obtained by Doppler technique.

maneuvers elicit changes in the pitch, and the amplitude increases.)

4. Competency. (Flow is in one direction only.)

5. Nonpulsatility. (The vein does not cycle with heartbeat.)

The sites of examination include the brachial, axillary, subclavian, and jugular veins bilaterally. Each site is examined for the five qualities. Normally, the spontaneous phasic venous signal is easily heard; compression distal to the vein provides augmentation and thereby demonstrates patency. In patients for whom compression maneuvers are not possible, the Valsalva maneuver produces the same effect. If thrombus formation occludes the vessel, the venous signal may be absent or there may be a continuous, high-pitched sound that will not augment. This is the "windstorm" effect, which is associated with collateral flow.

Duplex Scanner Technique

The duplex scanner with real-time imaging and spectral analysis provides an ideal method of examining the venous system. However, venous imaging is restricted in the upper extremity because of the overlying bony structures, which prohibit transmission of the beam. Therefore, we use a combined approach with the routine continuous-wave Doppler providing the baseline examination and the duplex scanner evaluating those venous vessels that are accessible. These include the jugular, proximal subclavian, and brachial veins.

The duplex scanner protocol includes the following:

1. *Visualization of the vessel lumen.* Identification of the patent sonolucent vessel with particle movement caused by blood flow (Fig. 22–45).

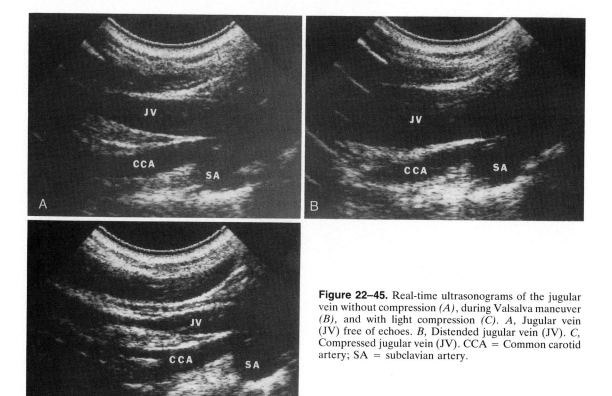

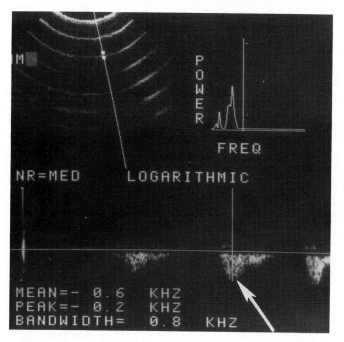

Figure 22–45. Real-time ultrasonograms of the jugular vein without compression (A), during Valsalva maneuver (B), and with light compression (C). A, Jugular vein (JV) free of echoes. B, Distended jugular vein (JV). C, Compressed jugular vein (JV). CCA = Common carotid artery; SA = subclavian artery.

Figure 22–46. Spectral analysis showing augmentation of venous signal (arrow) with distal compression, indicating patent vein.

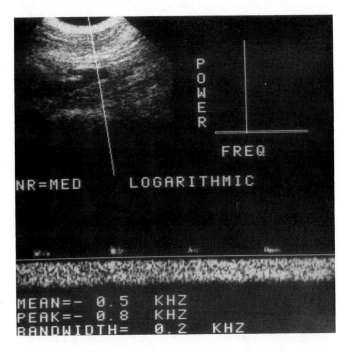

Figure 22–47. Spectral analysis demonstrating continuous flow pattern seen in the collateral veins secondary to obstruction.

2. *Spectral analysis and flow characteristics.* The characteristic venous qualities are verified. Normally, respiration motion will be seen with increased amplitude at augmentation (Fig. 22–46). In the presence of thrombus, there may be absence of flow or a continuous flow pattern with no augmentation because of collateral flow (Fig. 22–47).

3. *Compression maneuver measurements.* The anteroposterior diameter of the vein is measured while the patient is in a normal resting state. The vein is then compressed by the transducer, and a second measurement is obtained. If the vein is patent, the vein will collapse with compression. If there is thrombus occluding the vessel, there will be little or no compression (Figs. 22–48 and 22–49).

Thrombosis of the Axillary and Subclavian Veins

Thrombosis of the axillary and subclavian veins is an uncommon entity. It is classified as primary or secondary.

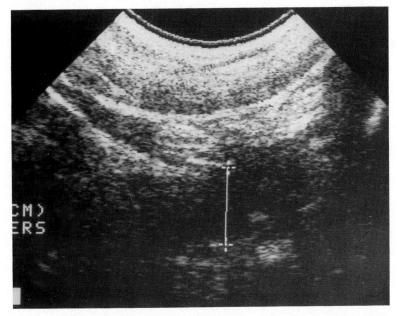

Figure 22–48. Real-time ultrasonogram showing thrombus occluding the vein.

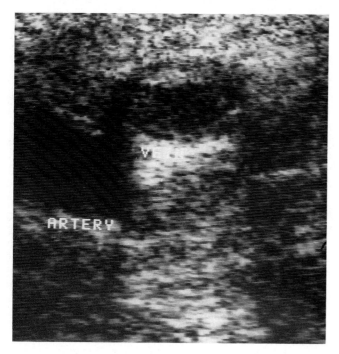

Figure 22–49. Cross-sectional view of the thrombosed filled lumen with compression. There is no decrease in size with compression, which is characteristic of a thrombosed filled lumen.

The primary disorder[38–42] occurs in fewer than 2% of cases of acute thrombophlebitis of deep veins of the extremities. The low frequency of this disorder may be due to three possible mechanisms in the upper extremity venous system:

1. Rapid emptying of blood from the arm.
2. A shorter course of blood flow.
3. Increased quantity of clot-resolving enzymes.

Thrombophlebitis usually occurs in males between 20 to 40 years of age but can be found in both sexes and at any age. The right arm is affected more frequently than the left arm. The etiology of the primary disorder is unknown. Several primary and secondary causes have been suggested.[38–42] These are listed in Tables 22–3 and 22–4.

Systemic manifestations of the disease are uncommon in the acute stage. The pulse and temperature are usually normal. An elevated sedimentation rate and leukocytosis may be present in some cases. Patients usually present with tightness and fullness of the affected upper extremity. This is associated with a dull ache in the shoulder, arm, and forearm; in some cases, severe pain may be present. Venous engorgement may be evident on the arm and anterior chest wall, and the extremity may be swollen from edema.

Although contrast venography remains the "gold standard" in the diagnosis of venous thrombosis, it is beginning to be replaced by duplex sonography. This is because duplex sonography, like contrast venography, actually displays an image of the thrombus within the vein lumen, which is necessary in making the diagnosis of venous thrombosis. How duplex sonography

Table 22–3. Primary Causes of Subclavian and Axillary Vein Thrombosis

Trauma
   Exercise
   Violent muscular effort
Spasm of the subclavian vein
Bony abnormalities
   High, horizontally curving first rib
Upward-directed and backward-directed clavicle
Idiopathic

Table 22–4. Secondary Causes of Subclavian and Axillary Vein Thrombosis

Polycythemia
Cachexia
Congestive heart failure
Mediastinal tumors
Aneurysms of ascending aorta
Trauma
   Indwelling catheter
   Intravenous drugs (irritating hypertonic solution, sclerosing solution)
Metastasis to axillary lymph nodes
Surgery
   Radical mastectomy
Neurovascular compression syndrome

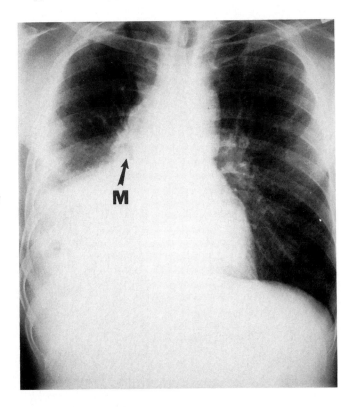

Figure 22–50. *Case XI.* Posteroanterior view of chest showing a mass (M) in the right hilum.

can be used to diagnose axillary and subclavian vein thrombosis is illustrated in the following cases.

Case XI

A 50-year-old man presented with the chief complaint of a painful, swollen arm. The upper extremity was very tender, edematous, and firm by palpation on physical examination. Chest x-ray (Fig. 22–50) and computed tomography (Fig. 22–51) revealed a neo-plastic mass in the right hilum and mediastinum. The right axillary vein showed absence of augmented Doppler velocity waveforms (Fig. 20–52) and thrombus in the axillary vein lumen on real-time ultrasonography (Fig. 22–53). The correlative contrast venogram is shown in Figure 22–54.

Case XII

A 60-year-old man was diagnosed with subclavian vein thrombosis by duplex sonography, as shown in

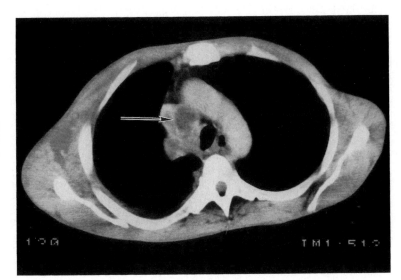

Figure 22–51. *Case XI.* Computed tomography demonstrating abnormal density in the mediastinum (arrow), indicating a neoplasm.

AXILLARY

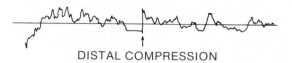

DISTAL COMPRESSION

Figure 22–52. *Case XI.* Doppler ultrasound waveform showing an absence of augmentation in the axillary vein, indicating the presence of thrombus.

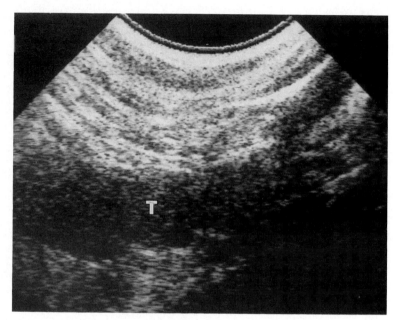

Figure 22–53. *Case XI.* Real-time ultrasonogram showing thrombus (T) in the axillary vein.

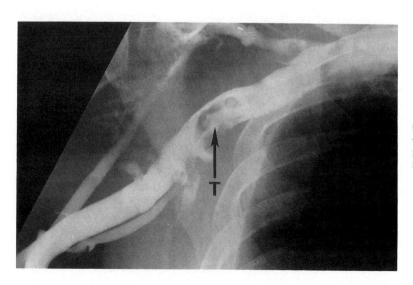

Figure 22–54. *Case XI.* Contrast venography of the upper extremity illustrating thrombus (T) in the axillary vein.

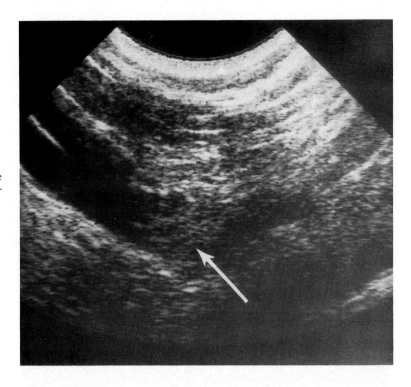

Figure 22–55. *Case XII.* Real-time ultrasonogram demonstrating thrombus (arrow) in the subclavian vein.

Figure 20–55. This figure demonstrates intraluminal echoes on the real-time ultrasound examination, which correlated with the site of subclavian vein thrombosis seen on the contrast venogram in Figure 22–56.

Case XIII

This case illustrates the total absence of Doppler shift frequencies from a sample volume placed in the lumen of the axillary vein (Fig. 22–57). The real-time

sonogram of this area explains why the Doppler shift frequencies are absent. Noncompressible, intraluminal echoes are present on both the transverse (Fig. 22–58A) and sagittal (Fig. 22–58B) real-time ultrasound freeze-frame images. Multiple collateral venous channels can be seen in the edematous soft tissues surrounding the thrombosed axillary vein (Fig. 22–58A). These channels correlate with the extensive network of collateral veins seen traversing the axillary vein thrombosis on the contrast venogram (Fig. 22–59).

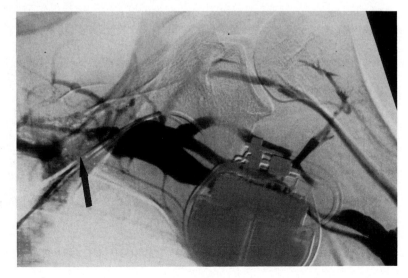

Figure 22–56. *Case XII.* Contrast venography of the upper extremity showing thrombus (arrow) in the subclavian vein.

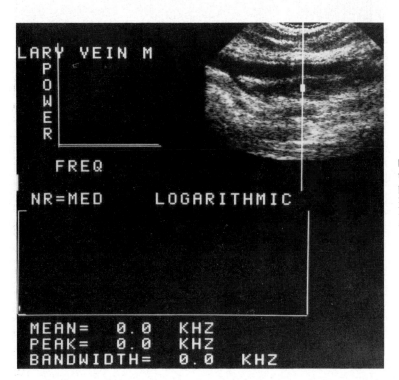

Figure 22–57. *Case XIII.* Axillary vein thrombosis. Spectral analysis from duplex scan showing no Doppler shift frequencies originating from the pulsed Doppler sample volume placed in the axillary vein lumen.

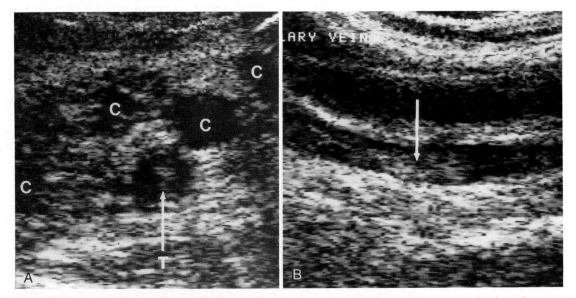

Figure 22–58. *Case XIII.* Real-time ultrasonogram of axillary vein thrombosis. *A,* Transverse projection of noncompressible thrombus (T) in axillary vein. Multiple collateral veins (C) are present in the surrounding soft tissues. *B,* Sagittal projection of echogenic thrombus (arrow) in axillary vein.

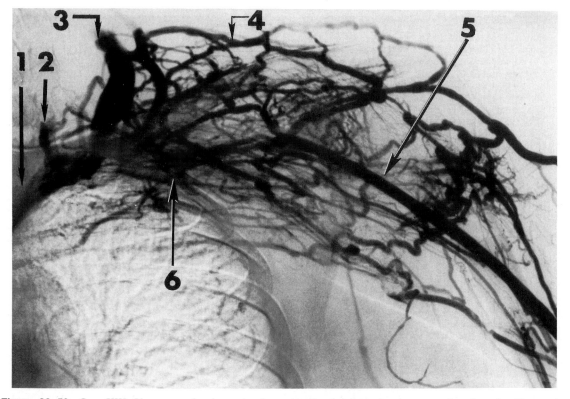

Figure 22–59. *Case XIII.* Venogram showing extensive network of collateral veins traversing site of axillary vein thrombosis. Large cephalic vein drains into patent subclavian vein. Both the brachial and basilic veins are also thrombosed. *1,* Innominate vein. *2,* Internal jugular (valve) vein. *3,* External jugular (valve) vein. *4,* Collaterals. *5,* Cephalic vein. *6,* Subclavian vein.

References

1. Gray H. The arteries of the upper extremity. *In* Goss CM (ed). Anatomy of the human body. 6th ed. Philadelphia, Lea & Febiger, 1964:641–665.
2. Bridges RA, Barnes RW. Segmental limb pressures. *In* Kempczinski RF, Yao JST (eds). Practical noninvasive vascular diagnosis. 3rd ed. Chicago, Year Book Medical Publishers, 1983:79–92.
3. Baker JD. Stress testing. *In* Kempczinski RF, Yao JST (eds) Practical noninvasive vascular diagnosis. 3rd ed. Chicago, Year Book Medical Publishers, 1983:93–103.
4. Carter SA. The role of pressure measurements in vascular disease. *In* Bernstein EF (ed). Noninvasive diagnostic techniques in vascular disease. 3rd ed. St Louis, CV Mosby Co, 1985:534.
5. Pierce WH, Ricco JB, Yao JST. Upper extremity vascular diagnosis using Doppler ultrasound. *In* Zwiebel WJ (ed) Introduction to vascular ultrasonography. 2nd ed. New York, Grune & Stratton, 1986:534.
6. Mulqueeney E, Yamada ET. Disorders of the peripheral vascular system. *In* Beyers M, Dudas S (eds). The clinical practice of medical surgical nursing. 2nd ed. Boston, Little, Brown & Co, 1984:590.
7. McCombs PR, Horwitz O. Disease of the arteries of the extremities. *In* Horwitz O, McCombs PR, Roberts B (eds). Disease of the blood vessels. Philadelphia, Lea & Febiger, 1985:203–227.
8. Spittell JA, Wallace RB. Aneurysms. *In* Fairbairn JF Jr, Juergens JL, Spittell JA (eds). Peripheral vascular diseases. 4th ed. Philadelphia, WB Saunders Co, 1972:281–302.
9. Cabelton S Jr, Gains TG, Monsivais JJ, et al. Brachial artery mycotic aneurysms: complications of cardiac catheterization. Milit Med 1986; 151:54–56.
10. Eshaghy B, Scanlon PJ, Amirpavix F, et al. Mycotic aneurysm of brachial artery: a complication of retrograde catheterization. JAMA 1974; 228:1574–1575.
11. Braunwald E, Swan HJC. Cooperative study on cardiac catheterization. Circulation 1968; 37 (Suppl):49–51.
12. Holleman JH, Martin BF, Parker JH. Giant cell arteritis causing brachial aneurysm in an eight year old child. J Miss State Med Assoc 1983; 24 (12):327–328.
13. Gasper MR. Arterial aneurysms. *In* Gasper MR, Baker WF (eds). Peripheral arterial disease. 3rd ed. Philadelphia, WB Saunders Co, 1981:176–227.
14. Baird RJ, Lajos TZ. Emboli to the arm. Ann Surg 1964; 160:905–909.
15. Haimovici H. Peripheral arterial embolism: a study of 330 unselected cases of embolism of the extremities. Angiology 1950; 1:20.
16. Strandness DE. Acute arterial obstruction. *In* Strandness ED (ed). Peripheral arterial disease: a physiologic approach. Boston, Little, Brown & Co, 1969:219–234.
17. Rich NM, Spencer FC. Forms of vascular injury: arterial trauma. Rich NM, Spencer FC (eds). Vascular

trauma. 9th ed. Philadelphia, WB Saunders Co, 1978:185–204.

18. Cohen A, Monion WC, Spencer FC, et al. Occlusive lesions of the great vessels of the aortic arch: Surgical and pathological aspects. Arch Surg 1962; 84:628.

19. Kolmanschn RB, Kalmansohn ROO. Thrombotic obliteration of the branches of the aortic arch. Circulation 1957; 15:237.

20. Upmalis IH. Collective review: The scalenus anticus and related syndromes. Surg Gynecol Obstet 1958; 107:521.

21. Crane C, Johnson R. Nerve conduction velocity and Doppler evaluations of thoracic outlet syndrome. South Med J 1974; 67:269–270.

22. Pisko-Dubienski ZA, Hollingsworth J. Clinical application of Doppler ultrasonography in the thoracic outlet syndrome. Can J Surg 1978; 21:145–150.

23. Rush MP, McNally DM, Rossman ME, Otis S. Noninvasive vascular diagnosis of thoracic outlet syndrome. Bruit 1983; 7:56–59.

24. McNamara MF, Takaki HS, Yao JST, et al. A systemic approach to severe hand ischemia. Surgery 1978; 83:1–11.

25. Strandness E. Vascular disease of the extremities. In Petersdorf RG, Adams RD, Braunwald E, Isselbacher KJ, Martin JB, Wilson JD (eds). Harrison's principles of internal medicine. 10th ed. New York, McGraw-Hill Book Co, 1982:1491–1497.

26. Porter J, River S, Anderson J, et al. Evaluation and management of the patient with Raynaud's syndrome. Am J Surg 1981; 142:182–196.

27. Thulesius O. Methods for the evaluation of peripheral vascular function in the upper extremities. Acta Chir Scand 1976;465(Suppl):53.

28. Thulesius O. Problems in the evaluation of hand ischemia. In Bernstein EF (ed). Noninvasive diagnostic techniques in vascular disease. 3rd ed. St. Louis, CV Mosby Co, 1985:639–651.

29. Hiral M. Cold sensitivity of the hand in arterial occlusive disease. Surgery 1979; 85:140–146.

30. Downs AR, Gaskell P, Morrow I, et al. Assessment of arterial obstruction in vessels supplying the fingers by measurement of local blood pressures and the skin temperature response test—correlation with angiographic evidence. Surgery 1975; 77:530–539.

31. Rivers SP, Porter JM. Clinical approach to Raynaud's syndrome. Vascular Diagnosis and Therapy Jan/Feb 1983.

32. Conrad MC. Vasospasm. In Functional anatomy of the circulation to the lower extremities. Chicago, Year Book Medical Publishers, 1971:158–164.

33. Conrad MC, Green HD. Hemodynamics of large and small vessels in peripheral vascular disease. Circulation 1964; 29:487.

34. Hertzman AB, Roth LW. The reaction of the digital artery and minute pad arteries to local cold. Am J Physiol 1942; 136:680.

35. Sumner DS, Strandness DE Jr. An abnormal finger pulse associated with cold sensitivity. Am Surg 1972; 175:294.

36. Strandness DE Jr. Episodic digital ischemia. In Peripheral arterial disease: A physiologic approach. Boston, Little, Brown & Co, 1969: 265–278.

37. Gray H. The veins of the upper extremity and thorax. In Goss CM (ed). Anatomy of the human body. 6th ed. Philadelphia, Lea & Febiger, 1964:742–745.

38. Abramson DI. Venous thrombosis: Involvement of deep venous system. In Abramson DI (ed). Vascular disorders of the extremities. 2nd ed. New York, Harper & Row, Publishers, 1974:557–585.

39. Adams JT, McEvoy RK, DeWeese JA. Primary deep venous thrombosis of the upper extremity. Arch Surg 1965; 91:29.

40. Hughs ESR. Venous obstruction in the upper extremity (Paget-Schroetter's syndrome). Surg Gynecol Obstet 1949; 88:89.

41. Ochsner A, DeBakey ME, DeCamp PT, et al. Thrombo-embolism: an analysis of cases at the Charity Hospital in New Orleans over a 12-year period. Ann Surg 1951; 134:1951.

42. McCleery RS, Kesterson JE, Kirtley JA, et al. Subclavius and anterior scalenus muscle compression as a cause of intermittent obstruction of the subclavian vein. Ann Surg 1951; 133:588.

23 • Subclavian Steal Syndrome

Introduction

The subclavian steal syndrome is characterized by the neurologic symptoms of vertigo, limb paresis, visual disturbances, ataxia, and syncope. These symptoms are associated with stenosis or occlusion of the left subclavian artery (Fig. 23–1A), the right subclavian artery proximal to the origin of the vertebral artery (Fig. 23–1B), or the innominate (brachiocephalic) artery (Fig. 23–2).

Atherosclerosis is the most common cause of the subclavian steal syndrome.[1, 2] Other causes include obstructive lesions of the aortic arch,[3] atresias,[4] embolic occlusions,[5] and Takayasu's arteritis.[6]

Fields and Lemak, reviewing 168 angiographically proven cases of subclavian steal syndrome, found involvement of the left subclavian artery in 70% of cases and of the right subclavian or innominate artery in 30% of cases.[1] Isolated innominate artery occlusion occurs in approximately 8% of the patients with subclavian steal syndrome.[7]

An understanding of the various blood flow patterns that may produce the subclavian steal phenomenon is vital for a correct diagnosis by means of duplex scanning. A stenosis or occlusion of the proximal left subclavian artery (Fig. 23–1A) can cause reduced blood pressure in the left upper extremity. This pressure may be reduced even further when the left upper extremity is exercised. Blood flow is then diverted away from the high pressure vertebrobasilar circulation into the low-pressure upper extremity circulation through a reversal of the blood flow direction in the left vertebral artery (Fig. 23–1A). This diversion, or stealing, of blood from the vertebrobasilar circulation has been reported to be associated with the symptoms of brain stem ischemia by Reivich and colleagues[8] and was entitled "the subclavian steal syndrome" by Fisher in 1961.[9] A similar collateral pathway may be found in the right vertebral artery when the stenotic or obstructive lesion involves the proximal portion of the right subclavian artery, as shown in Figure 23–1B.

A more complex form of the subclavian steal phenomenon occurs with lesions involving the innominate artery. Because of the many different collateral possibilities associated with an innominate artery occlusion that are not available with a subclavian artery occlusion, Blackmore and associates termed this clinical syndrome the "innominate artery steal" in 1965.[10] An innominate artery occlusion is more likely to cause symptoms because it reduces the total cerebral blood flow by 18%, whereas a subclavian artery occlusion reduces this blood flow by only 8%.[11]

The most common form of the innominate artery steal is shown in Figure 23–2A. It consists of reversed right vertebral artery blood flow with antegrade right subclavian and carotid artery blood flow. This form of innominate artery steal was originally described by Killen and Gobbel and was named the "carotid recovery phenomenon."[7] Should the right carotid artery not recover, it will have a reversed blood flow, as shown in Figure 23–2B. A third possibility implicates the presence of a right vertebral artery stenosis in addition to the innominate artery occlusion (Fig. 23–2C). The direction of the blood flow becomes reversed in the right carotid arteries but remains antegrade in the right vertebral artery.

Noninvasive Vascular Evaluation

Brachial Systolic Blood Pressure

A comparison of the right and left systolic brachial blood pressures is a simple method of detecting an underlying subclavian steal phenomenon. Fields and Lemak found in a series of 168

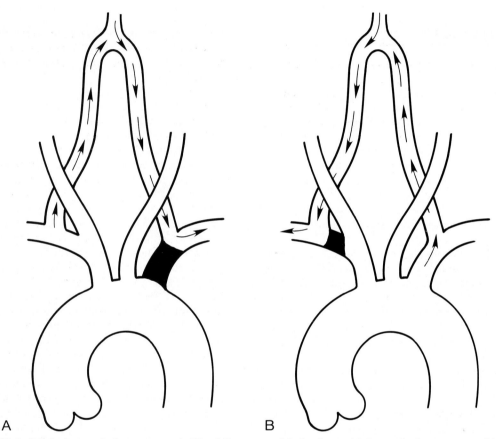

Figure 23–1. Subclavian steal phenomenon. *A,* Blood flow reversal in basilar and left vertebral artery caused by left subclavian artery occlusion. *B,* Blood flow reversal in basilar and right vertebral artery caused by right subclavian artery occlusion.

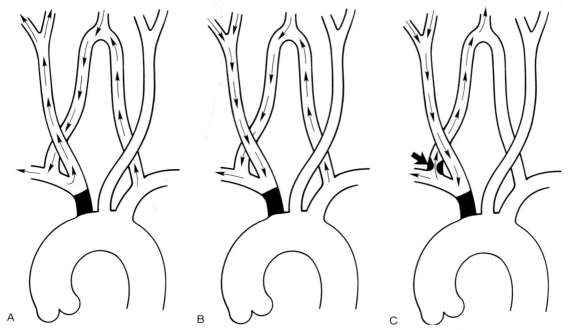

Figure 23–2. Innominate artery steal phenomenon. *A*, Carotid recovery phenomenon. *B*, Blood flow reversed in right vertebral and carotid arteries. *C*, Blood flow reversed in right carotid and antegrade in right vertebral arteries. Note right vertebral artery stenosis (large arrow).

cases of subclavian steal syndrome that the average difference in these pressure measurements was 45 mm Hg.[1] Rarely, there may be no difference in the brachial systolic pressures between the right and left upper extremities because of the presence of bilateral lesions. Reduced pressure in both brachial arteries should arouse the suspicion that bilateral lesions are present.

Generally, the brachial systolic blood pressures should be within 10 mm Hg of each other. A pressure difference greater than 10 mm Hg signifies innominate, subclavian, axillary, or brachial artery occlusion or stenosis. The patient whose angiogram is shown in Figure 23–3 had a right brachial systolic pressure of 108 mm Hg and a left pressure of 71 mm Hg. These pressures were obtained with the upper extremities at rest. There was a pressure difference of 37 mm Hg between the two upper extremities.

Indirect Noninvasive Modalities (Ocular Plethysmography and Periorbital Doppler Examinations)

As illustrated in Figure 23–2B and C, occlusive disease of the innominate artery may result in the "stealing" of blood from the carotid artery branches. With periorbital Doppler insonation, a pattern of reversed flow is obtained, which cannot be distinguished from the reversed flow pattern that occurs with occlusive disease of the internal carotid artery. Although these modalities do not have the capability of diagnosing the steal phenomenon, they can be helpful in the total cerebrovascular evaluation of patients with such a condition. Fields and Lemak found that 81% of patients in the Joint Study of Extracranial Arterial Occlusion with subclavian steal had disease of more than one extracranial vessel.[1] Only 50 of 168 patients with subclavian steal had disease limited to the subclavian and vertebral arteries. Therefore, the indirect noninvasive modalities may be used to detect the disease, which often exists in the other regions of the cerebrovascular circulation.

Digital Pulse Plethysmography

Conrad and colleagues used digital pulse plethysmography to monitor patients with the subclavian steal syndrome.[12] They found that the decreases in the digital artery pressures and pulse amplitudes, pulse delays, and abnormal pulse contours were present on the involved side. Such information only suggests that there is an arterial abnormality in the upper extremity and is not specific for the subclavian steal phenomenon.

Duplex Sonography

The diagnosis of subclavian steal syndrome has become a simple, noninvasive procedure with the use of duplex scanning. When a difference between the brachial systolic pressures suggests the presence of subclavian steal, real-time B-mode imaging can be used to locate the vertebral artery for Doppler probe placement on the affected side. The diagnosis of subclavian steal syndrome by means of ultrasonography can be established by demonstrating the retrograde flow in the vertebral artery on the abnormal side.

Accurate results have been described throughout the literature on the use of various probe positions to study the direction of blood flow in the vertebral artery. Corson and colleagues reported the reversal of vertebral artery flow in two patients with the probe positioned medially and inferiorly in the region of the sixth cervical vertebra.[13] Barnes and Wilson documented reversed vertebral artery flow with the probe directed cranially at the base of the neck.[14] At this position, the vertebral artery can be found supraclavicularly and laterally from the common carotid artery and the jugular vein. Liljeqvist and coworkers suggested positioning the probe below the transverse process of the atlas vertebra and in a cephalad direction.[15] At this level, the vertebral artery is not confused with the vessels that arise from the thyrocervical trunk. Reactive hyperemia of the affected upper extremity should be induced whenever a reversal of blood flow is not demonstrated in the vertebral artery. Reactive hyperemia is accomplished by inflation of the pressure cuff above the brachial systolic pressure for 5 minutes. The Doppler probe is used to examine the blood flow direction in the vertebral artery immediately after the pressure cuff is deflated.

Sound spectral analysis of retrograde left vertebral artery blood flow is shown in Figure 23–4. This analysis was obtained from the patient whose angiograms are shown in Figure 23–3. Percutaneous transluminal angioplasty was used to treat this lesion, and the immediate angiographic results of this procedure are shown in Figure 23–5. There is prompt visualization of the left subclavian artery, but numerous filling defects and irregularities persist within the lumen of the proximal left subclavian artery. These indicate either residual atherosclerotic disease not dilated by the procedure or intramural vessel hemorrhage and dissection caused by the procedure. Bilateral systolic brachial blood pressure measurements were obtained immediately following angioplasty and were found to be equal

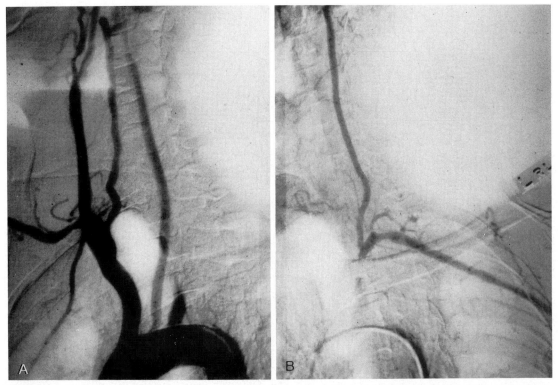

Figure 23–3. Angiogram of patient with subclavian steal syndrome. *A,* Early arterial phase showing absent left vertebral and subclavian arteries resulting from total occlusion of the proximal left subclavian artery. *B,* Late arterial phase showing the subclavian steal phenomenon and retrograde flow in the left vertebral artery.

Figure 23–4. Reversed left vertebral artery blood flow shown by sound spectral analysis. The main systolic and diastolic components are located below the zero baseline (arrows).

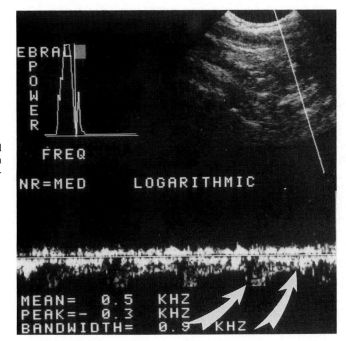
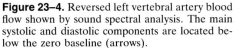

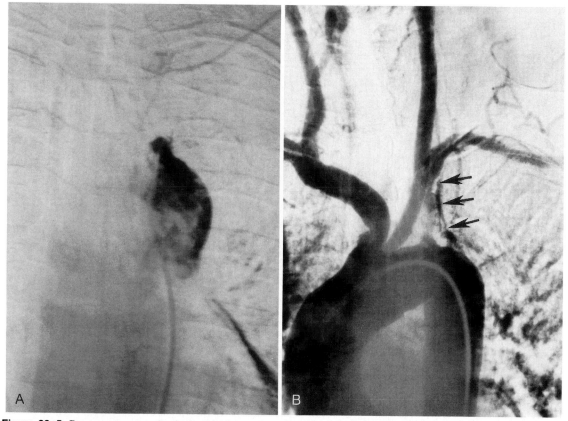

Figure 23–5. Percutaneous transluminal angioplasty of occluded proximal left subclavian artery segment. *A,* Catheter tip position prior to traversing occluded segment with guide wire. *B,* Post-angioplasty angiogram showing irregular appearance of dilated, previously occluded proximal subclavian artery segment (arrows).

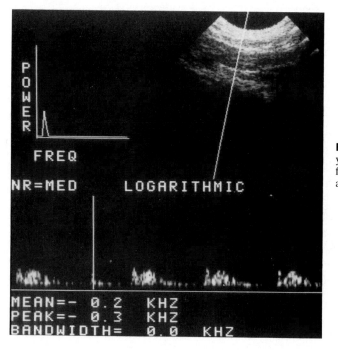

Figure 23–6. Post-angioplasty sound spectral analysis of left vertebral artery showing antegrade blood flow. Both the systolic and diastolic components are above the zero baseline.

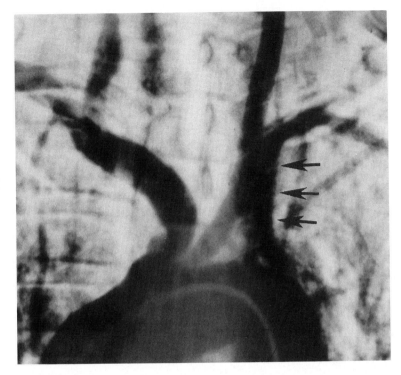

Figure 23–7. Follow-up angiogram showing healing of subclavian artery segment (arrows).

(115 mm Hg) in each arm. A duplex scan of the left vertebral artery was also obtained at this time. It revealed a patent left vertebral artery with antegrade blood flow on sound spectral analysis (Fig. 23–6). Although the patient's symptoms of brain stem and upper extremity ischemia resolved, a follow-up angiogram was used to evaluate the status of the irregular proximal subclavian artery segment. The angiogram was obtained 12 days after angioplasty and showed healing of this segment (Fig. 23–7). This case demonstrates how duplex scanning may be used both in the diagnosis and in the management of the subclavian steal syndrome.

Not all patients with the subclavian steal phenomenon will be symptomatic. Symptoms must exist in order for subclavian steal syndrome to be considered present.

References

1. Fields WS, Lemak NA. Joint study of extracranial arterial occlusion: VII. Subclavian steal—a review of 168 cases. JAMA 1972; 222:1139–1143.
2. Crawford ES, DeBakey ME, Morris GC, et al. Surgical treatment of occlusion of the innominate, common carotid, and subclavian arteries: A 10 year experience. Surgery 1969; 65:17–31.
3. Daves ML, Tregar A. Vertebral grand larceny. Circulation 1964; 29:911–913.
4. Massumi RA. The congenital variety of the "subclavian steal" syndrome. Circulation 1963; 28:1149–1152.
5. Bandyk DF. Innominate artery steal syndrome due to embolic occlusion. VD&T December/January 1981; 46–47.
6. Wood CPL, Meire HB. Intermittent bilateral subclavian steal detected by ultrasound arteriography. Br J Radiol 1980; 727–730.
7. Killen DA, Gobbel WG Jr. Subclavian steal–carotid recovery phenomenon. J Thorac Cardiovasc Surg 1965; 50:421–426.
8. Reivich M, Holling HE, Roberts B, et al. Reversal of blood flow through the vertebral artery and its effects on cerebral circulation. N Engl J Med 1961; 265:878–885.
9. Fisher CM. A new vascular syndrome, "subclavian steal." N Engl J Med 1961; 265:912–913.
10. Blackmore WS, Hardesty WH, Bevilacqua JE, et al. Reversal of blood flow in the right vertebral artery accompanying occlusion of the innominate artery. Ann Surg 1965; 161:353–356.
11. Handa J, Yosida K, Meyer JS. Hemodynamic effects of subclavian and innominate artery ligation. Surgery 1966; 59:1069–1078.
12. Conrad MC, Toole JF, Janeway R. Hemodynamics of the upper extremities in subclavian steal syndrome. Circulation 1965; 32:346–351.
13. Corson JD, Menzoian JO, LoGerfo FW. Reversal of vertebral artery blood flow demonstrated by Doppler ultrasound. Arch Surg 1977; 112:715–719.
14. Barnes RW, Wilson MR. Doppler ultrasonic evaluation of cerebrovascular disease. (A programmed audiovisual instruction.) Richmond, Va, The Medical College of Virginia, 1980.
15. Liljeqvist L, Ekestrom S, Nordhus O. Monitoring direction of vertebral artery blood flow by Doppler shift ultrasound in patients with suspected "subclavian steal." Acta Chir Scand 1981; 147:421–424.

Part VI • Miscellaneous

24 • Duplex Sonography of Superficial Masses

Introduction

This chapter describes how duplex sonography can be used in the initial evaluation of superficial mass lesions. The use of duplex sonography arises from the fact that it can be difficult to determine the vascularity of a mass on the physical examination. Because the duplex scanner is used to study both the anatomy and the blood flow characteristics of vessels, it can be used to decide whether or not a mass is either vascular, avascular, or of vascular origin. As illustrated in the following examples, this is of considerable importance because the decision to proceed with other examinations, such as angiography, often depends on this determination.

Buckling of the Brachiocephalic Vessels

Buckling or tortuosity of the brachiocephalic vessels can result in pulsatile masses at the base of the neck. These masses are generally located in the suprasternal and right supraclavicular fossa regions and are usually found in hypertensive women over 50 years of age. Hypertension causes dilatation, elongation, and tortuosity of the brachiocephalic vessels, which then present as pulsatile neck masses. A buckled right subclavian artery may occur alone or with other tortuous, elongated brachiocephalic vessels. Duplex sonography can be used to differentiate these buckled vessels from aneurysms or transmitted pulsations that are due to neck masses.[1, 2] The patient shown in Figure 24–1 was hypertensive and presented with palpable, pulsatile masses in both the right supraclavicular and suprasternal fossae at the base of the neck. Fullness in the right supraclavicular fossa may extend into the superior mediastinum and may appear as a mass on the chest radiograph. Duplex sonography showed that the

mass was caused by a dilated, tortuous right subclavian artery. Doppler velocity waveforms were used to confirm that the structures being investigated on the B-mode image were arterial in origin, as illustrated in Figure 24–2. This was useful information because buckling of the innominate, common carotid, and subclavian arteries is usually a benign condition.[3–5] The duplex sonographic findings were confirmed by the angiogram in Figure 24–3.

Extracranial Internal Carotid Artery Aneurysms

Most extracranial internal carotid artery (ICA) aneurysms occur in the region of the carotid bifurcation. Causes of aneurysms include atherosclerosis, syphilis, local infection, trauma, and previous carotid artery surgery.[6] Trauma is currently considered to be the most common cause of these aneurysms.[7] Although patients with extracranial ICA aneurysms usually present with pulsatile neck masses, there are reported instances in which biopsies of neck masses, mistaken for metastatic lesions, were performed, producing alarming hemorrhage.[8] Other cervical ICA aneurysms have presented as pharyngeal masses; these were excised as peritonsillar abscesses, with fatal results.[9]

An example of a patient with an extracranial ICA aneurysm presenting as a pulsatile neck mass is shown in Figure 24–4. The sonographic appearance of an aneurysm is correlated with the angiogram shown in Figure 24–5. An enlarged ICA lumen with a grossly irregular surface is seen on the angiogram. The corresponding sonographic sagittal image shows that the irregular luminal surface is due to thrombus formation in the wall of the aneurysm. This can also be appreciated on the transverse scan in Figure 24–6. A bi-directional Doppler probe was used to

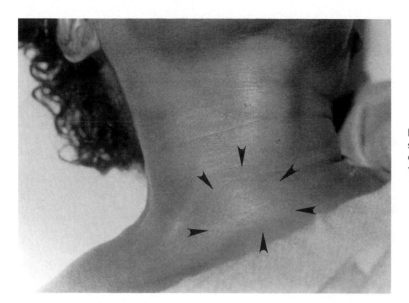

Figure 24–1. Pulsatile masses in right supraclavicular fossa (arrowheads) caused by tortuous brachiocephalic vessels.

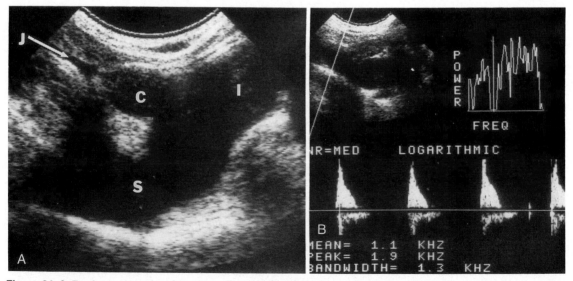

Figure 24–2. Duplex sonography of tortuous, dilated right subclavian artery. *A,* B-mode image. J = Jugular vein; S = subclavian artery; C = common carotid artery; I = innominate artery. *B,* Doppler velocity waveform.

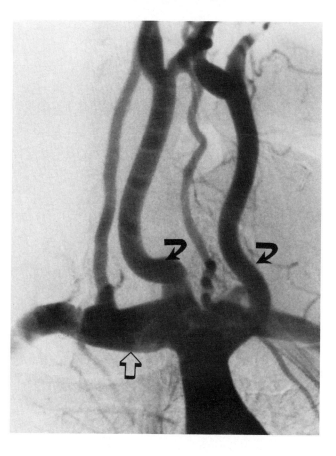

Figure 24–3. Brachiocephalic angiogram of tortuous common carotid arteries (curved arrows) and dilated, tortuous right subclavian artery (open arrow).

demonstrate blood flow in the structure under investigation during the sonographic examination. The Doppler velocity waveform obtained from the aneurysm is shown in Figure 24–7.

The irregular surface caused by the thrombus is of particular interest because it could be a source of intracerebral embolization. The aneurysms in the angiogram in Figure 24–8 were bilateral and were most likely atherosclerotic in etiology.

Sonography can readily be used to diagnose an extracranial ICA aneurysm by detecting its large size, thrombus in the aneurysm wall, and blood flow through the involved vessel lumen. The main limitation of sonography when used to image the neck is in delineating the cephalad extent of a high cervical ICA aneurysm that extends above the angle of the mandible.

External Carotid Artery Aneurysms

Like extracranial ICA aneurysms, external carotid artery (ECA) aneurysms are usually caused

by trauma.[10-14] Other causes include atherosclerosis, syphilis, cystic medial necrosis, Marfan's syndrome, and congenital predisposition.[15, 16] Traumatic ECA aneurysms may be caused by either blunt or penetrating trauma that perforates the arterial wall and results in extensive hemorrhage into the surrounding tissues.[12, 17] Generally, the perforation in the vessel wall closes and the hematoma resolves. If the perforation does not close spontaneously, the blood flow from the injured vessel may continue to pass back and forth between the vessel lumen and the surrounding hemorrhage, forming a pulsatile hematoma. The center of the hematoma remains liquid because blood is forced into it under arterial pressure during systole and returns to the injured vessel lumen during diastole. The hematoma is contained within the confines of the surrounding tissues and may not be palpable on the physical examination. An example is shown in Figure 24–9.

A patient sustained a gunshot wound to the face 3 days before the sonographic examination. There was extensive swelling about the angle of the mandible. There was no radiographic evidence of mandibular fracture, and no discrete

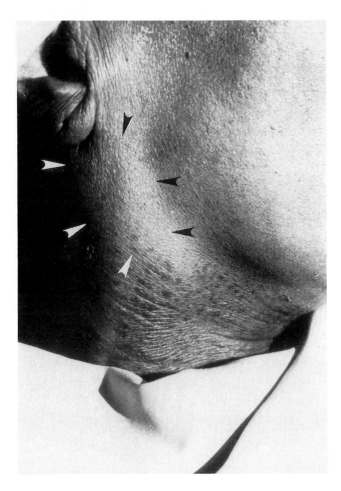

Figure 24–4. Pulsatile neck mass (arrowheads) caused by internal carotid artery aneurysm.

palpable, pulsatile mass could be found on the physical examination. The sonogram in Figure 24–9B was obtained to further evaluate the cause of the facial swelling and to rule out the presence of an underlying aneurysm. Sonography revealed a localized anechoic cavity within the area of the facial swelling that contained blood flow, indicating the presence of an aneurysm or a pulsatile hematoma. This was confirmed by the selective ECA angiogram, as shown in Figure 24–9A.

Pulsatile hematomas that go unrecognized can continue to enlarge; they can develop an inflammatory fibrotic reaction around the periphery that forms the outer wall. When the cavity of the hematoma continues to communicate with the vessel lumen, the hematoma becomes endothelialized, forming a false aneurysm or pseudoaneurysm. These are not true aneurysms because they do not contain all of the normal arterial wall layers. Instead, these fake aneurysms are composed of an inner endothelial surface and an outer wall formed from the surrounding inflammatory reaction. The development of a false

aneurysm may take days, months, or even years after the original injury and may be diagnosed erroneously as an abscess or a tumor when it finally presents. An example is shown in Figure 24–10.

The patient in this example continued to have nonpulsatile, painful facial swelling 2 months after mandibular surgery for what was earlier thought to be an abscess on the physical examination. Attempts to drain it, however, resulted in bleeding. The sutures in Figure 24–10 define the attempted drainage site. An angiogram was then obtained to rule out aneurysm formation. The angiogram showed a large false aneurysm arising from the ECA. A subselective ECA angiogram revealed the precise location of the false aneurysm—as arising from the facial branch of the left ECA, as shown in Figure 24–11. Although sonography was not used to diagnose the ECA false aneurysm in this particular example, the procedure was used in the follow-up evaluation after treatment.

Follow-up treatment consisted of isolating the

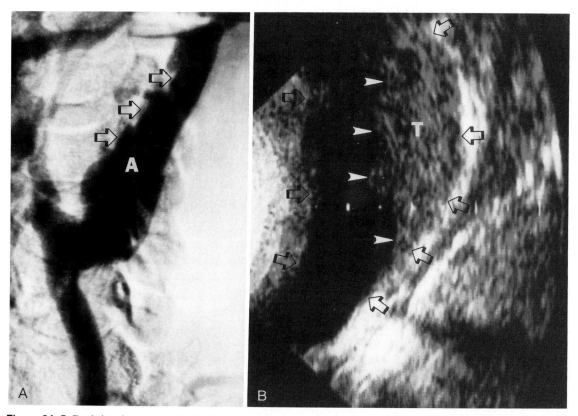

Figure 24–5. Real-time image correlated with angiogram of internal carotid artery aneurysm. *A,* Angiogram of irregular lumen surface (open arrows) of aneurysm (A). *B,* Sagittal real-time image of thrombus (T) in aneurysm (open arrows). Irregular lumen surface of thrombus (white arrowheads).

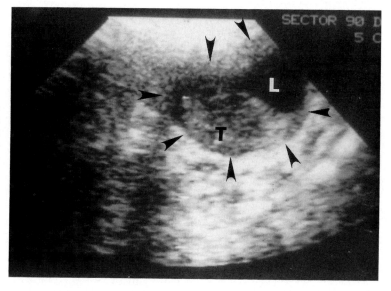

Figure 24–6. Transverse real-time image shows large amount of thrombus in aneurysm wall, which is greater than that seen on angiogram. L = Internal carotid artery lumen; T = thrombus in aneurysm; arrowheads outline the outer aneurysm margins.

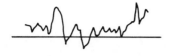

A

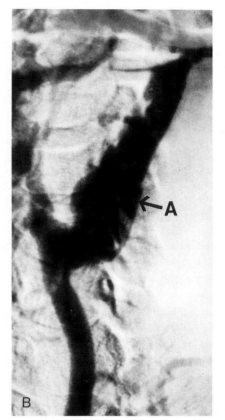

A

B

Figure 24–7. Doppler velocity waveform *(A)* of blood flow in aneurysm *(B)*. A = Aneurysm.

aneurysm from its blood supply by occluding the facial artery with a percutaneously placed wire coil. The pre-embolization angiogram in Figure 24–12A shows the catheter tip placed subselectively into the facial branch of the left ECA. Contrast media injected through the catheter filled the aneurysm and outlined a large thrombus lying in its lumen. A wire coil was then passed through the catheter to occlude the facial artery. The post-embolization angiogram in Figure 24–12B was made with the catheter tip positioned in the common carotid artery. The angiogram shows the wire coil in the occluded facial artery and non-opacification of the false aneurysm. Duplex sonography was used to follow up the aneurysm in order to make certain that it thrombosed and that the facial artery remained occluded.[17a] The follow-up procedures consisted of first obtaining the pre-embolization baseline duplex sonogram shown in Figures 24–13A and 24–14A. Real-time B-mode imaging prior to the embolization procedure demonstrated swirling echoes passing around the thrombus in the aneurysm wall. A freeze-frame image of this swirling pattern is shown in Figure 24–13A. Blood flow in the aneu-

rysm is shown by the sound spectral analysis waveforms in Figure 24–14A. The follow-up real-time B-mode examination performed 3 days after the embolization procedure showed absence of the previously noted swirling echoes and multiple low-level to high-level echoes of clot and thrombus formation filling the lumen of the aneurysm. A freeze-frame image from this examination is shown in Figure 24–13B. No blood flow was detected on the sound spectral analysis of the aneurysm after embolization, as shown in Figure 24–14B. Duplex sonograms of the occluded aneurysm obtained approximately 14 days after embolization began to appear sonolucent as a result of liquefaction of the thrombus. The process of liquefaction continued to occur until the whole aneurysm was occupied by a sonolucent area 26 days after embolization, as shown in Figure 24–13C. The liquid contents were then aspirated, decompressing the mass caused by the occluded aneurysm.

The figures just discussed illustrate how duplex sonography can be used to determine whether or not the embolization of a vascular mass like an aneurysm is successful. Because the duplex scan

Text continued on page 513

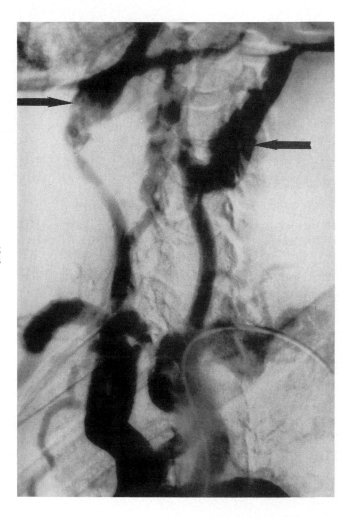

Figure 24–8. Brachiocephalic angiogram showing bilateral cervical internal carotid artery aneurysms (arrows).

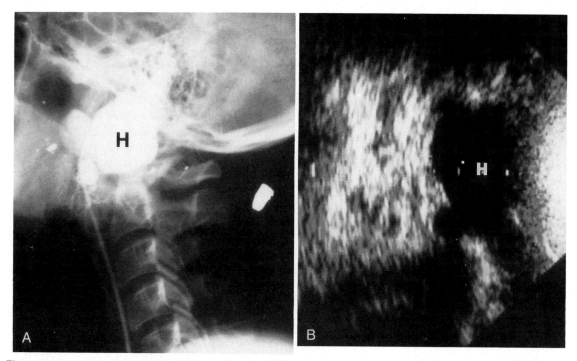

Figure 24–9. Traumatic external carotid artery pulsatile hematoma. *A,* Selective external carotid artery angiogram showing cavity of pulsatile hematoma (H). *B,* Sagittal real-time image showing the cavity in the pulsatile hematoma (H). (From Giyanani VL, Gerlock AJ, Mirfakhraee M, et al. Duplex sonography in embolus therapy of external carotid artery traumatic aneurysm. AJNR 1987; 8:1131–1133. © by American Society of Neuroradiology 1987, with permission.)

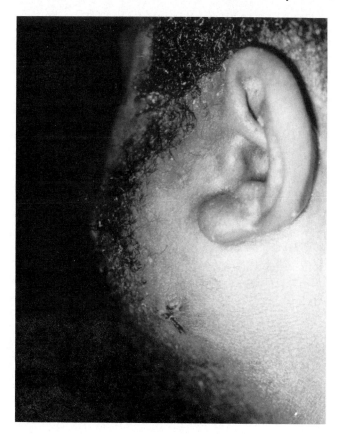

Figure 24–10. Nonpulsatile facial swelling, which persisted 2 months after mandibular surgery.

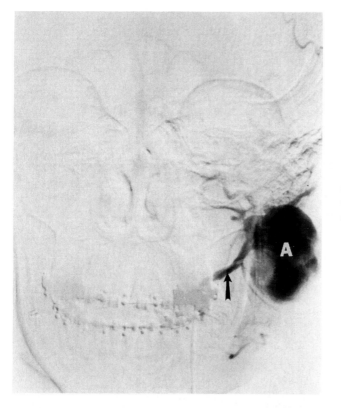

Figure 24–11. Subselective facial artery angiogram of pseudoaneurysm (A) in the anteroposterior projection. The arrow points to the facial artery.

Figure 24–12. Pre-embolization and post-embolization angiograms in the lateral view. *A,* Aneurysm filling from facial branch of external carotid artery (arrow) containing thrombus (T). *B,* Facial artery occluded by coil, eliminating blood flow to aneurysm (arrow). (From Giyanani VL, Gerlock AJ, Mirfakhraee M, et al. Duplex sonography in embolus therapy of external carotid artery traumatic aneurysm. AJNR 1987; 8:1131–1133. © by American Society of Neuroradiology 1987, with permission.)

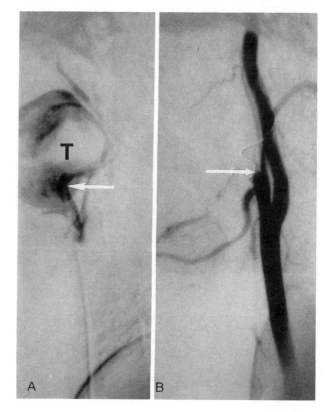

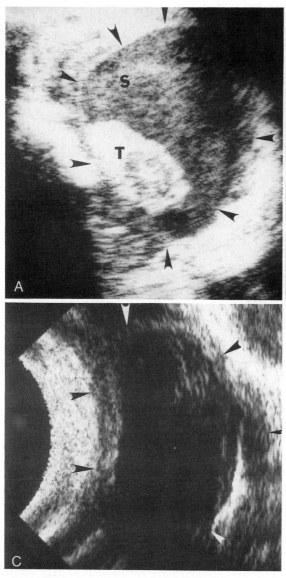

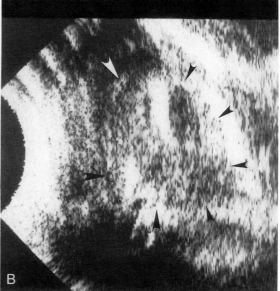

Figure 24–13. Follow-up serial B-mode images of aneurysm after embolization. Aneurysm is outlined by arrowheads. *A*, Pre-embolization B-mode image shows thrombus (T) and swirling echoes of slow blood flow (S) in the direction of the arrows, which were seen during real-time sonography. *B*, Real-time image 3 days post embolization shows nonswirling low-to-high level echoes of clot and thrombus formation. *C*, Real-time image 26 days post embolization shows sonolucency caused by liquefaction of the thrombus. (From Giyanani VL, Gerlock AJ, Mirfakhraee M, et al. Duplex sonography in embolus therapy of external carotid artery traumatic aneurysm. AJNR 1987; 8:1131–1133. © by American Society of Neuroradiology 1987, with permission.)

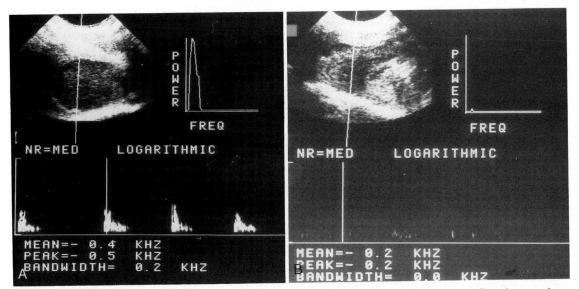

Figure 24–14. Continuous-wave Doppler velocity waveforms before and after embolization. *A,* Doppler waveforms showing blood flow in aneurysm before embolization. *B,* Blood flow absent after embolization.

can currently be used to determine whether or not there is still significant blood flow in the mass after embolization, there may be no need to use angiography in these types of follow-up evaluations. The B-mode image of an embolized mass can also be helpful in determining whether or not the mass can be aspirated for further decompression.

A lymph node metastasis surrounding a blood vessel may present as a palpable, pulsatile neck mass, which can be mistaken for an aneurysm on physical examination. Under these circumstances, duplex ultrasonography may assist in distinguishing a lymph node metastasis from an aneurysm. Usually, metastases demonstrate a homogeneous echotexture (Fig. 24–15*A*), whereas aneurysms often have an inhomogeneous echo pattern because of the combination of slow-flowing blood and thrombus (Figure 24–13*A*). Aneurysms will demonstrate pulsatility on duplex ultrasonography; pulsatility is absent when lymph node metastases are present. When Doppler ultrasonography is used, flow will usually be present within an aneurysm (Figure 24–14*A*), whereas the flow is usually absent within a lymph node metastasis (Fig. 24–15*B*). If blood flow is seen in a lymph node metastasis (Fig. 24–15*C*), the unusual circumstance of a single vessel that happens to be coursing through an otherwise avascular mass has been imaged, which should not be confused with an aneurysm. Angiography may further assist in differentiating these entities (Fig. 24–15*D*).

False Aneurysms of Aortofemoral Bypass Grafts

The angiographic anatomy of false aneurysms of aortofemoral bypass grafts is shown in Figure 24–16. This type of false aneurysm occurs mainly in the groin at the anastomotic site between the graft and the common femoral artery. The exact cause of false aneurysms remains unknown. In most cases, the graft appears to have pulled away from the artery so that one might suspect that there is shortening of the graft over a period of time, with increased tension at the anastomotic site. Ultimately, there is hemorrhage into the tissues surrounding the anastomosis, causing the false aneurysms shown in Figure 24–16. These aneurysms are termed "false" because they do not contain all the layers of the artery wall. Instead, the lumen is surrounded by thrombus formation and fibrous tissue, as shown in Figure 24–17. Because these aneurysms may rupture or thrombose, it is usually desirable to proceed with repair once they are identified.

The B-mode image in Figure 24–17 was obtained from the large false aneurysm arising from the anastomotic site between the right distal limb of the aortofemoral bypass graft and the common femoral artery. The B-mode image shows internal echoes, which swirled around inside the aneurysm lumen on real-time ultrasound imaging. These swirling internal echoes were not seen in the small false aneurysm involving the left distal limb of the graft, as shown in Figure 24–18.

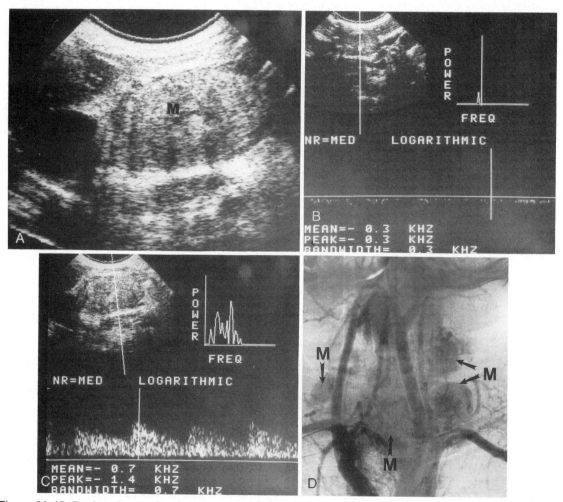

Figure 24–15. Duplex ultrasound and angiogram of lymph node metastasis. *A,* Real-time ultrasound image shows a solid mass (M) with homogeneous echotexture. *B,* Duplex ultrasound image demonstrating an absence of blood flow from the solid portion of a mass. *C,* Duplex ultrasound image showing the presence of blood flow obtained from the blood vessel coursing through the mass. *D,* Arteriogram showing multiple vascular masses (M).

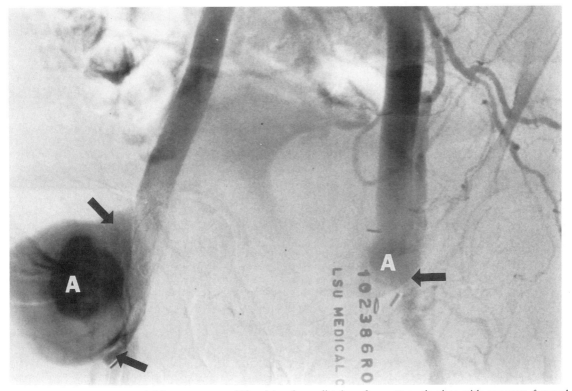

Figure 24–16. Angiogram of false aneurysms (A) arising from distal graft anastomotic sites with common femoral arteries (arrows).

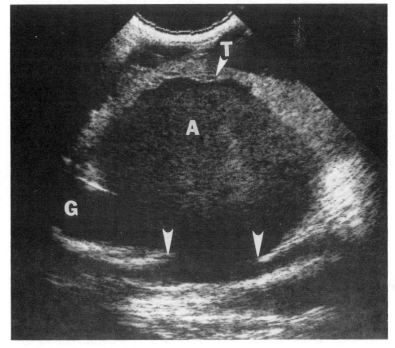

Figure 24–17. Sagittal real-time image of aortofemoral bypass graft false aneurysm. A = Swirling echoes seen in aneurysm on real-time ultrasound; G = graft (arrowheads point to site of graft anastomosis with common femoral artery); T = thrombus in aneurysm wall.

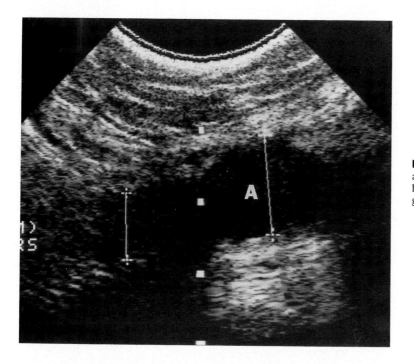

Figure 24–18. Sagittal real-time image of false aneurysm (A) involving limb of left distal aortofemoral bypass graft.

Echogenic arterial blood flow has been described previously.[18] The source of these echoes has been attributed to backscatter from red blood cells[19] or from microbubbles.[20-24] Both in vitro and in vivo experiments have indicated that red cell aggregation plays an important role in producing echogenicity of unclotted blood during stasis.[25-28] Other observations and experiments with moving blood have suggested that red cell aggregation may also cause echogenicity in flowing blood.[29, 30] Aggregation of red cells is dependent upon multiple factors, such as hematocrit

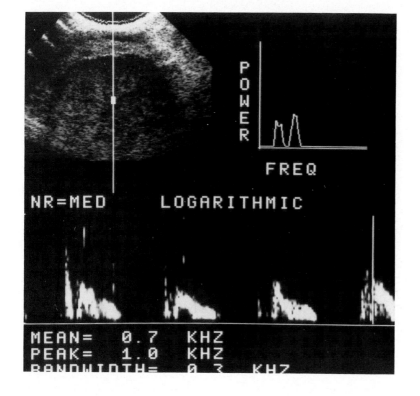

Figure 24–19. Doppler velocity waveform of false aneurysm.

level, erythrocyte membrane conditions, plasma macromolecules, and shear rate. Normal blood will demonstrate red cell aggregation at low shear rates. The aggregates are broken up into individual red cells at high shear rates. Shear rate is related to the velocity of flow and to the caliber of the blood vessel. Shear rate, not velocity per se, determines, the degree of red cell aggregation.[31] The low blood flow velocity and the large caliber of the false aneurysm in Figure 24–17 could decrease the shear rate and produce the swirling echoes seen on the real-time ultrasound examination of this aneurysm. The combination of an increased blood flow velocity and a small-caliber false aneurysm (Fig 24–17) could increase the shear rate, accounting for the absence of real-time ultrasonographic swirling echoes in this aneurysm.

Echogenicity of blood has been considered in terms of induced or spontaneously occurring microbubbles.[19–24] Induced microbubbles are caused by the injection of fluid or contrast media into the circulation. The frequent high velocity of such injections is believed to produce microbub-bles by cavitation. Such microbubbles, because of an extreme acoustical impedance mismatch between gas and blood, are intense reflectors of ultrasonic waves. Cavitation also might produce some spontaneous microbubbles (e.g., post-sten-otic areas in a rapid flow stream). Intestinal passage of gas via the portal circulation has been cited as a possible source of microbubbles in the blood under conditions of spontaneous flow.[23]

In any event, the finding of swirling echoes on real-time ultrasonography helps to make the diagnosis that the mass under investigation is an aneurysm. The presence of blood flow within the mass can also be detected by the Doppler velocity waveforms shown in Figure 24–19. These waveforms were obtained form the large false aneurysm shown in Figure 24–16.

Hemangiomas

Capillary hemangiomas are so designated because they are composed of blood vessels that conform to the caliber of normal capillaries.

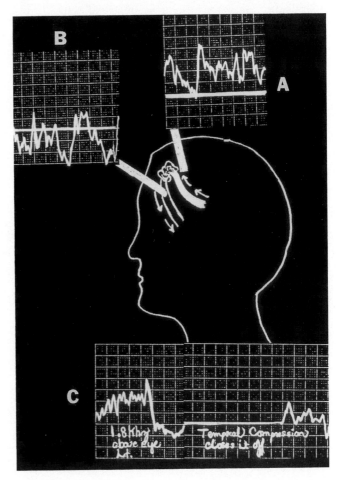

Figure 24–20. Bi-directional Doppler velocity waveform mapping scalp hemangioma. The waveform above the zero baseline *(A)* identifies the feeding artery; the waveform below the zero baseline *(B)* identifies the draining vein. Waveform *(C)* eliminated by manual compression of the superficial temporal artery.

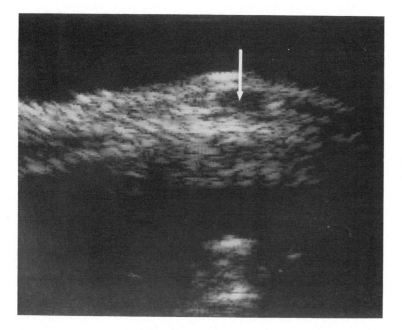

Figure 24–21. Real-time image of anechoic hemangioma nidus (arrow).

Cavernous hemangiomas are distinguished by the formation of large cavernous, vascular channels. Frequently, numerous small, capillary-like lumina are dispersed among the cavernous channels, and there is, in reality, no sharp line of distinction between the capillary and cavernous forms. Both forms may present as superficial mass lesions.

Because hemangiomas are composed of arteries feeding the vascular nidus of capillary or cavernous channels and veins draining the nidus, they may be detected by duplex sonography. An example is presented in Figures 24–20 through 24–22.

A positive velocity waveform is directed upward above the zero baseline, indicating that the blood flow direction in the artery being examined is towards the probe face. Because the vessel is directed towards a small scalp mass, it was suspected to be a feeding artery supplying the nidus

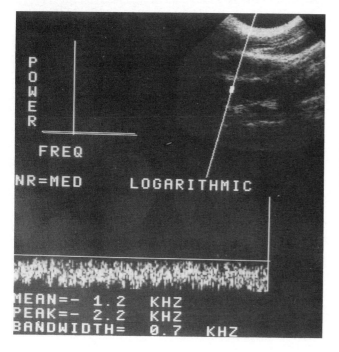

P
O
W
E
R

FREQ

NR=MED   LOGARITHMIC

MEAN=- 1.2 KHZ
PEAK=- 2.2 KHZ
BANDWIDTH= 0.7   KHZ

Figure 24–22. Spectral analysis of low-resistance continuous velocity blood flow in hemangioma nidus. Blood flow is directed away from the probe causing waveform below the zero baseline.

of a hemangioma. Compression of the superficial temporal artery eliminated this Doppler velocity waveform completely. This identified the feeding artery as arising from the superficial temporal artery, a branch of the external carotid artery. Further examination with the bi-directional Doppler probe revealed the blood flow to be in a vessel leading away from the scalp mass. This vessel was identified as a draining vein because the blood flow was directed away from the probe face, producing a negative velocity waveform deflection below the zero baseline level.

Duplex sonography of the scalp mass is shown in Figures 24–21 and 24–22. The sagittal real-time image shows the anechoic nidus of the scalp cavernous hemangioma (Fig. 24–21). The hemangioma is anechoic because it contains large, dilated vascular channels. These were identified as vascular channels because the sound spectral analysis revealed the continuous blood flow waveforms shown in Figure 24–22. This finding was confirmed by tissue diagnosis and by the angiogram shown in Figure 24–23 to be the nidus of a cavernous hemangioma of the scalp.

A cavernous hemangioma of the forearm is shown in Figure 24–24. An enlarged interosseous artery supplies a large vascular nidus with multiple draining veins. The enlarged, multiple vascular channels of the nidus appeared as circumscribed anechoic foci on the B-mode image (Fig. 24–25). They are separated from each other by soft tissue echoes. The circumscribed anechoic areas on the real-time image were identified as vascular channels because they contained blood flow, as shown by the sound spectral analysis Doppler shift frequencies in Figure 24–26.

Popliteal Artery Aneurysms

Several reports have demonstrated the usefulness of gray scale ultrasonography in the diagnosis of popliteal artery aneurysms.[32–36] The size of the normal popliteal artery by ultrasonographic scanning is reported to be 0.9 cm ($\pm$ 0.2 cm)[33] and 0.78 cm ($\pm$ 0.014 cm).[32] Aneurysms are suspected when ultrasonography reveals a focal enlargement of the popliteal artery, as shown in Figure 24–27. The scan may also help to detect thrombus within the aneurysm by the presence of internal echoes. This is an important finding because embolization to the distal arterial tree is a well-known complication of popliteal artery aneurysms. When such a clinical presentation is seen, a search must be made for the source of the emboli. Ultrasonography affords a quick, convenient way of excluding a popliteal artery aneurysm as the source of the emboli. The finding of thrombus within a popliteal aneurysm usually constitutes an indication for surgical intervention, regardless of the size of the aneurysm.

An advantage of ultrasonography over angiography is its ability to demonstrate a thrombosed popliteal aneurysm or one with a proximal occlusion. Angiography will not be helpful under these circumstances because the contrast material may not fill the aneurysm. Because popliteal aneurysms are bilateral in approximately half the cases[37] and because multiple aneurysms in the same patient are not uncommon, the presence of a popliteal aneurysm would suggest evaluation of other sites.

When a popliteal aneurysm is suspected, great

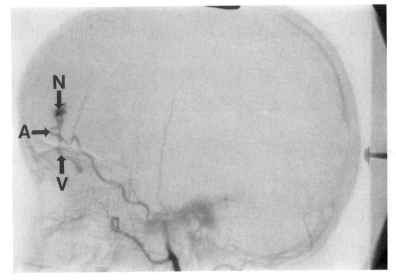

Figure 24–23. Angiogram of scalp hemangioma. N = Nidus; A = feeding artery; V = draining vein.

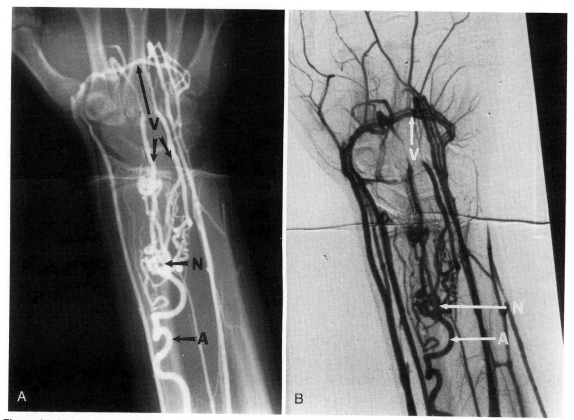

Figure 24–24. Angiogram of forearm hemangioma containing feeding artery (A), nidus (N), and draining veins (V). *A*, Arterial phase. *B*, Venous phase.

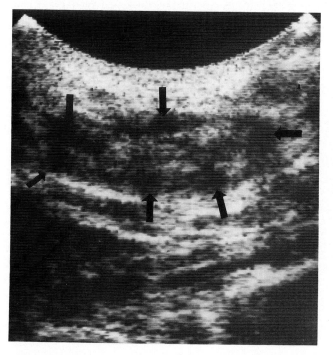

Figure 24–25. Real-time image of forearm hemangioma showing circumscribed foci of anechoic vascular channels in nidus (arrows).

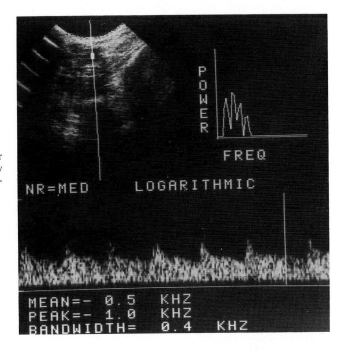

Figure 24–26. Spectral analysis showing Doppler shift frequencies of low-resistance blood flow through vascular channels in nidus of forearm hemangioma.

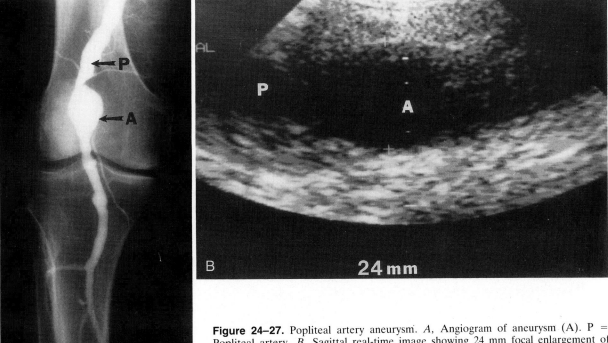

Figure 24–27. Popliteal artery aneurysm. *A*, Angiogram of aneurysm (A). P = Popliteal artery. *B*, Sagittal real-time image showing 24 mm focal enlargement of popliteal artery (P). A = Aneurysm.

care must be taken to demonstrate the vessel both proximal and distal to the suspected aneurysm. This maneuver simplifies the differentiation of a popliteal cyst from an aneurysm.[38, 39] In addition, duplex sonography confirms the vascular nature of the lesion and its continuity with the popliteal artery.

Popliteal artery aneurysms are most often encountered in male patients in the sixth and seventh decades of life. These aneurysms are second only to abdominal aortic aneurysms in frequency. Atherosclerosis remains the underlying cause in most popliteal aneurysms encountered. Complications of aneurysms include distal thromboembolization, expansion with impingement on adjacent neural structures, and compression of venous channels, which may cause discomfort and edema of the distal extremity. Rupture is a less common complication, occurring in about 5% of cases.

Calf Hematomas

Calf hematomas seem to occur predominantly in the gastrocnemius muscle. They may produce symptoms of calf pain, swelling, and a positive Homans sign (calf pain on passive dorsiflexion of the foot), suggesting the diagnosis of deep vein thrombosis.[40] Generally, once the diagnosis of deep vein thrombosis is excluded by venography, no further diagnostic studies are used to explain the patient's symptoms. At this point, the patient may be allowed to continue walking on the extremity or may be treated for suspected cellulitis. Usually, the hematoma resolves without any residual tissue alterations. If the hematoma is large, it may persist as a chronic expanding mass in the calf.[41] Continuing to walk on the extremity or anticoagulation therapy with heparin may lead to further extension of the hematoma as a result of recurrent bleeding episodes.[40]

Ultrasonography is useful in the detection of calf hematomas.[40] The sonographic appearance of the hematoma depends upon the age of the hematoma.[42] Hematomas in the early stage may be more echogenic; those in the chronic stage contain fewer internal echoes, as shown in Figures 24–28 and 24–30. The B-mode image in Figure 24–28 is of a 47-year-old woman with swelling of the calf, suggesting thrombophlebitis. There was a history of antecedent blunt trauma to the calf 1 week previously. The physical examination demonstrated tenderness of the calf, 2+ pitting edema, and a positive Homans sign. A venogram excluded the diagnosis of deep vein thrombosis but showed extrinsic compression of the soleus muscular plexus veins by a mass within the gastrocnemius muscle (Fig. 24–29). Needle aspiration of the mass yielded clotted blood, confirming the diagnosis of hematoma.

Another example is shown in Figure 24–30. A hematoma is approximately 2 weeks old. The venogram in Figure 24–31 shows the calf hematoma displacing the soleus muscular plexus veins anteriorly towards the tibia. This venogram showed negative results for deep vein thrombosis. Needle aspiration guided by ultrasonography demonstrated clotted blood from the mass shown in Figure 24–30, confirming the diagnosis of hematoma formation.

Either B-mode or duplex sonography may be

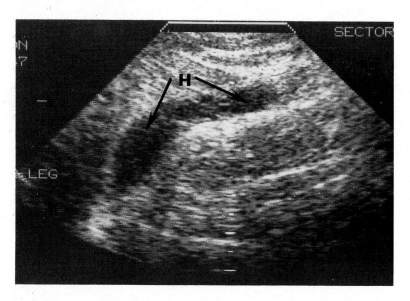

Figure 24–28. Transverse real-time image of 1-week-old hematoma of calf showing a crescent-shaped mass containing internal echoes in hematoma (H). The mass is hypoechoic relative to the contiguous muscles. (From Giyanani VL, Grozinger KT, Gerlock AJ Jr, et al. Calf hematoma mimicking thrombophlebitis. Radiology 1985; 154: 779–781, with permission.)

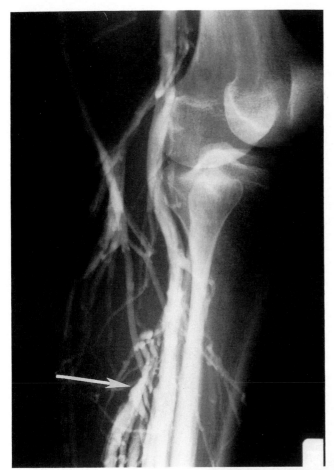

Figure 24–29. Venogram showing anterior and downward displacement of the soleus muscular plexus (arrow) by a mass in the calf region. There was no evidence of deep vein thrombosis on the venogram. (From Giyanani VL, Grozinger KT, Gerlock AJ Jr, et al. Calf hematoma mimicking thrombophlebitis. Radiology 1985; 154:779–781, with permission.)

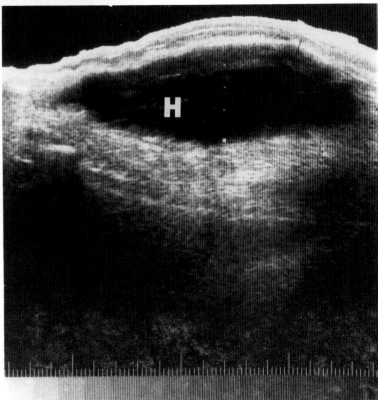

Figure 24–30. Sagittal real-time image of 2-week-old hematoma of calf showing transonic mass (H) containing only a few low-level echoes. (From Giyanani VL, Grozinger KT, Gerlock AJ Jr, et al. Calf hematoma mimicking thrombophlebitis. Radiology 1985; 154:779–781, with permission.)

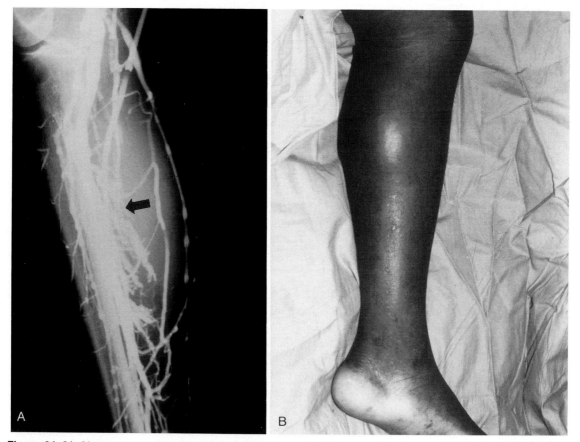

Figure 24–31. Venogram and photograph of calf hematoma. *A*, Venogram showing anterior displacement of soleus muscle plexus veins (arrow) by calf hematoma. (From Giyanani VL, Grozinger KT, Gerlock AJ Jr, et al. Calf hematoma mimicking thrombophlebitis. Radiology 1985; 154:779–781, with permission.)

used to exclude other underlying lesions that mimic deep vein thrombosis. These lesions include giant synovial cyst[43] associated with rheumatoid arthritis, large popliteal artery aneurysm, and Baker's cyst.

Giant Synovial Cyst. Giant synovial cysts are most commonly associated with rheumatoid arthritis, but they may occur with Reiter's syndrome, gouty arthritis, septic arthritis, and osteoarthritis. These may produce a "pseudo-thrombophlebitis syndrome" when the cyst ruptures, sending its contents down into the calf muscles. The arthrogram shows contrast material arising from either the popliteal bursa or the gastrocnemiosemimembranosus bursa and dissecting downward, usually between the soleus and gastrocnemius muscles. Rarely, thrombophlebitis may coexist with a ruptured giant synovial cyst. This unusual condition is referred to as *pseudopseudothrombophlebitis.* There is a distinct advantage of using duplex sonography arthrography in these instances because it may help

in diagnosing both the cyst and the deep vein thrombosis. Another advantage of ultrasonography is its capability of demonstrating cysts in the calf when they are sealed off from the knee joint itself.

Popliteal Artery Aneurysm. Popliteal artery aneurysms are diagnosed by (1) a close relationship with the popliteal artery and (2) the presence of blood flow on duplex sonography.

Baker's Cyst. What has become known as a popliteal cyst (Baker's cyst) is actually a filling of the gastrocnemiosemimembranosus bursa through a rupture into this normal structure from the popliteal bursa of the posterior knee. A popliteal cyst may be suspected when the duplex sonogram shows a hypo-echoic mass located in the popliteal fossa that contains no blood flow. Arthrography is used to confirm the diagnosis by demonstrating that the cyst communicates with the popliteal bursa of the knee joint.[44] Magnetic resonance imaging may also be used for this purpose.

References

1. Silver TM, Washburn R, Stanley JC, et al. Gray scale ultrasound evaluation of popliteal artery aneurysms. AJR 1977; 129:1003–1006.
2. Yeh HC, Mitty HA, Wolf BS, Jacobson JH. Ultrasonography of the brachiocephalic arteries. Radiology 1979; 132:403–408.
3. Hsu I, Kistin AD. Buckling of the great vessels: a clinical and angiocardiograpic study. Arch Intern Med 1956; 98:712–719.
4. Honig EI, Dubilier W Jr, Steinberg I. Significance of the buckled innominate artery. Ann Intern Med 1953; 39:74–80.
5. Deterling RA Jr. Tortuous right common carotid artery simulating aneurysm. Angiology 1952; 3:483–492.
6. Goldstone J. Aneurysms of the extracranial carotid artery. In Rutherford RB (ed). Vascular surgery. 2nd ed. Philadelphia, WB Saunders Co, 1984.
7. Rhodes EL, Stanley JC, Hoffman GL, et al. Aneurysms of extracranial carotid arteries. Arch Surg 1976; 111:339.
8. Weissman B, Rankow R. Traumatic aneurysm of the common carotid artery. Arch Otolaryng 1968; 88:543.
9. Wiaslow N. Extracranial aneurysms of the internal carotid artery. Arch Surg 1926; 13:689.
10. Beall AC, Crawford ES, Cooley DA, DeBakey ME. Extracranial aneurysms of the carotid artery. Postgrad Med 1962; 32:93.
11. Johnson JN, Helsby CR, Stell PM. Aneurysm of the external carotid artery. J Cardiovasc Surg 1980; 21:105–107.
12. Davis JM, Zimmerman RA. Injury of the carotid and vertebral arteries. Neuroradiol 1983; 25:55–69.
13. Hite SJ, Grores RA, Starkey PC. Superficial temporal artery aneurysms. Neurology 1966; 16:1044–1046.
14. Winslow N, Edwards M. Aneurysm of temporal artery: report of case. Bull School Med Univ Maryland 1934; 19:57–72.
15. Johns ME, Mentzer R, Fitz-Mugh GS. Mycotic carotid artery aneurysms. Otolaryngol Head Neck Surg 1979; 87:624–627.
16. Rittenhouse ER, Radkle HM. Carotid artery aneurysm. Review of the literature and report of a case with rupture into the oropharynx. Arch Surg 1972; 108:786–789.
17. Bresner M, Brekke J, Dubbit J, Finigio T. False aneurysms of the facial region. J Oral Surg 1972: 30:307–313.
17a. Giyanani VL, Gerlock AJ, Mirfakhraee M, et al. Duplex sonography in embolus therapy of external carotid artery traumatic aneurysm. AJNR 1987; 8:1131–1133.
18. King D, Van Natta RC, Thorsen K, Lechich RL. Spontaneously echogenic arterial blood flow in abdominal aortic aneurysms. AJR 1982; 138:350–352.
19. Wolverson MK, Nouri S, Joist JH, Sundaram M, Heiberg E. The direct visualization of blood flow by real-time ultrasound: clinical observation and underlying mechanism. Radiology 1981; 140:443–448.
20. Gramiak R, Shah PM, Framer DH. Ultrasound cardiography: contrast studies in anatomy and function. Radiology 1967; 92:939–948.
21. Kort A, Kronzon I. Microbubble formation: in vitro and in vivo observation. JCU 1982; 10:117–120.
22. Kremkau FW, Gramiak R, Carstensen EL, Shah PM, Kramer DH. Ultrasonic detection of cavitation of catheter tips. AJR 1970; 110:177–183.

23. Meltzer RS, Lancee CT, Swart GR, Roelandt J. Spontaneous echocardiographic contrast on the right side of the heart. JCU 1982; 10:240–242.
24. Meltzer RS, Tickner EG, Sahines TP, Popp RL. The source of ultrasound contrast effect. JCU 1980; 8:121–127.
25. Sigel B, Coelho JCU, Schade SG, Justin J, Spigos DG. Effect of plasma proteins and temperature on echogenicity of blood. Invest Radiol 1982; 17:29–33.
26. Sigel B, Coelho JCU, Spigos DG, et al. Ultrasonography of blood during stasis and coagulation. Invest Radiol 1981; 16:71–76.
27. Hanss M, Boynard M. Ultrasound backscattering from blood: hematocrit and erythrocyte aggregation dependence. In Linzer M (ed.) Ultrasonic Tissue Characterization II. National Bureau of Standards, Spec Publ 535 and Spec Publ 525. Washington, DC, US Government Printing Office, 1979:165–169.
28. Shung KK, Reid JM. Ultrasonic instrumentation for hematology. Ultrason Imaging 1979; 1:280–294.
29. Machi J, Sigel B, Beitler JC, Coelho JCU, Justin JR. Relation of in vivo blood flow to ultrasound echogenicity. JCU 1983; 11:3–10.
30. Sigel B, Machi J, Beitler JC, Justin JR, Coelho JCU. Variable ultrasound echogenicity in flowing blood. Science 1982; 218:1321–1323.
31. Wells RE Jr. Rheology of blood in the microvasculature. N Engl J Med 1964; 270:823, 889–893.
32. Collins GJ Jr, Rich NM, Phillips J, et al. Ultrasound diagnosis of popliteal arterial aneurysms. Am Surg 1976; 42:853–858.
33. Davis RP, Neiman HL, Yao JST, et al. Ultrasound scan in diagnosis of peripheral aneurysms. Arch Surg 1977; 113:55–58.
34. Sarti DA, Louie JS, Lindstrom RR, et al. Ultrasonic diagnosis of a popliteal artery aneurysm. Radiology 1976; 131:707–708.
35. Scott WW Jr, Scott PP, Sanders RC. B-scan ultrasound in the diagnosis of popliteal aneurysms. Surgery 1977; 81:436–441.
36. Silver TM, Washburn RL, Stanley JC, et al. Gray scale ultrasound evaluation of popliteal artery aneurysms. AJR 1977; 129:1003–1006.
37. Dent TL, Lindenauer SM, Ernst CB, et al. Multiple arteriosclerotic arterial aneurysms. Arch Surg 1972; 105:338–344.
38. Carpenter JR, Hattery RR, Hunder GG, et al. Ultrasound evaluation of popliteal space. Comparison with arthrography and physical examination. Mayo Clin Proc 1976; 51:498–503.
39. Moore CP, Santi DA, Louie JS. Ultrasonographic demonstration of popliteal cysts in rheumatoid arthritis. A noninvasive technique. Arthritis Rheum 1975; 18:577–580.
40. Giyanani VL, Grozinger KT, Gerlock AJ Jr, Mirfakhraee M, Husbands HS. Calf hematoma mimicking thrombophlebitis: Sonographic and computed tomographic appearance. Radiology 1985; 154:779–781.
41. Friedlander HL, Bump RS. Chronic expanding hematoma of the calf. J Bone Joint Surg (Am) 1968; 50:1237–1241.
42. Wicks JD, Silver TM, Bree RL. Gray scale features of hematomas: an ultrasonic spectrum. AJR 1978; 131:977–980.
43. Gordon GV, Edell S. Ultrasound evaluation of popliteal cysts. Arch Intern Med 1980; 140:1453–1455.
44. Freiberger RH, Kaye JY. Extrameniscal abnormality. In Spiller J (ed). Arthrography. New York, Appleton-Century-Crofts, 1979:109–110.

25 • Accuracy of Measurement Determinations

Introduction

Many questions may arise about the accuracy of the test results produced by the noninvasive vascular laboratory. Most of these questions come from the personnel in the laboratory who wish to know just how good they are in detecting a specific level of disease. The referring physicians also want to know the likelihood of their patients having disease when a test result is positive. The use of accuracy measurements offers one way to answer these questions. Another way is to review the published data concerning the accuracy of a given test. However, in the final analysis, it is the accuracy measurements of the test results produced by a local laboratory that really counts. The methods by which the accuracy measurements may be obtained and interpreted are reviewed in this chapter. Five accuracy measurements may be used in the evaluation of the laboratory's test results.

Sensitivity. The ability of a test to detect the disease level when the disease level exists on the gold standard.

Specificity. The ability of a test to establish the disease level absent when the disease level does not exist on the gold standard.

Positive Predictive Value. Given a positive test result, the percentage of those (patients or vessels) with the disease level present when it exists on the gold standard.

Negative Predictive Value. Given a negative test result, the percentage of those (patients or vessels) with an absent disease level when it does not exist on the gold standard.

Overall Accuracy. The percentage of all the results correctly predicted by the test as either positive or negative.

These accuracy measurements should answer most of the questions concerning the accuracy of the tests results from the noninvasive laboratory.

The next step is to organize the data so that they can be correctly analyzed.

Data Organization

Question Formation and Analysis

Begin by seeking a precise answer to a well-defined question. A well-defined question should contain three basic components: (1) the *disease level*, (2) a *gold standard*, and (3) the *test level*. The question may be constructed as shown in the following example.

Example I
In our laboratory, how accurate is a systolic peak frequency (SPF) of >4 kHz in the diagnosis of an internal carotid artery (ICA) stenosis >50% as seen on the angiogram?

The disease level in *Example I* is an ICA stenosis >50%, and the test level is an SPF >4 kHz. An SPF >4 kHz is a positive test result; an SPF <4 kHz is a negative test result. The positive test result means that an ICA stenosis >50% will be found on the angiogram. A negative test result means that either no stenosis or one <50% will be found on the angiogram. Again, it must be emphasized that a negative test result does not mean that no disease is present in the ICA; it means that the stated disease level does not exist in the ICA. The ICA may have an ulcerative plaque causing a 30% stenosis, but it should not contain a >50% stenotic lesion. The proof that a stenosis either greater than or less than 50% exists in the ICA will be provided by the angiogram of that ICA. Because the presence or absence of this disease level is to be determined by the angiogram, the angiogram constitutes the gold standard component of the example question.

Next, examine each of the three components

of the question to see how they might bias the results of the accuracy measurements.

Disease Level

The patient population containing the *disease level* to be evaluated will certainly bias the accuracy measurements. For instance, assume that all patients with a positive test result underwent angiography, whereas those with a negative test result did not. The positive predictive value will be correct because all positive tests, both true and false, will be in the comparison population. The other four accuracy measurements—sensitivity, specificity, negative predictive value, and overall accuracy (all partially or totally based on negative test results)—may be incorrect because patients with negative test results did not undergo a gold standard testing. This type of population bias can be avoided by including in the analysis only those patients in whom the gold standard studies were obtained, regardless of the testing results.

The population in *Example I* consisted of patients suspected of transient ischemic attacks (TIAs). Both SPF measurements and angiography were performed. Regardless of the results, this group may be used in the data analysis. This population is now free from biasing by the testing results because the accuracy statements are independent of the testing results. However, the population is still biased according to whether or not the patients actually had TIAs. This is because different examiners may disagree on the diagnosis of a TIA.[1] Also, the patient population may not be able to convey the history of disease as well as another patient population may. One population may be made up of mostly males (e.g., in a Veterans Administration Hospital) and may be different from that found in a community hospital. The age range of the population introduces another bias variable. Coexistent diseases like diabetes, hypertension, and cancer can also influence the observations. Body habitus (e.g., long, thin necks versus short, fat necks) can certainly influence the results of a carotid examination by duplex scanning. All of these factors are of particular importance when the accuracy measurements of two different patient populations are to be compared. This type of bias may also explain why the accuracy measurements obtained from a local laboratory do not match those found in the literature. One must understand the importance of population bias because it cannot be totally avoided in the data organization.

Gold Standard

The methods by which the *gold standard* was performed and interpreted offer another source of bias. Currently, there are several modalities used for carotid angiography. These consist of intravenous digital subtraction angiography, transarterial selective catheter digital subtraction angiography, and conventional transarterial selective catheter angiography. Each one of these modalities may produce different results and may introduce bias into the accuracy measurements.[2] Ideally, the same modality should be used for each patient in the data sample population. This would eliminate the bias introduced into the accuracy measurements by a mixture of all three of the modalities just mentioned.

Another source of bias arises from discrepancies in measuring and reporting the stenoses from the angiograms. Unfortunately, these may be measured by several different methods. Breslau and associates have measured the residual lumen and have estimated the true vessel width at that point.[3] The ratio of these two measurements is reported as a diameter stenosis. Baker and Hayes have measured the residual lumen and the lumen of the distal ICA beyond all disease and the tapering bulb. Thus, these two groups of authors disagree on the percentage of diameter stenosis from the same angiogram. Ideally, the stenoses should be measured by the same method throughout the sample population to eliminate this type of bias from the accuracy measurements. Taking the stenosis measurements directly from the operative specimen would appear to be another way to eliminate the introduction of bias into the gold standard measurement. However, it must be realized that during the noninvasive study the artery is evaluated in a pressurized state; unless the specimen is fixed under the same pressure prior to examination, resultant measurements may be considerably different. Mixing of the gold standards by using both operative specimens and angiography biases the accuracy measurements. Only a single form of gold standard should be used.

At the time of gold standard interpretation, it is important to know whether or not the interpreter was blinded from the noninvasive test results. A prior knowledge of the test results can influence the gold standard measurement. If the angiogram is suboptimal, the knowledge of the test results may be used to derive the angiographic report. Subsequent use of this report as the gold standard result will be erroneous because the test result has influenced the report.

One's personal opinions for or against the noninvasive test can influence the gold standard interpretation when the interpreter knows the test results. Therefore, it is best for the interpreter to be blinded and not to know the test results before making the gold standard interpretations. Any unblinded interpretation of the gold standard, especially in retrospect, has the potential of introducing considerable bias into the accuracy measurements.

Test Level

The *noninvasive test* results can also bias the accuracy measurements. This bias generally occurs when the noninvasive test result has completely failed to detect the disease process under investigation. Stimulated by such an event, the laboratory personnel immediately begin to review the testing methodology for mistakes. The correction of these mistakes constitutes the learning curve, which is an ongoing process in the laboratory. Unfortunately, the learning curve introduces bias into the accuracy measurements because the data obtained earlier in the learning curve are not as accurate as those obtained later in the learning curve. One way of eliminating this type of bias is not to use the data collected from the early learning curve phase of the test procedure. Instead, wait until this phase is completed and the laboratory personnel are comfortable with the testing methodology before applying the accuracy measurements to the test results.

Data Collection

Be sure that during the data collection process the test results are not altered in any way to meet the criteria set up by the gold standard. All of the test results must be used in the analysis, regardless of whether or not the results agree or disagree with the criteria set up by the gold standard. This entry of bias can be avoided only by a careful, honest review of the data.

The next step is to decide whether the study is to determine the disease level in each patient or in each individual artery examined. Many of the noninvasive carotid studies provide bilateral information, as do the angiogram. Two data points are then available in each patient. These may be used to evaluate the accuracy of the test to detect the disease level of either each individual artery or of each individual patient.

Because the proposed sample question specifically concerned ICA stenosis, each ICA in the population will be a data point for this investi-

Table 25–1. Sample Data Record

ICA Number	Test Result	Gold Standard Result
1	−	−
2	−	−
3	+	+
4	+	−
5	+	+

Key: + + = True positive; − − = true negative; + − = false positive; − + = false negative.

gation. Data points may be recorded, as shown in Table 25–1. This completed table shows that of the 100 ICAs examined, the results were 25 true positives, 58 true negatives, 12 false positives, and 5 false negatives. These are further defined as follows:

1. *True positive* (25): Patients show a positive test result, and angiograms show ICA stenosis >50%.

2. *True negative* (58): Patients show a negative test result, and angiograms show ICA stenosis <50%.

3. *False positive* (12): Patients show a positive test result, but angiograms show ICA stenosis <50%.

4. *False negative* (5): Patients show negative test results, but angiograms show ICA stenosis >50%.

The data are now organized and ready to be placed into the 2 × 2 Tables for analysis.

The 2 × 2 Tables

A 2 × 2 Table organizes the data for the accuracy measurement calculations. However, for the formulas to work, the 2 × 2 Table must be constructed exactly as shown by Table 25–2. The precise placement of the data within the 2 × 2 Table, and the results of the accuracy measurement calculations are shown in Table 25–3.

Interpretation of Results

As mentioned earlier, laboratory personnel wish to know how good they are in detecting a specific level of disease. Test results may mean either that the skills of laboratory personnel are good or poor or that the test is helpful or not helpful in the detection of the disease level under investigation. Such factors are determined by the accuracy measurement of sensitivity. Table 25–3 shows there were a total of 30 ICAs with a

Table 25–2. 2 × 2 Gold Standard

		NEG	POS
TEST	NEG	A True Negative	B False Negative
	POS	C False Positive	D True Positive

Key: Sensitivity = D/(B + D); specificity = A/(A + C); positive predictive value = D/(C + D); negative predictive value = A/(A + B); overall accuracy = (A + D)/(A + B + C + D).

Examine the following relationships in this 2 × 2 table.

1. A *decrease* in the number of false-negative test results "B" *increases* the test's sensitivity, negative predictive value, and overall accuracy.

2. An *increase* in the number of false-negative test results "B" *decreases* the test sensitivity, negative predictive value, and overall accuracy.

3. A *decrease* in the number of false-positive test results "C" *increases* the test specificity, positive predictive value, and overall accuracy.

4. An *increase* in the number of false-positive test results "C" *decreases* the test specificity, positive predictive value, and overall accuracy.

stenosis >50% on angiography. In other words, the angiogram showed positive results for the disease level in 30 ICAs (B + D = 30). The test showed positive results in 25 of these (D = 25). Sensitivity of the test to detect the disease level on the gold standard is D/(B + D), or 25/30, or 83%. Optimally, the laboratory personnel and the test should have a sensitivity of 100%, which would mean that all of the ICAs found positive by the gold standard also has positive test results. Under these circumstances, the sensitivity would be D/D, or 30/30, or 100%. The B result would be eliminated from the formula because a test with a sensitivity of 100% would have no false-negative results. It would indeed be an excellent test.

Unlike true statistical analyses, there is no *p* value for sensitivity and there is not a universally

Table 25–3. 2 × 2 Angiography

		NEG	POS
TEST	NEG	A 58	B 5
	POS	C 12	D 25

Key: Sensitivity = 83%; specificity = 82%; positive predictive value = 67%; negative predictive value = 92%; overall accuracy = 83%.

Table 25–4. 2 × 2 Gold Standard

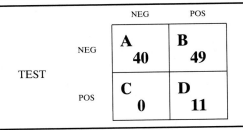

		NEG	POS
TEST	NEG	A 40	B 49
	POS	C 0	D 11

Key: Sensitivity = 11/60 = 18%; specificity = 40/40 = 100%; positive predictive value = 11/11 = 100%; negative predictive value = 40/89 = 44%; overall accuracy = 51/100 = 51%.

accepted level of sensitivity that denotes excellence. Thus, each person and laboratory must develop some innate feel for what is acceptable. It is possible to have a test with a low sensitivity and still have a very valuable test. An example of this is illustrated in Table 25–4. Note that the sensitivity value of this test is only 18% because it produces a huge number of *false-negative* results. In other words, the gold standard was positive in 60 cases (B + D = 60), but the test was positive in only 11 of these and negative in 49 of these. Sensitivity of this test to detect the disease level on the gold standard is D/(B+D), or 11/60, or 18%. Although its sensitivity is low, it is still a very valuable test, as will be described later in this chapter.

Referring physicians want to know the likelihood that a patient has a given level of disease when the test results are positive. This question is answered by the positive predictive value accuracy measurement. The positive predictive value for the test results in *Example I* is shown in Table 25–3 to be 67%; this means that when the test results are positive, the ICA under investigation has a 67% likelihood of having >50% stenosis on the angiogram. The positive predictive value is derived from the number of true-positive tests divided by the total number of all the positive tests, which equals D/(C+D), or, in this case, 25/37, or 67%. From these calculations, it can be seen that for a test to have a high positive predictive value it must have few false-positive results. Ideally, a test should have a positive predictive value of 100%, which would eliminate C from the formula entirely. In this case, it would then be D/D, or 37/37, or 100%. The positive predictive value then, is, the ability of a positive test result to indicate the given level of disease as found on the gold standard. This value was low in this case because there were too many false-positive test results (C=12).

Although the accuracy measurement test has only a fair positive predictive value, it does have an excellent negative predictive value, as shown in Table 25–3. This means that given a negative test result, the likelihood of an ICA not having >50% stenosis on the angiogram is 92%. This value is the number of true-negative tests divided by all the negative tests, which equals A/(A + B), or, in this case, 58/63, or 92%. The negative predictive value is high because there were few false-negative tests results (B = 5), (Table 25–3). Ideally, there would be no false-negative results and B would be eliminated from the formula entirely. Then the negative predictive value in this case would be A/A, or 58/58, or 100%.

The overall accuracy measurement means that of the 100 ICAs examined, 83 of them were correctly classified by the SPF >4 kHz measurement as having either an angiographic stenosis >50% (true positives = 25 ICAs) or an angiographic stenosis <50% (true negatives = 58 ICAs). The overall accuracy is calculated by adding the number of true positives and true negatives and then dividing by the total sample population, which in this case equals (25 + 58) ÷ 100, or 83%; thus, 17% of all ICAs examined using an SPF test level >4 kHz were incorrectly classified as compared with the angiographic findings and 83% of ICAs were correctly classified as compared with the angiographic findings.

Example II

In our laboratory how accurate is the reversal of blood flow in the supraorbital artery by periorbital Doppler testing in diagnosing a patient with >50% stenosis of the ICA as compared with angiography?

Data obtained from 100 patients indicated the following:
60 should >50% ICA stenosis on angiography
11 of these showed a positive test result
49 of these showed a negative test result

40 showed <50% ICA stenosis on angiography
0 of these showed a positive test result
40 of these showed a negative test result

From the data, the following results were derived: true positive = 11; true negative = 40; false positive = 0; and false negative = 49.

Refer to Table 25–4 for the accuracy measurement calculations for *Example II.*

The ability of the accuracy measurement test to indicate the stated disease level in our hypothetical laboratory is poor because the sensitivity of the test is only 18%. However, the ability of this test to determine that an ICA does not have a >50% stenosis when one is not found on the angiogram is excellent because the specificity of the test is 100%.

Although the sensitivity of the test is extremely poor, the reliability of the test is excellent when results are positive. The positive predictive value was 100%, which means that every time the test was positive, the patient had an ICA stenosis >50% on the angiogram. Despite the fact that this test has an excellent specificity, a negative test was of little value in ruling out the presence of a >50% stenosis in patients. In 49 of the patients with an ICA stenosis >50%, the test result was negative. There were too many false-negative results obtained with this test for it to have any significant negative predictive value. The low negative predictive value also reduced the overall accuracy of this test to 51%. As shown in this example, to reject the test based upon the single measurement of overall accuracy would be a mistake because its positive predictive power of 100% would be missed.

Summary

It is important to understand that the accuracy measurements of sensitivity and specificity define the ability of a test to either detect or rule out a specific disease level that is present or absent on the gold standard. These measurements say nothing about how accurate the test results are when they are positive or negative. Given a test with positive results, the accuracy of the measurements in diagnosing the disease level found on the gold standard is provided by the positive predictive value. Given negative results, the accuracy of this test in excluding the disease level not found on the gold standard is provided by the negative predictive value. Confusing these four different accuracy measurements can only lead to frustration and a misinterpretation of what the accuracy measurements actually mean.

References

1. Kraijeveld CL, Van Gijn J, Schouten HJA, Stall AL. Intraobserver agreement for the diagnosis of transient ischemic attacks. Stroke 1984; 15:723.
2. Russel JB, Watson TM, Modi JR, Lambeth A, Sumner DS. Digital subtraction angiography for evaluation of extracranial occlusive disease: Comparison and conventional arteriography. Surgery 1983; 94:604.
3. Breslau PJ, Know RA, Phillips DJ, Beach KW, Chikos PM, Thiele BL, Strandness DE. Ultrasonic duplex scanning with spectral analysis in extracranial carotid artery disease. Vasc Diag Ther 1982; 3:17.
4. Baker WH, Hayes AC. The Loyola Experience. *In* Baker WH (ed). Diagnosis and treatment of carotid artery disease. Mt Kisco, NY, Futura Publishing, 1979:82–89.

Index